Tuberculosis of the Central Nervous System

Mehmet Turgut • Ali Akhaddar
Ahmet T. Turgut • Ravindra K. Garg
Editors

Tuberculosis of the Central Nervous System

Pathogenesis, Imaging, and Management

Springer

Editors
Mehmet Turgut
Adnan Menderes University
School of Medicine
Aydın, Turkey

Ahmet T. Turgut
Hacettepe University
School of Medicine
Ankara, Turkey

Ali Akhaddar
Mohammed V University in Rabat
Avicenne Military Hospital of
Marrakech
Rabat, Morocco

Ravindra K. Garg
King George Medical University
Lucknow, UP, India

ISBN 978-3-319-50711-8   ISBN 978-3-319-50712-5 (eBook)
DOI 10.1007/978-3-319-50712-5

Library of Congress Control Number: 2017940255

Printed on acid-free paper

This Springer imprint is published by Springer Nature
The registered company is Springer International Publishing AG
The registered company address is: Gewerbestrasse 11, 6330 Cham, Switzerland

Preface

Tuberculosis is still a major public health challenge for most of the developing world and is increasingly recognized in developed countries due to mass immigration, refugee movements, international traveling, and immunocompromised patients. Known since ancient civilizations, it has received a great deal of attention among the various scientific communities. However, tuberculosis of the central nervous system and its covering did not receive a comparable large interest in the medical literature. In spite of all the advances in biological/infectious investigations, imaging techniques, and therapeutic methods, optimal management of neurotuberculosis is still controversial owing to the limited individual experience and the variable clinical course of the condition.

With the introduction of multidisciplinary team approach, a need has become evident for a timely and concise book that provides a comprehensive and updated review of basic, clinical, and therapeutic aspects of central nervous system tuberculosis that will be of value to the medical community and researchers involved in the care of patients affected by this old disease.

The format of the material presented is categorized into eight sections that include general considerations, tuberculosis of the brain and its coverings, tuberculosis of the spine and its coverings, tuberculosis of the cranial and peripheral nerves, laboratory studies in neurotuberculosis, therapy of tuberculosis of the nervous system and its coverings, an overview of tuberculosis disease, and further insights into tuberculosis.

This book of 39 chapters is written by more than 100 authors who are world-renowned specialists in their respective fields of interests. *Tuberculosis of the Central Nervous System: Pathogenesis, Imaging, and Management* would not have been possible without the enthusiastic response from these contributors who shared their expertise in this richly illustrated book. The editors sincerely thank all of them.

Our particular thanks go also to the Springer personnel for their patience and experienced advice in the production of this work. We also like to thank our families for their support and devotion. Finally, our gratitude goes to our patients for having given us the opportunity to be a part of their lives.

Aydın, Turkey — Mehmet Turgut, MD, PhD
Marrakech, Morocco — Ali Akhaddar, MD, IFAANS
Ankara, Turkey — Ahmet T. Turgut, MD
Lucknow, India — Ravindra K. Garg, MD, DM

Contents

Part I

General Considerations

Historical Preview and Epidemiology of Tuberculosis

1

Jaffar A. Al-Tawfiq and Ziad A. Memish

Contents

J.A. Al-Tawfiq, MD, FACP, FCCP, FRCP
Johns Hopkins Aramco Healthcare,
Dhahran, Kingdom of Saudi Arabia

Indiana University School of Medicine,
Indianapolis, IN, USA
e-mail: jaltawfi@yahoo.com; Jaffar.tawfiq@jhah.com

Z.A. Memish, MD, FRCPC (✉)
Ministry of Health,
Riyadh, Kingdom of Saudi Arabia

College of Medicine, Alfaisal University,
Riyadh, Kingdom of Saudi Arabia
e-mail: zmemish@yahoo.com

Abbreviations

AIDS	Acquired immunodeficiency syndrome
BCG	Bacillus Calmette-Guérin
CNS	Central nervous system
HIV	Human immunodeficiency virus
INH	Isoniazid
PAS	Para-aminosalicylic acid
PZA	Pyrazinamide
RIF	Rifampicin
STR	Streptomycin
TB	Tuberculosis
TBM	Tuberculous meningitis
USPHS	US Public Health Service

1.1 Introduction

Mycobacterium tuberculosis is a leading cause of morbidity and mortality around the globe. Tuberculosis (TB) was known to humans since early ages. It was stated that the genus *Mycobacterium* existed for >150 million years ago [1]. However, the specific time of *M. tuberculosis* to initialy cause infection in humans was about three million years ago and occurred in East Africa [2]. The significance of the disease is exemplified by the different names it had through history from consumption to phthisis pulmonalis and the white plague [3, 4]. The word consumptions refers to the significant weight loss that TB inflects on its victims and the development of extreme anemia resulting in

M. Turgut et al. (eds.), *Tuberculosis of the Central Nervous System*,
DOI 10.1007/978-3-319-50712-5_1

pallor (hence the white plague). TB was also called "the captain of all men of death" [3], and the emergence of human immunodeficiency virus (HIV) infection in the early 1980s gave the chance to TB to increase significantly in many areas around the globe. In this chapter, we review historical aspects of TB and epidemiology of the disease.

1.2 History

Using PCR techniques, *M. tuberculosis* complex was detected in the skeletal specimen in a fossil of a wiped-out long-horned bison dated back 17870 years ago[4]. In addition, TB was also detected in a human remain which is 9000 years old [5]. There was a clear similarity of the genetic signature between these and the current TB organism suggesting a long-term existence of TB and the human population [5]. This is further substantiated by the fact that only 10% of infected human population develop active infection [6]. The presence of vertebral TB infection (Pott's disease) (Fig. 1.1) was described in pre-

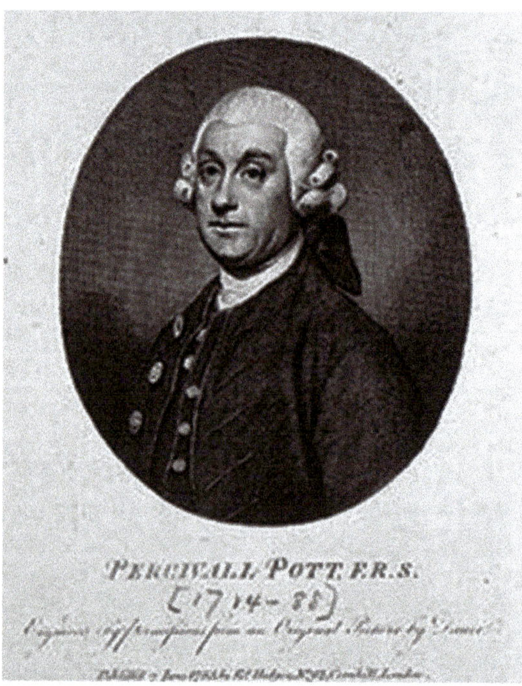

Fig. 1.1 A portrait of Percivall Pott (6 January 1714–22 December 1788), an English surgeon who was the first to describe tuberculosis (TB) of the spine (Pott's disease)

dynastic (3500–2650 BC) Egypt, and Neolithic (3200–2300 BC) Sweden racially linked to the first cattle breeders [7].

1.3 Epidemiology

It goes without saying that the global burden of TB is enormous. It is estimated that two billion people (33% of the world population) are infected with TB [8, 9]. Although certain countries harbor larger number of cases than other countries, these represent the high burden of TB countries. The appearance of HIV/acquired immunodeficiency syndrome (AIDS) resulted in an increase in the global burden of TB with a peak in the early 2000s and subsequent decrease over the last two decades [10]. These two diseases, TB and HIV infections, are the leading infectious disease agents to cause death worldwide (World Health Organization) [10]. It is estimated that the annual decline in the rate of TB worldwide is only 1·5% per year [10]. Of all the TB cases, 20% of cases are associated with HIV infection mainly in the sub-Saharan Africa [11]. Talking specifically about TB of the central nervous system (CNS), TB meningitis is considered to be rare constituting 1% of all cases of TB and 5% of extrapulmonary disease in patients with normal immunity [12, 13]. The main risk factors for the development of CNS TB include children and HIV infection [14–16], in addition to malnutrition, the use of immunosuppressive agents, and foreign-born individuals [17–19].

1.4 TB Vaccine

The widely used TB vaccine, the BCG, was initially started in 1908 by two French scientists Albert Calmette and Camille Guérin [20] (Fig. 1.2). They serially grew the "Koch's bacillus" (Fig. 1.3) to decrease the organism's virulence. The vaccine was later introduced in 1921 [20] after 230 culture times. Of particular importance is that the BCG was initially given orally to a child in Paris who was born to a mother with TB [20]. After that, BCG vaccine became the most

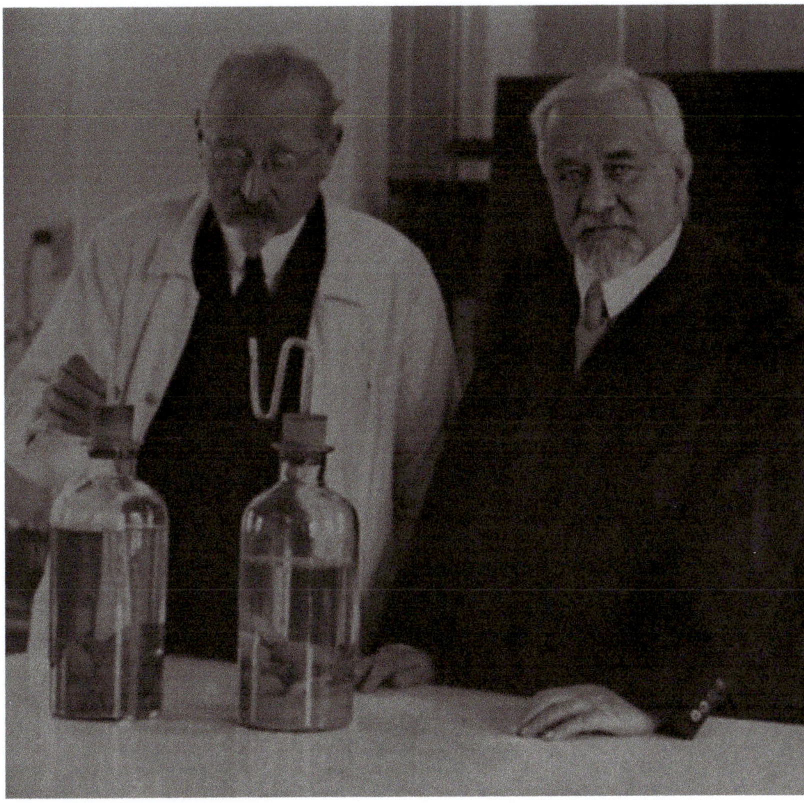

Fig. 1.2 Albert Calmette and Camille Guérin discovered that bovine TB bacilli can be used as a vaccine. They first used the BCG vaccine to vaccinate a child who lost his mother during delivery

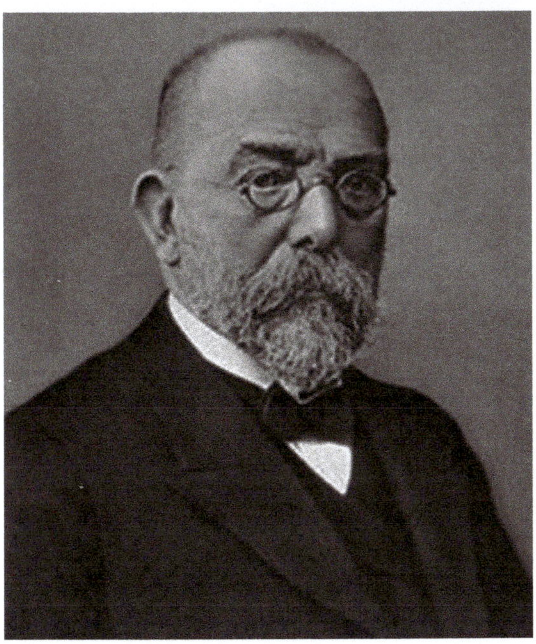

Fig. 1.3 Robert Heinrich Hermann Koch (11 December 1843–27 May 1910), a German physician who identified the specific causative agents of TB

frequently used vaccine worldwide. The effectiveness of the vaccine was variable from the 1920s to date, and one of the reasons for the observed variability is the use of different strains by different laboratories, thus accounting for what is known as different BCGs [21, 22]. These differences were elucidated using genomic comparison [21]. It had also been stated that BCG is a cost-effective intervention against severe pediatric TB in high-incidence countries [23]. However, it is important to keep in mind the possible dissemination of BCG vaccine strain in children with HIV infection which is estimated to be 992 per 100,000 children [24].

1.5 Surgical Therapy

The use of surgery to treat TB was started in 1821 by a Scottish physician, Dr. James Carson [25]. The surgery consisted of drainage of pleural effusion, inducing pneumothorax, or the plombage technique was used to treat TB [26]. The collapse therapy was initiated by the Italian physician Forlanini in 1888 [26]. In 1939, Hjaltested et al. published his experience with pneumothorax therapy in 191 TB cases [27]. Surgical therapy now is considered as an adjunct for treatment of MDR and XDR-TB [28].

1.6 Antimicrobial Therapy of TB

The use of anti-mycobacterial agents to treat TB was started with the discovery of streptomycin (STR) in 1944 [29]. The use of single agent, STR, resulted in considerable improvement in 51% compared with 8% in the bed rest group [30] (Fig. 1.4).

Subsequently, the use of a combination of STR and para-aminosalicylic acid (PAS) showed similar results with the reduction of resistance from 70% in STR compared to 9% in the combination therapy [31]. One additional advantage of PAS is being an oral medication. Subsequent studies utilized isoniazid (INH), STR, and PAS with an increase in the cure rate from 70 to 95% when the treatment was prolonged for 18–24 months [32]. The initial major study of a 6-month regimen of rifampicin (RIF) or pyrazinamide (PZA) with STR and INH showed better conversion rate to culture negative sputum and a reduced relapse rate [33–35]. Thus, a combination therapy became the standard therapy for the management of TB.

1.7 History of Therapy of CNS Tuberculosis

TB of the CNS was reported in 5–10% of patients with extrapulmonary TB [12] in 1963 to 1986. It was estimated that CNS TB developed in 1% of 82,764 TB cases in a Canadian cohort from 1970 to 2001 [13]. Tuberculous meningitis (TBM) was first described by Robert Whyth in 1768 in children [36], and subsequently in 1847, Charles Morehead described the autopsy findings in children with TBM followed by the description of tuberculoma by Ford [37]. The first attempt to cure CNS tuberculomas was done by Wernicke and Hahn in 1884 [38].

With the advent of modern therapy of TB, surgical interventions in patients with CNS TB are limited. Indications for neurosurgical referral include hydrocephalus, brain abscess, and vertebral TB with cord compression [39]. Initial surgical therapy was associated with 10% operative mortality and 40% mortality secondary to postoperative meningitis [40]. Surgical resection of intracranial tuberculoma was compared with anti-TB therapy with INH, ethambutol, and RIF. Anti-TB therapy was associated with improvement or a return to baseline activity [41]. This study was not randomized and uncontrolled trial of 20 cases of intracranial tuberculoma [41].

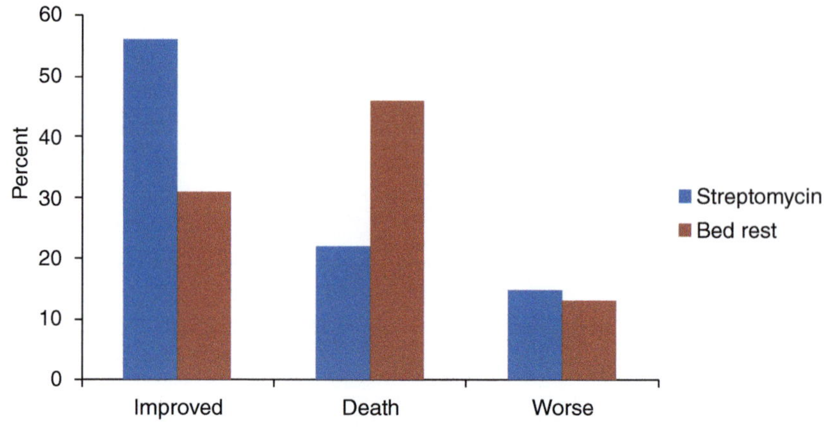

Fig. 1.4 Early study of streptomycin vs. bed rest in the treatment of pulmonary TB (Adapted from Ref. [30])

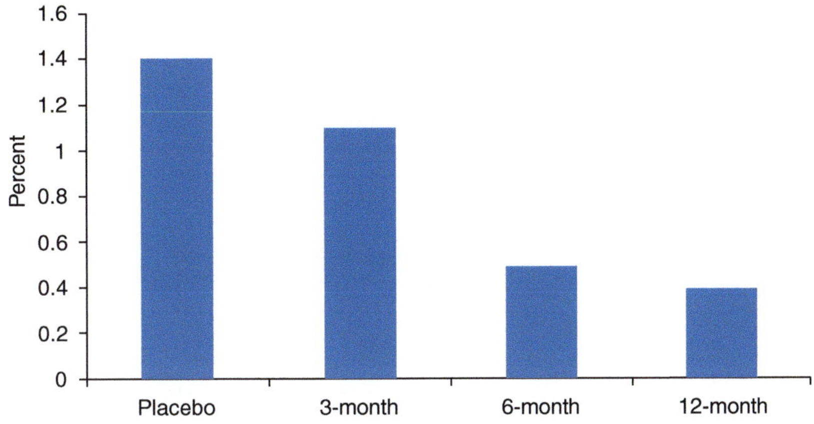

Fig. 1.5 A direct comparison of 3-, 6-, and 12-month regimens of INH showed a lower rate of active TB (Adapted from Ref. [45])

1.8 History of TB Preventive Therapy

There is a large population of patients with latent TB. Thus, the treatment of those patients makes an opportunity to reduce the global burden of TB. An initial study of the use of INH was done in children exposed to TB in the 1950s [42]. The study by the US Public Health Service (USPHS) in 1958 among Alaskan boarding school children (5–20 years of age) compared the use of 1.25 versus 5 mg/kg INH once a day or five times a week for 6 months [43]. The rate of active TB was 1.9% (10 of 513) of the higher-dose arm and was 5.8% (31/536) of the lower-dose arm [43]. Further studies showed that a longer duration of 24-month therapy was not better than a 6-month therapy [42, 44]. A direct comparison of 3-, 6-, and 12-month regimens of INH showed a lower rate of active TB among the longest duration (Fig. 1.5) [45]. Subsequently, RIF-PZA short-course therapy was effective for latent TB treatment with the rate of active TB of 2.4% in the RIF and PZA and 3.3% in the INH group corresponding to rates of 0.8 and 1.1 per 100 person-years, respectively [46]. This combination later was associated with increased hepatotoxicity [47].

Conclusion

TB is an antique disease and continues to be a main public health concern worldwide. The disease was described in Egyptian mummies and infected humans about three million years back. The development of the current therapeutic modalities passed through multiple stages since the introduction of STR. The introduction of BCG vaccines had initially resulted in wide use of this vaccine, and later the vaccine showed variable efficacy.

References

1. Hayman J (1984) Mycobacterium ulcerans: an infection from Jurassic time? Lancet (London, England) 2:1015–1016
2. Gutierrez MC, Brisse S, Brosch R, Fabre M, Omaïs B, Marmiesse M, Supply P, Vincent V (2005) Ancient origin and gene mosaicism of the progenitor of Mycobacterium tuberculosis. PLoS Pathog 1:e5
3. Mack RB (1984) Mimi, Violetta and the "captain of all the men of death" INH (isoniazid) poisoning. N C Med J 45:321–322
4. Rothschild B, Martin L, Lev G, Bercovier H, Kahila Bar-Gal G, Greenblatt C, Donoghue H, Spigelman M, Brittain D (2001) Mycobacterium tuberculosis complex DNA from an extinct bison dated 17,000 years before the present. Clin Infect Dis 33:305–311

5. Hershkovitz I, Donoghue HD, Minnikin DE, Besra GS, Lee OY, Gernaey AM, Galili E, Eshed V, Greenblatt CL, Lemma E, Bar-Gal GK, Spigelman M (2008) Detection and molecular characterization of 9,000-year-old Mycobacterium tuberculosis from a Neolithic settlement in the Eastern Mediterranean. PLoS One 2008:3
6. Hirsh AE, Tsolaki AG, DeRiemer K, Feldman MW, Small PM (2004) Stable association between strains of Mycobacterium tuberculosis and their human host populations. Proc Natl Acad Sci U S A 101:4871–4876
7. Zink A, Haas CJ, Reischl U, Szeimies U, Nerlich AG (2001) Molecular analysis of skeletal tuberculosis in an ancient Egyptian population. J Med Microbiol 50:355–366
8. Lönnroth K, Raviglione M (2008) Global epidemiology of tuberculosis: prospects for control. Semin Respir Crit Care Med 429:481–491
9. Dheda K, Barry CE, Maartens G (2015) Tuberculosis. Lancet 387(10024):1211–1226
10. WHO (2015) Global tuberculosis report 2015 Available at: http://apps.who.int/iris/bitstream/10665/191102/1/9789241565059_eng.pdf. Accesed 20 Mar 2016
11. Waaler HT (2002) Tuberculosis and poverty. Int J Tuberc Lung Dis 6:745–746
12. Rieder HL, Snider DE, Cauthen GM (1990) Extrapulmonary tuberculosis in the United States. Am Rev Respir Dis 141:347–351
13. Phypers M, Harris T, Power C (2006) CNS tuberculosis: a longitudinal analysis of epidemiological and clinical features. Int J Tuberc Lung Dis 10:99–103
14. Farer LS, Lowell AM, Meador MP (1979) Extrapulmonary tuberculosis in the United States. Am J Epidemiol 109:205–217
15. Berenguer J, Moreno S, Laguna F, Vicente T, Adrados M, Ortega A, González-LaHoz J, Bouza E (1992) Tuberculous meningitis in patients infected with the human immunodeficiency virus. N Engl J Med 326:668–672
16. Dubé MP, Holtom PD, Larsen RA (1992) Tuberculous meningitis in patients with and without human immunodeficiency virus infection. Am J Med 93:520–524
17. Klein NC, Damsker B, Hirschman SZ (1985) Mycobacterial meningitis. Retrospective analysis from 1970 to 1983. Am J Med 79:29–34
18. Ogawa SK, Smith MA, Brennessel DJ, Lowy FD (1987) Tuberculous meningitis in an urban medical center. Medicine (Baltimore) 66:317–326
19. Verdon R, Chevret S, Laissy JP, Wolff M (1996) Tuberculous meningitis in adults: review of 48 cases. Clin Infect Dis 22:982–988
20. Calmette A (1931) Preventive vaccination against tuberculosis with BCG. Proc R Soc Med 24:1481–1490
21. Behr MA (2002) BCG–different strains, different vaccines? Lancet Infect Dis 2:86–92
22. Kernodle DS (2010) Decrease in the effectiveness of Bacille Calmette-Guérin vaccine against pulmonary tuberculosis: a consequence of increased immune suppression by microbial antioxidants, not overattenuation. Clin Infect Dis 51:177–184
23. Trunz BB, Fine P, Dye C (2006) Effect of BCG vaccination on childhood tuberculous meningitis and miliary tuberculosis worldwide: a meta-analysis and assessment of cost-effectiveness. Lancet 367:1173–1180
24. Hesseling AC, Johnson LF, Jaspan H, Cotton MF, Whitelaw A, Schaaf HS, Fine PE, Eley BS, Marais BJ, Nuttall J, Beyers N, Godfrey-Faussett P (2009) Disseminated bacille Calmette-Guérin disease in HIV-infected South African infants. Bull World Health Organ 87:505–511
25. Dubovsky H (1992) Artificial pneumothorax in the treatment of lung tuberculosis. S Afr Med J 81:372–375
26. Wolfart W (1990) Surgical treatment of tuberculosis and its modifications–collapse therapy and resection treatment and their present-day sequelae. Offentl Gesundheitswes 52:506–511
27. Oli Hjaltested KT (1939) No Title. Br J Tuberc 33:4–16
28. Fox GJ, Mitnick CD, Benedetti A, Chan ED, Becerra M, Chiang CY, Keshavjee S, Koh WJ, Shiraishi Y, Viiklepp P, Yim JJ, Pasvol G, Robert J, Shim TS, Shin SS, Menzies D, Collaborative Group for Meta-Analysis of Individual Patient Data in MDR-TB (2016) Surgery as an adjunctive treatment for multidrug-resistant tuberculosis: an individual patient data metaanalysis. Clin Infect Dis 62(7):887–895
29. Waksman SA (1954) Tenth anniversary of the discovery of streptomycin, the first chemotherapeutic agent found to be effective against tuberculosis in humans. Am Rev Tuberc 70:1–8
30. [No authors listed] (1948) Streptomycin treatment of pulmonary tuberculosis. Br Med J 2:769–782
31. [No authors listed] (1949) PAS and streptomycin. Br Med J 2:1515–1516
32. Council MR (1962) Long-term chemotherapy in the treatment of chronic pulmonary tuberculosis with cavitations. Tubercle 43:201
33. [No authors listed] (1973) Controlled clinical trial of four short-course (6-month) regimens of chemotherapy for treatment of pulmonary tuberculosis. Second report. Lancet 1:1331–1338
34. [No authors listed] (1974) Controlled clinical trial of four short-course (6-month) regimens of chemotherapy for treatment of pulmonary tuberculosis. Lancet 2:1100–1106
35. [No authors listed] (1974) Controlled clinical trial of four short-course (6-month) regimens of chemotherapy for treatment of pulmonary tuberculosis. Third report. East African-British Medical Research Councils. Lancet 2:237–240
36. Gupta SKC (1981) Tuberculosis meningitis in children. Indian J Tuberc 28:3–11
37. Ramamurthi B, Ramamurthi R, Vasudevan MC, Sridhar K (1993) The changing face of tuberculomas. Ann Acad Med Singapore 22:852–855
38. Buchstein HFAA (1940) Tuberculoma of the brain. Arch Neur Psych 43:635–648

39. Cherian A, Thomas SV (2011) Central nervous system tuberculosis. Afr Health Sci 11:116–127
40. Yaramiş A, Gurkan F, Elevli M, Söker M, Haspolat K, Kirbaş G, Taş MA (1998) Central nervous system tuberculosis in children: a review of 214 cases. Pediatrics 102:E49
41. Harder E, Al-Kawi MZ, Carney P (1983) Intracranial tuberculoma: conservative management. Am J Med 74:570–576
42. Comstock GW, Baum C, Snider DE (1979) Isoniazid prophylaxis among Alaskan Eskimos: a final report of the bethel isoniazid studies. Am Rev Respir Dis 119:827–830
43. Comstock GW (1999) How much isoniazid is needed for prevention of tuberculosis among immunocompetent adults? Int J Tuberc Lung Dis 3:847–850
44. Comstock GW, Ferebee SH (1970) How much isoniazid is needed for prophylaxis? Am Rev Respir Dis 101:780–782
45. [No authors listed] (1982) Efficacy of various durations of isoniazid preventive therapy for tuberculosis: five years of follow-up in the IUAT trial. International Union Against Tuberculosis Committee on Prophylaxis. Bull World Health Organ 60:555–564
46. Gordin F, Chaisson RE, Matts JP, Miller C, de Lourdes GM, Hafner R, Valdespino JL, Coberly J, Schechter M, Klukowicz AJ, Barry MA, O'Brien RJ (2000) Rifampin and pyrazinamide vs isoniazid for prevention of tuberculosis in HIV-infected persons: an international randomized trial. Terry Beirn Community Programs for Clinical Research on AIDS, the Adult AIDS Clinical Trials Group, the Pan American Health O. JAMA 283:1445–1450
47. Centers for Disease Control and Prevention (CDC) (2001) Fatal and severe hepatitis associated with rifampin and pyrazinamide for the treatment of latent tuberculosis infection–New York and Georgia, 2000. MMWR Morb Mortal Wkly Rep 50:289–2891

Human Genetics of Tuberculosis of the Nervous System

2

Jamila El Baghdadi, Safa El Azbaoui, Fatima Ailal, Ali Akhaddar, Ayoub Sabri, Xiao-Fei Kong, Ahmed Aziz Bousfiha, Jean Laurent Casanova, Laurent Abel, and Stéphanie Boisson-Dupuis

Contents

J. El Baghdadi, PhD (✉)
Genetics Unit, Military Hospital Mohammed V, Hay Riad, 10100 Rabat, Morocco
e-mail: baghdadijamila@yahoo.fr

S. El Azbaoui, PhD student • A. Sabri, PhD student
Genetics Unit, Military Hospital Mohammed V, Hay Riad, 10100 Rabat, Morocco

Faculty of Sciences – Kenitra, IbnTofail University, Kenitra, Morocco
e-mail: safa.elazbaoui@gmail.com; ayoub.sabri@gmail.com

F. Ailal, MD
Department of Pediatrics P1, Clinical Immmunology Unit, Casablanca Children Hospital, Medical and Pharmacy School of Casablanca, King Hassan II University, Casablanca, Morocco
e-mail: drailalfatima@gmail.com

A. Akhaddar, MD, IFAANS
Department of Neurosurgery, Avicenne Military Hospital, Marrakech, Morocco
Mohammed V University, Rabat, Morocco
e-mail: akhaddar@hotmail.fr

X.-F. Kong, MD, PhD
St. Giles Laboratory of Human Genetics of Infectious Disease, Rockefeller Branch, Rockefeller University Hospital, The Rockefeller University, 1230 York Avenue, New York, NY 10065, USA
e-mail: xiko262@rockefeller.edu

A.A. Bousfiha, MD
Clinical Immunology Unit, Casablanca Children's Hospital, Ibn Rochd Medical School, King Hassan II University, Casablanca, Morocco
e-mail: profbousfiha@gmail.com

J.L. Casanova, MD, PhD
St. Giles Laboratory of Human Genetics of Infectious Disease, Rockefeller Branch, Rockefeller University Hospital, The Rockefeller University, 1230 York Avenue, New York, NY 10065, USA

Laboratory of Human Genetics of Infectious Diseases, Necker Branch, INSERM U1163, Necker Hospital for Sick Children, Paris, France

Paris Descartes University, Imagine Institute, Paris, France

Pediatric Hematology-Immunology Unit, Assistance Publique-Hôpitaux de Paris, Necker Hospital for Sick Children, Paris, France

Howard Hughes Medical Institute, New York, NY, USA
e-mail: jean-laurent.casanova@rockefeller.edu

L. Abel, MD, PhD • S. Boisson-Dupuis, PhD
St. Giles Laboratory of Human Genetics of Infectious Disease, Rockefeller Branch,

M. Turgut et al. (eds.), *Tuberculosis of the Central Nervous System*,
DOI 10.1007/978-3-319-50712-5_2

Rockefeller University Hospital, The Rockefeller University, 1230 York Avenue, New York, NY 10065, USA

Laboratory of Human Genetics of Infectious Diseases, Necker Branch, INSERM U1163, Necker Hospital for Sick Children, Paris, France

Paris Descartes University, Imagine Institute, Paris, France
e-mail: laurent.abel@inserm.fr; stbo603@rockefeller.edu

Abbreviations

BCG	Bacillus Calmette-Guérin vaccine
CADD	Combined Annotation-Dependent Depletion is a tool for scoring the deleteriousness of single-nucleotide variants as well as insertion/deletion variants in the human genome (http://cadd.gs.washington.edu)
CNS	Central nervous system
CSF	Cerebrospinal fluid
CT scan	Computed tomography scan
DNA	Deoxyribonucleic acid
EBV	Epstein-Barr virus
EMSA	Electrophoretic mobility shift assay
GAF	Gamma-activating factor
GAS	Gamma-activating sequences
GOF	Gain of function
HIES	Hyper IgE syndrome
IFN-γ	Interferon gamma
IL-12	Interleukin 12
INH	Isoniazid
ISGF3	Interferon-stimulated gene factor 3
LIF	Leukemia inhibitory factor
LOF	Loss of function
MRI	Magnetic resonance imaging
MSMD	Syndrome of Mendelian susceptibility to mycobacterial diseases
NK	Natural killer cell
rh	Recombinant human
RIF	Rifampin
SNP	Single-nucleotide polymorphism
TB	Tuberculosis
TBM	Tuberculous meningitis
WES	Whole exome sequencing

2.1 Introduction

Tuberculosis (TB) remains a major public health problem, as *Mycobacterium tuberculosis* infects about one third of the world's population, with >9 million new cases and ~1.5 million deaths from TB in 2014 [1]. The burden of TB in children is also very high, with an estimated number of ~1 million new cases of TB in children and 136,000 deaths reported in 2014 [1]. However, only a small fraction of infected subjects develop clinical TB [2, 3]. Most subjects (~95%) contain the initial infection, and a minority of latently infected subjects (~5%) subsequently develop active disease after an interval of many years, typically due to the reactivation of pulmonary TB [4]. The remaining infected subjects (~5%) develop clinical TB within 2 years of infection, either without latency or after a short latent phase. This "primary" TB is common in children, runs an acute course, and is often associated with extrapulmonary disease [2]. BCG vaccination provides some protection against disseminated TB in childhood, but this protection is incomplete [5]. One of the fundamental questions in the field of childhood TB therefore concerns the causes of the predisposition to the development of severe forms in only a minority of infected children.

Among disseminated extrapulmonary forms of the diseases, central nervous system (CNS) TB is the most devastating manifestation of the infection [6]. The main pathological manifestations include meningitis, tuberculomas, and brain abscesses [6, 7]. CNS TB accounts for up to 10% of all cases of extrapulmonary TB and carries high neurological morbidity and mortality rates [8]. CNS TB is more frequent and virulent in children than in adults [9]. Hydrocephalus is more common in children, while vasculitis that develops due to the inflammatory process is the most serious consequence of tuberculous meningitis (TBM) [10]. The most common parenchymal lesions in TB of CNS are tuberculomas. Tuberculous abscesses are different from tuberculomas as they contain central caseation [11]. The clinical manifestations of CNS TB are nonspecific and may initially include cough, headache, fever, vomiting, stiff neck, focal seizures, convulsions, focal neurological deficits, loss of consciousness, and coma. The diagnosis of CNS TB remains challenging because of the common absence of bacteriological confirmation and is usually based on a combination of epidemiological, clinical, radiological, and biological features, in particular cerebrospinal fluid (CSF) analysis.

Despite the severity of CNS TB, the cellular mechanisms underlying its pathophysiology are poorly understood [7]. The findings obtained in the last decade have provided the first clues for the involved mechanisms, by showing that at least some severe TB cases can be explained by single-gene inborn errors of immunity [2]. In particular, these studies have highlighted the central role of the IL-12/IL-23-IFN-γ pathway in some children who presented with disseminated TB as their sole clinical phenotype [12–15]. Upon *M. tuberculosis* infection, primary host response cells such as macrophages release a range of cytokines including IL-12, which stimulate the production of IFN-γ by T and NK cells [15] (Fig. 2.1). This cytokine activates macrophages to kill intracellular pathogens such as *M. tuberculosis* and enhances the differentiation of IFN-γ-producing T helper cells [16]. Genetic defects leading to an impairment of production of (e.g., mutations in *IL12B*, *IL12RB1*, *ISG15*) or response to (e.g., mutations in *IFNGR1*, *IFNGR2*, *STAT1*) IFN-γ were found initially in patients who had disseminated infections by weakly virulent mycobacteria as the BCG vaccine in the context of the syndrome of Mendelian susceptibility to mycobacterial diseases (MSMD) [2, 17, 18]. Several cases of severe TB children were subsequently shown to be explained by mutations in some MSMD genes such as *IL12B*, *STAT1*, and *IFNGR1* [2, 15] with the most common defect being IL-12Rβ1 deficiency (due to *IL12RB1* mutations) [13] including in several Moroccan children [14]. Those children had disseminated TB, with several extrapulmonary manifestations, but none of them were clearly reported with CNS TB yet.

TB is still highly endemic in Morocco, with ~28,000 new TB cases in 2013, including 2051 (7%) in children under the age of 15 years [1]. Few studies have reported series of CNS TB patients in Morocco. In a large series of 465 Moroccan TB children reported in the late

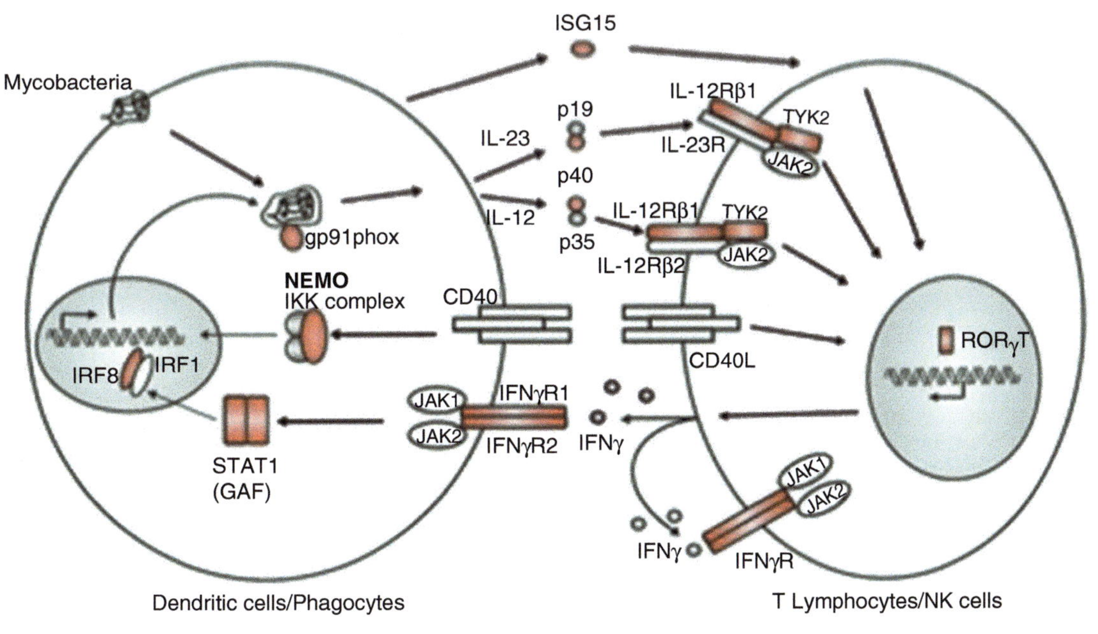

Fig. 2.1 Schematic representation of the interaction between phagocytes/dendritic cells and T lymphocytes/NK cells upon mycobacterial infection. Molecules in red are mutated in patients with mycobacterial diseases

1980s from the Pediatric Rabat Hospital, about 50% (234) had extrapulmonary TB [19]. Among those 234 patients with extrapulmonary forms, 43 (18%) had TBM, and the CSF was bacteriologically positive in 18% of these 43 patients. Anti-TB treatment was 18 months associated with corticosteroids in 30 patients, and the proportion of fatal outcomes was 21% (9/43) [19]. A more recent report described the clinical features of 22 Moroccan adult patients with CNS TB [20]. CSF analysis was abnormal in 82.2% cases, and magnetic resonance imaging (MRI) was abnormal in 12 patients with hydrocephalus, intracerebral tuberculomas, meningitis, cerebral infarction, and/or spinal cord involvement [20]. In the present review, we describe two Moroccan children with CNS TB in whom we recently identified mutations in two genes of the IL-12/IFN-γ circuit, *TYK2* and *STAT1*.

2.2 Patients

2.2.1 Family 1

The index case P1 is a young girl, born in 1992 to a Moroccan first-degree consanguineous family. She was BCG vaccinated at birth according to the national immunization program. At the age of 13 years, she was diagnosed with peritoneal TB. She was treated with anti-mycobacterial treatment for 6 months: rifampin (RIF), isoniazid (INH), and pyrazinamide for 2 months, followed by 4 months with RIF and INH. At 1-month follow-up from end of treatment, she suffered from intermittent fever and abdominal pain. She presented with an extra-articular flessum of the right hip and an abdominal mass. Echography of the abdomen showed a psoas abscess associated with deep abdominal adenopathy. X-ray showed no involvement of the spine and chest. The echocardiography revealed a constricted pericarditis. The culture on Lowenstein-Jensen from the pus of psoas abscess identified *M. tuberculosis*, and the anatomopathologic examination showed some epithelioid cells and inflammatory lesions without granulomatous or necrosis. She was again treated with anti-TB treatment with good clinical and radiological outcomes. Four months after the end of treatment, P1 was hospitalized for acute febrile meningitis. CSF hypoglycorrhachia and decreased levels of chlorides raised the suspicion of TB meningitis. Despite a treatment associating cephalosporin, ciprofloxacin, amikacin, and anti-TB drugs with corticosteroids, neurological complications occurred leading to coma and death. Her young brother, denoted as P2, was hospitalized at the age of 8 months for meningitis of unknown etiology. He suffered from recurrent otitis and urinary tract infections and presented asthma and eczema of the ear canal. P2 is now 15 years old, has no treatment, and is followed in Pediatric Hospital in Casablanca.

2.2.2 Family 2

The patient P3 is a young girl born in 1994, to a Moroccan first-degree consanguineous family. She was BCG vaccinated at birth and was healthy until 2011. At the age of 17 years, she was hospitalized with clinical symptoms including fever, headache, night sweats, weight loss, weakness, vomiting, cough, and tetraplegia. She had cervical lymphadenopathy, and the pathological analysis from a lymph-node biopsy revealed typical caseating necrosis tuberculous granulomas which were culture negative for *M. tuberculosis*. She developed triventricular aggressive hydrocephalus. Cranial MRI revealed multiple lesions throughout the cerebral hemispheres, cerebellum, and brain stem suggestive of tuberculomas [21]. The patient received anti-TB therapy for 1 year with 2 months of corticosteroids. She recovered and a follow-up MRI showed that all lesions were resolved. Six months after the end of treatment, the contrast-enhanced brain CT scan revealed a solitary brain abscess, and surgical intervention was performed. The pus from the brain abscess was microscopy positive (Ziehl-Neelsen staining) with identification of *M. tuberculosis* by culture. The patient died despite anti-TB and intensive care treatments.

2.3 Genetic and Functional Analyses

Whole exome sequencing (WES) analysis was performed on P1 and P3 as described elsewhere [22]. All calls with a coverage ≤4X and a phred-scaled quality ≤30 were filtered out. WES data were filtered based on the frequency of the variations: at first unknown variations, not described in public databases, particularly in genes known to be part of the IL-12/IFN-γ signaling pathway were considered.

The patient P1 displays a homozygous frame-shift insertion of one base pair in exon 23 of *TYK2*, 3315_3316insC [23]. The mutation is predicted to cause a premature stop codon at position 1109 (T1105HfsX4). Familial segregation reveals that both parents are heterozygous and healthy (Fig. 2.2a). Her younger brother, P2, is also homozygous for the rare *TYK2* mutation and suffered from meningitis at 8 months of age, from unknown etiology. These results suggest an autosomal recessive TYK2 deficiency in this family. TYK2 is a member of the Janus kinase family (JAK) and part of the JAK-STAT signaling pathways (Fig. 2.1). Briefly, following ligand binding to the receptors, the JAKs are activated by auto- and transphosphorylation (on tyrosines), and they phosphorylate the intracellular part of the receptor to which they are associated. This created a docking site for latent cytoplasmic STATs protein. The STATs are then recruited to the receptor, phosphorylated by the JAKs, and then dissociate from the receptors to form homo-/heterodimers or heterotrimers, translocate to the nucleus, and modulate the transcription of target genes. At this time, human TYK2 deficiency had already been identified in two different families [24, 25]. The first description in 2006 identifies *TYK2* as a new genetic etiology of the hyper IgE syndrome. Indeed, the Japanese patient suffered from atopic dermatitis, high IgE serum level, and staphylococcal abscesses [24]. This patient also displayed mycobacterial and viral diseases. The second patient identified was Turkish and suffered only from mycobacterial and viral diseases [25]. Altogether, *TYK2* was a good candidate gene for this family.

At the cellular level, a complete and thorough analysis was performed in order to understand the differences in clinical phenotypes of the patients described and to highlight TYK2-dependent signaling pathways, in humans. Western blot analysis showed that TYK2 expression was not detectable on immortalized EBV-transformed B cells derived from P1, compared to a healthy control. TYK2-deficient patients displayed impaired but not abolished cellular responses to IL-12, as illustrated in Fig. 2.2b. The response to IL-12 was tested in the context of a whole blood assay. Briefly, blood from the patient as well as healthy travel controls, healthy controls, and IL-12Rβ1-deficient patients were either not stimulated or stimulated with BCG and BCG+IL-12. As a readout, the production of IFN-γ was tested 48 h later. As expected, patients with a complete IL-12Rβ1 deficiency were unable to respond to a stimulation with IL-12, as compared to healthy controls and healthy travel controls. TYK2-deficient patients display a significantly impaired response, as compared to the healthy travel controls. This demonstrates that TYK2 is required for a normal IL-12 response; however, a TYK2-independent response is also visible, explaining the impaired but not abolished IL-12 response. The response to IFN-α was also tested. After IFN-α stimulation, phosphorylation of STAT1 and STAT3 is observed in control cells. However, in cells from the TYK2-deficient patient, the phosphorylation of STAT1 was impaired, and the phosphorylation of STAT3 was abolished (Fig. 2.2c). The STAT3 phosphorylation after IFN-α/IFN-β stimulation was rescued by transduction of the WT allele of *TYK2* within the cells. These results show that TYK2 is required for IFN-α/IFN-β signaling, but, as for IL-12, a TYK2-independent response to IFN-α/IFN-β is also visible. Other functional assessments showed that TYK2-deficient cells display an impaired response to IL-23, with normal proportions of circulating IL-17+ T cells, and an impaired IL-10 response [23]. Cellular responses to IL-21, IL-27, IFN-γ, IL-28/IL-29 (IFN-l), and leukemia inhibitory factor (LIF) were normal.

WES of patient P3 was analyzed following the same criteria as P1. In P3, a heterozygous unreported

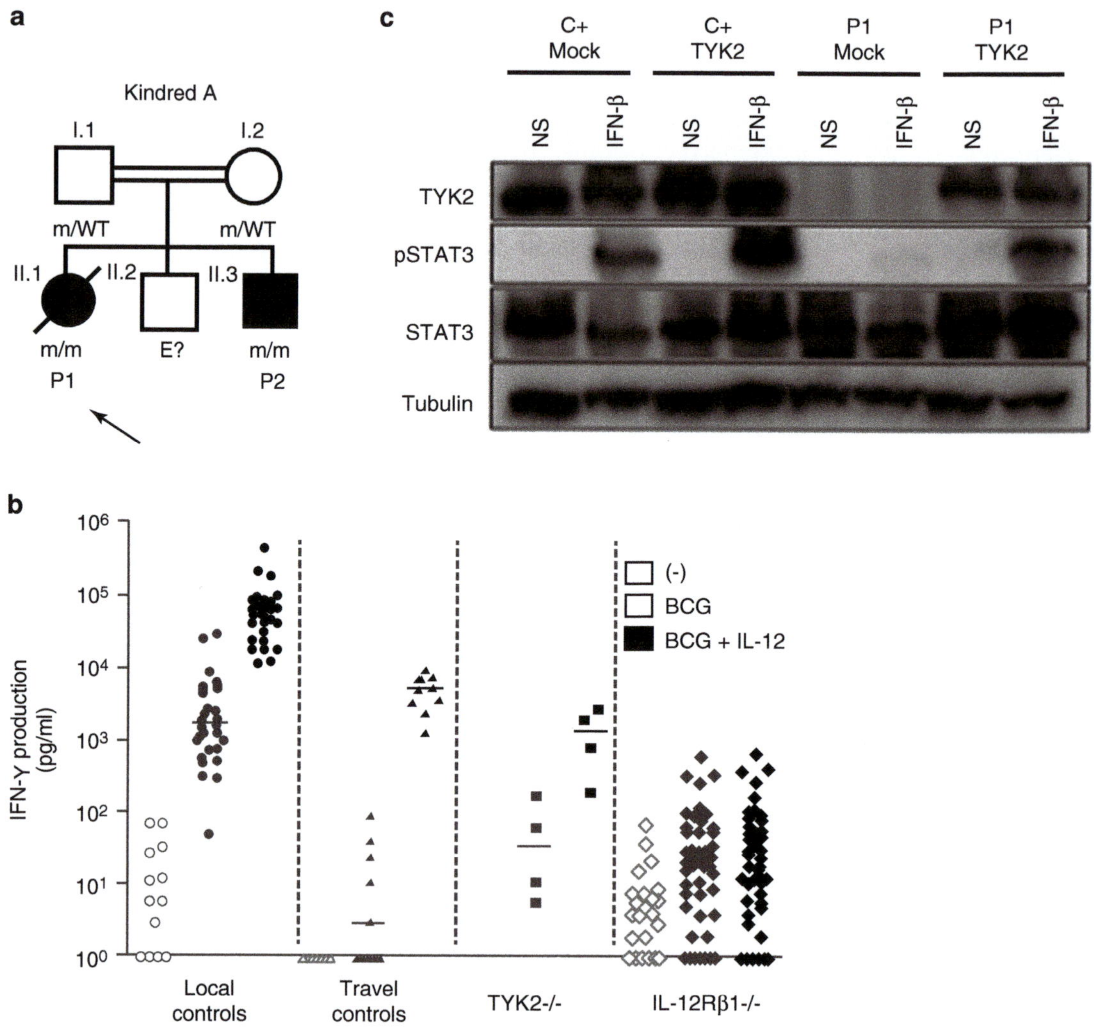

Fig. 2.2 Genetic and functional characterization of TYK2-deficient patient P1. (**a**) Pedigree of the TYK2-deficient family. The generations are indicated by a Roman numeral (I–II) and the individuals by an Arabic numeral. A double line between the parents means consanguinity. The arrow points to the proband (P1). *Black* shapes indicate disease status. "m" indicates a mutated allele. (**b**) Impaired response to IL-12 in TYK2-deficient patients. Blood was stimulated for 48 h with BCG alone (MOI = 20) or BCG and 20 ng/ml IL-12. The IFN-γ production was assessed by ELISA on supernatants from healthy individuals (local controls, LC), patients, healthy relatives (travel controls, TC, to whom the patients should be compared), TYK2-deficient patients including P1, and negative controls (IL-12Rβ1-/-). Mean values for each set of conditions are indicated by solid lines. (**c**) Impaired IFN-α/IFN-β signaling pathway, rescued by transduction of *WT-TYK2*. Western blot detecting pSTAT3 in mock-transduced (Mock) or TYK2-transduced (TYK2) EBV-B cells from a healthy control (C+) and P1, without (NS) and with (IFN-β) stimulation for 30 min with 10^5 IU/ml IFN-β. The following specific antibodies were used: anti-TYK2, anti-pSTAT3, anti-STAT3, and anti-tubulin as a loading control

variation was detected in *STAT1*. The familial segregation is currently unknown (Fig. 2.3a). The variation is a missense mutation replacing a leucine in position 498 to a valine (L498V). The leucine at position 498 is highly conserved in other species and predicted to be damaging with a CADD score at 24. It locates in the linker domain of STAT1, and surprisingly no mutations in this domain of the protein have been described. STAT1 is a transcription factor of the STAT family, activated as described before. Schematically, STAT1 is involved in different signaling pathways: IFN-γ (and IL-27) and IFN-α/IFN-β (and IL-29). Activation by IFN-γ (and IL-27) leads to the activation of STAT1 homodi-

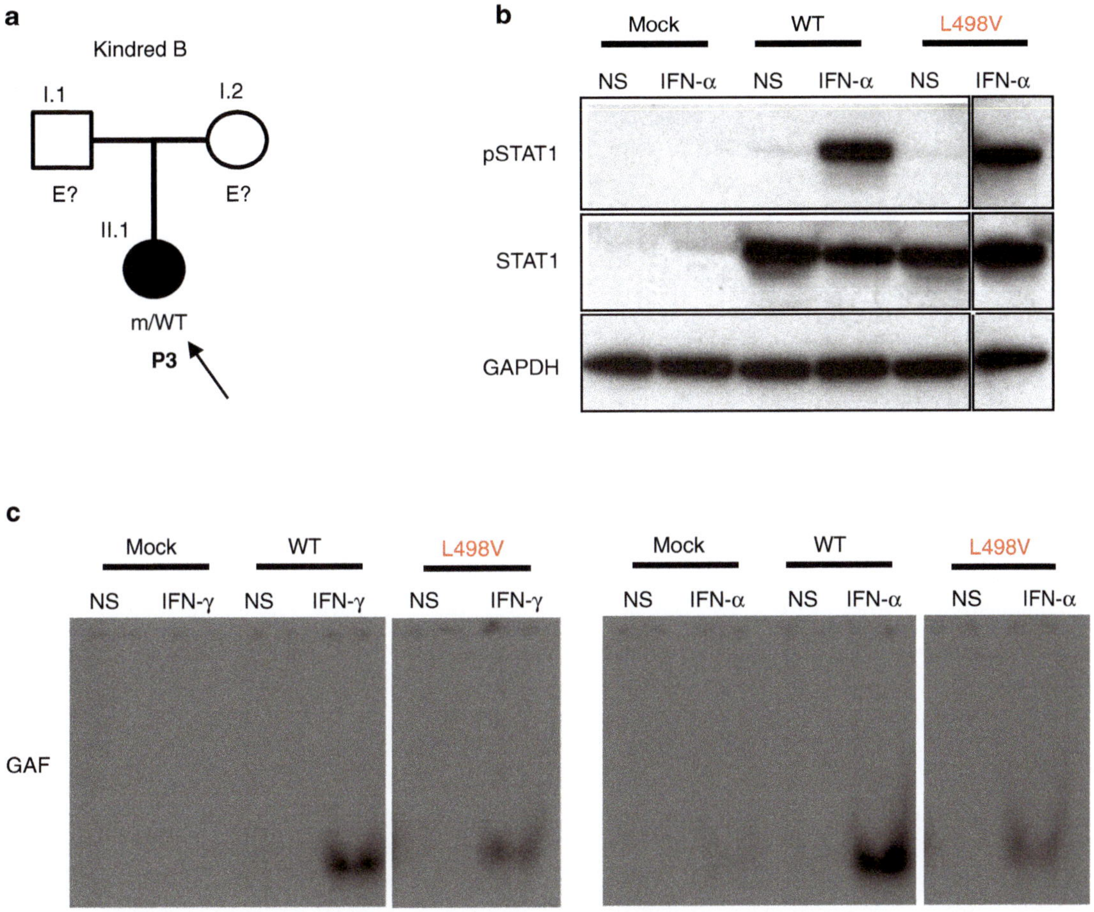

Fig. 2.3 Genetic and cellular investigation of STAT1-deficient patient P3. (**a**) Familial segregation of the mutant *STAT1* allele. The generations are indicated by a Roman numeral (I–II) and the individuals by an Arabic numeral. The *arrow* points to the proband. *Black shapes* indicate disease status. "E" means no genetic data available and "m" indicates a mutated allele. (**b**) L498V *STAT1* allele is normally phosphorylated. Western blot detecting pSTAT1 in mock-transduced (Mock), wild-type STAT1-transduced (WT), or L498V-STAT1-transduced (L498V) U3C cell line (deficient for STAT1) without (NS) and with (IFN-α) stimulation for 30 min with 10^5 IU/ml IFN-α. The following specific antibodies were used: anti-STAT1, anti-pSTAT1, and anti-GAPDH as a loading control. (**c**) L498V *STAT1* allele impairs DNA-binding activity. EMSA performed on mock-transduced (Mock), wild-type STAT1-transduced (WT), or L498V-STAT1-transduced (L498V) U3C cell line (deficient for STAT1) without (NS) or with stimulation with IFN-γ (10^5 IU/ml)(*left*) or IFN-α (10^5 IU/ml)(*right*) for 30 min, with a GAS probe

mers, named GAF for gamma-activating factor, that bind GAS (gamma-activated sequences) in the promoter of target genes. GAF activation also occurs following IFN-α/IFN-β stimulation. The main transcription factor activated by IFN-α/IFN-β and IL-29 is a heterotrimer consisting of STAT1/STAT2 and p48 and named ISGF3 (interferon-stimulated gene factor 3) that subsequently binds to ISRE sequences in the promoter of target genes. It was shown previously that GAF-IFN-γ and ISGF3-IFN-α/IFN-β signaling mediate anti-mycobacterial and antiviral immunity, respectively [26, 27]. Different types of autosomal dominant *STAT1* mutations have been described [26, 28–30]. The first ones are loss-of-function (LOF) mutations with a dominant negative effect over the wild type [26, 28, 31–33]. They alter either the phosphorylation or the DNA-binding activity of STAT1. The patients suffered from mycobacterial disease due to a lack of IFN-γ responses, via STAT1. The others are gain-of-function (GOF) *STAT1* mutations and have been described extensively in patients with chronic mucocutaneous candidiasis [29, 30]. However, mycobacterial disease is also observed in a minority of patients even though the cellular mechanism remains unexplained [34–37].

To differentiate between these two possibilities, Western blotting and electrophoretic mobility shift assays (EMSA), looking at the phosphorylation and DNA-binding activity of STAT1 homodimers (GAF, gamma-activating factor), respectively, were performed. In human cells deficient for STAT1, the functional effect of the mutation was assessed. As shown in Fig. 2.3b, by the Western blotting, the *STAT1* L498V allele displayed normal phosphorylation (comparable to the wild-type allele) after IFN-α/IFN-β stimulation. GOF alleles previously tested and reported in the literature exhibit an increased phosphorylation as compared to the wild-type allele [29]. In addition, a decreased (but not abolished) intensity of the GAS-binding complexes is observed in Fig. 2.3c by EMSA compared to the wild-type allele. The complexes were shown to be specific and formed of STAT1 by adding an excess of cold probe and by super-shift experiments (adding specific antibodies) (not shown). These results suggest that L498V allele is hypomorphic and results in AD LOF STAT1 deficiency. As for the other AD LOF STAT1 mutations, GAF DNA-binding activity is also impaired after IFN-α/IFN-β stimulation; however, the DNA-binding activity of ISGF3, interferon-stimulated gene factor 3 (composed of STAT1/STAT2/p48), is maintained, certainly explaining the absence of viral diseases in these patients. Altogether, we describe here another genetic etiology for childhood TB, AD LOF STAT1 deficiency, that should be considered in patients, in particular with CNS TB.

2.4 Discussion

We described the first Moroccan patients with inherited TYK2 deficiency. The proband P1 had multifocal TB disease (lymphadenopathy, abdominal, and meningitis TB) leading to her death. Her younger brother P2 had meningitis from unknown etiology at 8 months of age and did not suffer from any other infectious diseases since. The clinical phenotype of these two TYK2-deficient patients is similar to the six other TYK2-deficient patients described [23–25]. The core clinical phenotype shared by all the patients with TYK2 deficiency is mycobacterial disease (either BCG or *M. tuberculosis*) and/or viral diseases (mainly from herpes viruses), due to impaired IL-12 and IFN-α/IFN-β responses, respectively. All TYK2-deficient patients but one exhibit a normal response to IL-6 and did not display any clinical signs of hyper IgE (atopic dermatitis, high serum IgE level, and staphylococcal abscesses) [23]. This contrasts with the first Japanese TYK2-deficient patient described who presented the classical clinical signs of hyper IgE associated with mycobacterial and viral diseases [24]. It has been shown that the response to IL-6 is independent of TYK2 and that reintroduction of a WT *TYK2* into the Japanese cells did not rescue the impaired response to IL-6 [23]. Altogether, this suggests that the impaired response to IL-6 in this patient may be TYK2 independent and responsible for some of the clinical features of HIES. All the TYK2-deficient patients were BCG vaccinated, but only four developed BCG-osis, consistent with an impaired but not abolished response to IL-12/IL-23. Indeed, incomplete clinical penetrance is also observed in patients with complete IL-12Rβ1 deficiency presenting with an abolished response to both IL-12 and IL-23. Finally, an Iranian TYK2-deficient patient has also been identified, and the patient suffered from pulmonary TB as the sole clinical phenotype [23]. These cases show clearly that complete TYK2 deficiency is a genetic etiology of TB.

We are also reporting the first Moroccan patient (P3) with inherited STAT1 deficiency presenting with multifocal TB disease including lymphadenopathy, meningoencephalitis, tuberculomas, and brain abscesses. The first identification of MSMD-causing mutations of *STAT1* was described in a 33-year-old French patient, who developed a disseminated infection by BCG in her infancy [26]. To date, eight heterozygous LOF *STAT1* mutations have been reported in nine unrelated families (including ours) originating from different countries

(France, Saudi Arabia, Japan, the United States of America, Germany) [26, 28, 31–33]. These mutations are heterozygous missense mutations affecting mainly the C-terminal part of STAT1, i.e., the SH2 domain and the tail segment of STAT1 (L706S, Y701C, K673R, M654K, and K637E). Two additional mutations are located in the DNA-binding domain of STAT1 (E320Q and Q463H). The mutation we are presently reporting is located in the linker domain of STAT1 (in between the DNA-binding and the SH2 domains). The mutations affect either phosphorylation (L706S, Y701C, K673R, and M654K) or DNA binding (E320Q, Q463H, L498V) or both (K637E) and exert a dominant negative effect over the WT allele. As a consequence, patients are vulnerable to mycobacterial disease due to an impaired response to IFN-γ. In a family with AD LOF *STAT1* mutation and MSMD, the grandfather of the proband was shown to carry the heterozygous mutation and had suffered from TB when he was younger, suggesting that AD LOF *STAT1* mutations can predispose to TB [28]. Here, we provide the proof of principle that AD LOF STAT1 deficiency is a genetic etiology of TB and should be suspected in patients with low response to IFN-γ even in the absence of MSMD.

In the present review, we showed that CNS TB of two Moroccan children were explained by single-gene inborn errors of the IL-12/IL-23-IFN-γ pathway affecting *TYK2* and *STAT1* (Fig. 2.4). To our knowledge, these are the first cases of genetic defects in patients with clearly documented CNS TB. More generally, these observations support the general hypothesis that severe TB of childhood is not only an infectious disease but also a genetic disorder, at least in some patients [3, 5, 15, 38]. These recent genetic findings have provided us with some clues to understand TB pathogenesis which is still barely understood. A number of genetic defects impairing IFN-γ immunity lead to a vulnerability to mycobacterial infections and in particular to severe TB of childhood. These findings have major medical implications, as they could pave the way for novel treatments based on physiopathology. The best example is for patients with

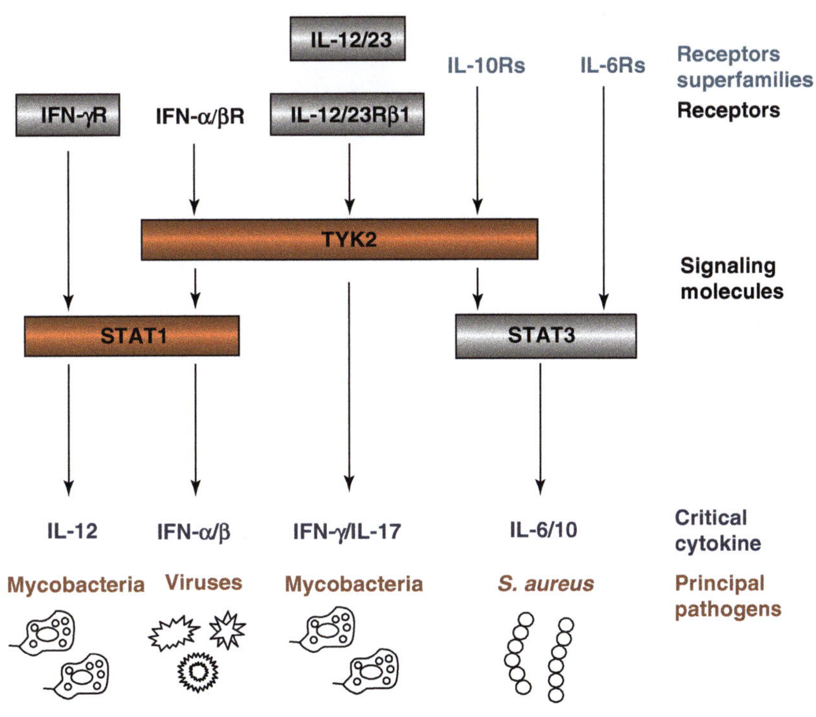

Fig. 2.4 Schematic representation of TYK2 and STAT1 in cytokine signaling. Cytokine receptors for IFN-γ, IFN-α/IFN-β, IL-12/IL-23, IL-6, and IL-10 are shown with TYK2 involvement and STATs. The principal secreted cytokines and the resulting resistance to the pathogens are shown. TYK2 and STAT1 are highlighted in *red*

impaired IFN-γ production, such as those with IL-12Rβ1 (and possibly TYK2) deficiency, for whom treatment with recombinant human (rh) IFN-γ, in addition to anti-mycobacterial drugs, seems to be effective [39–41]. Interestingly, patients with AD STAT1 deficiency with partial response to IFN-γ, like patients with partial IFN-γR1 deficiency, may also benefit from rhIFN-γ, as successfully done recently [32].

Conclusion

We illustrated in this review the genetic, immunological analyses of patients with CNS TB. They were explained by single-gene inborn errors of IL-12/IL-23-IFN-γ pathway and IFN-γ-dependent immunity affecting *TYK2* and *STAT1*.

References

1. WHO (2014) Global tuberculosis report 2014. World Health Organization, Geneva. http://www.who.int/tb/publications/global_report
2. Abel L, El-Baghdadi J, Bousfiha AA, Casanova JL, Schurr E (2014) Human genetics of tuberculosis: a long and winding road. Philos Trans R Soc Lond B Biol Sci 369:20130428
3. Alcais A, Fieschi C, Abel L, Casanova JL (2005) Tuberculosis in children and adults: two distinct genetic diseases. J Exp Med 202:1617–1621
4. O'Garra A, Redford PS, McNab FW, Bloom CI, Wilkinson RJ, Berry MP (2013) The immune response in tuberculosis. Annu Rev Immunol 31:475–527
5. Maartens G, Wilkinson RJ (2007) Tuberculosis. Lancet (London, England) 370:2030–2043
6. Vadivelu S, Effendi S, Starke JR, Luerssen TG, Jea A (2013) A review of the neurological and neurosurgical implications of tuberculosis in children. Clin Pediatr (Phila) 52:1135–1143
7. Rock RB, Olin M, Baker CA, Molitor TW, Peterson PK (2008) Central nervous system tuberculosis: pathogenesis and clinical aspects. Clin Microbiol Rev 21:243–261
8. Chatterjee S (2011) Brain tuberculomas, tubercular meningitis, and post-tubercular hydrocephalus in children. J Pediatr Neurosci 6:S96–S100
9. Thwaites GE, van Toorn R, Schoeman J (2013) Tuberculous meningitis: more questions, still too few answers. Lancet Neurol 12:999–1010
10. Figaji AA, Fieggen AG (2010) The neurosurgical and acute care management of tuberculous meningitis: evidence and current practice. Tuberculosis (Edinb) 90:393–400
11. Sanei Taheri M, Karimi MA, Haghighatkhah H, Pourghorban R, Samadian M, Delavar Kasmaei H (2015) Central nervous system tuberculosis: an imaging-focused review of a reemerging disease. Radiol Res Pract 2015:202806
12. El Azbaoui S, Alaoui Mrani N, Sabri A, Jouhadi Z, Ailal F, Bousfiha AA, Najib J, El Hafidi N, Deswarte C, Schurr E, Bustamante J, Boisson-Dupuis S, Casanova JL, Abel L, El Baghdadi J (2015) Pott's disease in Moroccan children: clinical features and investigation of the interleukin-12/interferon-gamma pathway. Int J Tuberc Lung Dis 19:1455–1462
13. de Beaucoudrey L, Samarina A, Bustamante J, Cobat A, Boisson-Dupuis S, Feinberg J, Al-Muhsen S, Janniere L, Rose Y, de Suremain M, Kong XF, Filipe-Santos O, Chapgier A, Picard C, Fischer A, Dogu F, Ikinciogullari A, Tanir G, Al-Hajjar S, Al-Jumaah S, Frayha HH, AlSum Z, Al-Ajaji S, Alangari A, Al-Ghonaium A, Adimi P, Mansouri D, Ben-Mustapha I, Yancoski J, Garty BZ, Rodriguez-Gallego C, Caragol I, Kutukculer N, Kumararatne DS, Patel S, Doffinger R, Exley A, Jeppsson O, Reichenbach J, Nadal D, Boyko Y, Pietrucha B, Anderson S, Levin M, Schandene L, Schepers K, Efira A, Mascart F, Matsuoka M, Sakai T, Siegrist CA, Frecerova K, Bluetters-Sawatzki R, Bernhoft J, Freihorst J, Baumann U, Richter D, Haerynck F, De Baets F, Novelli V, Lammas D, Vermylen C, Tuerlinckx D, Nieuwhof C, Pac M, Haas WH, Muller-Fleckenstein I, Fleckenstein B, Levy J, Raj R, Cohen AC, Lewis DB, Holland SM, Yang KD, Wang X, Wang X, Jiang L, Yang X, Zhu C, Xie Y, Lee PP, Chan KW, Chen TX, Castro G, Natera I, Codoceo A, King A, Bezrodnik L, Di Giovani D, Gaillard MI, de Moraes-Vasconcelos D, Grumach AS, da Silva Duarte AJ, Aldana R, Espinosa-Rosales FJ, Bejaoui M, Bousfiha AA, Baghdadi JE, Ozbek N, Aksu G, Keser M, Somer A, Hatipoglu N, Aydogmus C, Asilsoy S, Camcioglu Y, Gulle S, Ozgur TT, Ozen M, Oleastro M, Bernasconi A, Mamishi S, Parvaneh N, Rosenzweig S, Barbouche R, Pedraza S, Lau YL, Ehlayel MS, Fieschi C, Abel L, Sanal O, Casanova JL (2010) Revisiting human IL-12Rbeta1 deficiency: a survey of 141 patients from 30 countries. Medicine 89:381–402
14. Boisson-Dupuis S, El Baghdadi J, Parvaneh N, Bousfiha A, Bustamante J, Feinberg J, Samarina A, Grant AV, Janniere L, El Hafidi N, Hassani A, Nolan D, Najib J, Camcioglu Y, Hatipoglu N, Aydogmus C, Tanir G, Aytekin C, Keser M, Somer A, Aksu G, Kutukculer N, Mansouri D, Mahdaviani A, Mamishi S, Alcais A, Abel L, Casanova JL (2011) IL-12Rbeta1 deficiency in two of fifty children with severe tuberculosis from Iran, Morocco, and Turkey. PLoS One 6:e18524
15. Boisson-Dupuis S, Bustamante J, El-Baghdadi J, Camcioglu Y, Parvaneh N, El Azbaoui S, Agader A, Hassani A, El Hafidi N, Mrani NA, Jouhadi Z, Ailal F, Najib J, Reisli I, Zamani A, Yosunkaya S, Gulle-Girit S, Yildiran A, Cipe FE, Torun SH, Metin A, Atikan

BY, Hatipoglu N, Aydogmus C, Kilic SS, Dogu F, Karaca N, Aksu G, Kutukculer N, Keser-Emiroglu M, Somer A, Tanir G, Aytekin C, Adimi P, Mahdaviani SA, Mamishi S, Bousfiha A, Sanal O, Mansouri D, Casanova JL, Abel L (2015) Inherited and acquired immunodeficiencies underlying tuberculosis in childhood. Immunol Rev 264:103–120
16. van Crevel R, Ottenhoff TH, van der Meer JW (2003) Innate immunity to Mycobacterium tuberculosis. Adv Exp Med Biol 531:241–247
17. Bustamante J, Boisson-Dupuis S, Abel L, Casanova JL (2014) Mendelian susceptibility to mycobacterial disease: genetic, immunological, and clinical features of inborn errors of IFN-gamma immunity. Semin Immunol 26:454–470
18. Okada S, Markle JG, Deenick EK, Mele F, Averbuch D, Lagos M, Alzahrani M, Al-Muhsen S, Halwani R, Ma CS, Wong N, Soudais C, Henderson LA, Marzouqa H, Shamma J, Gonzalez M, Martinez-Barricarte R, Okada C, Avery DT, Latorre D, Deswarte C, Jabot-Hanin F, Torrado E, Fountain J, Belkadi A, Itan Y, Boisson B, Migaud M, Arlehamn CS, Sette A, Breton S, McCluskey J, Rossjohn J, de Villartay JP, Moshous D, Hambleton S, Latour S, Arkwright PD, Picard C, Lantz O, Engelhard D, Kobayashi M, Abel L, Cooper AM, Notarangelo LD, Boisson-Dupuis S, Puel A, Sallusto F, Bustamante J, Tangye SG, Casanova JL (2015) IMMUNODEFICIENCIES. Impairment of immunity to Candida and *Mycobacterium* in humans with bi-allelic RORC mutations. Science (New York, NY) 349:606–613
19. El Harim RL, El Matar A, Jorio M, El Malki Tazi A (2007) Aspects de la tuberculose de l'enfant à propos de 465 cas. Maroc Med 29:1–12
20. El Midaoui A, Messouak O, ELOuali ouarda O, Belahsen MF (2012) La tuberculose du système nerveux central: Étude clinique et neuroradiologique de 22 cas. RMNSCI.NET http://www.rmnsci.info/document.php?id=894
21. Akhaddar A, Boucetta M (2011) Images in clinical medicine. Multiple intracranial tuberculomas. N Engl J Med 365:1527
22. Byun M, Abhyankar A, Lelarge V, Plancoulaine S, Palanduz A, Telhan L, Boisson B, Picard C, Dewell S, Zhao C, Jouanguy E, Feske S, Abel L, Casanova JL (2010) Whole-exome sequencing-based discovery of STIM1 deficiency in a child with fatal classic Kaposi sarcoma. J Exp Med 207:2307–2312
23. Kreins AY, Ciancanelli MJ, Okada S, Kong XF, Ramirez-Alejo N, Kilic SS, El Baghdadi J, Nonoyama S, Mahdaviani SA, Ailal F, Bousfiha A, Mansouri D, Nievas E, Ma CS, Rao G, Bernasconi A, Sun Kuehn H, Niemela J, Stoddard J, Deveau P, Cobat A, El Azbaoui S, Sabri A, Lim CK, Sundin M, Avery DT, Halwani R, Grant AV, Boisson B, Bogunovic D, Itan Y, Moncada-Velez M, Martinez-Barricarte R, Migaud M, Deswarte C, Alsina L, Kotlarz D, Klein C, Muller-Fleckenstein I, Fleckenstein B, Cormier-Daire V, Rose-John S, Picard C, Hammarstrom L, Puel A, Al-Muhsen S, Abel L, Chaussabel D, Rosenzweig SD, Minegishi Y, Tangye SG, Bustamante J, Casanova JL, Boisson-Dupuis S (2015) Human TYK2 deficiency: mycobacterial and viral infections without hyper-IgE syndrome. J Exp Med 212:1641–1662
24. Minegishi Y, Saito M, Morio T, Watanabe K, Agematsu K, Tsuchiya S, Takada H, Hara T, Kawamura N, Ariga T, Kaneko H, Kondo N, Tsuge I, Yachie A, Sakiyama Y, Iwata T, Bessho F, Ohishi T, Joh K, Imai K, Kogawa K, Shinohara M, Fujieda M, Wakiguchi H, Pasic S, Abinun M, Ochs HD, Renner ED, Jansson A, Belohradsky BH, Metin A, Shimizu N, Mizutani S, Miyawaki T, Nonoyama S, Karasuyama H (2006) Human tyrosine kinase 2 deficiency reveals its requisite roles in multiple cytokine signals involved in innate and acquired immunity. Immunity 25:745–755
25. Kilic SS, Hacimustafaoglu M, Boisson-Dupuis S, Kreins AY, Grant AV, Abel L, Casanova JL (2012) A patient with tyrosine kinase 2 deficiency without hyper-IgE syndrome. J Pediatr 160:1055–1057
26. Dupuis S, Dargemont C, Fieschi C, Thomassin N, Rosenzweig S, Harris J, Holland SM, Schreiber RD, Casanova JL (2001) Impairment of mycobacterial but not viral immunity by a germline human STAT1 mutation. Science (New York, NY) 293: 300–303
27. Dupuis S, Jouanguy E, Al-Hajjar S, Fieschi C, Al-Mohsen IZ, Al-Jumaah S, Yang K, Chapgier A, Eidenschenk C, Eid P, Al Ghonaium A, Tufenkeji H, Frayha H, Al-Gazlan S, Al-Rayes H, Schreiber RD, Gresser I, Casanova JL (2003) Impaired response to interferon-alpha/beta and lethal viral disease in human STAT1 deficiency. Nat Genet 33:388–391
28. Chapgier A, Boisson-Dupuis S, Jouanguy E, Vogt G, Feinberg J, Prochnicka-Chalufour A, Casrouge A, Yang K, Soudais C, Fieschi C, Santos OF, Bustamante J, Picard C, de Beaucoudrey L, Emile JF, Arkwright PD, Schreiber RD, Rolinck-Werninghaus C, Rosen-Wolff A, Magdorf K, Roesler J, Casanova JL (2006) Novel STAT1 alleles in otherwise healthy patients with mycobacterial disease. PLoS Genet 2:e131
29. Liu L, Okada S, Kong XF, Kreins AY, Cypowyj S, Abhyankar A, Toubiana J, Itan Y, Audry M, Nitschke P, Masson C, Toth B, Flatot J, Migaud M, Chrabieh M, Kochetkov T, Bolze A, Borghesi A, Toulon A, Hiller J, Eyerich S, Eyerich K, Gulacsy V, Chernyshova L, Chernyshov V, Bondarenko A, Grimaldo RM, Blancas-Galicia L, Beas IM, Roesler J, Magdorf K, Engelhard D, Thumerelle C, Burgel PR, Hoernes M, Drexel B, Seger R, Kusuma T, Jansson AF, Sawalle-Belohradsky J, Belohradsky B, Jouanguy E, Bustamante J, Bue M, Karin N, Wildbaum G, Bodemer C, Lortholary O, Fischer A, Blanche S, Al-Muhsen S, Reichenbach J, Kobayashi M, Rosales FE, Lozano CT, Kilic SS, Oleastro M, Etzioni A, Traidl-Hoffmann C, Renner ED, Abel L, Picard C, Marodi L, Boisson-Dupuis S, Puel A, Casanova JL (2011) Gain-of-function human STAT1 mutations

impair IL-17 immunity and underlie chronic mucocutaneous candidiasis. J Exp Med 208:1635–1648
30. van de Veerdonk FL, Plantinga TS, Hoischen A, Smeekens SP, Joosten LA, Gilissen C, Arts P, Rosentul DC, Carmichael AJ, Smits-van der Graaf CA, Kullberg BJ, van der Meer JW, Lilic D, Veltman JA, Netea MG (2011) STAT1 mutations in autosomal dominant chronic mucocutaneous candidiasis. N Engl J Med 365:54–61
31. Tsumura M, Okada S, Sakai H, Yasunaga S, Ohtsubo M, Murata T, Obata H, Yasumi T, Kong XF, Abhyankar A, Heike T, Nakahata T, Nishikomori R, Al-Muhsen S, Boisson-Dupuis S, Casanova JL, Alzahrani M, Shehri MA, Elghazali G, Takihara Y, Kobayashi M (2012) Dominant-negative STAT1 SH2 domain mutations in unrelated patients with Mendelian susceptibility to mycobacterial disease. Hum Mutat 33:1377–1387
32. Sampaio EP, Bax HI, Hsu AP, Kristosturyan E, Pechacek J, Chandrasekaran P, Paulson ML, Dias DL, Spalding C, Uzel G, Ding L, McFarland E, Holland SM (2012) A novel STAT1 mutation associated with disseminated mycobacterial disease. J Clin Immunol 32:681–689
33. Hirata O, Okada S, Tsumura M, Kagawa R, Miki M, Kawaguchi H, Nakamura K, Boisson-Dupuis S, Casanova JL, Takihara Y, Kobayashi M (2013) Heterozygosity for the Y701C STAT1 mutation in a multiplex kindred with multifocal osteomyelitis. Haematologica 98:1641–1649
34. Uzel G, Sampaio EP, Lawrence MG, Hsu AP, Hackett M, Dorsey MJ, Noel RJ, Verbsky JW, Freeman AF, Janssen E, Bonilla FA, Pechacek J, Chandrasekaran P, Browne SK, Agharahimi A, Gharib AM, Mannurita SC, Yim JJ, Gambineri E, Torgerson T, Tran DQ, Milner JD, Holland SM (2013) Dominant gain-of-function STAT1 mutations in FOXP3 wild-type immune dysregulation-polyendocrinopathy-enteropathy-X-linked-like syndrome. J Allergy Clin Immunol 131:1611–1623
35. Romberg N, Morbach H, Lawrence MG, Kim S, Kang I, Holland SM, Milner JD, Meffre E (2013) Gain-of-function STAT1 mutations are associated with PD-L1 overexpression and a defect in B-cell survival. J Allergy Clin Immunol 131:1691–1693
36. Kataoka S, Muramatsu H, Okuno Y, Hayashi Y, Mizoguchi Y, Tsumura M, Okada S, Kobayashi M, Sano C, Sato H, Oh-Iwa I, Ito M, Kojima D, Hama A, Takahashi Y, Kojima S (2016) Extrapulmonary tuberculosis mimicking Mendelian susceptibility to mycobacterial disease in a patient with signal transducer and activator of transcription 1 (STAT1) gain-of-function mutation. J Allergy Clin Immunol 137:619–622 e611
37. Sharfe N, Nahum A, Newell A, Dadi H, Ngan B, Pereira SL, Herbrick JA, Roifman CM (2014) Fatal combined immunodeficiency associated with heterozygous mutation in STAT1. J Allergy Clin Immunol 133:807–817
38. Casanova JL, Abel L (2002) Genetic dissection of immunity to mycobacteria: the human model. Annu Rev Immunol 20:581–620
39. Alangari AA, Al-Zamil F, Al-Mazrou A, Al-Muhsen S, Boisson-Dupuis S, Awadallah S, Kambal A, Casanova JL (2011) Treatment of disseminated mycobacterial infection with high-dose IFN-gamma in a patient with IL-12Rbeta1 deficiency. Clin Dev Immunol 2011:691956
40. Holland SM (2001) Immunotherapy of mycobacterial infections. Semin Respir Infect 16:47–59
41. Holland SM, Eisenstein EM, Kuhns DB, Turner ML, Fleisher TA, Strober W, Gallin JI (1994) Treatment of refractory disseminated nontuberculous mycobacterial infection with interferon gamma. A preliminary report. N Engl J Med 330:1348–1355

Pathogenesis of Tuberculosis of the Nervous System

3

Mohammad A. Bosaeed and Adel Alothman

Contents

M.A. Bosaeed, MD, MB, SB-Med (✉)
Division of Infectious Diseases, Department of Medicine, King Abdulaziz Medical City, Riyadh, Saudi Arabia

King Abdullah International Medical Research Center, Riyadh, Saudi Arabia
e-mail: dr.bosaeed@live.com

A. Alothman, MB, FRCPC, FACP
Division of Infectious Diseases, Department of Medicine, King Abdulaziz Medical City, Riyadh, Saudi Arabia

College of Medicine, King Saud bin Abdulaziz University for Health Sciences, Riyadh, Saudi Arabia

King Abdullah International Medical Research Center, Riyadh, Saudi Arabia
e-mail: othmanaf@hotmail.com

Abbreviations

BBB	Blood-brain barrier
CNS	Central nervous system
CSF	Cerebrospinal fluid
TB	Tuberculosis
TBM	Tuberculous meningitis
TNF	Tumor necrosis factor

3.1 Introduction

Mycobacterium tuberculosis is a slow-growing intracellular pathogen, and it is an acid-fast bacterium because the cell wall consists mainly of hydrophobic mycolic acids. This is a specific component of the cell wall of *M. tuberculosis*, which makes up 50% of its dry weight. Due to this thick layer of mycolic acids, the entry of nutrients is impaired, which causes slow growth of mycobacteria but also increases cellular resistance to degradation through lysosomal enzymes [1, 2] (Fig. 3.1).

Some components of the cell wall are important virulence factors of *M. tuberculosis*. They are characteristic for pathogenic mycobacteria but not present on less pathogenic fast-growing mycobacterial strains. It is always expected to

M. Turgut et al. (eds.), *Tuberculosis of the Central Nervous System*,
DOI 10.1007/978-3-319-50712-5_3

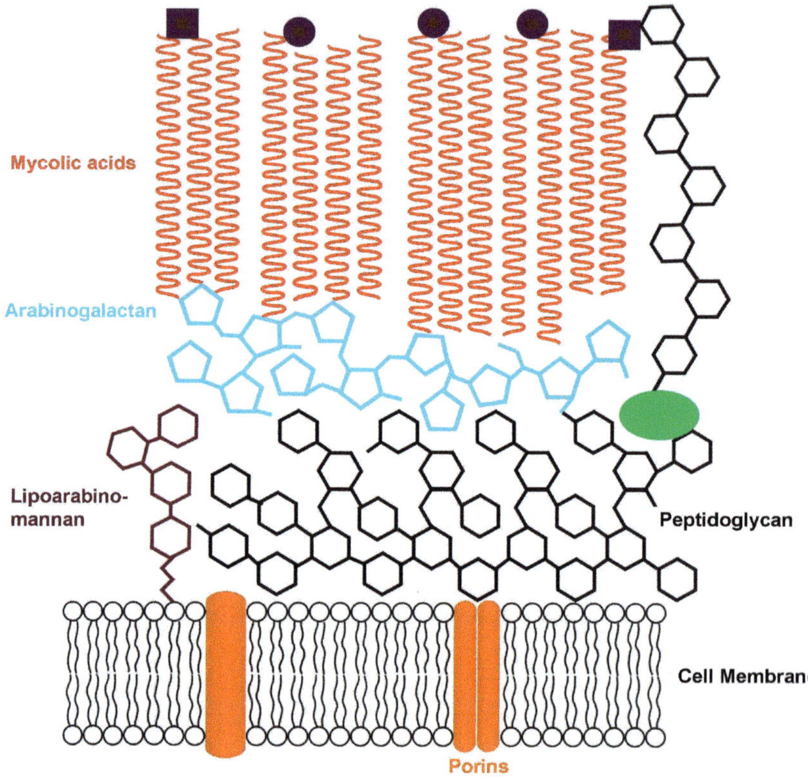

Fig. 3.1 The structure of the *Mycobacterium tuberculosis* cell wall

have predisposing factors for developing tuberculosis (TB), including overcrowding, malnutrition, drug abuse, immunosuppressive treatment, chronic diseases, and human immunodeficiency virus (HIV) infection.

It is believed that extrapulmonary TB infection including the central nervous system (CNS) starts with respiratory infection followed by hematogenous dissemination to other sites. The first interaction between *M. tuberculosis* and the host immune system occurs after inhalation of tubercle bacilli to the distal respiratory tract and reaching the alveoli where multiplication will start. This interaction between *M. tuberculosis* and host cells is complex and extensively studied, but until now, it is not completely understood. Other sources of infection like the skin, intestine, oropharynx, or the genitalia are very rare and all associated with foci in regional lymph nodes.

3.2 Immune Response in Tuberculosis

In pulmonary TB, innate immunity is primarily carried out by macrophages and dendritic cells in the alveoli, which recognize diverse bacterial moieties or pathogen-associated molecular patterns using specific receptors, such as Toll-like receptors (TLR2, TLR4, TLR9), mannose, C3, or IgG Fc receptors among others [3–8]. Some of these receptors also participate in macrophage activation mediated by cytokines or chemokines. Also airway epithelial cells respond rapidly to mycobacterial bacilli and produce murine b-defensin-3 (mBD3) and murine b-defensin-4 (mBD4), which probably contribute to the killing of mycobacteria [2, 9, 10].

However, bacterial multiplication tends to be mostly unimpeded by destroying the macrophages (lysosomal acidification) or avoiding their death inside the infected alveolar macrophage by apoptosis [11, 12]. This apoptosis mechanism during *M. tuberculosis* infection has been demonstrated in multiple in vitro [9, 13] and in vivo [14–19] studies. It also showed differences according to the virulence of the *M. tuberculosis* strain which may suppress this mechanism favoring bacterial survival [20].

Adaptive immunity against mycobacterial bacilli starts in the lung and regional lymph nodes. Dendritic cells (not macrophages) transport the bacilli from the lung to the mediastinal lymph nodes [21]; this pathway is controlled by chemokines and chemokine receptors (CCR5 and CCR7). Activation and proliferation of T lymphocytes and monocytes by dendritic cells with the participation of cytokines (including tumor necrosis factor alpha (TNFα), interleukin-1 (IL-1), and IL-12) may produce extensive inflammation, which can cause local tissue damage. To protect against tissue damage, anti-inflammatory cytokines (including IL-10 and transforming growth factor beta {TGF- β}) will be produced to limit the inflammation and may also contribute to downregulating the protective, immunity-facilitating bacilli proliferation [22, 23].

Immune reaction in the CNS was described as being selective and modified to limit tissue damage within the brain parenchyma, as it is poorly regenerative [24–26]. The studies about the immune response in CNS TB are limited. Studies that reported high concentrations of cytokines such as IFN-γ, TNFα, IL-1β, IL-6, IL-8, and IL-10 did not find a relation with the activity or severity of the disease and suggest the persistence of CNS inflammation [27, 28]. Other studies showed that cerebrospinal fluid (CSF) gamma interferon (IFN-γ) and TNFα were elevated before treatment but non-detectable after 6 months of therapy when antibiotics were administrated with corticosteroids during the first 2 months of treatment [29–31]. One of these studies suggested that high levels of IFN-γ measured at 1 month of therapy predicted more likelihood to have an intracranial granuloma detected [29]. Earlier studies with a small number of tuberculous meningitis (TBM) patients showed the presence of other pro-inflammatory and anti-inflammatory cytokines (IL-10 and TNFα soluble receptors) in the CSF [32, 33].

3.3 Mycobacterium Tuberculosis in the Brain

The blood-brain barrier (BBB) is the primary physiological protector of the CNS from hematogenous pathogens. It is principally composed of tightly apposed human brain microvascular endothelial cells, and despite the integrity of this barrier, there are some bacterial and viral pathogens capable of crossing the BBB and causing subsequent infection of brain parenchyma and meninges (Fig. 3.2).

M. tuberculosis showed the ability in vitro to invade and traverse the human brain microvascular endothelial cell monolayer mainly by virulent mycobacteria [34]. This in vitro model does not include cells that form the brain side of the BBB (mainly astrocytes), and the role of these cells in defense against entry into the brain parenchyma is still unclear [35]. Previously, it was believed that *M. tuberculosis* can cross the BBB as a free

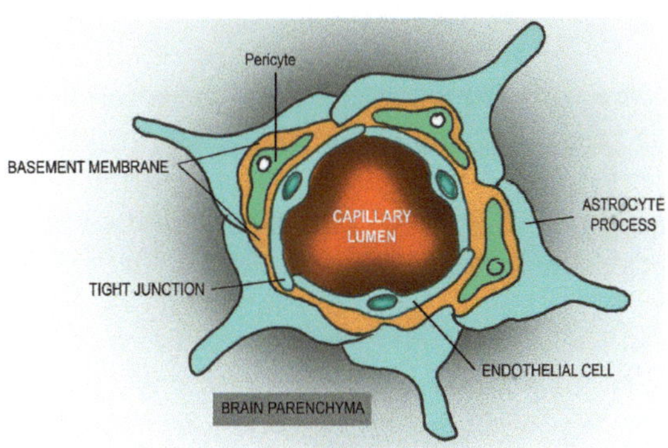

Fig. 3.2 The blood-brain barrier (BBB) is composed essentially of brain microvascular endothelial cells, the basal portions of which are supported by astrocyte processes. These endothelial cells provide protection by limiting the access to the CNS. Such limited access is aided by tight junctions and minimal transcytosis, thereby significantly reducing paracellular and transcellular movement

(extracellular) organism or via infected monocytes/neutrophils. While the following review about CNS infection, such cellular traffic, is severely restricted to the CNS before the invasion by the offending pathogen [24], one report utilizing CD18 (-/-) leukocyte adhesion deficient mice suggests that free mycobacteria (*M. avium*) via intravenous inoculation may traverse the BBB independence of leukocytes or macrophages, which develop a chronic, but not acute, CNS infection [36].

An understanding of the pathogenesis of TB of CNS was developed early in 1933 when Rich and McCordock published their experimental observations of TBM. Using animal modules (rabbits and guinea pigs), they were able to prove that the intravenous injection of *M. tuberculosis* did not result in immediate meningitis in any of the animals. They also suggested that during or after bacteremia due to the primary tuberculous infection, tuberculous lesions (Rich's foci) will develop in the meninges, the subpial or subependymal surfaces of the brain, and may remain dormant for years. Ruptures of the foci and mycobacteria release into subarachnoid space or the ventricular system can cause meningitis depending on the virulence of the bacilli, ruptured foci number, and the immune status of the host [37].

These two stages of CNS TB development were also demonstrated in later articles, but the specific stimulus for the rupture or growth of Rich foci is not known [38–40]. If this progression of the disease occurs in the brain parenchyma and meninges, different forms of CNS TB can develop (Table 3.1). A recent experimental study in BALB/c mice suggested that mycobacterial strains with a distinctive genotype can disseminate extensively after the respiratory infection and infect the brain. In meningeal TB, mycobacteria reach the CNS by the hematogenous route secondary to pulmonary infection [42].

Table 3.1 Various manifestations of cerebral tuberculosis

Tuberculoma
Tuberculous abscess
Cerebral miliary tuberculosis
Tuberculous encephalopathy/encephalitis
Tuberculous meningitis
Tuberculous vasculopathy

The table is modified from Katti [41]

3.4 Tuberculous Meningitis (TBM)

TBM is characterized as a meningoencephalitis as it affects both the meninges and the brain's parenchyma and its vasculature. After the release of tubercle bacilli from granulomatous lesions into the subarachnoid space, a dense gelatinous exudate forms; it is florid in the interpeduncular fossa and suprasellar region anteriorly, and it may extend throughout the prepontine cistern and surround the spinal cord. Microscopically diffuse exudates consist of polymorphonuclear leukocytes, macrophages, lymphocytes, and erythrocytes with a variable number of bacilli within a loose fibrin network [39, 41]. With the disease progression, lymphocytes and connective tissue elements predominate. Small and medium arteries, as well as other blood vessels (capillaries and veins) adjacent to and traversing the exudates, become inflamed. This vasculitis, leading to vascular occlusion and thus cerebral ischemia, is a common sequela of tuberculous arteritis. The most serious consequence of TBM is vasculitis in the vessels of the circle of Willis, the vertebrobasilar system, and the perforating branches of the middle cerebral artery, resulting in infarctions in the distribution of these vessels. Hydrocephalus, often the communicating type associated with chronic infection, results from a disturbance in the flow of CSF because of obstruction of the basal cisterns, an outflow of the fourth ventricle, or the occlusion of the cerebral aqueduct by the exudates [43]. Chronic hydrocephalus may lead to atrophy of the gray and white matter if untreated. "Border-zone encephalitis" describes a tissue reaction commonly seen in brain tissue adjacent to zones of thick adherent exudate which will cause edema, perivascular infiltration, and microglial reaction.

3.5 Intracranial Tuberculoma

Tuberculoma is avascular spherical granulomatous mass of small tubercles. The exact route of entry of tubercle bacilli into the ventricles is controversial. Hematogenous spread through the choroid plexus is the most likely mechanism. Inside the tuberculoma mass, TB bacilli could be demonstrated within a necrotic area composed of caseous material. Intracranial tuberculomas can occur at any age, and the presenting symptoms are related to their location. Infratentorial tuberculomas are more frequent in children and may present with brainstem syndromes, cerebellar manifestations, and multiple cranial nerve palsies [44–47].

Tuberculoma is considered to be a likely source of diffuse meningitis. Also, paradoxical enlargement or development of tuberculomas during anti-TB treatment can occur [48].

3.6 Intracranial Tuberculous Abscess

Intracranial abscess formation is a rare manifestation of CNS TB but has greater mass effect and edema compared to tuberculoma. TB abscesses have frank pus with a large number of polymorphonuclear leukocytes and a large number of bacilli. Tuberculous brain abscess develops either from parenchymal tubercular granulomas or through the spread of tuberculous foci from the meninges. It can present as solitary or multiple lesions [49, 50].

3.7 Tuberculous Encephalopathy

It consists of diffuse edema of cerebral white matter with fewer neurons in gray matter. The pathogenesis of "tuberculous encephalopathy" was described exclusively in infants and in children by Dastur and Udani [51, 52] who suggested that it was an allergic delayed type IV hypersensitivity reaction due to cell-mediated immunity to tuberculin protein. It was seen in Indian children with pulmonary TB who developed neurological symptoms in the form of convulsions, stupor, and coma without signs of meningeal irritation or focal neurological deficit. TB encephalopathy is a rare entity and develops as a complication of pulmonary TB and extensive cerebral demyelination.

3.8 Tuberculous Spondylitis (Pott's Disease)

It is usually secondary to an extra-spinal source of infection and represents a combination of osteomyelitis and arthritis that usually involves more than one vertebra. It spreads either via the arterial or the venous route. An arterial arcade, in the subchondral region of each vertebra, is derived from anterior and posterior spinal arteries; this arcade forms a rich vascular plexus. This vascular plexus facilitates the hematogenous spread of the infection in the paradiskal regions. The spread of the infection via the intraosseous venous system may be responsible for central vertebral body lesions [53]. The anterior aspect of the vertebral body adjacent to the subchondral plate is usually affected. TB may spread from that area to adjacent intervertebral disks. In adults, disk disease is secondary to the spread of infection from the vertebral body. In children, the disk, because it is vascularized, can be the primary site [54].

Vertebral destruction leads to a collapse of the body of the vertebra along with anterior wedging. Spinal cord compression in Pott's spine is mainly caused by pressure from a paraspinal abscess, which is retropharyngeal in the cervical region and spindle-shaped in thoracic and thoracolumbar regions. Neurological deficits may also result from dural invasion by granulation tissue and compression from the debris of sequestrated bone, a destroyed intervertebral disk, or a dislocated vertebra. Rarely, vascular insufficiency in the territory of the anterior spinal artery has also been suggested [41].

In spinal TB, with the involvement of more than one vertebra because of segmental arteries that bifurcate to supply two adjacent vertebrae, the spread of the disease beneath the anterior or posterior longitudinal ligaments involves multiple contiguous vertebrae. A lack of proteolytic enzymes in

Table 3.2 Mechanisms of paraplegia/tetraplegia in spinal tuberculosis

Causes of neurological involvement	
Early-onset paraplegia	
Mechanical pressure	By tuberculous debris, sequestrum of bone or disk, abscess, subluxation and dislocations, concertina collapse, and internal gibbus
Tuberculous granuloma	Tuberculoma in extradural, intradural, or intramedullary regions
Tuberculous myelitis	May involve spinal cord parenchyma
Spinal artery thrombosis	Infective thrombosis of anterior spinal artery
Tuberculous arachnoiditis	Meningeal inflammation and fibrosis
Late-onset paraplegia	
Transection of spinal cord by bony bridge	Transverse ridge of bone produced by severe kyphosis
Fibrosis of dura (pachymeningitis)	Formation of tough, fibrous membrane encircling the cord

The table is modified from Garg and Somvanshi [53]

mycobacterial infections has been suggested as the cause of the subligamentous spread of infection unlike in the case of pyogenic infections [55–58].

The upper lumbar and lower thoracic spine are the most frequently involved sites. More than one vertebra is typically affected, and the vertebral body is more commonly affected than the posterior arch [59]. The distortion of the spinal column leads to spinal deformities [53, 60] (Table 3.2). Paraplegia is the most devastating complication of spinal TB. In a classical paper, Hodgson [60] classified paraplegia into two groups according to the activity of the TB infection. These two groups were paraplegia of active disease (early-onset paraplegia) and paraplegia of healed disease (late-onset paraplegia).

The kyphotic deformity is more likely to be caused by lesions in the thoracic spine than by those in the lumbar spine. A cold abscess can occur if the infection extends to adjacent ligaments and soft tissues. Abscesses in the lumbar region may descend to the sheath of the psoas to the femoral trigone region and eventually erode into the skin [61].

3.9 Tuberculous Arachnoiditis

Tuberculous arachnoiditis is a cause of myeloradiculopathy in countries endemic for TB. The inflammatory exudate surrounds the spinal cord and nerve roots without infiltration. Frequently, there is vascular involvement with periarteritis and occlusion of small vessels. Neuronal structures are damaged by direct compression as well as by ischemia. The changes of arachnoiditis may be focal, multifocal, or diffuse. In TB arachnoiditis, features of spinal cord or nerve root involvement may predominate, but most often, there is a mixed picture [44].

3.10 Non-osseous Spinal Cord Tuberculosis

Intramedullary tuberculomas are extremely rarely reported, and reports from developing countries have also been sporadic. This was seen by Dastur in 1983, when he reviewed cases with tuberculous paraplegia without evidence of Pott's disease [62]. It was observed that extradural tuberculomas, arachnoid lesions without dural involvement, and subdural/extramedullary lesions were present in a significant number of patients.

Conclusion

In summary, despite the fact that it has been long since the discovery of *M. tuberculosis*, remarkably little is known about the pathogenesis of CNS TB. Understanding how *M. tuberculosis* invades and survives in the CNS would be very helpful to developing better preventive and management strategies. Future studies on *M. tuberculosis* and their interactions with the host immune system and the BBB will lead to a better understanding of CNS TB, with the aim to overcome the considerable challenges in diagnosing, treating, and managing this disease.

References

1. Brennan PJ, Nikaido H (1995) The envelope of mycobacteria. Annu Rev Biochem 64:29–63
2. Kleinnijenhuis J, Oosting M, Joosten LA, Netea MG, Van Crevel R (2011) Innate immune recognition of Mycobacterium tuberculosis. Clin Dev Immunol 2011:405310
3. Tapping RI, Tobias PS (2003) Mycobacterial lipoarabinomannan mediates physical interactions between TLR1 and TLR2 to induce signaling. J Endotoxin Res 9:264–268
4. Means TK, Wang S, Lien E, Yoshimura A, Golenbock DT, Fenton MJ (1999) Human toll-like receptors mediate cellular activation by Mycobacterium tuberculosis. J Immunol 163:3920–3927
5. Bulut Y, Michelsen KS, Hayrapetian L, Naiki Y, Spallek R, Singh M, Arditi M (2005) Mycobacterium tuberculosis heat shock proteins use diverse Toll-like receptor pathways to activate pro-inflammatory signals. J Biol Chem 280:20961–20967
6. Bafica A, Scanga CA, Feng CG, Leifer C, Cheever A, Sher A (2005) TLR9 regulates Th1 responses and cooperates with TLR2 in mediating optimal resistance to Mycobacterium tuberculosis. J Exp Med 202:1715–1724
7. Means TK, Jones BW, Schromm AB, Shurtleff BA, Smith JA, Keane J, Golenbock DT, Vogel SN, Fenton MJ (2001) Differential effects of a Toll-like receptor antagonist on Mycobacterium tuberculosis-induced macrophage responses. J Immunol 166:4074–4082
8. Davila S, Hibberd ML, HariDass R, Wong HE, Sahiratmadja E, Bonnard C, Alisjahbana B, Szeszko JS, Balabanova Y, Drobniewski F, van Crevel R, van de Vosse E, Nejentsev S, Ottenhoff TH, Seielstad M (2008) Genetic association and expression studies indicate a role of toll-like receptor 8 in pulmonary tuberculosis. PLoS Genet 4:e1000218
9. Rivas-Santiago B, Sada E, Tsutsumi V, Aguilar-Leon D, Contreras JL, Hernandez-Pando R (2006) beta-Defensin gene expression during the course of experimental tuberculosis infection. J Infect Dis 194:697–701
10. Isabel BE, Rogelio HP (2014) Pathogenesis and immune response in tuberculous meningitis. Malays J Med Sci 21:4–10
11. Divangahi M, Behar SM, Remold H (2013) Dying to live: how the death modality of the infected macrophage affects immunity to tuberculosis. Adv Exp Med Biol 783:103–120
12. Behar SM, Divangahi M, Remold HG (2010) Evasion of innate immunity by Mycobacterium tuberculosis: is death an exit strategy? Nat Rev Microbiol 8:668–674
13. Rios-Barrera VA, Campos-Pena V, Aguilar-Leon D, Lascurain LR, Meraz-Rios MA, Moreno J, Figueroa-Granados V, Hernández-Pando R (2006) Macrophage and T lymphocyte apoptosis during experimental pulmonary tuberculosis: their relationship to mycobacterial virulence. Eur J Immunol 36:345–353
14. Oddo M, Renno T, Attinger A, Bakker T, MacDonald HR, Meylan PR (1998) Fas ligand-induced apoptosis of infected human macrophages reduces the viability of intracellular Mycobacterium tuberculosis. J Immunol 160:5448–5454
15. Kremer L, Estaquier J, Brandt E, Ameisen JC, Locht C (1997) Mycobacterium bovis Bacillus Calmette Guerin infection prevents apoptosis of resting human monocytes. Eur J Immunol 27:2450–2456
16. Keane J, Remold HG, Kornfeld H (2000) Virulent Mycobacterium tuberculosis strains evade apoptosis of infected alveolar macrophages. J Immunol 164:2016–2020
17. Spira A, Carroll JD, Liu G, Aziz Z, Shah V, Kornfeld H, Keane J (2003) Apoptosis genes in human alveolar macrophages infected with virulent or attenuated Mycobacterium tuberculosis: a pivotal role for tumor necrosis factor. Am J Respir Cell Mol Biol 29:545–551
18. Rojas M, Barrera LF, Puzo G, Garcia LF (1997) Differential induction of apoptosis by virulent Mycobacterium tuberculosis in resistant and susceptible murine macrophages: role of nitric oxide and mycobacterial products. J Immunol 159:1352–1361
19. Klingler K, Tchou-Wong KM, Brandli O, Aston C, Kim R, Chi C, Rom WN (1997) Effects of mycobacteria on regulation of apoptosis in mononuclear phagocytes. Infect Immun 65:5272–5278
20. Parandhaman DK, Narayanan S (2014) Cell death paradigms in the pathogenesis of Mycobacterium tuberculosis infection. Front Cell Infect Microbiol 4:31
21. Salgame P (2005) Host innate and Th1 responses and the bacterial factors that control Mycobacterium tuberculosis infection. Curr Opin Immunol 17:374–380
22. Hernandez-Pando R, Orozco H, Aguilar D (2009) Factors that deregulate the protective immune response in tuberculosis. Arch Immunol Ther Exp (Warsz) 57:355–367
23. Sahiratmadja E, Alisjahbana B, de Boer T, Adnan I, Maya A, Danusantoso H, Nelwan RH, Marzuki S, van der Meer JW, van Crevel R, van de Vosse E, Ottenhoff TH (2007) Dynamic changes in pro- and anti-inflammatory cytokine profiles and gamma interferon receptor signaling integrity correlate with tuberculosis disease activity and response to curative treatment. Infect Immun 75:820–829
24. Ransohoff RM, Kivisakk P, Kidd G (2003) Three or more routes for leukocyte migration into the central nervous system. Nat Rev Immunol 3:569–581
25. Galea I, Bechmann I, Perry VH (2007) What is immune privilege (not)? Trends Immunol 28:12–18
26. Be NA, Kim KS, Bishai WR, Jain SK (2009) Pathogenesis of central nervous system tuberculosis. Curr Mol Med 9:94–99
27. Nagesh Babu G, Kumar A, Kalita J, Misra UK (2008) Proinflammatory cytokine levels in the serum and cerebrospinal fluid of tuberculous meningitis patients. Neurosci Lett 436:48–51

28. Misra UK, Kalita J, Srivastava R, Nair PP, Mishra MK, Basu A (2010) A study of cytokines in tuberculous meningitis: clinical and MRI correlation. Neurosci Lett 483:6–10
29. Mansour AM, Frenck RW Jr, Darville T, Nakhla IA, Wierzba TF, Sultan Y, Bassiouny MI, McCarthy K, Jacobs RF (2005) Relationship between intracranial granulomas and cerebrospinal fluid levels of gamma interferon and interleukin-10 in patients with tuberculous meningitis. Clin Diagn Lab Immunol 12:363–365
30. Tobin DM, Roca FJ, Oh SF, McFarland R, Vickery TW, Ray JP, Ko DC, Zou Y, Bang ND, Chau TT, Vary JC, Hawn TR, Dunstan SJ, Farrar JJ, Thwaites GE, King MC, Serhan CN, Ramakrishnan L (2012) Host genotype-specific therapies can optimize the inflammatory response to mycobacterial infections. Cell 148:434–446
31. Vanden Driessche K, Persson A, Marais BJ, Fink PJ, Urdahl KB (2013) Immune vulnerability of infants to tuberculosis. Clin Dev Immunol 2013:781320
32. Akalin H, Akdis AC, Mistik R, Helvaci S, Kilicturgay K (1994) Cerebrospinal fluid interleukin-1 beta/interleukin-1 receptor antagonist balance and tumor necrosis factor-alpha concentrations in tuberculous, viral and acute bacterial meningitis. Scand J Infect Dis 26:667–674
33. Mastroianni CM, Lancella L, Mengoni F, Lichtner M, Santopadre P, D'Agostino C, Ticca F, Vullo V (1998) Chemokine profiles in the cerebrospinal fluid (CSF) during the course of pyogenic and tuberculous meningitis. Clin Exp Immunol 114:210–214
34. Jain SK, Paul-Satyaseela M, Lamichhane G, Kim KS, Bishai WR (2006) Mycobacterium tuberculosis invasion and traversal across an in vitro human blood-brain barrier as a pathogenic mechanism for central nervous system tuberculosis. J Infect Dis 193:1287–1295
35. Rock RB, Olin M, Baker CA, Molitor TW, Peterson PK (2008) Central nervous system tuberculosis: pathogenesis and clinical aspects. Clin Microbiol Rev 21:243–261
36. Wu HS, Kolonoski P, Chang YY, Bermudez LE (2000) Invasion of the brain and chronic central nervous system infection after systemic Mycobacterium avium complex infection in mice. Infect Immun 68:2979–2984
37. Rich AR, McCordock HA (1933) Pathogenesis of tubercular meningitis. Bull John Hopkins Hosp 52:5–13
38. Ray H, Riggs HE, Rupp C (1956) Clinicopathologic study of tuberculous meningitis in adults. Am Rev Tuberc 74:830–834
39. Dastur DK, Manghani DK, Udani PM (1995) Pathology and pathogenetic mechanisms in neurotuberculosis. Radiol Clin North Am 33:733–752
40. al-Deeb SM, Yaqub BA, Sharif HS, Motaery KR (1992) Neurotuberculosis: a review. Clin Neurol Neurosurg 94(Suppl):S30–S33
41. Katti MK (2004) Pathogenesis, diagnosis, treatment, and outcome aspects of cerebral tuberculosis. Med Sci Monit 10:RA215–RA229
42. Hernandez Pando R, Aguilar D, Cohen I, Guerrero M, Ribon W, Acosta P, Orozco H, Marquina B, Salinas C, Rembao D, Espitia C (2010) Specific bacterial genotypes of Mycobacterium tuberculosis cause extensive dissemination and brain infection in an experimental model. Tuberculosis (Edinb) 90:268–277
43. Tandon PN, Rao MAP, Banerji AK, Pathak SN, Dhar J (1975) Isotope scanning of the cerebrospinal fluid pathways in tuberculous meningitis. J Neurol Sci 25:401
44. Garg RK (1999) Tuberculosis of the central nervous system. Postgrad Med J 75:133–140
45. Talamas O, Del Brutto OH, Garcia-Ramos G (1989) Brain-stem tuberculoma. An analysis of 11 patients. Arch Neurol 46:529–535
46. Rajshekhar V, Chandy MJ (1997) Tuberculomas presenting as isolated intrinsic brain stem masses. Br J Neurosurg 11:127–133
47. Vengsarkar US, Pisipaty RP, Parekh B, Panchal VG, Shetty MN (1986) Intracranial tuberculoma and the CT scan. J Neurosurg 64:568–574
48. Zein TM, Fletcher PS, Mirghani ZM (2000) Intracranial tuberculoma. Saudi Med J 21:196–199
49. Mohindra S, Savardekar A, Gupta R, Tripathi M, Rane S (2016) Tuberculous brain abscesses in immunocompetent patients: a decade long experience with nine patients. Neurol India 64:66–74
50. Menon S, Bharadwaj R, Chowdhary A, Kaundinya D, Palande D (2011) Tuberculous brain abscesses: case series and review of literature. J Neurosci Rural Pract 2:153–157
51. Dastur DK, Udani PM (1966) The pathology and pathogenesis of tuberculous encephalopathy. Acta Neuropathol 6:311–326
52. Udani PM, Dastur DK (1970) Tuberculous encephalopathy with and without meningitis. Clinical features and pathological correlations. J Neurol Sci 10:541–561
53. Garg RK, Somvanshi DS (2011) Spinal tuberculosis: a review. J Spinal Cord Med 34:440–454
54. Davidson PT, Le HQ (1999) Tuberculosis and nontuberculous mycobacterial infections. In: Schlossberg D (ed) Musculoskeletal tuberculosis, 4th edn. W B Saunders, Saint Louis, pp 204–220
55. Jain AK, Dhammi IK (2007) Tuberculosis of the spine: a review. Clin Orthop Relat Res 460:39–49
56. McLain RF, Isada C (2004) Spinal tuberculosis deserves a place on the radar screen. Cleve Clin J Med 71:537–539
57. Quinones-Hinojosa A, Jun P, Jacobs R, Rosenberg WS, Weinstein PR (2004) General principles in the medical and surgical management of spinal infections: a multidisciplinary approach. Neurosurg Focus 17:E1
58. Lee KY (2014) Comparison of pyogenic spondylitis and tuberculous spondylitis. Asian Spine J 8:216–223

59. Moon MS (1997) Tuberculosis of the spine. Controversies and a new challenge. Spine (Phila Pa 1976) 22:1791–1797
60. Hodgson AR, Yau A (1967) Pott's paraplegia: a classification based upon the living pathology. Paraplegia 5:1–16
61. Pott disease: background, pathophysiology, epidemiology. http://emedicine.medscape.com/article/226141-overview. Accessed 17 Mar 2016
62. Dastur HM (1983) Diagnosis and neurosurgical treatment of tuberculous disease of the CNS. Neurosurg Rev 6:111–117

Pathology of Tuberculosis of the Nervous System (Tuberculous Meningitis, Tuberculoma, Tuberculous Abscess)

4

Kiran Preet Malhotra and Dinkar Kulshreshtha

Contents

K.P. Malhotra, MD, DNB, PDCC (✉)
Department of Pathology, Dr. Ram Manohar Lohia Institute of Medical Sciences, Lucknow, UP, India
e-mail: drkiranpreetmalhotra@yahoo.co.in

D. Kulshreshtha, MBBS, DM
Department of Neurology, Dr. Ram Manohar Lohia Institute of Medical Sciences, Lucknow, UP, India
e-mail: dinkar.kulshreshtha@rediffmail.com

Abbreviations

ADA	Adenosine deaminase
AFB	Acid-fast bacilli
AIDS	Acquired immunodeficiency syndrome
CNS	Central nervous system
CSF	Cerebrospinal fluid
CSW	Cerebral salt wasting
CT	Computed tomography
CVST	Cortical venous sinus thrombosis
HIV	Human immunodeficiency virus
MAC	*Mycobacterium avium* complex
MRI	Magnetic resonance imaging
NAA	Nucleic acid amplification assay
NTM	Nontubercular mycobacteria
PCR	Polymerase chain reaction
SIADH	Syndrome of inappropriate antidiuretic hormone secretion
TB	Tuberculosis
TBA	Tuberculous brain abscess
TBM	Tuberculous meningitis

4.1 Introduction

The scourge of tuberculosis (TB) is borne profoundly by the nervous system. The frequently subtle clinical presentation, varied sensitivity of noninvasive diagnostic tests, and the understandable resistance of the clinician to biopsy brain tissue heightens the malady of TB of the central

M. Turgut et al. (eds.), *Tuberculosis of the Central Nervous System*,
DOI 10.1007/978-3-319-50712-5_4

nervous system (CNS). TB can cause diverse lesions in the brain and spine and mimic a large number of infective and noninfective disorders. The current chapter discusses in detail the various pathologic manifestations of TB of CNS, the modalities used for diagnosis, and the differentials to be considered before diagnosing a lesion as tubercular in origin.

4.2 Pathogenesis of CNS Tuberculosis: Infection to Organ Dissemination

The infection typically begins when tubercle bacilli are inhaled and reach a terminal airway forming a pulmonary parenchymal (Ghon's) focus. The lymphatics in the vicinity of the Ghon's focus spread the infection to the regional lymph nodes and contribute to the primary complex in TB. The interplay between the hosts' immunity and the bacterial virulence decides the future course of the disease. In the early phase, the infection is contained by nonspecific immunity, and 4–8 weeks later, cell-mediated immunity eliminates the infection or leads to the formation of an inactive focus. In the natural course of the disease, the bacilli disseminate from the primary complex via hematogenous route and reach the target organs where they may survive for prolonged periods [1]. Wallgren documented the clinical and pathological spectrum after primary infection with TB and formulated the timetable for childhood TB which is composed of five phases [2]. The period of highest risk for miliary TB and tuberculous meningitis (TBM) is 1 to 3 months after primary infection [2].

In adults, after 10–30 years of initial infection, secondary or postprimary TB occurs when the bacteria are reactivated, or the person gets reinfected to develop characteristic upper zone lung cavities with proliferation of mycobacteria [1, 3]. It is rather surprising that immunocompetent adult patients suffer worse from postprimary TB. This is a mechanism to control the infection locally, mainly in the upper lung zone as cavitary lesions that shed large numbers of organisms into bronchi that are subsequently coughed out from the air passages. Extrapulmonary spread of infection is on the other hand commoner in immunosuppressed and aged patients who develop disseminated disease. In immunocompetent adults, extrapulmonary TB constitutes 15–20% cases of TB, while in immunosuppressed patients, 50% cases of TB are extrapulmonary. Almost any organ can be involved in extrapulmonary TB, especially in HIV coinfection or other immunosuppressed states. Table 4.1 enlists the extrapulmonary organs involved in TB [4, 5].

Table 4.1 Organs involved in extrapulmonary tuberculosis

Site of involvement	Manifestation
Lymph nodes	Tubercular lymphadenitis
Central nervous system	Tubercular meningitis, tuberculomas, abscesses, radiculomyelitis
Pleura	Tubercular pleuritis
Skeletal	Tubercular osteomyelitis and spondylitis
Intra-abdominal	Gastrointestinal and genitourinary tuberculosis, tubercular peritonitis
Heart	Tubercular pericarditis
Skin	Cutaneous tuberculosis
Disseminated tuberculosis	Involving two or more organs

4.3 Nervous System Involvement in Tuberculosis

TB of CNS occurs in about 10–15% of patients with TB [5]. According to the two-step model of Rich and McCordock, at the time of initial pulmonary infection, the bacteria reach the oxygen-rich CNS via the systemic circulation within 2–4 weeks and get lodged in the parenchyma of the brain, meninges, and adjacent tissues. These sites eventually develop variable-sized granulomas (Rich focus). Such foci may home in the meninges or subpial or subependymal brain parenchyma. After periods of dormancy, these foci may rupture or grow to produce different manifestations of CNS TB. TBM occurs with the involvement of meninges which is usually due to the rupture of such foci into the subarachnoid space or ventricles and less frequently secondary to rupture into a blood vessel. When tubercles enlarge in the substance of the brain but do not rupture into the subarachnoid space, tuberculomas result. Impaired cell-mediated immunity underlies the development of CNS TB, and the risk factors include old age, alcohol abuse, iatrogenic immunosuppression, human immunodeficiency virus (HIV) coinfection, and lymphomas [6–11].

Resultant manifestations of the dissemination of tubercle bacilli in the CNS include TBM, tuberculomas, and tuberculous abscess. The pathology of these lesions is detailed in this section. Involvement of the spinal cord and cranial and peripheral nerves is also common and will be discussed in later chapters. Most of the present-day understanding of the pathology of tubercular lesions is based on studies on autopsy specimens from patients with CNS TB. Most of the CNS TB is caused by *Mycobacterium tuberculosis*; the nontuberculous mycobacteria species (atypical mycobacteria) cause infections in immunosuppressed individuals and are dealt with in Sect. 4.3.6 [12].

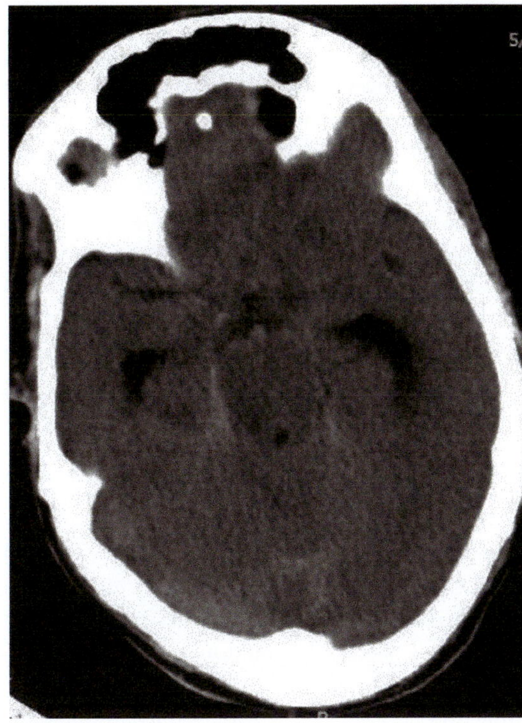

Fig. 4.1 Contrast-enhanced CT scan of the head showing basal exudates causing obstructive hydrocephalus in a patient of tuberculous meningitis (TBM)

4.3.1 Tuberculous Meningitis

4.3.1.1 Introduction

Meningitis is the commonest manifestation of CNS TB; it is also the most severe [13]. Children are affected more frequently than adults, as noted in 78 of the 100 autopsied cases of TBM in a seminal study by Dastur et al. [14]. As earlier discussed, hematogenous dissemination of TB bacilli to the CNS leads to formation of a focus at the site where the bacilli lodge. This focus is known as the Rich's focus, the rupture of which into the subarachnoid space largely accounts for meningitis. The lesion is usually suspected in cases with chronic meningitic symptoms and a lymphocytic pleocytosis of the cerebrospinal fluid (CSF). Basal meningeal enhancement and hydrocephalus are the usual findings noted on computed tomography (CT) done in patients with TBM (Fig. 4.1). Conventional magnetic resonance imaging (MRI) sequences in early stages may not show any abnormality; in such a situation, magnetization transfer sequences are considered superior in detecting abnormal meninges. Common sites of meningeal involvement, as noted on post-contrast T1-weighted sequences, are interpeduncular fossa, pontine cistern, perimesencephalic cistern, suprasellar cistern, and Sylvian fissures, with occasional involvement of sulci over the convexities [15, 16].

4.3.1.2 Gross Pathology

TBM lesions predominate in the leptomeninges at the base of the brain. Autopsy studies of brain specimens from patients with TBM reveal cerebral edema, increased brain weight, and flattening of gyri. Herniation of tonsils and uncus may occur as a result of the edema. The basal arachnoiditis presents as opacity and thick surface exudates, extending into the cisterns and around Sylvian fissures, optic chiasm, cerebellum, and brainstem. On cut sections of the brain, the ventricles appear dilated, and communicating or obstructive hydrocephalus may be present [17].

The distal internal carotid artery, proximal middle cerebral artery, proximal anterior cerebral artery, and perforating vessels of the basal ganglion are encased in the exudates. The lumina of the encased arteries are narrowed and eventually occluded. Areas of gray and white matter infarction especially involving the Sylvian fissure, basal ganglia, and internal capsular region may be present. Tubercles associated with TBM appear as small focal opacities, 3–5 mm in diameter [16, 19–21]. The infection may track down from the posterior fossa and lead to spinal TBM or myeloradiculopathy [21].

4.3.1.3 Microscopic Pathology

The exudates in the leptomeninges are serofibrinous with extensive caseous necrosis [16, 18] (Fig. 4.2). An infiltrate of lymphocytes, plasma cells, and epithelioid histiocytes is prominent by the second week of infection [22]. Occasional giant cells of Langhans type may be present. Well-formed epithelioid granulomas are the hallmark of tubercular lesions but usually are few and ill defined in TBM [17] (Fig. 4.3). Similar chronic inflammation may be seen in the ependyma and choroid plexus. The underlying brain parenchyma is edematous with reactive gliosis and areas of ischemic infarction. The vessels may show infiltrative, necrotizing, or proliferative lesions or any combination of these on histology [17]. Infiltrative transmural lymphocytic inflammation may be noted in sections from the encased basal arteries [16, 18, 23]. Fibrinoid necrosis of vascular intima and media is seen in necrotizing lesions. Proliferative lesions comprise proliferation of intima, atrophy of medial layer, and fragmentation of elastic lamina (Fig. 4.4). Meningeal veins also show phlebitis and luminal thrombi. Vascular lesions are usually resistant to anti-TB treatment. Acid-fast bacilli (AFB) are found in areas of caseous necrosis and can be demonstrated in about 70–80% of cases [17] (Fig. 4.5).

4.3.2 CNS Tuberculoma

4.3.2.1 Introduction

Tuberculomas are caseous foci which result from tubercles lying deep in the brain parenchyma. Wakeley, in his observations on tuberculomas, summarized the reported incidence of tuberculomas of the brain to range between 2% and 33% [24]. Brain tuberculomas may be seen in 15–50% of all intracranial lesions in the developing world and 4% of all intracranial lesions in developed countries and account for a high morbidity and

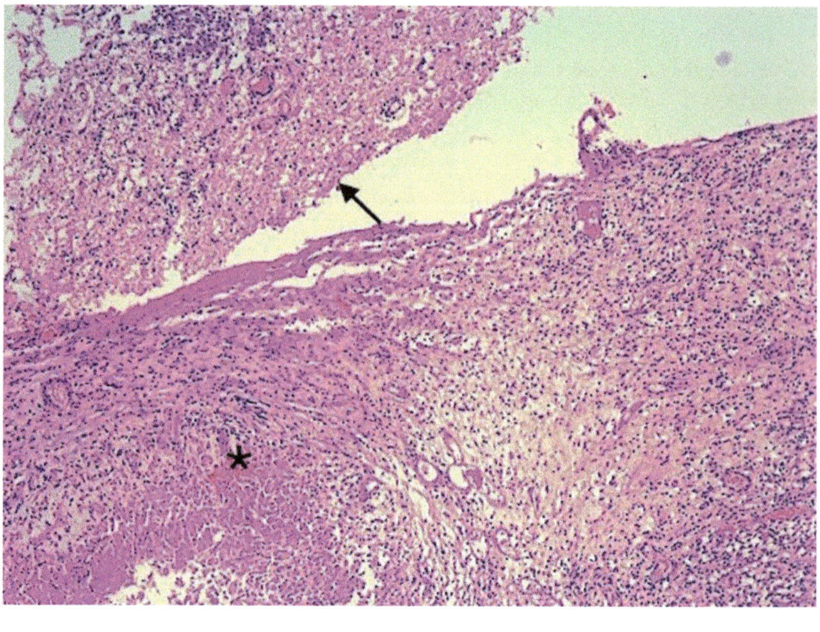

Fig. 4.2 Meningeal exudate (*arrow*) and underlying granuloma (*asterisk*) in a case of TBM (hematoxylin and eosin, ×50)

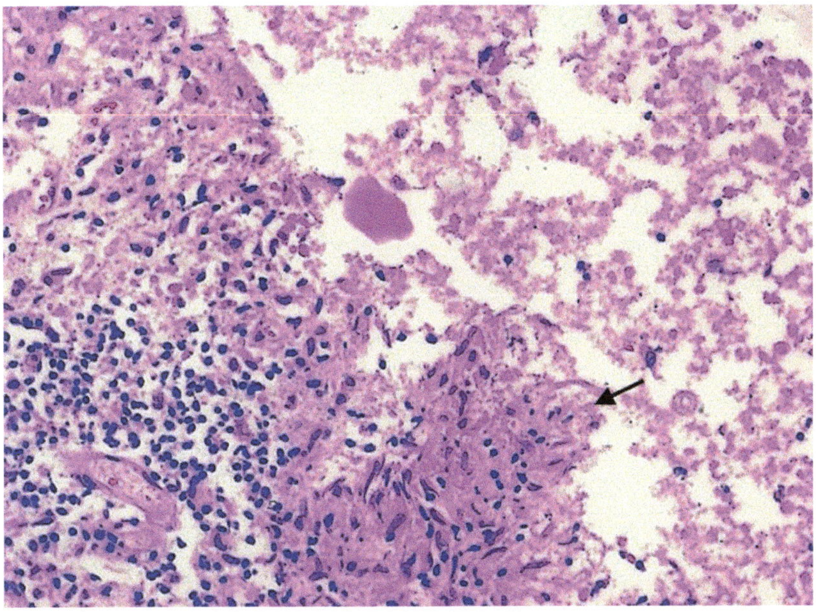

Fig. 4.3 The meningeal exudate comprising of lymphocytes and a collection of epithelioid histiocytes (*arrow*) (hematoxylin and eosin, ×200)

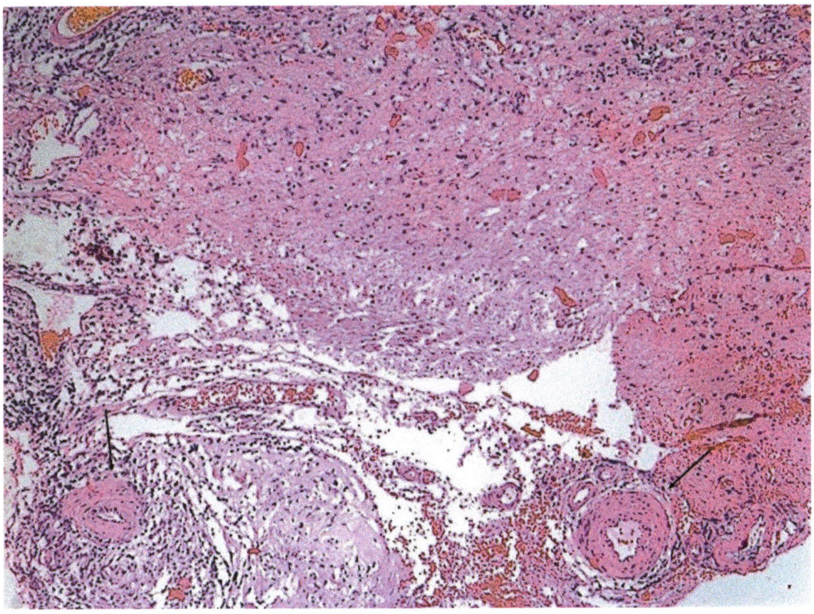

Fig. 4.4 Meningeal exudate with fibrointimal proliferation of vessel walls (*arrows*) (hematoxylin and eosin, ×100)

mortality [22]. Way back in the late 1950s, Arseni described the features in 201 cases of operated tuberculomas [25]. The highest incidence was seen in patients less than 30 years of age [25]. Infratentorial involvement was found to be more common in adolescent age group, while supratentorial tuberculomas predominated in adult males [25]. Dastur et al. noted a high incidence of tuberculomas in children compared to adults with infratentorial location being the favored site in the younger age group [26]. The relatively high frequency of tuberculomas in children, presumably, is due to the fact that TB infection is relatively commoner during childhood, and children are particularly susceptible to extrapulmonary TB because they are unable to contain the infection at sites beyond the lung. Brain tuberculomas are usually single; multiple tuberculomas are seen in

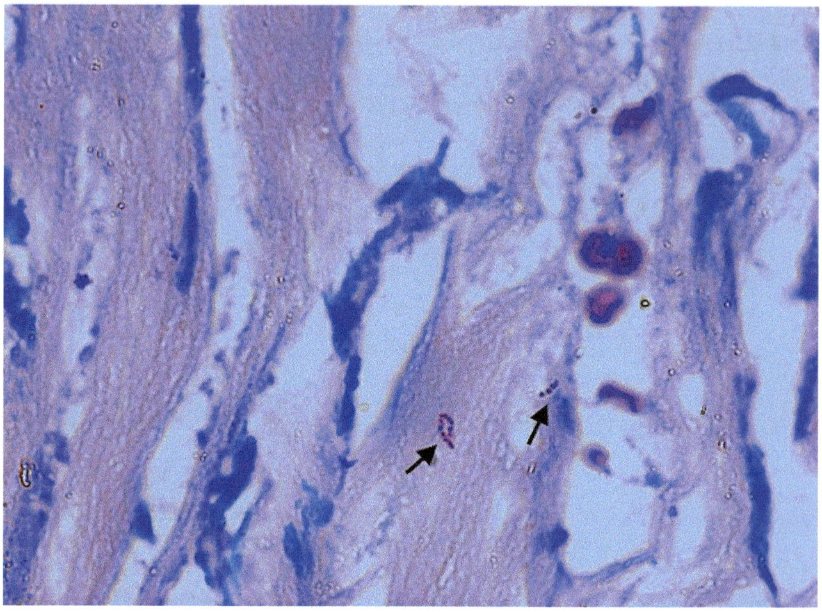

Fig. 4.5 Acid-fast tubercle bacilli (*arrows*) in a biopsy from a case of TBM (Ziehl-Neelsen, ×1000)

15–34% of cases. The size varies between 1 mm and 12 cm [22, 27, 28]. Tuberculoma patients may present with signs and symptoms of raised intracranial pressure mimicking other space-occupying lesions. Thus, headache, vomiting, drowsiness, papilledema, hemiparesis, or seizures can be the presenting feature/s in such patients [29]. On contrast-enhanced CT scan and MRI of the brain, tuberculomas are seen as ring-enhancing lesions usually with a conglomerate appearance (Fig. 4.6).

4.3.2.2 Gross Pathology

Mature tuberculomas are firm, grayish white, lobulated nodules without a capsule and contain a central area of caseation. Satellite lesions often surround a larger granuloma. Most tuberculomas vary in size from 2 to 40 mm in diameter but can reach up to 12 cm in diameter. Tuberculomas have a predilection for frontal lobes in adults and cerebellum in children, but this is not always true, and they can occur anywhere supra- or infratentorially. Less common features include calcification or invasion of the bone surrounding the tuberculoma [30].

4.3.2.3 Microscopic Pathology

A classic tubercle, as seen on microscopy, is a central area of necrosis surrounded by inflammatory cells comprising lymphocytes, epithelioid histiocytes, and Langhans giant cells, with an encircling rich vascular zone (Fig. 4.7). These lesions begin as a cluster of microgranulomas which join to form a noncaseating tuberculoma. Reactivation or further evolution of these lesions leads to caseation within the center of this tuberculoma. The caseation is initially solid surrounded by a rim of granulomatous infiltrate comprising of epithelioid histiocytes, multinucleate giant cells, and mononuclear inflammatory cells. The central core is cheesy and has high lipid content, with macrophage infiltration, regional fibrosis, and perilesional cellular infiltrates with a few bacilli in the center (Figs. 4.8 and 4.9). Liquefaction of the solid caseation slowly begins from the center. The capsule consists of granulation tissue and compressed glial tissue. There is associated perilesional edema with some proliferation of astrocytes in the surrounding brain parenchyma [16, 22, 31]. There may be evidence of calcification in inactive lesions. Rarely, tuberculomas may occur as a plaque-like meningeal covering without exudation. This leads to formation of a solid mass without calcification or caseation. This is called an *en plaque* tuberculoma and was first described by Pardee and Knox in 1927. The commonest location of *en plaque* tuberculoma is reportedly in the frontoparietal region [32].

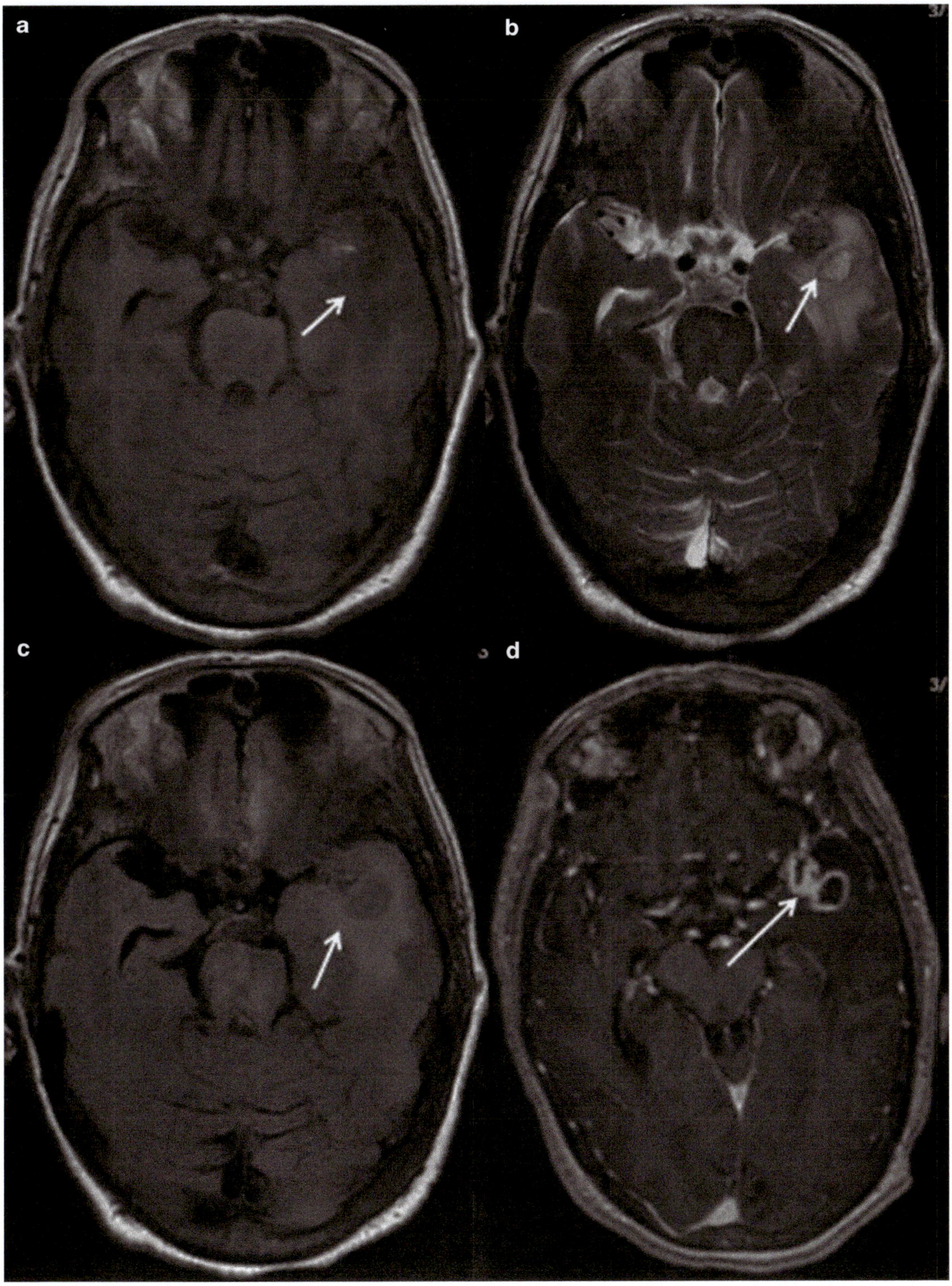

Fig. 4.6 A left temporal tuberculoma exhibiting an iso- to hypointense lesion with mild perilesional edema on T1-W image (**a**), T2-W (**b**), and fluid-attenuated inversion recovery (**c**) images showing areas of mixed intensity surrounded by edema. Post-contrast T1-W image (**d**) shows ring enhancement and conglomerate appearance of the granuloma

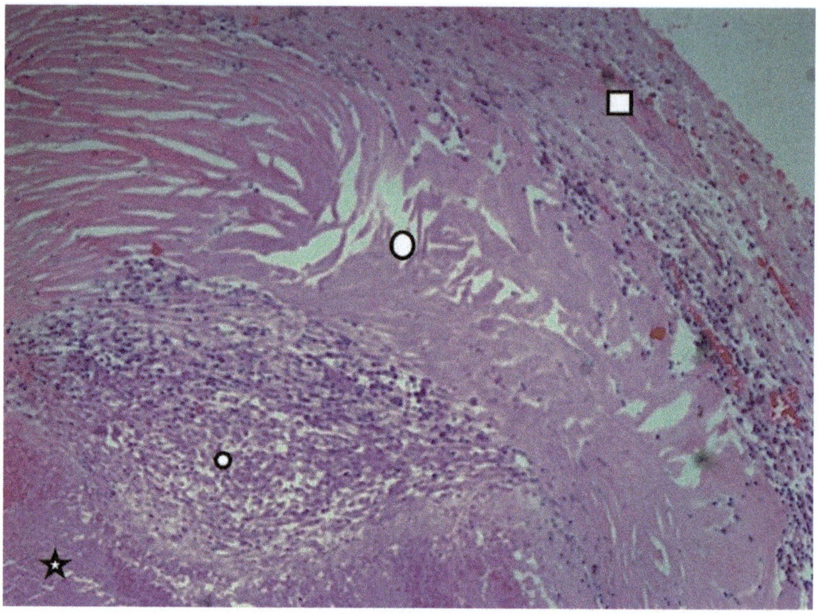

Fig. 4.7 Low-power view of a tuberculoma showing areas of caseous necrosis (*asterisk*), granuloma formation (*circle*), hyalinization (*oval*), and inflamed glial tissue (*square*) (hematoxylin and eosin, ×50)

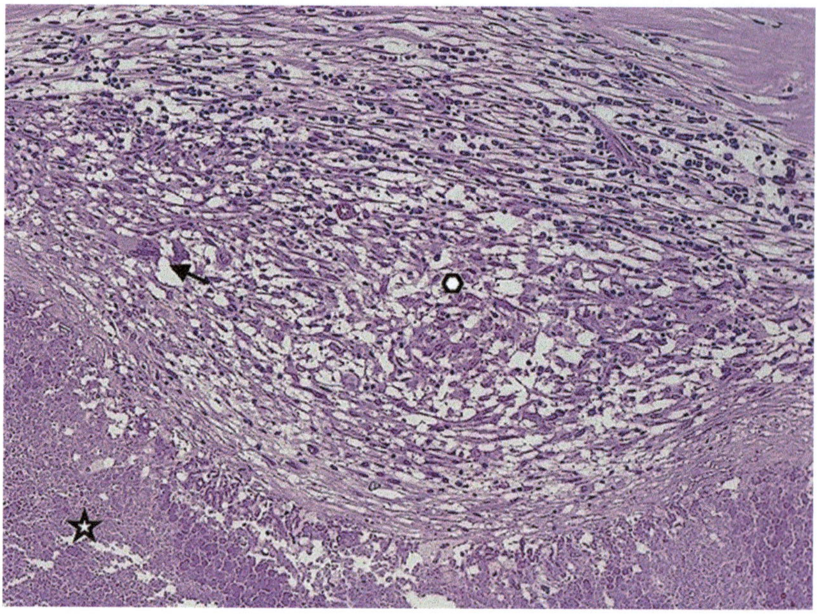

Fig. 4.8 Caseous necrosis (*asterisk*) in the center of a granuloma (*circle*). Few giant cells are noted (*arrow*) (hematoxylin and eosin, ×200)

4.3.3 Tuberculous Abscess

4.3.3.1 Introduction

Tuberculous brain abscess (TBA) is a rarer manifestation of CNS TB, compared with TBM and tuberculoma. Whitener analyzed verified cases of TBA from the literature prior to 1978 and concluded that their presentation is acute, often occurring in the third and fourth decades of life. Abscesses are usually supratentorial in location, and their common mode of presentation is with focal neurologic signs. Associated evidence on history and laboratory findings is present. He proposed the criteria for the diagnosis of TB abscess as (1) the presence of a cavity in brain parenchyma with pus

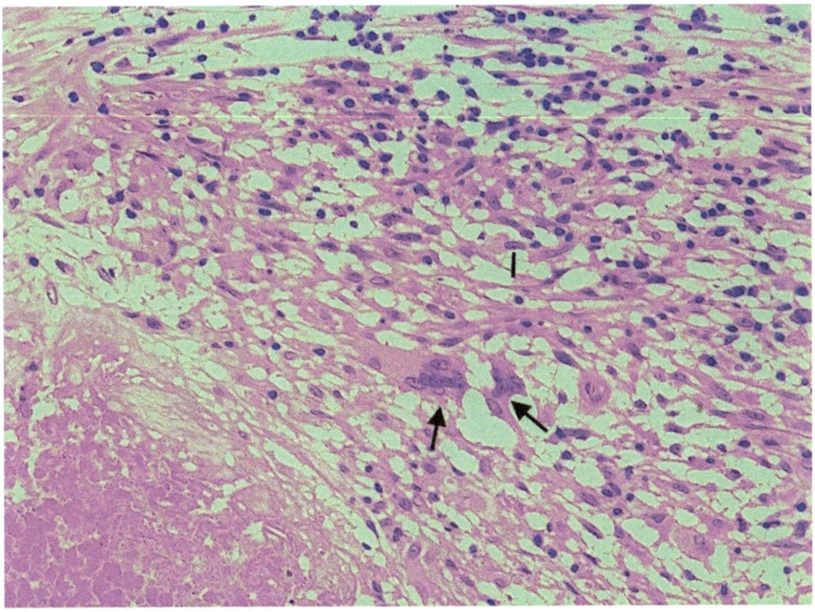

Fig. 4.9 Langhans giant cells (*arrows*) and epithelioid cells (*line*) in a tubercular granuloma (hematoxylin and eosin, ×400)

in the center, as revealed on autopsy or surgical material, (2) microscopic evidence of mixed inflammation with a predominance of neutrophils and vascular granulation tissue, and (3) the presence of tubercle bacilli in the pus or wall of the abscess or a positive culture for *M. tuberculosis* [33].

The exact pathogenesis of TBA is unknown. It is hypothesized that the abscess arises from liquefaction and caseous necrosis of tuberculomas. The TB bacilli in TBA, as in other forms of CNS TB, reach the brain via hematogenous spread from foci in the lungs or other sites of primary infection. The deficiency in the host immune status, bacterial load, virulence of the organism, and route of infection plays a central role in formation of TBA after the primary infection. On MRI, TB abscesses vary form 3–20 mL in volume. They are hypointense on T1-weighted and hyperintense on T2-weighted images and show distinct rim enhancement on contrast administration (Fig. 4.10). The wall of the abscess is smooth or lobulated in majority of cases. On routine sequences, it is difficult to differentiate pyogenic from TBA; newer sequences, like magnetization transfer MRI, in vivo MR spectroscopy, and diffusion-weighted imaging, may be useful in differentiating them [34].

4.3.3.2 Gross Pathology

TBA may be solitary or multiple. In a study on 110 patients comparing pyogenic, TB and fungal brain abscesses, of the eleven culture-proven TB abscesses, six were solitary and five multiple. Three of eleven cases showed satellite lesions [35]. On macroscopic examination, TBAs are discrete lesions with central liquefactive necrosis surrounded by a fibrous reaction and edema [36].

4.3.3.3 Microscopic Pathology

The classical histomorphological features of TBA have been well described. A TBA is a localized collection of pus admixed with TB bacilli and surrounded by a capsule. A TBA does not show typical tubercular granulomas. It closely resembles a pyogenic abscess, and hence the diagnosis of a TBA relies on the identification of TB bacilli in the pus or wall of the abscess and presence of a predominantly neutrophilic infiltrate. The presence of epithelioid and giant cells which are a characteristic feature of tubercular granuloma is lacking in TBA [37].

Microscopically, the outermost wall of the abscess is composed of gliotic parenchyma with perivascular lymphocytic infiltrates and edema surrounded in most cases by a collagenous capsule and a rim of granulation tissue (Fig.

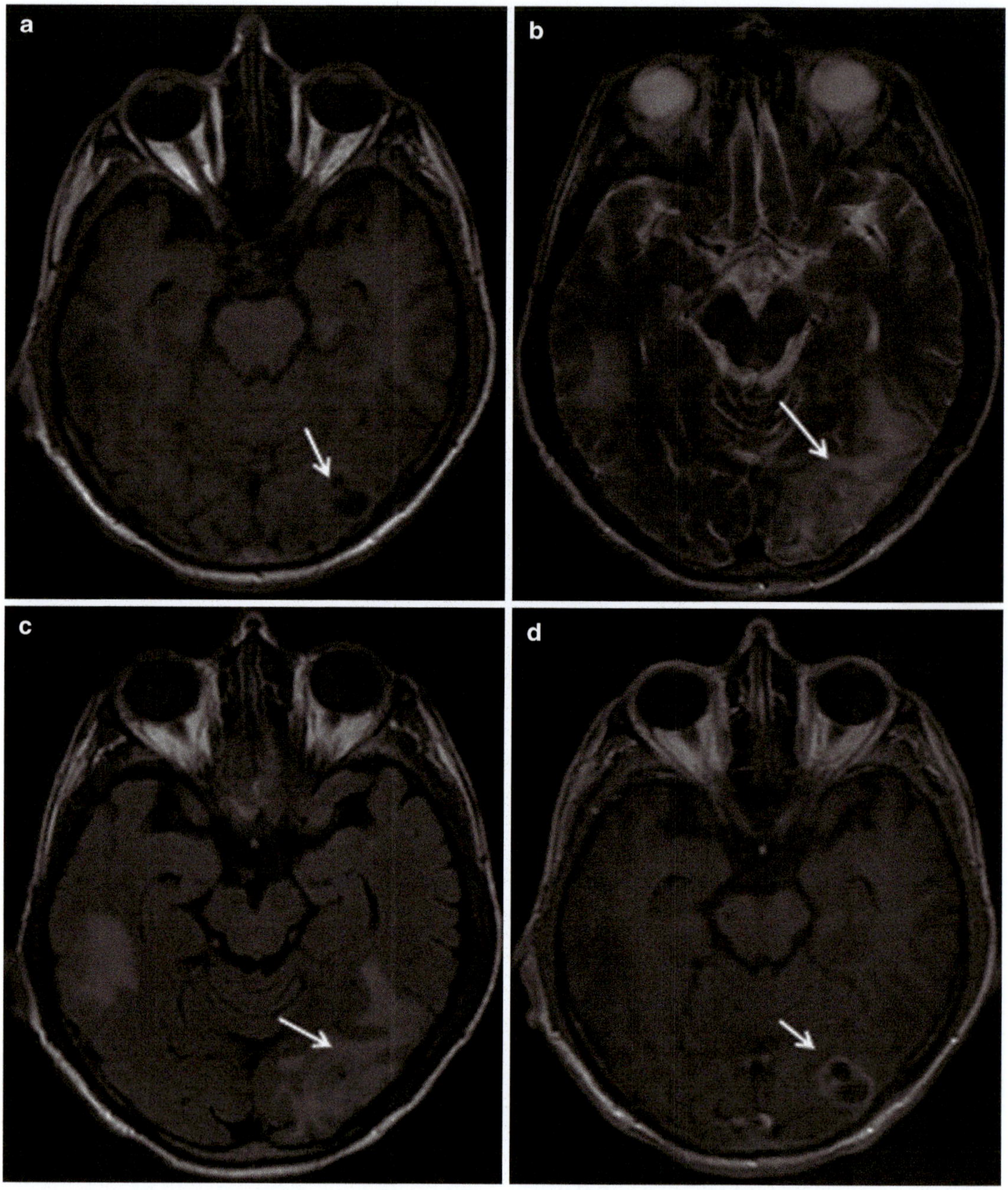

Fig. 4.10 MR imaging findings in case of a tuberculous brain abscess (TBA) with perilesional edema in left parieto-occipital region (*arrows*). T1-W image shows a hypointense lesion with a hyperintense wall (**a**). Mixed intensity lesion with irregular walls is seen on T2-W (**b**) and fluid-attenuated inversion recovery sequences (**c**). Post-contrast T1-W image (**d**) shows rim enhancement

4.11). This is followed by sheets of histiocytes and foamy macrophages with interspersed aggregates of neutrophilic infiltrate (Figs. 4.12 and 4.13). Luminal necrosis differs from caseous necrosis by its richer content of fibrin and the presence of neutrophils. Epithelioid granulomas which are so typical of tuberculomas are ill formed or resemble palisades around the necrotic

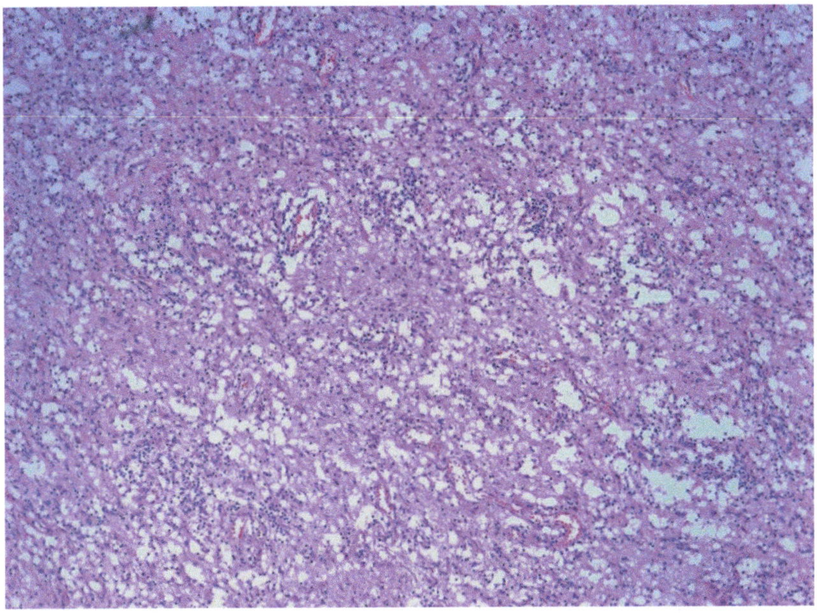

Fig. 4.11 Intense glial inflammatory infiltrate in a case of TBA (hematoxylin and eosin, ×50)

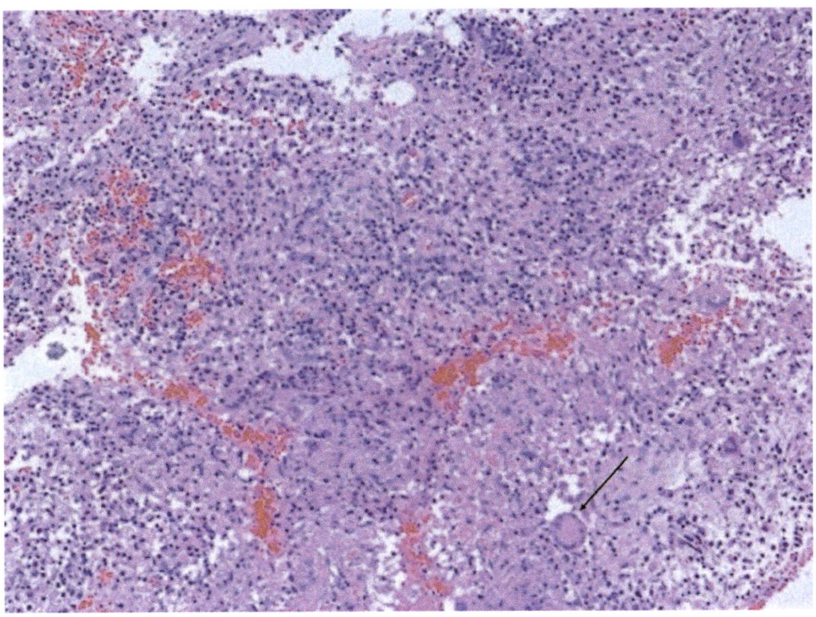

Fig. 4.12 Intense mixed inflammation and occasional giant cells (*arrow*) in a section from TBA (hematoxylin and eosin, ×100)

center [36–38]. Chakraborty et al. found that AFB could be identified using Ziehl-Neelsen staining in 62% cases and immunohistochemical staining for mycobacterial antigen in 83% cases of TBA [36] (Fig. 4.14). They could demonstrate mycobacterial antigen within the epithelioid cells, foamy macrophages, and Langhans giant cells on immunohistochemical staining [36].

4.3.4 Complications of Tuberculous Meningitis

Apart from tuberculomas and abscesses which complicate TBM, there can be other life-threatening complications that may occur despite anti-TB treatment. These complications are briefly discussed below.

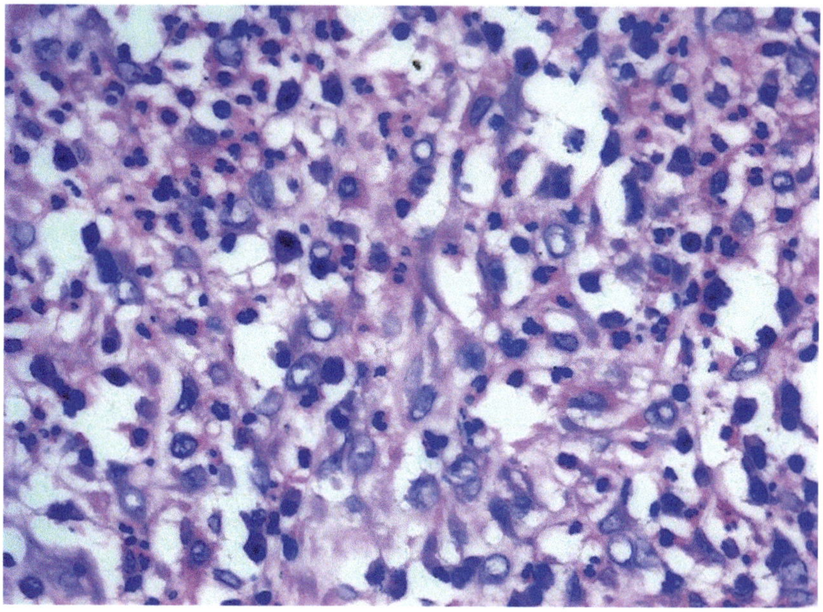

Fig. 4.13 Inflammatory infiltrate in TBA comprising numerous polymorphs with few lymphocytes (hematoxylin and eosin, ×400)

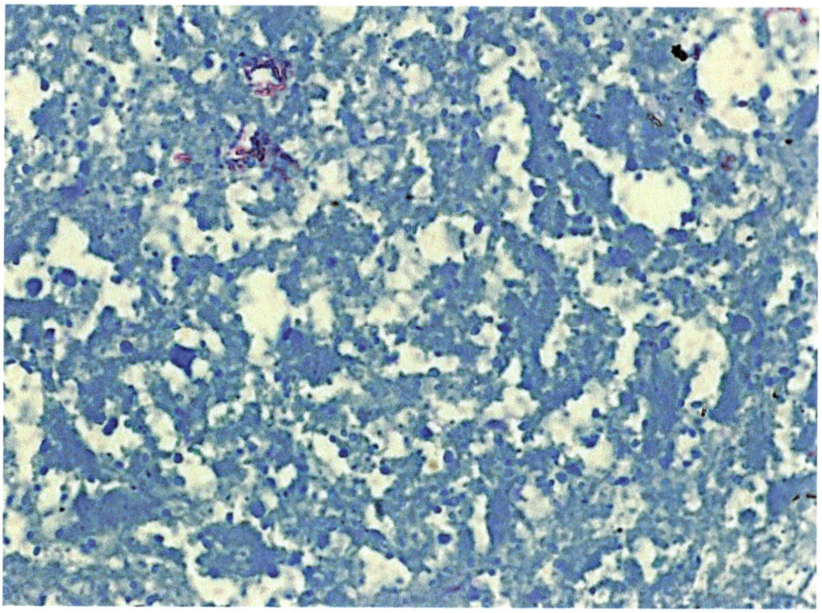

Fig. 4.14 Numerous tubercle bacilli in a TBA (Ziehl-Neelsen, ×1000)

Hydrocephalus

Hydrocephalus is the most common complication of TBM and can occur any time during the course of the disease, as well as either before or after commencement of therapy. Hydrocephalus in patients with TBM is usually of communicating type (Fig. 4.15). Hydrocephalus occurs due to the blockage of the subarachnoid space or the ventricular pathways by the inflammatory exudates. Obstructive hydrocephalus develops when the aqueduct or the fourth ventricular outlets are clogged by exudates [39, 40].

Stroke

As discussed earlier, basal exudates spread anteriorly encompassing the optic chiasm and ante-

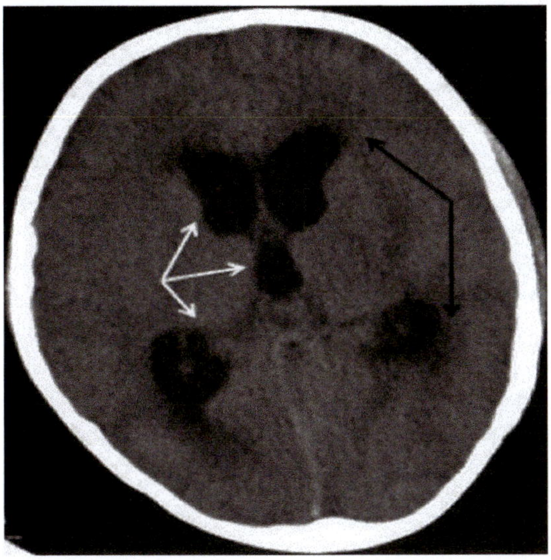

Fig. 4.15 Dilated lateral and third ventricles in a patient with TBM and hydrocephalus (*white arrows*). Mild periventricular lucency can be seen around the frontal and occipital horns of lateral ventricles (*black arrows*)

rior cerebral vessels and extend laterally into the Sylvian fissures around the carotid artery, middle cerebral trunks, and their penetrating branches. Cortical infarcts in TBM are believed to result from any or all of vasculitis, intimal proliferation of vessel walls and thrombosis. These infarcts occur most commonly in the territory of small- or medium-sized vessels [41, 42]. Cortical venous sinus thrombosis (CVST) or venous infarcts are a lesser known complication of TBM. There are isolated reports of CVST in TBM, usually occurring secondary to endothelial injury due to an inflammatory response, sluggish venous flow, and increase in platelet aggregation [43, 44]

Ventriculitis

Ventriculitis or ependymitis is a more common complication of bacterial meningitis but does occur in TBM as well. It requires long-term anti-TB treatment or surgical intervention in resistant or acutely deteriorating cases. As reported by Singh et al., the most common feature of tubercular ventriculitis is hydrocephalus along with contrast enhancement of ependymal lining of one or more of ventricle walls, with or without ventricular sludge in lateral ventricles [45].

Cranial Neuropathies

Evidence of cranial nerve involvement is seen in about one-fourth of TBM patients. The most common affliction is seen in the sixth cranial nerve. In a retrospective analysis of 158 cases with TBM, 38% of patients had cranial nerve involvement, with abducens being the one most commonly involved; 10% had multiple cranial nerve involvement. Involvement of the first, fourth, fifth, or eighth nerves was not observed. Cranial nerve involvement is due to basal exudates, vasculitis of arteries supplying the midbrain region, optochiasmatic arachnoiditis, and infiltration either directly by exudates or by fibrous bands compressing the nerves [46].

Tuberculous Encephalopathy

Dastur and Udani described the clinicopathological features of 20 cases of diffuse brain damage in patients with TB [47]. They coined the term "tuberculous encephalopathy," and the most striking abnormality on autopsy was edema predominantly of the white matter. It was originally proposed that the diffuse brain damage is immune mediated, though later studies suggested that hypoxic ischemic damage was also contributory [47, 48].

Hyponatremia

Hyponatremia is one of the more common complications in TBM seen in about 50% cases. Two physiologically distinct conditions which can lead to hyponatremia in TBM are syndrome of inappropriate antidiuretic hormone secretion (SIADH) and cerebral salt-wasting (CSW) syndrome. Hyponatremia in the setting of SIADH is dilutional as the total body sodium remains normal, while in CSW, urinary sodium excretion is increased, and the urine output is inappropriately high despite the presence of dehydration. While fluid restriction can be detrimental for patients with CSW, it is beneficial in SIADH; exact diagnosis of the etiology of hyponatremia hence becomes important. The electrolyte and hydration status of these patients require close monitoring [49, 50].

Optochiasmatic Arachnoiditis

Optochiasmatic arachnoiditis is the foremost cause of visual impairment in TBM. This is a consequence of basal exudates in the interpeduncular, suprasellar, and Sylvian cisterns. An Indian study related younger age, female sex, and raised CSF proteins with optochiasmatic arachnoiditis. This devastating condition is thought to be a result of the exaggerated host response against proteins of TB bacilli [51, 52].

4.3.5 HIV and CNS Tuberculosis

With the increasing incidence of acquired immunodeficiency syndrome (AIDS), a concomitant increase in the incidence of extrapulmonary TB, especially TBM, has been noted. Worldwide, TB is among the leading causes of death in people infected by HIV. CNS involvement has been reported in 10–20% of patients with AIDS-related TB. A high mortality of around 80% has been reported for TB of CNS among HIV-infected patients [53].

TB of CNS may present in HIV-infected individuals as meningitis, tuberculoma, abscess, encephalitis, or radiculomyelitis. Treatment in cases coinfected by HIV is complicated by HIV-TB drug-drug interactions, interrelated drug toxicities, and immune reconstitution inflammatory syndrome. Generally, HIV-infected CNS TB patients have a poorer outcome compared to non-HIV patients. Impaired T cell-mediated immunity and decline in CD4 T cells in HIV-infected persons increase the risk of CNS TB. There is a heightened risk of dissemination and extrapulmonary TB during the stage of reactivation or of primary progression after TB infection [54, 55].

Pathology

Though HIV infection does not modify the presentation of TBM or tuberculoma, the likelihood of opportunistic intracranial infections and malignancies should be excluded. An Indian study demonstrated that HIV-positive patients with TBM have fewer basal exudates which are thin and serous. The inflammatory response is minimal with few epithelioid histiocytes and no Langhans type of giant cells. On the contrary, cerebral parenchyma and meninges are full of AFB, and infarcts are common [56]. Tubercular granulomas are less common in HIV-infected individuals, and the most common etiology for granulomatous lesions in HIV infection is cerebral toxoplasmosis. It has been postulated that a severe degree of immunosuppression impairs the granulomatous inflammatory response to mycobacteria. TBAs occur in a greater proportion of HIV-positive patients than in the population in general [38]. In the absence of a strong immune response, the foci of cerebritis develop into abscess in the presence of HIV infection. A higher yield of AFB on smear (69%) and culture (87.9%) of CSF has been reported from HIV-positive patients rather than HIV-negative ones [57].

4.3.6 Nontubercular Mycobacterial CNS Infection

Nontubercular mycobacteria (NTM) are a rare but serious cause of meningitis, especially in immunosuppressed states. The pathogenic potential of these organisms can be made out with increasing incidence of NTM with the advent of AIDS pandemic. Flor et al., in 1996, described the clinical details on reviewing all cases of NTM described in English literature. Of the 52 reported cases, 31 were caused by *Mycobacterium avium* complex (MAC), 9 were caused by *scotochromogens*, 6 by *Mycobacterium kansasii*, and 6 by *Mycobacterium fortuitum* [58]. Apart from meningitis, there have been reports of abscesses, both single and multiple, caused by atypical mycobacteria, most notably, MAC and *M. fortuitum* [59, 60]. Table 4.2 lists the atypical mycobacteria that cause CNS infections [61, 62]. On histopathology, low-grade inflammation, perivascular lesions, ill-formed granulomas without giant cells, and the presence of AFB are the characteristic features of CNS involvement [58].

The importance of identifying NTM species in cases of meningitis/abscess lies in the fact that these agents are nonresponsive to the first-line drugs used to treat TBM. The choice of antibiotics and duration of treatment are based on the species identified. An apt clinical scenario and a high degree of suspicion are required to diagnose CNS infection with atypical mycobacteria.

Table 4.2 Atypical Mycobacteria causing CNS infections

Mycobacterium abscessus
Mycobacterium avium complex
Mycobacterium celatum
Mycobacterium fortuitum
Mycobacterium gordonae
Mycobacterium haemophilum
Mycobacterium kansasii
Mycobacterium mucogenicum
Mycobacterium scrofulaceum

4.4 Histopathologic Differential Diagnoses of CNS Tuberculosis

4.4.1 Acute Inflammatory Pathology

TBM may have an acute presentation. This is relatively frequent in HIV-positive patients with TBM. The CSF may show a neutrophilic predominance. The exclusion of bacterial pyogenic meningitis is of utmost importance in such cases. Examination of CSF sediment for the presence of acid-fast TB bacilli and other bacteria is essential. The use of CSF culture and molecular methods like PCR for identifying specific bacterial or TB antigens is noteworthy [63].

4.4.2 Chronic Inflammatory Pathology

A variety of lesions may mimic TBM or tuberculomas, both clinically and on radiologic assessment. Such lesions may range from infections with neurotropic fungi and viruses to partially treated pyogenic meningitis, sarcoidosis, and involvement of meninges with metastatic tumor deposits. CSF may also show a lymphocytic pleocytosis in most of these. The differential diagnosis is aided by molecular tests for specific antigens in CSF and serum. In cases where a noninvasive battery of tests does not lead to a conclusive diagnosis, a biopsy of the lesion becomes necessary. Many chronic lesions, especially fungal meningitis, produce granulomatous lesions in the brain. Utility of special cytochemical stains, including those for tubercle bacilli (Ziehl-Neelsen), fungi (periodic acid-Schiff, Gomori's methenamine silver, India ink staining), and other bacteria (Grams), cannot be overemphasized [64]. The time taken for culture of CSF or biopsied tissue limits its utility as a diagnostic modality. Important differentials to be considered in the workup of a patient with TB of CNS are listed in Table 4.3 [17, 22, 63, 65–67]. Neurosarcoidosis deserves a special mention in being a great mimicker of TB both clinically and on biopsy. Sarcoid granulomas show subtle differences from TB ones. The presence of caseation necrosis and a lymphocytic cuff around the epithelioid cells favors a TB granuloma. Schaumann and asteroid bodies may accompany sarcoid granulomas but are nonspecific and can be seen in TB lesions too [67]. In lesions where a definitive diagnosis cannot be made, empiric antimicrobial therapy may be instituted depending on the clinical scenario [68].

4.5 Diagnostic Tests

Biopsies of parenchymal brain lesions are rarely necessary to make a diagnosis of TB of CNS. The diagnosis is usually made with the help of radiological findings in adjunct with evidence of TB at other sites, usually the lung [30]. Evaluation of the CSF is an invaluable aid in the diagnosis of TB of CNS. Various tests can be done on CSF samples in cases of TB of CNS. An overview of the tests is provided here. These will be detailed in Sect. V of the book.

4.5.1 Cerebrospinal Fluid Aspiration

Cytology and Chemistry The CSF obtained in TBM is usually at an elevated opening pressure. A cobweb coagulum may be present. CSF protein is elevated and usually ranges between 100 and 500 mg/dl. Grossly raised protein levels associated with xanthochromia may be seen

Table 4.3 Differential diagnoses of CNS tuberculosis

Cause	Gross	Microscopy	Diagnostic tests
Fungal			
Cryptococcosis	Basal meningitis, midbrain and basal ganglia lesions	Chronic inflammation, granulomas, foreign-body giant cells, encapsulated budding yeast	CSF cryptococcal capsular polysaccharide antigen (CRAg), India ink preparation
Aspergillosis	Basal meningitis, vascular infarcts and necrosis, fungal abscess	Granulomas, uniform septate hyphae, branching at 45° angles	Galactomannan ELISA and PCR for fungal components in CSF/serum, CSF culture
Histoplasmosis	Basal meningitis, lesions at gray-white matter interface, vasculitis	Necrotizing granulomas, intracellular yeast in macrophages	Specific CSF polysaccharide antigen, fungal culture, urine histoplasma antigen
Coccidioidomycosis	Basal meningitis, abscess, infarction	Necrotizing granulomas, dimorphic fungus with branched septate hyphae and endosporulating spherules	CSF complement fixation test, fungal culture
Blastomycosis	Meningitis, subdural and parenchymal abscesses	Granulomas, dimorphic fungus with broad-based budding	CSF fungal culture, serology not helpful
Viral	Panencephalitis, with or without meningitis	Hemorrhagic encephalitis, microglial nodules, intracellular inclusions	Molecular tests for viral DNA in CSF or serum; plasma, CSF bromide partition test
Partially treated bacterial meningitis	Exudate over cerebral surface, basal surface spared, cortical venous thrombosis	Mixed inflammatory infiltrate, subpial gliosis	Latex agglutination test, counter immunoelectrophoresis, PCR for specific bacterial antigens
Neurosarcoidosis	Single or multiple mass lesions in parenchyma	Noncaseating granulomas, absence of lymphocytic cuffing of granulomas, Schaumann and asteroid bodies	Angiotensin-converting enzyme (ACE) in CSF and serum (nonspecific)
Neoplastic meningitis	Superficial parenchymal and intradural metastatic nodules, thickened meninges	Atypical lymphoma or carcinoma cells in meningeal biopsy	Examination of centrifuged CSF sediment for malignant cells, biochemical tumor markers in CSF (nonspecific), tumor-specific sequences on CSF PCR

in cases with subarachnoid block. Glucose levels are low and generally less than 45 mg/dl [69]. A centrifuged sediment shows an elevated cell count with a majority of lymphocytes (Fig. 4.16). Adenosine deaminase (ADA) is a marker of T cell-mediated immune response, and ADA levels are elevated in TBM in comparison to aseptic meningitis. But the utility of ADA as a test diagnostic for TBM is limited by its low specificity [70, 71]

Microbiology Demonstration of AFB in CSF gives definitive evidence of TBM. However, results of a Ziehl-Neelsen stain on a centrifuged CSF deposit are not very encouraging, and positivity rates as low as 10% have been reported (Fig. 4.17). The probability of detecting bacilli in the CSF increases with examination of repeat samples, of large CSF volumes, or in ventricular CSF samples [18]. The use of fluorescent stains like auramine-rhodamine has also been reported to be of help [72]. Culture of CSF is time consuming and may take 4–8 weeks to reveal a growth [63]. Conventional Lowenstein-Jensen culture positivity for TB bacilli has been reported to range between 25 and 70% [73]. Rapid techniques for

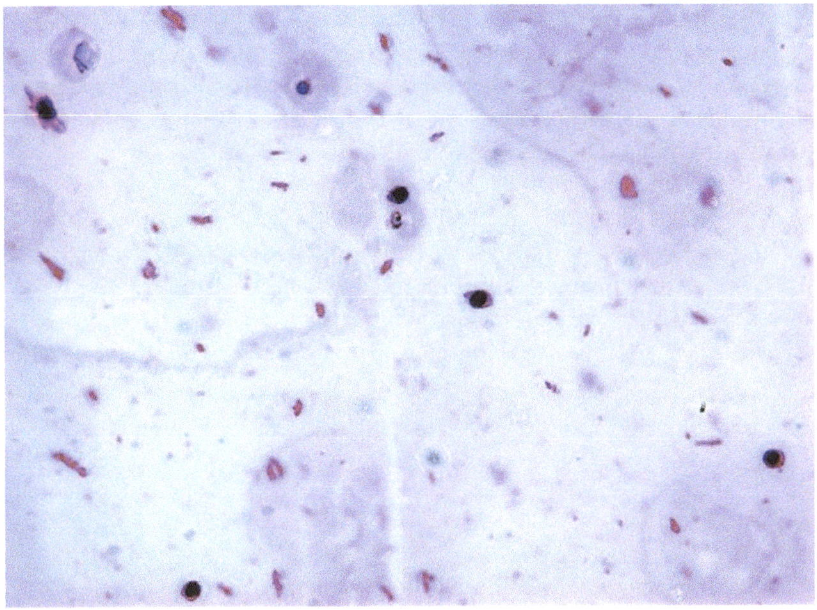

Fig. 4.16 Lymphocytic pleocytosis in a centrifuged cerebrospinal fluid (CSF) sediment (hematoxylin and eosin, ×200)

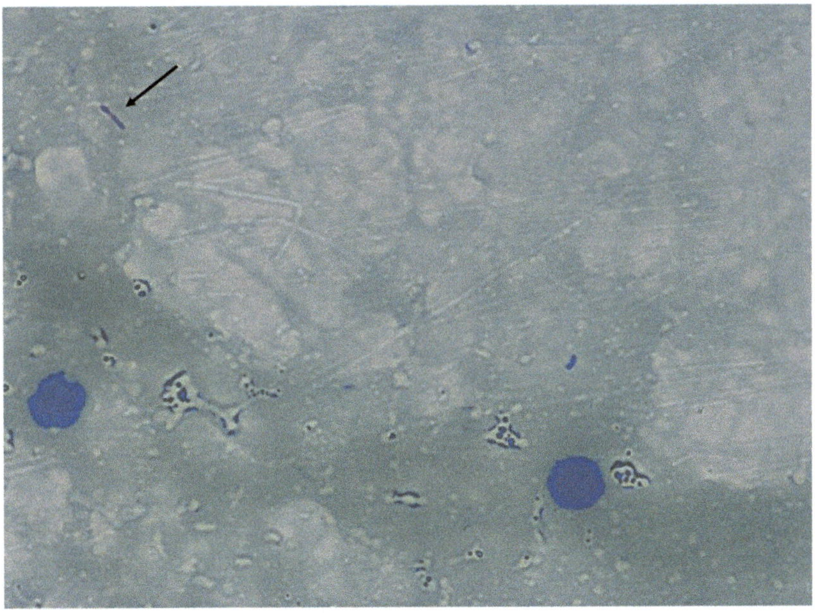

Fig. 4.17 Centrifuged CSF showing a tubercle bacillus (*arrow*) (Ziehl-Neelsen, ×1000)"

culture including the radiometric BACTEC method take 7–10 days for diagnosis [74]. CSF samples from cases of tuberculomas or TB abscess usually do not show a specific change. The definitive diagnosis in these cases can be made using histopathologic or culture demonstration of bacilli on biopsy tissue [75].

Immunopathology Tests detecting specific TB antigens or antibodies include Hemagglutination, Enzyme-linked immunosorbent assay, Immunofluorescence assay, Radioimmunoassay, and Western blotting. These give rapid results, but the outcome is dependent on proper standardization and type of probe used in the assay [75, 76].

Nuclei Acid Amplification The polymerase chain reaction (PCR) amplifies and detects a specific sequence of the DNA of TB bacilli. Though promising, a meta-analysis has shown limited sensitivity (56%) and specificity (98%) for these tests [77]. Conventional bacteriologic detection may be better than nucleic acid amplification (NAA) assays in initial disease detection; however, the NAA may be more helpful in detecting disease in patients already under treatment. It should nevertheless be borne in mind that negative results on bacteriology and PCR do not exclude the diagnosis of TBM [68].

4.5.2 Biopsy

Histopathological confirmation on biopsy tissue sample is the gold standard for the diagnosis of CNS TB. Stereotactic, meningeal, or open biopsy approach is used depending on the accessibility of the lesion. Noninvasive diagnostic modalities are the preferred diagnostic approaches. However, biopsy becomes necessary in certain cases. Indications for performing a biopsy in suspected TB of CNS are detailed in Table 4.4.

4.5.3 Fine Needle Aspirates

Ancillary diagnosis of TB of CNS can be made using material aspirated from a paraspinal abscess, an enlarged peripheral lymph node, or a mass in the lung. The aspirated material is usually thick and creamy white. It is spread onto glass slides, stained appropriately, and examined. The procedure is relatively noninvasive and painless, and results can be obtained promptly since unlike biopsy tissue, tissue processing is not required.

Table 4.4 Indications for biopsy in CNS tuberculosis

Clinical	No clinical improvement
	Deterioration in clinical status
	Possibility of an alternative diagnosis
Radiological	Lesion/changes not responding to treatment
	Increase in size of lesion (not attributable to paradoxical reaction)
	Atypical changes in the morphology of lesion
	Polymorphic lesions

Conclusion

TB of CNS is the most dreaded expression of extrapulmonary TB. Host-pathogen interactions determine to a large extent the pathologic expression in the CNS. The diagnostic armamentarium for neuro-TB includes an in-depth assessment of clinical manifestations, radiologic images, serology, CSF findings, and tissue morphology. It is imperative to remember the pathologic manifestations of TB of CNS in order to correctly interpret the diagnostic test results and judiciously treat the patient.

References

1. Marais BJ, Gie RP, Schaaf HS, Hesseling AC, Obihara CC, Starke JJ, Enarson DA, Donald PR, Beyers N (2004) The natural history of childhood intra-thoracic tuberculosis: a critical review of literature from the pre-chemotherapy era. Int J Tuberc Lung Dis 8:392–402
2. Wallgren A (1948) The time-table of tuberculosis. Tubercle 29:245–251
3. Hunter RL (2011) Pathology of post primary tuberculosis of the lung: an illustrated critical review. Tuberculosis 91:497–509
4. Gupta SD, Ray R, Gill SS (2009) Pathology. In: Sharma SK (ed) Tuberculosis. Jaypee, New Delhi, pp 66–101
5. Sharma SK, Mohan A (2004) Extra pulmonary tuberculosis. Indian J Med Res 120:316–353
6. Macgregor AR, Green CA (1937) Tuberculosis of the central nervous system, with special reference to tuberculous meningitis. J. Pathol. Bacteriol. 45:613–645
7. Rich AR, MacCordock HA (1933) The pathogenesis of tuberculosis. Bull Johns Hopkins Hosp 52:5–37
8. Gupta RK, Kohli A, Gaur V, Lal JH, Kishore J (1997) MRI of the brain in patients with miliary pulmonary tuberculosis without symptoms or signs of central nervous system involvement. Neuroradiology 39:699–670
9. Donald PR, Schaaf HS, Schoeman JF (2005) Tuberculous meningitis and military tuberculosis: the "Rich" focus revisited. J Infect 50:193–195

10. Thwaites GE, Schoeman JF (2009) Update on tuberculosis of the central nervous system: pathogenesis, diagnosis, and treatment. Clin Chest Med 30:745–754
11. Isabel BE, Rogelio HP (2014) Pathogenesis and immune response in tuberculous meningitis. Malays J Med Sci 21:4–10
12. Jacob CN, Henein SS, Heurich AE, Kamholz S (1993) Non-tuberculous mycobacterial infection of the central nervous system in patients with AIDS. South African Med J 86:638–640
13. Garcia-Monco JC (1999) Central nervous system tuberculosis. Neurol Clin 17:737–759
14. Dastur DK, Lalitha VS, Udani PM, Parikh U (1970) The brain and meninges in tuberculous meningitis: gross pathology in 100 cases and pathogenesis. Neurol India 18:86–100
15. Etlik O, Evirgen O, Bay A, Yilmaz N, Temizoz O, Irmak H, Dogan E (2004) Radiologic and clinical findings in tuberculous meningitis. Eur J Gen Med 1:19–24
16. Gupta RK, Kumar S (2011) Central nervous system tuberculosis. Neuroimaging Clin N Am 21:795–814
17. Prabhakar S, Modi M, Heemskerk D, Van TTT, Thwaites G, Radotra B, Ahuja C, Khandelwal N, Singla N, Mathuriya SN (2016) Tuberculous meningitis. In: Chopra JS, Sawhney IMS (eds) Neurology in tropics. Elsevier, New Delhi, pp 185–188
18. Garg RK (1999) Classic diseases revisited: tuberculosis of the central nervous system. Postgrad Med J 75:133–140
19. Udani PM, Parekh UC, Dastur DK (1971) Neurological and related syndromes in CNS tuberculosis. Clinical features and pathogenesis. J Neurol Sci 14:341–357
20. Lindsay I, Scholtz CL (1978) Recent presentations of neurological tuberculosis. J R Soc Med 71:223–227
21. Dastur DK, Manghani DK, Udani PM (1995) Pathogenetic mechanisms in neurotuberculosis. Radiol Clin North Am 33:733–752
22. Husain N, Kumar P (2011) Pathology of tropical diseases. Neuroimaging Clin N Am 21:757–775
23. Lammie GA, Hewlett RH, Schoeman JF, Donald PR (2009) Tuberculous cerebrovascular disease: a review. J Infect 59:156–166
24. Wakeley CPG (1939) Some observations on tuberculomas of the brain. Br J Tuberc 33:75–79
25. Arseni C (1958) Two hundred and one cases of intracranial tuberculoma treated surgically. J Neurol Neurosurg Psychiatry 21:308–311
26. Dastur DK, Lalitha VS, Prabhakar V (1968) Pathological analysis of intracranial space-occupying lesions in 1000 cases including children: part 1. Age, sex and pattern; and the tuberculomas. J Neurol Sci 6:575–592
27. Jinkins JR (1991) Computed tomography of intracranial tuberculosis. Neuroradiology 33:126–135
28. Salaskar AL, Hassaneen W, Keenan CH, Suki D (2015) Intracranial tuberculoma mimicking brain metastasis. J Cancer Res Ther 11:653
29. DeLance AR, Safaee M, Oh MC, Clark AJ, Kaur G, Sun MZ, Bollen AW, Phillips JJ, Parsa AT (2013) Tuberculoma of the central nervous system. J Clin Neurosci 20:1333–1341
30. Starke JR (1999) Tuberculosis of the central nervous system in children. Semin Pediatr Neurol 6:318–331
31. Patkar D, Narang J, Yanamandala R, Lawande M, Shah GV (2012) Central nervous system tuberculosis: pathophysiology and imaging findings. Neuroimaging Clin N Am 22:677–705
32. Agarwal A, Patra DP, Gupta K, Sodhi HB (2016) Dural tuberculoma mimicking meningioma: a clinicoradiologic review of dural en-plaque lesions. World Neurosurg 88:686 e1-7
33. Whitener DR (1978) Tuberculous brain abscess: report of a case and review of the literature. Arch Neurol 35:148–155
34. Gupta RK, Vatsal DK, Husain N, Chawla S, Prasad KN, Roy R, Kumar R, Jha D, Husain M (2001) Differentiation of tuberculous from pyogenic brain abscesses with in vivo proton MR spectroscopy and magnetization transfer MR imaging. Am J Neuroradiol 22:1503–1509
35. Luthra G, Parihar A, Nath K, Jaiswal S, Prasad KN, Husain N, Husain M, Singh S, Behari S, Gupta RK (2007) Comparative evaluation of fungal, tubercular, and pyogenic brain abscesses with conventional and diffusion MR imaging and proton MR spectroscopy. AJNR Am J Neuroradiol 28:1332–1338
36. Chakraborti S, Mahadevan A, Govindan A, Nagarathna S, Santosh V, Yasha TC, Devi BI, Chandramouli BA, Kovoor JM, Chandramuki A, Shankar SK (2009) Clinicopathological study of tuberculous brain abscess. Pathol Res Pract 205:815–822
37. Prakash B, Mehta G, Gondal R, Kumar S, Malhotra V (1989) Tuberculous abscess of the brain stem. Surg Neurol 32:445–448
38. Farrar DJ, Flanigan TP, Gordon NM, Gold RL, Rich JD (1997) Tuberculous brain abscess in a patient with HIV infection: case report and review. Am J Med 102:297–301
39. Rajshekhar V (2009) Management of hydrocephalus in patients with tuberculous meningitis. Neurol India 57:368–374
40. Chan KH, Cheung RT, Fong CY, Tsang KL, Mak W, Ho SL (2003) Clinical relevance of hydrocephalus as a presenting feature of tuberculous meningitis. QJM 96:643–648
41. Del Brutto OH (1998) Infections and stroke. In: Ginsberg MD, Bogousslavsky J (eds) Cerebrovascular disease. Pathophysiology, diagnosis, and management. Blackwell Science, Malden, pp 1628–1646
42. Misra UK, Kalita J, Maurya PK (2011) Stroke in tuberculous meningitis. J Neurol Sci 303:22–30
43. Uesugi T, Takizawa S, Morita Y, Takahashi H, Takagi S (2006) Hemorrhagic infarction in tuberculous meningitis. Intern Med 45:1193–1194

44. Verma R, Lalla R, Patil TB, Tiwari N (2013) A rare presentation of cerebral venous sinus thrombosis associated with tubercular meningitis. BMJ Case Rep 2013
45. Singh P, Paliwal VK, Neyaz Z, Srivastava AK, Verma R, Mohan S (2014) Clinical and magnetic resonance imaging characteristics of tubercular ventriculitis: an under-recognized complication of tubercular meningitis. J Neurol Sci 342:137–140
46. Sharma P, Garg RK, Verma R, Singh MK, Shukla R (2011) Incidence, predictors and prognostic value of cranial nerve involvement in patients with tuberculous meningitis: a retrospective evaluation. Eur J Intern Med 22:289–295
47. Dastur DK, Udani PM (1966) The pathology and pathogenesis of tuberculous encephalopathy. Acta Neuropathol 6:311–326
48. Lammie GA, Hewlett RH, Schoeman JF, Donald PR (2007) Tuberculous encephalopathy: a reappraisal. Acta Neuropathol 113:227–234
49. Benson SM, Narasimhamurthy R (2013) Severe hyponatremia and MRI point to diagnosis of tuberculous meningitis in the Southwest USA. BMJ Case Rep 2013
50. Celik U, Celik T, Tolunay O, Baspınar H, Komur M, Levent F (2015) Cerebral salt wasting in tuberculous meningitis: two cases and review of the literature: case report. Neuro Endocrinol Lett 36:306–310
51. Anupriya A, Sunithi M, Maya T, Goel M, Alexander M, Aaron S, Mathew V (2010) Tuberculous optochiasmatic arachnoiditis. Neurol India 58:732–735
52. Garg RK, Paliwal V, Malhotra HS (2011) Tuberculous optochiasmatic arachnoiditis: a devastating form of tuberculous meningitis. Expert Rev Anti Infect Ther 9:719–729
53. Whiteman M, Espinoza L, Post MJ, Bell MD, Falcone S (1995) Central nervous system tuberculosis in HIV-infected patients: clinical and radiographic findings. AJNR Am J Neuroradiol 16:1319–1327
54. Thwaites GE, Duc Bang N, Huy Dung N, Thi Quy H, Thi Tuong Oanh D, Thi Cam Thoa N, Quang Hien N, Tri Thuc N, Ngoc Hai N, Thi Ngoc Lan N, Ngoc Lan N, Hong Duc N, Ngoc Tuan V, Huu Hiep C, Thi Hong Chau T, Phuong Mai P, Thi Dung N, Stepniewska K, Simmons CP, White NJ, Tinh Hien T, Farrar JJ (2005) The influence of HIV infection on clinical presentation, response to treatment, and outcome in adults with tuberculous meningitis. J Infect Dis 192:2134–2141
55. Chamie G, Marquez C, Luetkemeyer A (2014) HIV-associated central nervous system tuberculosis. Semin Neurol 34:103–115
56. Katrak SM, Shembalkar PK, Bijwe SR, Bhandarkar LD (2000) The clinical, radiological and pathological profile of tuberculous meningitis in patients with and without human immunodeficiency virus infection. J Neurol Sci 181:118–126
57. Torok ME, Chau TT, Mai PP, Phong ND, Dung NT, Chuong LV, Lee SJ, Caws M, de Jong MD, Hien TT, Farrar JJ (2008) Clinical and microbiological features of HIV-associated tuberculous meningitis in Vietnamese adults. PLoS One 3:e1772
58. Flor A, Capdevila JA, Martin N, Gavalda J, Pahissa A (1996) Nontuberculous mycobacterial meningitis: report of two cases and review. Clin Infect Dis 23:1266–1273
59. Marie I, Heron F, Lecomte F, Jarlier V, Truffot-Pernot C, Laquerriere A, Huerre M, Levesque H, Courtois H (2003) Multiple cerebral abscesses as a complication of Mycobacterium fortuitum infection. Eur J Intern Med 14:386–389
60. Begley C, Amaraneni A, Lutwick L (2014) Mycobacterium avium-intracellulare brain abscesses in an HIV-infected patient. IDCases 2:19–21
61. French AL, Benator DA, Gordin FM (1997) Non tuberculous mycobacterial infections. Med Clin North Am 81:361–379
62. Talati NJ, Rouphael N, Kuppalli K, Franco-Paredes C (2008) Spectrum of CNS disease caused by rapidly growing mycobacteria. Lancet Infect Dis 8:390–398
63. Garcia-Monco JC (2014). Tuberculosis. Handb Clin Neurol 121:148–1499
64. Suvarna KS, Layton C, Bancroft JD (eds) (2013) Bancroft's theory and practice of histological techniques, 7th edn. Churchill Livingstone, China
65. Martins SJ, Azevedo CR, Chinen LT, Cruz MR, Peterlevitz MA, Gimenes DL (2011) Meningeal carcinomatosis in solid tumors. Arq Neuropsiquiatr 69:973–980
66. Baldwin KJ, Zunt JR (2014) Evaluation and treatment of chronic meningitis. Neurohospitalist 4:185–195
67. Kumar V, Abbas AK, Aster JC, Robbins SL (2013) Robbins & cotran pathologic basis of disease, 9th edn. Elsevier Saunders, Philadelphia
68. Thwaites GE, Tran TH (2005) Tuberculous meningitis: many questions, too few answers. Lancet Neurol 4:160–170
69. Leonard JM (2014) Tuberculosis of central nervous system. In: Aminoff MA, Josephson SA (eds) Aminoff's neurology and general medicine. Elsevier, London
70. Lopez-Cortes LF, Cruz-Ruiz M, Gomez-Mateos J, Jimenez-Hernandez D, Jimenez-Mejias E, Pachon J, Castillo J (1995) Adenosine deaminase activity in the CSF of patients with aseptic meningitis: utility in the diagnosis of tuberculous meningitis or neurobrucellosis. Clin Infect Dis 20:525–530
71. Choi SH, Kim YS, Bae IG, Chung JW, Lee MS, Kang JM, Ryu J, Woo JH (2002) The possible role of cerebrospinal fluid adenosine deaminase activity in diagnosis of tuberculous meningitis in adults. Clin Neurol Neurosurg 104:10–15
72. Jain A, Bhargava A, Agarwal SK (2002) A comparative study of two commonly used staining techniques for acid fast bacilli in clinical specimens. Indian J Tub 49:161–162
73. Kent SJ, Crowe SM, Yung A, Lucas CR, Mijch AM (1993) Tuberculous meningitis: a 30 year review. Clin Infect Dis 17:987–994

74. Watterson SA, Drobniewski FA (2000) Modern laboratory diagnosis of mycobacterial infections. J Clin Pathol 53:727–732
75. Katti MK (2001) Are enzyme-linked immunosorbent assay and immunoblot assay independent in immunodiagnosis of infectious diseases? Clin Infect Dis 32:1114
76. Katti MK (2004) Pathogenesis, diagnosis, treatment, and outcome aspects of cerebral tuberculosis. Med Sci Monit 10:RA 215–RA 229
77. Pai M, Flores LL, Pai N, Hubbard A, Riley LW, Colford JM Jr (2003) Diagnostic accuracy of nucleic acid amplification tests for tuberculous meningitis: a systematic review and meta-analysis. Lancet Infect Dis 3:633–643

Part II

Tuberculosis of the Brain and Its Coverings

5 Scalp and the Calvarium

Prasad Krishnan

Contents

P. Krishnan, MD
Department of Neurosurgery, National Neurosciences Centre, Peerless Hospital Complex, IInd Floor, 360, Panchasayar, Garia, Kolkata 700094, India
e-mail: prasad.krishnan@rediffmail.com

Abbreviations

AFB	Acid-fast bacilli
CNS	Central nervous system
CRP	C-reactive protein
CT	Computed tomography
DNA	Deoxyribonucleic acid
ESR	Erythrocyte sedimentation rate
FNAC	Fine needle aspiration cytology
HIV	Human immunodeficiency virus
IICP	Increased intracranial pressure
MRI	Magnetic resonance imaging
PCR	Polymerase chain reaction
RIF	Rifampicin
TB	Tuberculosis
TBM	Tubercular meningitis

5.1 Introduction

Tuberculosis (TB) is a disease of antiquity [1]. Mention of this disease has been found as far back as the Rig Veda, and evidence of the disease has been found in Egyptian mummies dating to 3000 BC [2]. Though it can affect any organ system of the body, central nervous system (CNS) TB is a particularly dangerous form with high mortality and morbidity [2]. Though the commonly encountered variants of CNS TB are tubercular meningitis (TBM), intracranial tuberculomas or abscesses, and spinal TB, occasionally patients may present with TB affliction of the scalp and skull bones as well.

M. Turgut et al. (eds.), *Tuberculosis of the Central Nervous System*,
DOI 10.1007/978-3-319-50712-5_5

5.2 Scalp Tuberculosis

Cutaneous affliction by TB can be of three types – lupus vulgaris, TB verrucosa cutis, and scrofuloderma. However, the scalp is an uncommon site of occurrence of all three. Lupus is the Latin word for wolf and is a generic name for diseases causing erosive, erythematous ulceration of the face ravaging it like the bites of a wolf [3]. The suffix vulgaris was used to denote its common occurrence. It was first described by Erasmus Wilson in 1865 [4]. Manifesting as reddish brown papules that later coalesce into elevated plaques, it is caused by hematogenous dissemination of TB bacilli from a primary site of infection [3]. It usually occurs in the face. It has an indolent course and rarely may progress to squamous cell carcinoma. "Apple-jelly" appearance of the papules is found on diascopy [3]. It is diagnosed by the clinical features and skin biopsy. It responds well to anti-TB drugs.

TB verrucosa cutis (also called warty TB or prosector's wart) is a paucibacillary TB infection of the superficial layers of the skin in an individual who has a high degree of immunity [3–5]. It was first described by Laennec in 1826, based on his own disease that he contracted in the autopsy room [4]. As it was thought to be contracted from corpses, it was termed verruca necrogenica by Wilks and Poland in 1862 [4]. It commonly occurs at the distal extremities, dorsal aspects of joints, and buttocks after trivial penetrating injury [3, 6]. These warts tend to enlarge centrifugally with central healing. Ulceration is not a prominent feature. Diagnosis is made by positive tuberculin skin test and histology. They regress with anti-TB drugs.

The last variant, scrofuloderma, is the commonest type of cutaneous TB. It usually occurs following secondary involvement of the skin following liquefactive necrosis of the afflicted lymph nodes lying underneath [3]. The neck is the commonest site of involvement. Painless fistula formation with pus discharge is the main clinical feature – a finding in most cases of calvarial TB too. Diagnosis is made on clinical grounds as well as by detection of the organism on staining, culture, or polymerase chain reaction (PCR) testing. Under treatment the fistula heals with scarring [3].

5.3 Calvarial Tuberculosis

5.3.1 Introduction

Calvarial TB is a rare disease [7–9], infrequently encountered, and not always considered as a first differential diagnosis. It was first reported by Reid in 1842 from Germany [9, 10]. Though recent years have seen a spurt of publications on calvarial TB, these tend to be in the nature of single case reports rather than large series.

5.3.2 Epidemiology

The majority of cases of calvarial TB are reported from developing countries where systemic TB is endemic [7–22]. While 1% of cases of TB occur in the bone [23], calvarial involvement accounts for only 0.2–1.3% of these [7, 23], i.e., approximately 1 in 10,000 cases of TB. Literature states that the frontal and parietal bones having greater amount of diploic space (and hence receiving more blood flow) are more commonly affected than bones like occipital or temporal which are less vascularized [7, 8, 23]. Conversely, it has also been stated that muscular attachments to the temporal and occipital bones render them vascular with higher flow rates where a TB nidus cannot gain a foothold unlike the frontal and parietal bones which have a slow flowing diploic emissary circulation that allows deposition of mycobacteria and growth of the TB focus [12].

The disease is rare in infants [23], as the skull is poor in cancellous bone [10]. Despite this, it has been described in children [24] – the youngest described being only 10 months old [19]. This condition is predominantly encountered in younger individuals, and 75–90% cases have been reported to occur in patients less than

20 years and 50% in children less than 10 years old [23]. It affects both sexes equally though certain series show a predilection toward females or males [13–15].

5.3.3 Pathogenesis

The disease follows hematogenous seeding of TB bacilli in the marrow spaces [7, 8, 13]. It can occur rarely by lymphatic or contiguous local spread from the face, paranasal sinuses, orbit, or cervical lymph nodes [10, 13]. Infrequency of calvarial TB is due to paucity of cancellous component in the flat bones of the skull and also due to lack of lymphatics in them [7, 12]. Mukherjee et al. have used the term primary calvarial TB when there is no evidence of TB detected anywhere else in the body [12].

In the setting of depressed host immunity, deposition of the bacilli in the diploic spaces of the skull is followed by proliferation of bacteria, capillary obliteration, replacement of the bone by granulation tissue and finally abscess formation with destruction of the cortex. Destruction of the outer table occurs and subgaleal collection of pus and granulation tissue results in a boggy swelling without increased temperature, tenderness, induration, or systemic symptoms like fever. On occasion this may erode through the scalp and present as a non-healing sinus. The inner table is relatively resistant but when eroded results in the development of an epidural collection [9]. The dura is usually a resistant barrier to further intracranial spread [8, 22]. However, sutures do not prevent spread of the disease [8, 23]. It is unclear if any of the tables is more likely to get eroded than the other. While Strauss held that the inner table was more likely to be initially involved [25], others [9, 13] believe that the outer table is more likely to be destroyed first, and still others [26] found both tables to be equally affected. In the series of Raut et al. [18], 85% of patients had bony destruction, and epidural collections were seen in 52%.

5.3.4 Role of Trauma and Immune Suppression

Several case reports of calvarial TB report a past history of trauma [17] to the involved bone. It has been speculated that these areas have focal immunosuppression with increased vascularity that predisposes to the genesis of TB here at a later date [12, 13]. Inflammatory cells that are attracted to the site of trauma are also held to act as vectors aiding transmission [15]. Several authorities, however, hold that trauma is probably coincidental rather than causal [26, 27]. Immune-suppressed states like human immunodeficiency virus (HIV) infection are also implicated in its causation [13, 20] as extrapulmonary TB has a higher incidence in such patients (70% in HIV-infected versus 15% in noninfected patients).

5.3.5 Presentation

The common presenting complaints are painless, boggy swelling of the scalp and which may occasionally spontaneously erode the skin (Fig. 5.1) and form a discharging sinus [13, 17, 19, 28]. The underlying bone may or may not be visible. Inflammatory signs are markedly absent even in the presence of pus. Skin discoloration (Fig. 5.2) is a late feature [13]. Unlike Pott's puffy tumor, it may have a firmly attached base, and deficient outer table of the skull may be palpable. Rarely, headache may be present and is usually localized to the site of infection [13]. Concomitant intracranial pathologies (like epidural or cerebral abscess, tuberculoma, or meningitis) may occur due to which occasional patients have been reported with drowsiness, seizures, hemiparesis, and even increased intracranial pressure (IICP) [13, 15, 21, 29]. There is a case report of occlusion of sigmoid sinus following TBC mastoiditis with IICP and formation of an encephalocele [30] as well as one of occlusion of the superior sagittal sinus [17]. Systemic manifestations like weight loss, evening rise of temperature, decreasing appetite, etc. are rare.

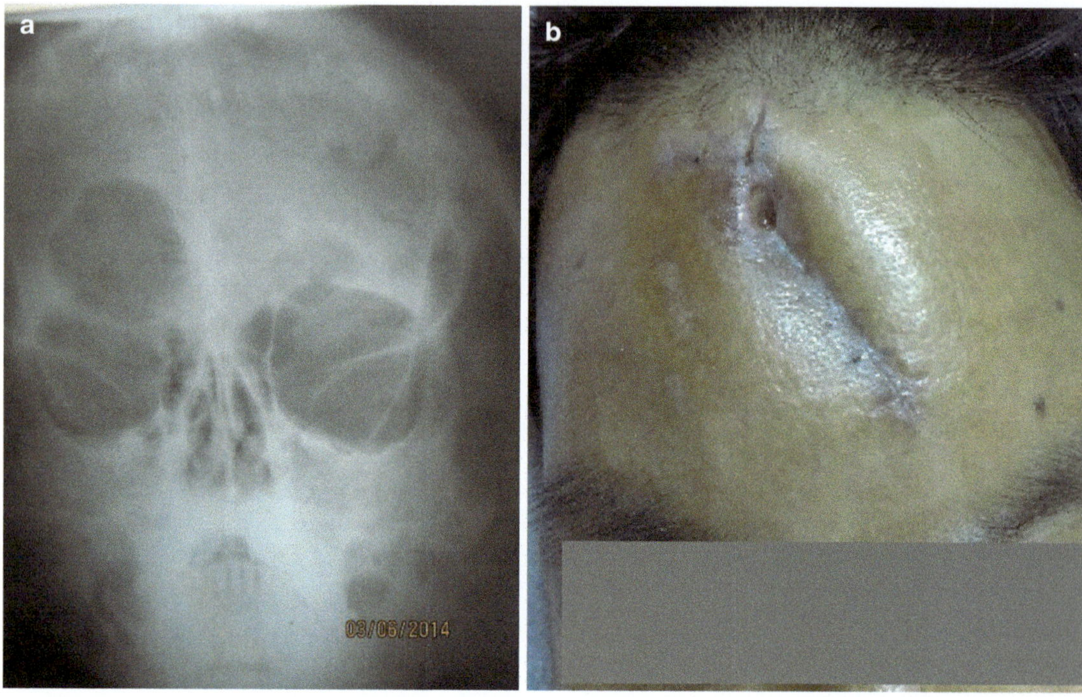

Fig. 5.1 (**a**) Plain radiograph showing erosion of the right frontal bone in a 34-year-old male that had been twice unsuccessfully operated and treated with broad-spectrum antibiotics assuming swelling was due to an infected sebaceous cyst and (**b**) a discharging sinus showing skin changes overlying sequestered bone

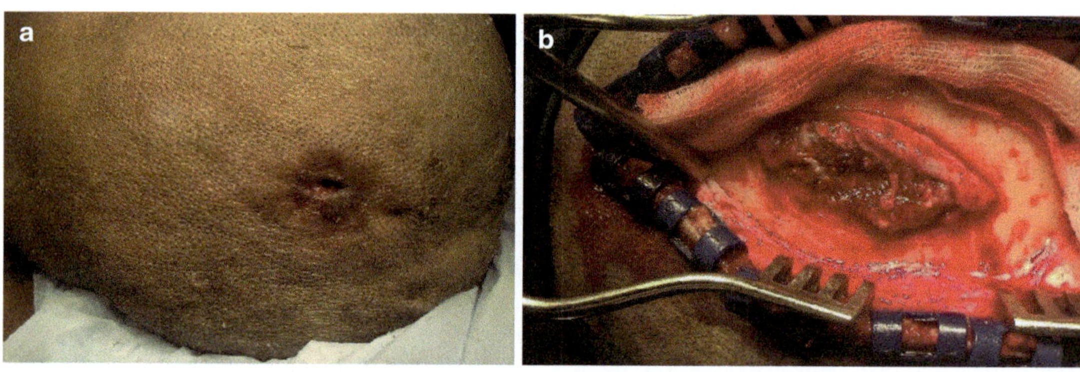

Fig. 5.2 (**a**) Preoperative clinical photograph showing a spontaneously ruptured draining sinus in a 26-year-old lady with skin changes and (**b**) intraoperative photograph showing granulation tissue pouting out of the eroded parietal bone in a 26-year-old lady

5.3.6 Investigations

Raised erythrocyte sedimentation rate (ESR) and C-reactive protein (CRP) values and also positive Mantoux test may give a clue for diagnosis of skull TB. Mantoux test may not be positive in 10% of calvarial TB patients [23] and is of doubtful value when positive in countries having a vaccination program with attenuated TB bacilli. Likewise, ESR and CRP levels are not always raised and also are not specific for TB. Routine culture of the discharge is not regularly reported in literature and is probably not useful to clinch the diagnosis. Some series have reported sterile or polymicrobial cultures [12], and on occasion, it may even mislead the clinician into assuming the case to be one of pyogenic osteomyelitis [12].

Plain radiographs of skull are helpful in finding the bony changes which commonly manifest as punched-out lesions [23]. Computed tomography (CT) scans are useful in identifying the extent of damage to the skull bone, involvement and breach of dura, size of the swelling and associated intracranial pathologies [18]. Skull defects are usually single, but on occasion multiple punched-out lesions have been described [16, 29].

Radiologically, three variants are described – circumscribed sclerotic, lytic, and spreading [18]. The lytic variant (Fig. 5.3), also called "perforating TB of the skull" by Volkmann [13, 18], is the most common. In these areas of rarefaction are seen initially that later developing into punched-out defects. There is no periosteal reaction. Rarely these may have a central sequestrum ("button sequestrum" or "bone sand") within [12]. The second variant is a defect having a margin of sclerotic bone. Its presence may indicate secondary infection [12] or may represent evidence of healing and is caused by new bone formation on the edges. The third variant is the "spreading type" where there is widespread destruction of the diploic spaces with abundant granulation tissue. This was called "diffuse TB of the cranium" by Konig [18]. This classification has been disputed by some authors who feel that the types are not separable [12]. It must be remembered that the radiological picture is nonspecific [18], and usual differential diagnoses include skull metastasis, myeloma, hemangioma, aneurysmal bone cyst, pyogenic osteomyelitis, and Langerhans cell histiocytosis [12, 13].

Finally, magnetic resonance imaging (MRI) is a sensitive tool in bringing out any associated intracranial pathology (changes in meninges, ventricular walls, or parenchymal foci of infec-

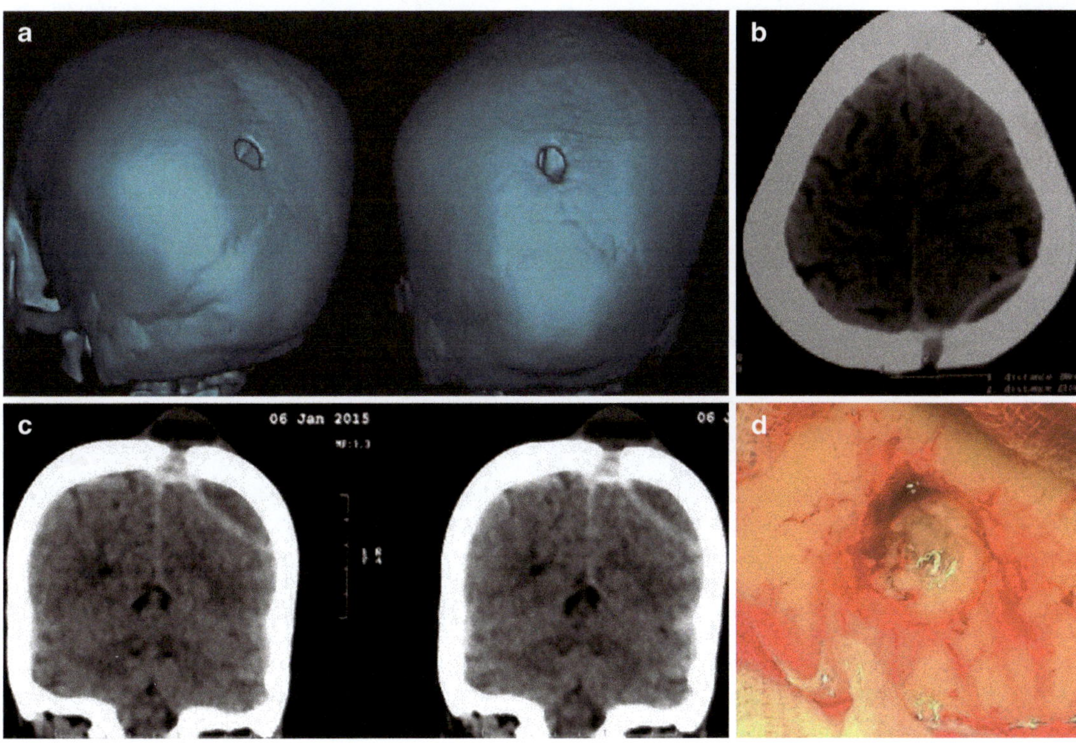

Fig. 5.3 (**a**) 3D reconstructed CT scan showing a punched-out lesion involving both tables of the skull in a 40-year-old lady (lytic tuberculosis) almost near the midline, (**b**, **c**) coronal and axial CT images with contrast showing skull defect, and an epidural collection and (**d**) intraoperative picture showing a punched-out lesion with serous fluid mixed with pus coming out of it. The surrounding bone margins are hyperemic

tion) [18], epidural abscess, or venous sinus involvement (Fig. 5.4). The extent of bone involvement beyond the margins of the punched-out lesion can also be appreciated as bone edema on MRI sequences and may help to determine the extent of craniotomy.

The gold standard for diagnosis is the demonstration of acid-fast bacilli (AFB) on microscopy and growth on culture, but this may not be always possible [7, 8]. The presence of characteristic granuloma (epitheloid cells, plasma cells, and Langhans-type giant cells with central caseous

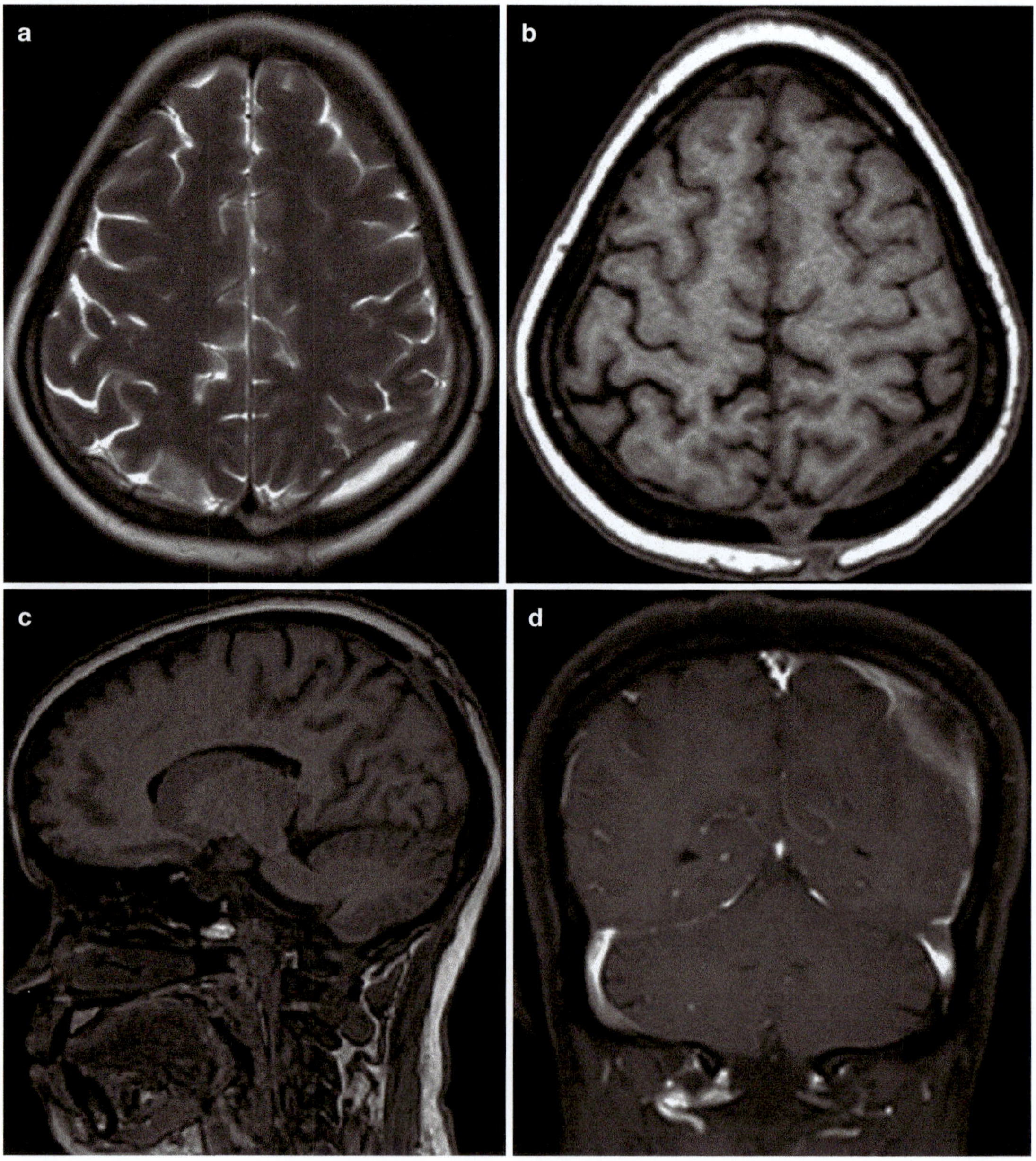

Fig. 5.4 (**a**) T2 axial imaging showing an hyperintense collection below the bone pushing dura inward, (**b**, **c**) T1 axial and sagittal imaging showing isointense collection showing perforation of the skull but there is as yet no scalp collection and (**d**) coronal contrast imaging showing that there is enhancing soft tissue representing granulation tissue. There is as yet no intradural involvement

necrosis) on histology with response to empirical anti-TB drugs is then considered to be proof that the infection is TB [8, 11]. Usually, this tissue is obtained by craniotomy of the involved bone or by curettage and debridement. Some authors have advocated fine needle aspiration cytology (FNAC) to obtain tissue as a means of avoiding surgery [7, 12]. They have, however, cautioned that FNAC may not yield the correct diagnosis in the presence of secondary infection [12]. In situations with low bacillary load where detection on conventional staining and culture are difficult, automated nested PCR test using a platform for rapid nucleic acid amplification is a valid investigation to detect both mycobacterial DNA and rifampicin (RIF) resistance and can clinch the diagnosis [11].

5.3.7 Treatment

The mainstay of treatment is anti-TB drugs [22]. This consists of an intensive phase of therapy with four drugs – RIF, isoniazid, ethambutol, and pyrazinamide – and a continuation phase with two drugs. While the World Health Organization recommendation is to give the former for 2 months and the latter for 4 months in most cases of extrapulmonary TB, they have suggested continuing the latter for longer periods in special situations like CNS TB. Our institute protocol is to give the same for 18 months in calvarial TB – a practice followed by other centers as well [9, 14, 15, 28]. Some authorities have advocated giving anti-TB drugs for up to 24 months as well [18]. Steroids are not indicated unless there is evidence of concomitant meningitis as well. Likewise, anticonvulsants are also not required unless there is a history of seizures [18].

Surgery is indicated when diagnosis is uncertain [23], there is presence of epidural abscess, there are lesions with mass effect and to remove sequestrated bone [10, 28]. Craniotomy may be done to ensure removal of the diseased bone beyond the boundaries of the defect, but it is unclear what margins would be considered acceptable. We would think that freshening margins with a nibbler till there is bleeding from the raw edges to be acceptable. The fibrosed walls and mouth of any sinus can be dealt with at the same sitting [13]. Tension of the suture line is to be avoided to prevent necrosis of skin margins. The question of cranioplasty to repair the craniectomy defect has not been discussed in published literature [12] – particularly with respect to timing. Some authors advocate waiting for microbiological cure before cranioplasty [28]. As it is often unclear if the lesion is TB or pyogenic at the time of surgery, we too would advocate interval cranioplasty rather than primary repair.

Conclusion

The calvarium and scalp are uncommon locations of TB. These patients present with an indolent history and protean features. The clinician must bear this possibility in the back of his mind so that time is not wasted on futile therapies and further CNS involvement is arrested. Calvarial TB is a kind of CNS TB, and extended duration of anti-TB drugs is mandated.

References

1. Daniel TM (2006) The history of tuberculosis. Respir Med 100:1862–1870
2. Tandon PN, Pande A (2012) Tuberculosis of the central nervous system. In: Tandon PN, Ramamurthy R (eds) Textbook of neurosurgery, 1st edn. Jaypee Brothers Medical Publishers (P) Ltd., New Delhi, pp 725–741
3. Shimizu H (2007) Mycobacterial infections. In: Shimizu H (ed) Shimizu's textbook of dermatology. Nakayama Shoten Publishers, Hokkaido, pp 484–488
4. Padmavathy L, Lakshmana Rao L, Pari T, Ethirajan N, Krishnaswamy B (2008) Lupus vulgaris and tuberculosis verrucosa cutis (TBVC) – a clinical, pathological and epidemiological study of 71 cases. Indian J Tuberc 55:203–209
5. Aliağaoğlu C, Atasoy M, Güleç AI, Özdemir S, Erdem T, Engin RI (2009) Tuberculosis verrucosa cutis. Eur J Gen Med 6:268–273
6. Rajan J, Mathai AT, Prasad PVS, Kaviarasan PK (2011) Multifocal tuberculosis verrucosa cutis. Indian J Dermatol 56:332–334
7. Khare P, Gupta R, Chand P, Agarwal S (2015) Calvarial tuberculosis presenting as cystic lesion: an unusual presentation in two patients. J Cytol 32:176–180

8. Rajmohan BP, Anto D, Alappat JP (2004) Calvarial tuberculosis. Neurol India 52:278–279
9. Nair AP, Mehrotra A, Das KK, Kumar B, Srivastav AK, Sahu RN, Kumar R (2015) Calvarial tuberculosis of the parietal bone: a rare complication after dental extraction. Asian J Neurosurg 10:219–221
10. Zaki S, Dadge D, Shanbag P (2010) Calvarial tuberculosis. Int J Infect Dis 14:e86–e87
11. Krishnan P, Sanyal S, Gupta D (2015) Primary lytic calvarial tuberculosis: a report of two cases. Acta Neurochir 157:2223–2225
12. Mukherjee KK, Kaushik R, Nada R, Khosla VK, Khandelwal N, Kak VK (2002) Calvarial tuberculosis. Surg Neurol 57:195–202
13. Diyora B, Kumar R, Modgi R, Sharma A (2009) Calvarial tuberculosis: a report of eleven patients. Neurol India 57:607–612
14. Ramdurg SR, Gupta DK, Suri A, Sharma BS, Mahapatra AK (2010) Calvarial tuberculosis: uncommon manifestation of common disease – a series of 21 cases. Br J Neurosurg 24:572–577
15. Jadhav RN, Palande DA (1999) Calvarial tuberculosis. Neurosurgery 45:1345–1349
16. Samson SK, Kulkarni V, Chacko AG (2002) An unusual presentation of calvarial tuberculosis. Postgrad Med J 78:184
17. Sundaram PK, Sayed F (2007) Superior sagittal sinus thrombosis caused by calvarial tuberculosis: case report. Neurosurgery 60:E776
18. Raut AA, Nagar AM, Muzumdar D, Chawla AJ, Narlawar RS, Fattepurkar S, Bhatgadde VL (2004) Imaging features of calvarial tuberculosis: a study of 42 cases. AJNR Am J Neuroradiol 25:409–414
19. Dawar P, Gupta DK, Sharma BS, Jyakumar A, Gamanagatti S (2013) Extensive calvarial tuberculosis presenting as exophytic ulcerated growth on scalp in an infant: an interesting case report with review of literature. Childs Nerv Syst 29:1215–1218
20. Rajesh A, Purohit AK, Lakshmi V (2009) Calvarial tubercular osteomyelitic abscess. Indian J Med Microbiol 27:380–381
21. Patankar T, Varma R, Krishnan A, Prasad S, Desai K, Castillo M (2000) Radiographic findings in tuberculosis of the calvarium. Neuroradiology 42:518–521
22. Dawar P, Satyarthee GD, Sharma BS (2015) Total resolution of large scalp swelling due to calvarial tuberculosis with medical management only: case report and review of the literature. Turk Neurosurg 25:313–316
23. Rosli FJ, Haron R (2016) Tuberculosis of the skull mimicking a bony tumor. Asian J Neurosurg 11:68
24. Stones DK, Schoeman CJ (2004) Calvarial tuberculosis. J Trop Pediatr 50:361–364
25. Strauss DC (1933) Tuberculosis of the flat bones of the vault of skull. Surg Gynaecol Obstet 57:384–398
26. Meng CM, Wu YK (1942) Tuberculosis of the flat bones of the vault of the skull. J Bone Joint Surg 34:341–353
27. Barton CJ (1961) Tuberculosis of the vault of skull. Br J Radiol 34:286–290
28. de Lima Fde M, Pessoa LA, da Silva JC, Jungman P, Maranhão S (2003) Calvarial tuberculosis: case report. Arq Neuropsiquiatr 61:144–145
29. García-García C, Ibarra V, Azcona-Gutiérrez JM, Oteo JA (2013) Calvarial tuberculosis with parenchymal involvement. Travel Med Infect Dis 11:329–331
30. Vitali AM (2008) Acquired encephalocele attributable to tuberculous osteitis: case report. Neurosurgery 62:E976

Dura Mater and Epidural Space

6

Erdal Kalkan, Fatih Erdi, Yaşar Karataş,
and Bülent Kaya

Contents

E. Kalkan, MD (✉) • F. Erdi, MD
Y. Karataş, MD • B. Kaya, MD
Department of Neurosurgery, Necmettin Erbakan University, Meram Faculty of Medicine, 42080 Akyokus, Konya, Turkey
e-mail: erdalkalkan62@yahoo.com; mfatiherdi@hotmail.com; yasarkrts@gmail.com; drbulentkaya1977@gmail.com

Abbreviations

CNS	Central nervous system
CSF	Cerebrospinal fluid
CT	Computed tomography
MRI	Magnetic resonance imaging
TB	Tuberculosis
TBM	Tuberculous meningitis

6.1 Introduction

Tuberculosis (TB) remains as a major public health issue along the world, in particular, in the underdeveloped and some developing countries. It causes over 1.7 million deaths mondial in 2007 with a 5–24% reported global case fatality [1]. Risk factors including human immunodeficiency virus coinfection, anti-TB drug resistance, advanced age with different comorbidities [1] and factors leading to immunodeficiency such as solid organ transplantation [2] increase the incidence and mortality/morbidity of TB along the world.

Extrapulmonary TB constitutes approximately 25% of all TB lesions [3]. TB of the central nervous system (CNS) occurs in 5–10% of extrapulmonary TB cases and accounts for almost 1% of all patients with TB [4]. Although it is rare, TB of CNS is the most hazardous form of the disease with associated mortality and morbidity such as serious neurological sequelae [5].

M. Turgut et al. (eds.), *Tuberculosis of the Central Nervous System*,
DOI 10.1007/978-3-319-50712-5_6

Dura mater and epidural space TB contains epidural tuberculoma, empyema and hypertrophic pachymeningeal TB [6, 7]. Isolated dural-epidural TB is exceptionally rare [8]. Our knowledge on this subject generally depends on the previous single or small group case reports [9]. Hypertrophic pachymeningitis is an unusual chronic fibrosing inflammatory disorder characterised by thickening of dura mater, leptomeninges and tentorium with various aetiologies including TB [10]. Pachymeningeal TB has diffuse or focal forms, and focal en plaque thickening of the dura is the most encountered form [11].

6.2 Pathogenesis

Dura mater has a good blood supply [9] and also could act as a barrier for invasion with its tenacious connective tissue composition [12]. Some different mechanisms including contiguous and haematogenous spreading have been proposed to explain the partially unclear pathogenesis of isolated dural-epidural TB. Local severe inflammation at the skull and related structures such as temporalis muscle [12], paranasal sinuses and orbits [3] could lead to contiguous spreading and secondary dural invasion. Haematogenous dissemination of the TB to the leptomeninges and brain tissue was suspected for the development of pachymeningeal form. Haematogenous bacilli seeding could lead to tubercle formation which can enlarge and coalesce. These tubercles can stay limited to the meninges and form fibrous aggregates that are adherent to the dura, or they rupture into the subarachnoid space and form subependymal or subpial granuloma, which is usually referred as the 'Rich focus'. The surrounding cerebral tissue around the tuberculoma creates a dense fibrous capsule which may expand substantially prior to become symptomatic [13].

6.3 Diagnosis

A high index of doubt is critical for early diagnosis and avoidance from associated significant morbidity and mortality. Previous medical history of the patient or the patient's close relatives should take into consideration. Extra-neural TB coexistence is reported within 50% of neuro-TB patients which may facilitate the diagnosis as a clue [14, 15]. Frequently, the absence of fever or other systemic symptoms and lack of a distinctive imaging appearance make the preoperative diagnosis difficult.

With the presence of tuberculous meningitis (TBM), cerebrospinal fluid (CSF) examination becomes important, and the typical CSF shows elevated protein, low glucose and elevated white blood cell with lymphocytic pleocytosis. High CSF adenosine deaminase levels and determination of acid-fast bacilli in CSF smears may be initial indicators; nevertheless, a certain diagnosis could only be designated after positive *Mycobacterium tuberculosis* culture. Nowadays, CSF polymerase chain reaction testing promises high sensitiveness for TB, but false-positive results remain as a major concern in cases of TBM [5]. In most cases, the need for stereotaxic, open or needle biopsy persists after suspicious findings.

6.4 Imaging

Magnetic resonance imaging (MRI) with gadolinium is the most favourite imaging modality and considered to be superior to computed tomography (CT) in the detection and evaluation of all forms of CNS TB [14]. Concomitant craniospinal multifocal [16] involvement can be seen; thus, neuroimaging should include all neuroaxis [14, 15, 17].

In general, epidural tuberculoma and empyema have a hypointense core on T1-weighted MRI with a peripherical hyperintensity (Fig. 6.1). On T2-weighted MRI, both the core and peripherical zone show hyperintensity, but the core has a more pronounced hyperintense signal (Fig. 6.2) [6]. In the case of epidural empyema, the displaced and edged dura mater seems as a hypointense rim on T2-weighted MRI that gives a clue about the epidural location of the lesion (Fig. 6.2) [19]. Concomitant osteomyelitis is a common feature of isolated epidural form which often involves the sphenoid bone (Fig. 6.3) [21].

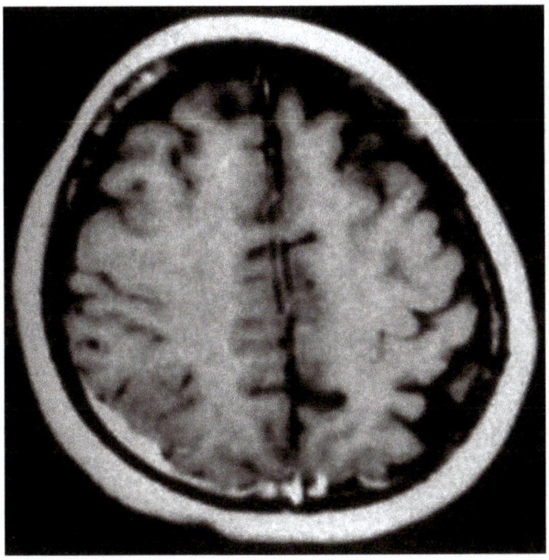

Fig. 6.1 Tl-weighted gadolinium-enhanced MRI showing an enhanced en plaque dural tuberculoma at the parietal region with adjacent hypointense brain (From Tseng et al. [9] with permission)

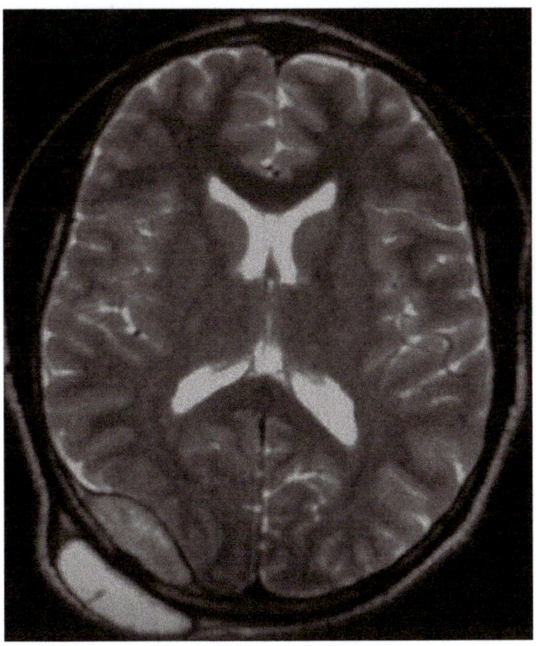

Fig. 6.2 T2-weighted axial MRI section demonstrates an epidural TB abscess in the right occipital region with skull and subcutaneous involvement (From O'Brien et al. [18] with permission)

Specific imaging features of leptomeningeal TB involvement are lacking, and a number of disorders including leptomeningeal carcinomatosis, intracranial fibromatosis, lymphoma, meningioma, sarcoidosis and syphilis even with idiopathic factors need to be considered in the differential diagnosis list (Fig. 6.4) [14].

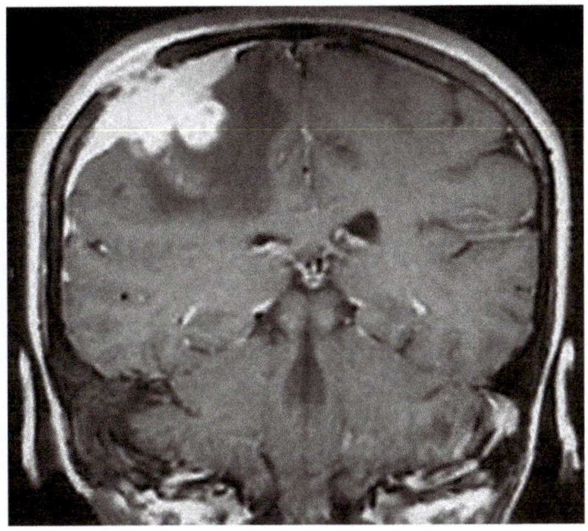

Fig. 6.3 T1-weighted gadolinium-enhanced coronal MRI image showing right parietal epidural tuberculoma with diffuse enhancement. Also note the associated lytic skull lesion (From Sencer et al. [20] with permission)

Focal lesions of pachymeningeal TB can be seen as en plaque, homogenous, uniformly enhanced, dural-based masses which mimic meningiomas [8, 23]. Hyperdense, thickened and enhanced dura mater can be seen in diffuse lesions on axial CT scans. Affected dura mater looks isointense on T1-weighted MRI and iso-hypointense on T2-weighted MRI with diffuse contrast enhancement (Fig. 6.4) [14].

6.5 Management

Medical anti-TB treatment is the mainstay of the management. The lesions which cause significant compression on neural tissue or the lesions which have calvarial or subgaleal involvement may require surgical drainage and debridement either with craniotomy or craniectomy. The relapsing rate is high after treatment, and the radiological evanescence of the lesions takes a long time; thus, imminent follow-up with proper neuroimaging is crucial, particularly in immunocompromised cases [24].

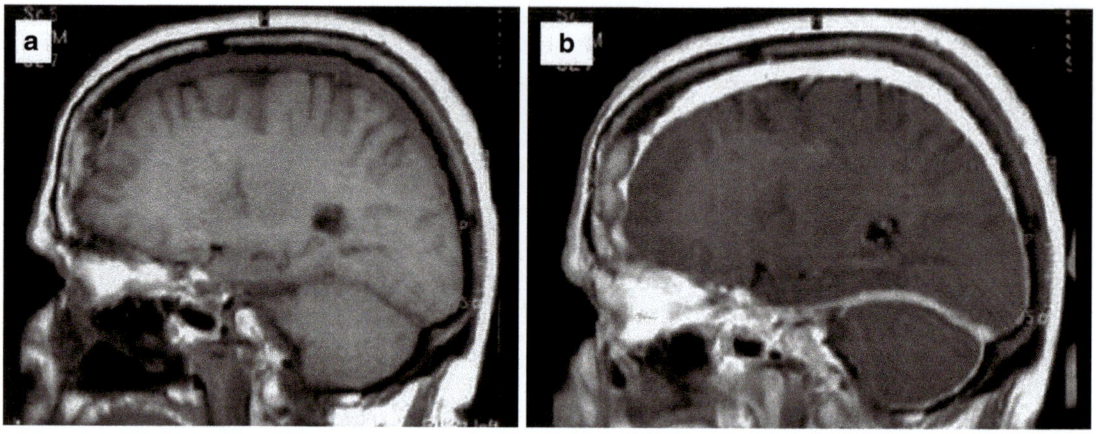

Fig. 6.4 T1-weighted pre-gadolinium (**a**) and post-gadolinium (**b**) sagittal MRI sections showing diffuse pachymeningitis (From D'Andrea et al. [22] with permission)

6.6 Follow-Up

Patients with dural-epidural TB should follow up closely due to high relapsing rate of the disease. When the signs of elevated intracranial pressure occur or new neurological appears, these patients should undergo new neuroimaging tests. The degree of contrast enhancement on CT or MRI may reflect the activity of a tuberculoma during follow-up [14]. Infrequently discharged tuberculoprotein from the destructed bacilli creates an inflammatory reaction and swelling at the infectious focus which causes fresh developing or expanded tuberculomas despite appropriate treatment. Calcifications and regional atrophy can be seen at long-term period although a great deal of lesions don't leave any radiological sign after successful treatment [14, 21].

Conclusion

- Dura mater and epidural TB are a very rare but severe infection.
- A high index of doubt is critical for early diagnosis and avoidance from associated significant morbidity and mortality.
- Patients with dural-epidural TB should follow up closely.
- When the signs of raised intracranial pressure or new neurological findings determined, these patients should undergo urgent radiological evaluation to exclude the possibility of newly developed or enlarged tuberculomas at eloquent areas.
- Dural-epidural TB must be remembered in the differential diagnosis of cranial epidural lesions, particularly in endemic countries.
- Unfortunately the relapsing rate of the disease is high despite successful medication.

References

1. Horne DJ, Hubbard R, Narita M, Exarchos A, Park DR, Goss CH (2010) Factors associated with mortality in patients with tuberculosis. BMC Infect Dis 10:258
2. Lopez de Castilla D, Schluger NW (2010) Tuberculosis following solid organ transplantation. Transpl Infect Dis 12:106–112
3. Vaid S, Lee YYP, Rawat S, Luthra A, Shah D, Ahuja AT (2010) Tuberculosis in the head and neck–a forgotten differential diagnosis. Clin Radiol 65:73–81
4. Cherian A, Thomas SV (2011) Central nervous system tuberculosis. Afr Health Sci 11:116–127
5. Zou H, Pan KH, Pan HY, Huang DS, Zheng MH (2015) Cerebral hemorrhage due to tuberculosis meningitis: a rare case report and literature review. Oncotarget 6:45005–45009. doi:10.18632/oncotarget.6528
6. Jacques C, Boukobza M, Polivka M, Ferrario A, George B, Merland JJ (2000) Cranial epidural tuberculoma. A case report. Acta Radiol 41:367–370
7. Khawcharoenporn T, Apisarnthanarak A, Apisarnthanarak P, Rakskul P, Warnnissorn N, Kiratisin P, Mundy LM (2008) Diffuse pachymeningitis due to Mycobacterium tuberculosis: a case report and review of the literature. Hawaii Med J 67:100–103

8. Lindner A, Schneider C, Hofmann E, Soerensen N, Toyka KV (1995) Isolated meningeal tuberculoma mimicking meningioma: case report. Surg Neurol 43:81–83
9. Tseng SH, Chen Y, Shun CT (1997) Isolated dural tuberculoma. Acta Neurochir 139:263–264
10. Tariq R, Ahmed R (2012) Tuberculous hypertrophic pachymeningitis presenting as visual blurring and headaches. J Pak Med Assoc 62:966–968
11. Goyal M, Sharma A, Mishra NK, Gaikwad SB, Sharma MC (1997) Imaging appearance of pachymeningeal tuberculosis. AJR Am J Roentgenol 169:1421–1424
12. Yan JL, Wei KC (2013) Tubercular temporalis abscess with skull and dural invasion. Surg Infect (Larchmt) 14:473–475
13. Kocaeli H, Taşkapılıoğlu O, Başaran E, Karaoğlu A, Bekar A (2011) Multiple dural tuberculomas presenting as leptomeningeal carcinomatosis. Case Rep Neurol Med 2011:581230
14. Bernaerts A, Vanhoenacker FM, Parizel PM, Van Goethem JWM, Van Altena R, Laridon A, De Roeck J, Coeman V, De Schepper AM (2003) Tuberculosis of the central nervous system: overview of neuroradiological findings. Eur Radiol 13:1876–1890
15. Kumar R, Jain R, Kaur A, Chhabra DK (2000) Brain stem tuberculosis in children. Br J Neurosurg 14:356–361
16. Turgut M (2001) Multifocal extensive spinal tuberculosis (Pott's disease) involving cervical, thoracic and lumbar vertebrae. Br J Neurosurg 15:142–146
17. Turgut M (2001) Spinal tuberculosis (Pott's disease): its clinical presentation, surgical management, and outcome. A survey study on 694 patients. Neurosurg Rev 24:8–13
18. O'Brien J, Buckley O, Persaud T, Colhoun E (2007) Calvarial tuberculosis: an unusual presentation (2007: 8b). Eur Radiol 17:3014–3015
19. Goasdoué P, Dubayle P, Boyer B, Debord T, Le Clainche P, Pharaboz C (1997) Disseminated tuberculosis of unusual locations. J Radiol 78:659–661
20. Sencer S, Sencer A, Aydin K, Hepgül K, Poyanli A, Minareci O (2003) Imaging in tuberculosis of the skull and skull-base: case report. Neuroradiology 45:160–163
21. Gupta RK, Kohli A, Gaur V, Lal JH, Kishore J (1997) MRI of the brain in patients with miliary pulmonary tuberculosis without symptoms or signs of central nervous system involvement. Neuroradiology 39:699–704
22. D'Andrea G, Trillò G, Celli P, Roperto R, Crispo F, Ferrante L (2004) Idiopathic intracranial hypertrophic pachymeningitis: two case reports and review of the literature. Neurosurg Rev 27:199–204
23. Aggarwal A, Patra DP, Gupta K, Sodhi HB (2016) Dural tuberculoma mimicking meningioma: a clinicoradiologic review of dural en-plaque lesions. World Neurosurg 88:686. doi:10.1016/j.wneu.2015.10.097
24. Dastur DK, Manghani DK, Udani PM (1995) Pathology and pathogenetic mechanisms in neurotuberculosis. Radiol Clin North Am 33:733–752

Subdural Space of the Brain and Its Coverings

7

Sailike Duishanbai, Mohammad Sami, Geng Dangmurenjiafu, and Mehmet Turgut

Contents

S. Duishanbai, MD, PhD (✉) • M. Sami, MD • G. Dangmurenjiafu, MD, PhD
Neurosurgery Center, Xinjiang Neurosurgical Research Institute, First Affiliated Hospital of Xinjiang Medical University, No137 Liyushan South Road, Xinshi District, Urumqi, Xinjiang, China
e-mail: serickd@yahoo.com; mohammad.sami37@yahoo.com; serickd@sina.com

M. Turgut, MD, PhD
Department of Neurosurgery, Adnan Menderes University School of Medicine, Aydın, Turkey
e-mail: drmturgut@yahoo.com

Abbreviations

CNS	Central nervous system
CSF	Cerebrospinal fluid
CT	Computed tomography
ELISPOT	Enzyme-linked immunospot assay
INH	Isoniazid
MRI	Magnetic resonance imaging
NAAT	Nucleic acid amplification test
PCR	Polymerase chain reaction
PZA	Pyrazinamide
RIF	Rifampicin
SIADH	Syndrome of inappropriate antidiuretic hormone secretion
TB	Tuberculosis
TBM	Tuberculous meningitis

7.1 Introduction

Tuberculosis (TB) is among the oldest and most disturbing infectious diseases worldwide. Approximately one-third of the world's population has active or latent disease, resulting in 1.5

M. Turgut et al. (eds.), *Tuberculosis of the Central Nervous System*,
DOI 10.1007/978-3-319-50712-5_7

million deaths annually. Central nervous system (CNS) involvement, while rare, is the most severe form of TB. Manifestations include tuberculoma and tuberculous meningitis (TBM), with the majority of cases occurring in children and immunocompromised patients. Despite advances in imaging and laboratory diagnostics, tuberculomas of the CNS remain a diagnostic challenge because of their insidious nature and nonspecific findings. Subdural intracranial TB is a subtype of intracranial TB; its clinical characteristics, diagnosis, and treatment are very important for understanding the disease process and improving patients' outcomes.

7.2 Brief Anatomy of the Intradural Space of the Brain and Its Coverings

There are three layers of meninges around the brain and spinal cord. The outer layer, the dura mater, consists of tough, fibrous, white connective tissue. The middle layer is the arachnoid, a thin layer that looks like a cobweb, with numerous threadlike strands attaching it to the innermost layer. The space under the arachnoid, the subarachnoid space, is filled with cerebrospinal fluid (CSF) and contains blood vessels. The innermost layer of the meninges is the pia mater. This thin, delicate membrane is tightly bound to the surface of the brain and spinal cord and cannot be dissected away without damaging the brain surface (Fig. 7.1).

7.3 Tuberculosis of the Subdural Space of the Brain and Its Coverings

7.3.1 Tuberculous Meningitis

Meningitis (from Greek "membrane" and the suffix "-itis, "inflammation") is an acute inflammation of the meninges, the protective membranes that cover the brain and spinal cord [1]. The inflammation may be caused by infection with viruses, bacteria, or other microorganisms, and less commonly it may be caused by certain drugs [2–4]. Tuberculous meningitis (TBM) can be life-threatening because of the proximity of the inflammation to the brain and spinal cord; thus, the condition is classified as a medical emergency [4, 5].

Headache and fever are the most common features of TBM; confusion and coma appear later and indicate a poor prognosis. However, signs and symptoms are absent in one-fifth of patients with TBM. Patients may also show neck stiffness and focal neurological deficits. In adults, the most common symptom of TBM is a severe headache, which occurs in around 90% of patients with bacterial meningitis, followed in frequency by nuchal rigidity (inability to flex the neck forward passively due to increased neck muscle tone and neck stiffness). The distinctive triplet of diagnostic signs consists of nuchal rigidity, rapid high fever, and altered mental status, although all three features are present in only 44–46% of patients with bacterial meningitis [3, 6–8]. Other signs usually linked with meningitis are photophobia (intolerance of bright light) and phono-

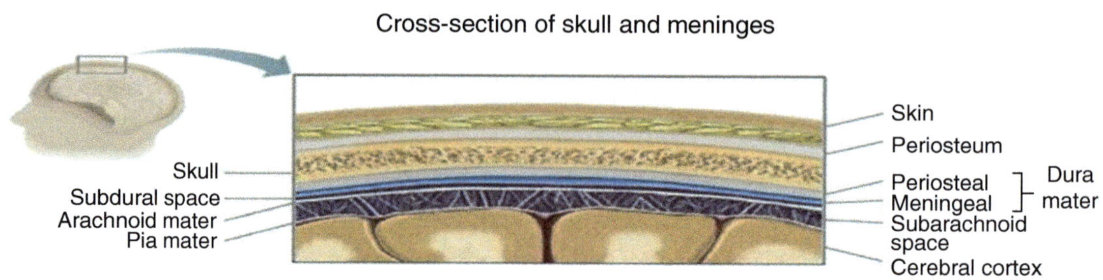

Fig. 7.1 The illustration shows a diagram of the anatomy of the intradural space of the brain and its coverings

phobia (intolerance of loud noises). Small children often do not exhibit the aforementioned signs and symptoms, and may only be irritable and looks abnormal. The fontanel (the soft spot on the top of a baby's head) can bulge in infants younger than 6 months. Other features that differentiate meningitis from less severe illnesses in youngsters are leg pain, cold extremities, and an abnormal skin color [9, 10].

7.3.2 Etiology

TBM caused by *Mycobacterium tuberculosis* infection is the most common form of CNS TB, with *M. tuberculosis* infection of the meninges being the cardinal feature, and the inflammation being near the base of the brain [4, 11]. When the inflammation is found in the brain stem subarachnoid area, cranial nerve roots may be affected. The symptoms will be similar to those of space-occupying lesions. Blood-borne spread certainly occurs, presumably by the organism crossing the blood-brain barrier (BBB); but a proportion of patients may contract TBM from the rupture of a cortical focus in the brain [4], while an even smaller proportion contract it from the rupture of a bony focus in the spine. As noted above, meningitis is typically caused by infection with microorganisms. Viral infections are the most common cause, with bacterial, fungal, and protozoal infections being the next most common causes; the condition may also have various noninfectious causes [3, 4].

The pathophysiology of TBM is characterized by the bacilli attaching to the brain parenchyma, causing small subpial tubercles to form. Then the Rich focus increases in size until the tubercles rupture. This rupturing in the subarachnoid area causes TBM.

7.3.3 Diagnosis

7.3.4 Lumbar Puncture

A lumbar puncture can be used to diagnose TBM. The CSF sample collected from the lumbar puncture can be removed from the spinal canal with a needle that passes through the three membranes that envelop the brain and spinal cord; the sample is examined in a medical laboratory [10]. TBM causes severe lasting consequences, such as epilepsy, deafness, hydrocephalus, and cognitive deficits if it is not treated or if treatment is delayed.

The diagnosis of TBM is completed by analysis of the CSF collected from the lumbar puncture. A minimum of 1 ml of CSF should be taken during lumbar puncture for CSF collection (preferably 5–10 ml). In TBM, usually protein in CSF is high, glucose is low, and the number of lymphocytes is elevated (see Table 7.1). Acid-fast bacilli are sometimes seen on a CSF smear, but more commonly, *M. tuberculosis* is grown in culture [12, 13]. A spider web clot in the collected CSF is characteristic of TBM, but is a rare outcome. An enzyme-linked immunospot assay (ELISPOT) test is not useful for the diagnosis of acute TBM and the result is often a false negative [13], but it may, paradoxically, become positive after treatment has started, which aids in confirming the diagnosis.

7.3.5 Radiological Findings

X-Ray, computed tomography (CT), and magnetic resonance imaging (MRI) are usually useful tools for investigating TBM. X-rays may show a calcified lesion in the lungs and

Table 7.1 CSF analysis in different types of meningitis

Meningitis type	Glucose	Protein	Cell type
Acute bacterial	Low↓	High↑	PMNs; often >300/mm^3
Acute viral	Normal	Normal or high↑	Mononuclear; <300 mm^3
Tuberculous	Low↓	High↑	Mononuclear and PMNs <300/mm^3
Fungal	Low↓	High↑	<300/mm^3
Malignant	Low↓	High↑	Usually: mononuclear

CSF Cerebrospinal fluid, *PMNs* polymorphonuclear leukocytes intracranial space. Non-contrast CT scans may be normal at the beginning of this disease, but later complications, such as hydrocephalus and cerebellar infarcts due to arteritis (especially in children), may be visible on follow-up images. On contrast CT scans, basal cisternal and leptomeningeal enhancement may be seen (Fig. 7.2). Plain MRI appears normal initially, but later, on contrast MRI scans, basal cisternal and leptomeningeal enhancement may be seen (Fig. 7.3).

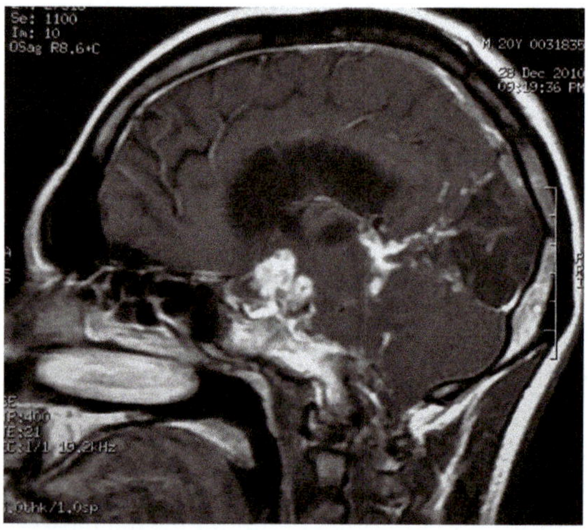

Fig. 7.2 Contrast-enhanced magnetic resonance imaging (MRI) shows prominent exudates in basilar regions (Courtesy of R. K. Garg)

7.3.6 Amplification of Nucleic Acid Tests

Polymerase chain reactions (PCRs) are used to detect mycobacterial nucleic acid. These tests vary in the nucleic acid sequence they detect and they vary in accuracy; two commercially available tests are the amplified *M. tuberculosis* direct test (AMTD; Gen-Probe) and the Amplicor Mycobacterium tuberculosis Test (Roche Molecular Diagnostics, California, USA). A 2007 review stated that for diagnosing TBM: "Individually the AMTD test appears to perform the best (sensitivity 74% and specificity 98%)"; the pooled prevalence of TBM was found to be only 29% [14].

7.3.7 CSF Findings

If there is a suspicion of meningitis in a patient, blood inflammatory markers should be tested (C-reactive protein or complete blood count), or blood cultures should be done [10, 12]. CSF examination is most important for diagnosis and for ruling out the disease [15]. However, lumbar puncture is contraindicated if there is a mass in the brain (tumor or abscess) or if the intracranial pressure (ICP) is elevated, as the procedure may lead to brain herniation. If someone is at risk for

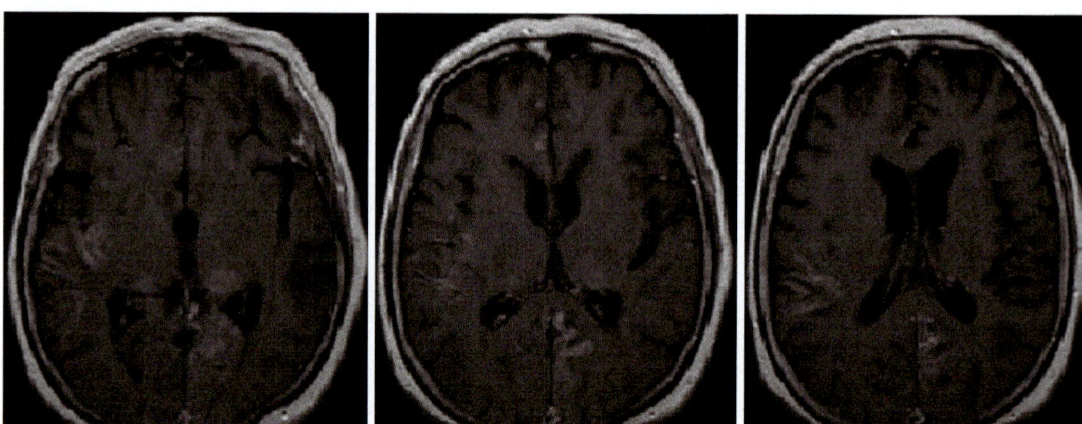

Fig. 7.3 Contrast MRI scan showed leptomeningeal enhancement in the temporal and occipital area in a patient with tuberculous meningitis (TBM)

either a mass or raised ICP (recent head injury, a known immune system problem, localizing neurological signs, or evidence on investigation of a raised ICP), CT or MRI is recommended before lumbar puncture [10, 12]. It can only apply in 45% of adult patients. If CT or MRI is required before lumbar puncture or if lumbar puncture is difficult, an antibiotic should be administered first to prevent postponement of treatment, and then CT, MRI, or lumbar puncture can be performed [10, 12]. Often, for assessing the complications of meningitis, CT or MRI can be performed later [14].

It is important to monitor blood electrolytes in severe forms of meningitis; instant hypothermia can occur with bacterial meningitis, due to a combination of dehydration, the syndrome of inappropriate secretion of anti-diuretic hormone (SIADH), or aggressive intravenous fluid infusion.

7.3.8 Treatment

TBM is treated with rifampicin (RIF), isoniazid (INH), pyrazinamide (PZA), and ethambutol (EMB) for 2 months, followed by INH and RIF only for an additional 10 months. In HIV patients with neurological defects, steroid reduces the risk of death. For the first 6 weeks of treatment in these patients we can use steroids [16]. Some patients need thalidomide, an immunomodulatory agent, while one-third of patients with TBM will develop hydrocephalus. Aspirin can delay or reduce mortality and complications such as infarction.

We should start treatment without an exact diagnosis (empirical antibiotics), even before the CSF results are available. Antibiotics can be selected based on the kind of bacteria and the particular geographical place of infection and the population. For example, empirical treatment in the United Kingdom consists of ceftriaxone or cefotaxime (third-generation cephalosporins) [17]. Streptococci resistant to cephalosporins have been progressively found in the United States, so vancomycin is recommended as the initial treatment [12, 18]. An ampicillin combination with chloramphenicol appears to work well, and chloramphenicol only works equally well [19].

Empirical treatment is chosen on the basis of the patient's age, infection of the head injury, whether they have had recent neurosurgery, or whether a cerebral shunt exists [17, 28]. In patients who are immunocompromised, those aged over 50 years, or very young children the addition of ampicillin is recommended to cover *Listeria monocytogenes* [12, 18]. Once the diagnosis is conformed via gram stain we can select the antibiotic for the presumed group of pathogens [19]. It takes about 24–48 h for CSF results. So we start empirical therapy, and after getting the CSF results, we change to a specific antibiotic therapy targeted to the causative organism. The antibiotic should not only be based on the findings of pathogenic bacteria but also on its capacity to reach the meninges in adequate quantities. Some antibiotics show inadequate penetration and so are less effective in meningitis. Antibiotics used in meningitis have not been tested directly on meningitis patients in clinical trials. The relevant knowledge of these antibiotics is obtained from laboratory studies on rabbits [14]. Patients with pulmonary TB need to be treated with antibiotics for 6 months, but TBM needs to be treated for 1 year or more [4].

Nowadays professional guidelines recommend the administration of dexamethasone or a similar corticosteroid before the first dose of antibiotic is given; the recommendation is to continue the steroid for 4 days; it is most effective in the treatment of pneumococcal meningitis, and some guidelines suggest that dexamethasone be discontinued if another cause of meningitis is diagnosed—dexamethasone suppresses excessive inflammation and that is why guidelines suggest its use at the beginning of treatment [13].

Further treatments of corticosteroids is different in children than adults but the corticosteroid demonstrate as beneficial as in children from developing countries, the uses of corticosteroids not supported by low income countries, because discrepancy is not known. The benefits of corticosteroids are only seen when they are used before the first dose of antibiotic is given; the benefits are highest in *Haemophilus influenzae* meningitis [2]. After the introduction of the Hib (*Haemophilus influenzae* type b) vaccine the incidence of pediatric meningitis decreased dramatically; it is now recommended that if the cause of pediatric meningitis is *H. influenzae*, treatment with corticosteroid should be given only before the first dose of antibiotic, as other uses are controversial.

7.3.9 Prognosis

Bacterial meningitis can be fatal if untreated, while viral meningitis is rarely fatal; in contrast with bacterial meningitis it tends to resolve spontaneously after treatment. Mortality in bacterial meningitis depends on the underlying causes and the age of the patient—20 to 30% of newborns with bacterial meningitis are at risk of dying, but the risk is lower in older children, whose mortality is about 2%, whereas the risk increases to 19–37% in adults. There are various risk factors apart from age and the causative pathogens; e.g., the time taken to eradicate the pathogen from the CSF, the severity of the illness, the level of consciousness, and an abnormally low WBC in the CSF. *H. influenzae* meningitis and meningococcal meningitis have a better outcome than meningitis caused by pneumococcal bacteria, *Streptococcus pneumoniae*, group B streptococci, or coliforms in adults; the mortality is lower in meningococcal meningitis (3–7%) than in meningitis caused by pneumococcal bacteria [9, 10].

CNS damage leads to several potential disabilities in children, including behavioral and learning difficulties, epilepsy, and sensorineural hearing loss, as well as cognitive impairment in 50% of those who survive; in adults hearing loss is variable and all cases are emergence without disability ;40% of adult survivors show deafness or cognitive impairment [9].

Children with TBM are associated with a high risk of death; even with treatment 19% of survivors have ongoing neurological problems. In many countries meningitis is epidemiologically notifiable, but the precise incidence is not known [16]. In 2013 there were 303,000 deaths of meningitis patients worldwide, down from 464,000 in 1990, and in 2010, it was estimated that there were 420,000 deaths because of meningitis, excluding that caused by Cryptococci [18]. In Western countries 3 bacterial meningitis deaths per 100,000 population have been reported, while viral meningitis is more common in population-wide studies, at an incidence of 10.9 per 100,000 population, and it occurs more often in the summer. In Brazil, the incidence of bacterial meningitis is greater, at 45.8 per 100,000 population annually. Sub-Saharan Africa has been plagued by large epidemics of meningococcal meningitis for over a century, leading to it being labeled the "meningitis belt" [5]. Epidemics typically occur in the dry season (December to June), and an epidemic wave can last 2–3 years, dying out during the overruling rainy seasons. Incidence rates of 100–800 cases per 100,000 population are encountered in this area, which is poorly served by medical care; these cases are predominantly caused by meningococci. The largest epidemic ever recorded in the history of the area swept across the entire region in 1996–1997, causing over 250,000 cases and 25,000 deaths [9].

Meningococcal disease occurs in epidemics in areas where many people live together for the first time, such as army barracks during mobilization, college campuses, and the annual Hajj pilgrimage. Although the pattern of epidemic cycles in Africa is not well understood, several factors have been associated with the development of epidemics in the meningitis belt. They include: medical conditions (immunological susceptibility of the population), demographic conditions (travel and large population displacements), socioeconomic conditions (overcrowding and poor living conditions), climatic circumstances (drought and dust storms), and concurrent infections (acute respiratory infections) [10].

Bacterial meningitis shows significant differences in local distribution. For example, in Europe and Asia most disease episodes are caused by meningitis groups B and C, while group A continues to predominate in Africa, where it causes most of the major epidemics in the meningitis belt, accounting for about 80–85% of documented meningococcal meningitis cases.

7.4 Tuberculous Arachnoiditis

In TB arachnoiditis the arachnoid mater is inflamed; this inflammation is called arachnoiditis. The CNS, spinal cord, and brain are surrounded by membranes called meninges, which protect the nerves. Arachnoiditis can be caused by adverse reactions to chemicals, infection with bacteria or viruses, straight to the brain [15].

7.4.1 Signs and Symptoms

TB arachnoiditis can lead to many painful and debilitating symptoms that can vary greatly in each case; chronic pain (including neuralgia) is the most common symptom, while numbness and tingling of the extremities can occur with spinal cord involvement, and bowel, bladder, and sexual functioning can be affected if the lower part of the spinal cord is involved. While arachnoiditis has no consistent pattern of symptoms, it mostly affects the nerves that supply the legs and lower back, and many patients experience difficulty sitting for long or short periods of time due to discomfort or pain, or because of efferent neurological or other motor symptoms, such as difficulties controlling limbs [15].

7.4.2 Diagnosis

For the diagnosis of TB arachnoiditis, arachnoid ossification may be detected better on unenhanced CT, which is more specific than MRI, showing calcification or hemosiderin deposits which are unclear on MRI. MRI is less specific in the diagnosis of TB arachnoiditis [15].

7.4.3 Treatment

The treatment of arachnoiditis is difficult, and is generally based on the severity of the pain and the symptoms. Thus, arachnoiditis is not yet curable, and can be life-threatening. Management includes medication, physical therapy, and psychotherapy. Surgical intervention decreases a bad outcome and gives temporary relief of pain [15].

7.5 Intracranial Subdural Tuberculous Empyema

Intracranial subdural TB empyema is an extremely rare form of CNS TB and is extremely uncommon. Subdural empyema in the subdural space is mostly pyogenic.

The co-occurrence of TB brain abscess and subdural TB empyema has been reported in the literature. Although chronic otitis media is commonly seen in children with TB empyema, TB empyema of otogenic origin is rare and is often misdiagnosed as pyogenic abscess; in the etiologic analysis of 75 cases of brain abscess, TB etiology was found in only 4% of the cases [19–22].

7.5.1 Diagnosis

7.5.2 Imaging

The primary approach to the diagnosis of intracranial subdural TB empyema mainly depends on imaging techniques such as CT and MRI. Newer technologies described below have significantly improved our ability to diagnose as well as to localize lesions and monitor them for response or progression during treatment. With the application of CT technology, both the ease of diagnosis and the prognosis have dramatically improved [14].

7.5.3 Treatment

The surgical treatment of intracranial subdural TB empyema needs individualization. Anti-TB treatment is the mainstay of the treatment. Surgical evacuation is advocated, depending on the severity of the neurological symptoms. Craniotomy is advisable in drug-resistant intracranial subdural TB empyema that shows no healing. Burr hole draining was not successful at the first attempt in an

8-year-old Kazakh patient diagnosed with intracranial subdural TB empyema, and the evacuation of TB pus, and draining, was done after the subsequent performance of a craniectomy [17, 23].

References

1. Lapeyssonnie L (1963) Cerebrospinal meningitis in Africa. Bull World Health Organ 28:1–114
2. Logan SA, MacMahon E (2008) Viral meningitis. BMJ 336:36–40
3. Swartz MN (2004) Bacterial meningitis—a view of the past 90 years. N Engl J Med 351:1826–1828
4. Thwaites G, Chau TT, Mai NT, Drobniewski F, McAdam K, Farrar J (2000) Tuberculous meningitis. J Neurol Neurosurg Psychiatry 68:289–299
5. Leach RM (2010) Acute and critical care medicine at a glance. New Jersey: John Wiley & Sons, USA. p 101
6. Tunkel AR, Hartman BJ, Kaplan SL (2004) Practice guidelines for the management of bacterial meningitis. Clin Infect Dis 39:1267–1284
7. World Health Organization (1998) Control of epidemic meningococcal disease, practical guidelines, 2nd edn. World Health Organization, Geneva . WHO/EMC/BA/98 (PDF) 3, pp 1–83
8. WHO (2003) Detecting meningococcal meningitis epidemics in highly-endemic African countries. Wkly Epidemiol Rec 78:294–296
9. Chiang SS, Khan FA, Milstein MB, Tolman AW, Benedetti A, Starke JR, Becerra MC (2014) Treatment outcomes of childhood tuberculous meningitis: a systematic review and meta-analysis. Lancet Infect Dis 14:947–957
10. Greenwood B (2006) One Hundred years of epidemic meningitis in West Africa — has anything changed? Trop Med Int Health 11:773–780
11. Weichselbaum A (1887) Ueber die Aetiologie der akuten Meningitis cerebro-spinalis. Fortschrift der Medizin (in German) 5:573–583
12. Behera D (2010) Textbook of pulmonary medicine. Jaypee Brothers Publishers, p 505; Christodoulides M (2013) Meningitis New Delhi: cellular and molecular basis. CABI, India. p 154
13. Dinnes J, Deeks J, Kunst H, Gibson A, Cummins E, Waugh N, Drobniewski F, Lalvani A (2007) A systematic review of rapid diagnostic tests for the detection of tuberculosis infection. Health Technol Assess 11:85–87
14. Britt RH, Enzmann DR, Yeager AS (1981) Neuropathological and computerized tomographic findings in experimental brain abscess. J Neurosurg 55:590–603
15. NINDS Arachnoiditis Information Page. National Institute of Neurological Disorders and Stroke, National Institutes of Health. Accessed 23 Oct 2015.
16. Heyderman RS, Lambert HP, O'Sullivan I, Stuart JM, Taylor BL, Wall RA (2003) Early management of suspected bacterial meningitis and meningococcal septicaemia in adults. J Infect 46:75–77
17. Flexner S (1913) The results of the serum treatment in thirteen hundred cases of epidemic meningitis. J Exp Med 17:553–576
18. Harrison J, Kulkarni K, Baguneid M, Prendergast B (2009) Oxford handbook of key clinical evidence (Oxford handbooks). Oxford University Press, Oxford
19. Chaudhuri A, Martinez–Martin P, Martin PM (2008) EFNS guideline on the management of community-acquired bacterial meningitis: report of an EFNS Task Force on acute bacterial meningitis in older children and adults. Eur J Neurol 15:649–659
20. Attia J, Hatala R, Cook DJ, Wong JG (1999) The rational clinical examination. Does this adult patient have acute meningitis? JAMA 282:175–181
21. Walker AE, Laws ER, Udvarhelyi GB (1998) Infections and inflammatory involvement of the CNS. The Genesis of Neuroscience, Thieme, pp 219–221
22. Peltola H (2000) Worldwide *Haemophilus influenzae* type b disease at the beginning of the 21st century: global analysis of the disease burden 25 years after the use of the polysaccharide vaccine and a decade after the advent of conjugates. Clin Microbiol Rev 13:302–317
23. Greenwood B (2006) 100 years of epidemic meningitis in West Africa – has anything changed? Tropical Flexner S (1913) The results of the serum treatment in thirteen hundred cases of epidemic meningitis. J Exp Med 17:553–576

8 Cerebrum, Cerebellum, and Deep Structures of the Brain

Forhad Hossain Chowdhury,
Mohammod Raziul Haque,
and Mainul Haque Sarker

Contents

Abbreviations

ADA	Adenosine deaminases
AFB	Acid-fast bacillus
AIDS	Acquired immunodeficiency syndrome
BCG	Bacillus Calmette and Guerin
CNS	Central nervous system
CPA	Cerebellopontine angle
CSF	Cerebrospinal fluid
CT	Computed tomography
DNA	Deoxyribose nucleic acid
ETV	Endoscopic third ventriculostomy
HIV	Human immunodeficiency virus
ICP	Intracranial pressure
INH	Isoniazid
MDR	Multidrug resistant
MRI	Magnetic resonance imaging
NNA	Nucleic acid amplification
PCR	Polymerase chain reaction
RIF	Rifampin
TB	Tuberculosis
TBA	Tuberculous brain abscess
TBM	Tubercular meningitis
VPS	Ventriculoperitoneal shunt
XDR	Extensive drug resistance

F.H. Chowdhury, FCPS, MS (✉)
Department of Neurosurgery,
National Institute of Neurosciences and Hospital,
Room no. 635 Sher-e-bangla nagar, Dhaka 1207,
Bangladesh
e-mail: forhadchowdhury74@yahoo.com

M.R. Haque, FCPS, MS • M.H. Sarker, MS
Department of Neurosurgery, Dhaka Medical College
and Hospital, Dhaka, Bangladesh
e-mail: raziulhaque@yahoo.co.in; mhsarker@gmail.com

M. Turgut et al. (eds.), *Tuberculosis of the Central Nervous System*,
DOI 10.1007/978-3-319-50712-5_8

8.1 Introduction, Incidences, and Predisposing Factors

With the increasing number of tuberculosis (TB) patients, central nervous system (CNS) TB is also increasing [1]. The CNS involvement comprises approximately 10–15% of all TB infections [2] and is seen most commonly in the developing countries. The World Health Organization reported that 8–10 million new cases of TB are diagnosed all over the world, each year. Incidence of TB is eight cases per 100,000 annually, in the United States. In the late 1980s, the rate of TB increased mostly due to HIV infection in countries where TB is common and where AIDS continues to be a pandemic disease with a high mortality and morbidity rate, especially in Asia and Africa. In endemic areas CNS TB is considered to follow the 10% rule [3]. There are an estimated 10 million new cases of TB worldwide, nearly 10% of all patients with TB tend to have CNS involvement either as tuberculous meningitis (TBM) or as intracranial tuberculomas, and till date the reported literature suggested that the two conditions may coexist in up to 10% of patients. In endemic areas, 10% of all intracranial space occupying lesions are tuberculomas and the mortality of intracranial tuberculomas has also been reported at around 10%. Almost 70% of patients have multiple tuberculomas [4].

The prevalence of tuberculomas varies in different countries and age groups. The incidence of TB also varies among different socioeconomic classes. Tuberculomas can occur at any site in the brain. Arvind et al. reported in a series of 1247 cases that the parietal hemisphere accounted for 47% of intracranial tuberculomas and that left-sided lesions were more common than right-sided ones [5].

In the reported studies following conditions such as HIV infection, [6] intravenous drug use, immunosuppression from increasing age, alcoholism, malnutrition, poverty, transplantation, aggressive chemotherapy, immigration, [7] homelessness, and crowding are mainly considered to be responsible for the development and for the annual increase of disease. The age range of neuro-TB is between 25 and 45 years [8–10], but authors found this to be 2–68 years in their series of 78 cases. Neuro-TB is mostly hemispheric [5]. Tuberculoma is encountered in only 15–30% cases of CNS TB [11].

8.2 TB of the Cerebral Hemisphere

8.2.1 Common Sites

TB granuloma (tuberculoma) is the most common form of parenchymal lesion [12]. Tuberculoma can occur at all age group; however, its incidence is higher in pediatric population [13]. TB lesions can involve any part of the cerebral hemisphere. These are usually located at the corticomedullary junction and periventricular region, as expected for hematogenous dissemination. They are mostly supratentorial (i.e., hemispheric) in adults, and in children the cerebral hemisphere is less commonly involved than the cerebellum [14, 15]. Common sites for tuberculomas are cerebral hemispheres and basal ganglia in adults due to the large blood supply to these areas [5]. Distribution of brain tuberculoma reported by Turgut et al. [16] was as follows: cerebral hemisphere 41%, cerebellum 35%, brain stem 6%, intraspinal 6%, and multiple 12%.

8.2.2 Pathology

Mycobacterium tuberculosis is an aerobic, nonmotile, nonspore-forming, acid/alcohol-fast bacillus (AFB) that infects primarily humans. Its doubling time is quite slow (15–20 h) [17]. *Mycobacterium bovis* and atypical *Mycobacterium* spp. can also involve in cerebral TB. The acquisition of *M. tuberculosis* infection occurs through the inhalation of droplet nuclei containing the bacilli, eventually leading to deposition in the lung alveoli. Due to host immune response, the activation of a type 1 T-helper cell-mediated immune response occurs, and, ultimately, a granuloma is formed. Early in this process, prior to the actual containment of the infection, bacilli are filtered into draining lymph nodes, and there exists a low-level bacteremia in which *M. tuberculosis* disseminates to distant sites in the body [18]. This hematogenous seeding occurs most frequently in regions of the body that are highly oxygenated such as the brain and in the brain cerebral and cerebellar hemispheres and basal ganglia that are highly oxygenated parts of the brain [19]. A complex interplay of host immune factors and *M. tuberculosis* virulence factors in the end determines whether or not the infection is contained and whether, or to what extent, the dissemination of the bacilli leads to clinical disease [18]. Macroglias are the key cells of the pathogenesis of neuro-TB [17]. For cerebral or other CNS TB, the disease begins with the development of small TB foci (rich foci) in the brain, spinal cord, or meninges. The location of these foci and the capacity to control them ultimately determine which form of CNS TB to occur [20]. Forms of cerebral TB are like that of CNS TB involvement. It can be in the form of tuberculoma (including hard or soft granulomas) and tubercular abscess (including TB cerebritis) [21, 22]. These forms of TB can occur with or without tubercular meningitis (TBM).

8.2.3 Clinical Features

Clinical manifestations of parenchymal tuberculoma or tuberculous brain abscess (TBA) depend largely on their location. Patients often present with headache, seizures, papilledema, or other signs of increased intracranial pressure. The pace of symptom development usually is measured in weeks to months with cerebral TB. The presentation of brain abscess is more acute (1 week–3 months) than tuberculoma but slower in onset than pyogenic brain abscesses. TBA is associated with fever, headaches, and focal neurological deficits (i.e., visual disturbances, limb weakness, dysphasia, memory disturbances, etc.) [23]. The clinical presentation of cerebral tuberculoma may be delayed months to years after the infection [24]. When associated with TBM, clinical features of TBM (i.e., classic meningitis symptoms of fever, headache, and stiff neck) along with focal neurological deficits, behavioral changes, seizures, and alterations in consciousness may present [25]. Low-grade fever and night sweat may present specially in children. Abnormal movement disorders may occur in the form of chorea or hemiballismus, athetosis, tremors, and myoclonic jerks [26]. Patients with CNS TB may or may not associate with other systemic TB.

8.2.4 Diagnosis

Definitive diagnosis Definitive diagnosis depends on detection of TB bacilli in CSF either by smear examination or bacterial culture [27]. Histopathological identification of TB granuloma is the hallmark of TB and is considered as confirmatory for TB.

Neuroimaging Neuroradiological findings can only be suggestive of neuro-TB but not confirmatory [17]. Tuberculomas are normally defined as single or multiple, low or high density, and round or lobulated masses with irregular walls and show homogenous or ring enhancement after administering contrast on CT scan [11, 28]. The magnetic resonance imaging (MRI) features of individual tuberculoma will depend on whether the lesion is noncaseating, caseating with a solid center, or caseating with a liquid center [29, 30]. The noncaseating granuloma is usually hypointense on T1-weighted images (T1WI) and hyperintense on T2-weighted images (T2WI) and shows homogenous nodular enhancement on post-gadolinium images. The caseating granuloma(s) with solid center appears hypointense to isointense on T1WI (may have a slight hyperintense rim) and strikingly hypointense on T2W images. On contrast administration, the lesion shows peripheral rim enhancement [31–33]. On MRI, focal tuberculous cerebritis appears hypointense on T1 and hyperintense on T2 and shows small areas of patchy contrast enhancement on post-gadolinium images [34]. On imaging, a TB abscess may be indistinguishable from a caseous tuberculoma with central liquefaction or a pyogenic abscess. However, a TB abscess is usually solitary and larger than tuberculoma.

Perilesional edema and mass effect are more as compared to tuberculoma. On CT and MRI, it is often multinucleated and shows thin, smooth peripheral wall enhancement on post-contrast images [35]. Commonly identified neuroradiological features of TBM (i.e., basal meningeal enhancement, hydrocephalus, and infarctions in the supratentorial brain parenchyma and brain stem) may be associated findings in cerebral parenchymal TB [22, 31, 36] (Fig. 8.1). On MRI contrast enhancing, high-intensity (in T2WI) CNS miliary TB lesions are small, are less than 5 mm in size, and located at the corticomedullary junction and in the distribution of perforating vessels [37] (Figs. 8.2 and 8.3).

CSF Study Cytological study, microbiological study, and molecular and biochemical analysis techniques include commercially available nucleic acid amplification (NAA) methods and other PCR (polymerase chain reaction)-based methods, antibody detection, antigen detection, or chemical assays such as adenosine deaminase (ADA), and tuberculostearic acid measurements of CSF sometimes can help significantly but cannot confirm TB [17].

Differential Diagnosis of Cerebral TB The main differential diagnosis of brain parenchymal TB is glial, meningeal, and ependymal tumors; neuroectodermal tumor; metastases; lymphoma; chordoma; brain abscess; fungal infection; neurocysticercosis; hydatidosis; sarcoidosis; etc. [36, 38].

8.2.5 Treatment

Drug Therapy (Anti-TB, Steroid, and Antiepileptics) The standard approach to CNS TB, endorsed by the Infectious Diseases Society of America, Centers for Disease Control and

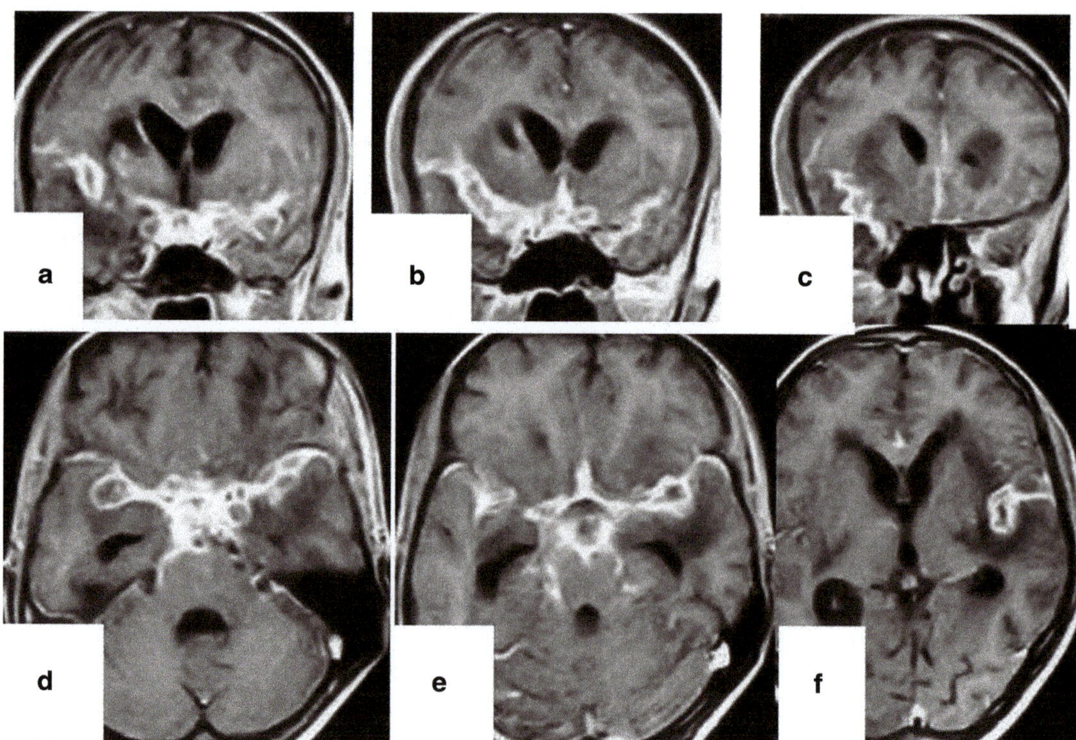

Fig. 8.1 Contrast MRI of the brain; (**a–c**) coronal images; (**d–f**) axial images showing numerous tubercular lesions in subarachnoid spaces (both Sylvian fissures, basal cisterns, prepontine cistern, etc., i.e., granulomatous basal meningitis)

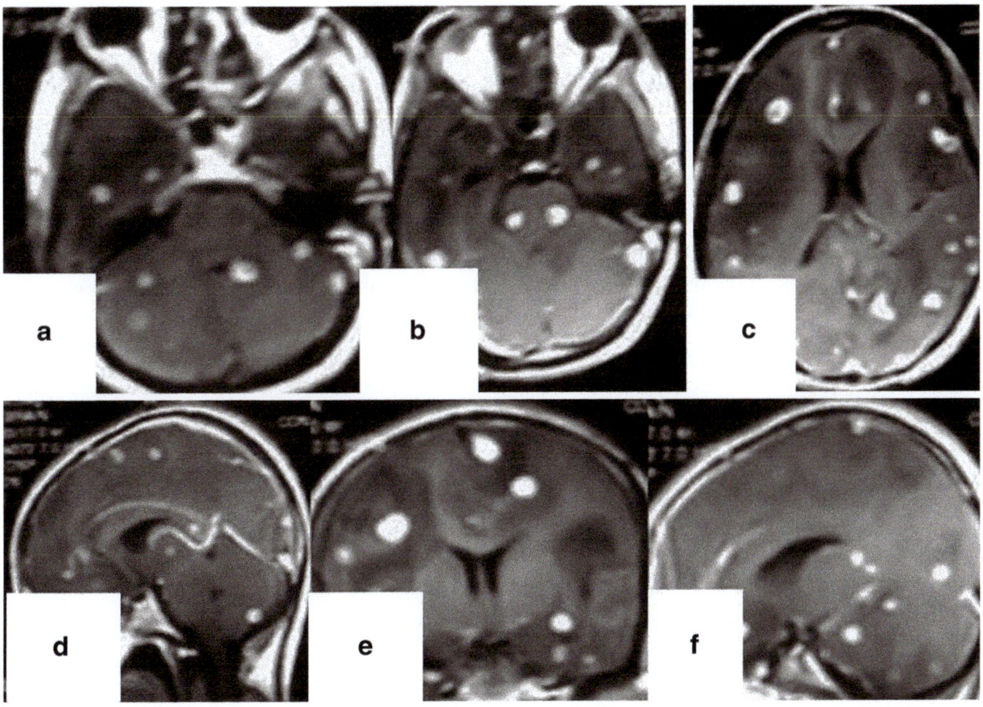

Fig. 8.2 Contrast MRI of the brain, (**a**–**c**) axial images; (**d**) sagittal and (**e**, **f**) coronal images showing "panencephalic miliary tuberculomatosis"

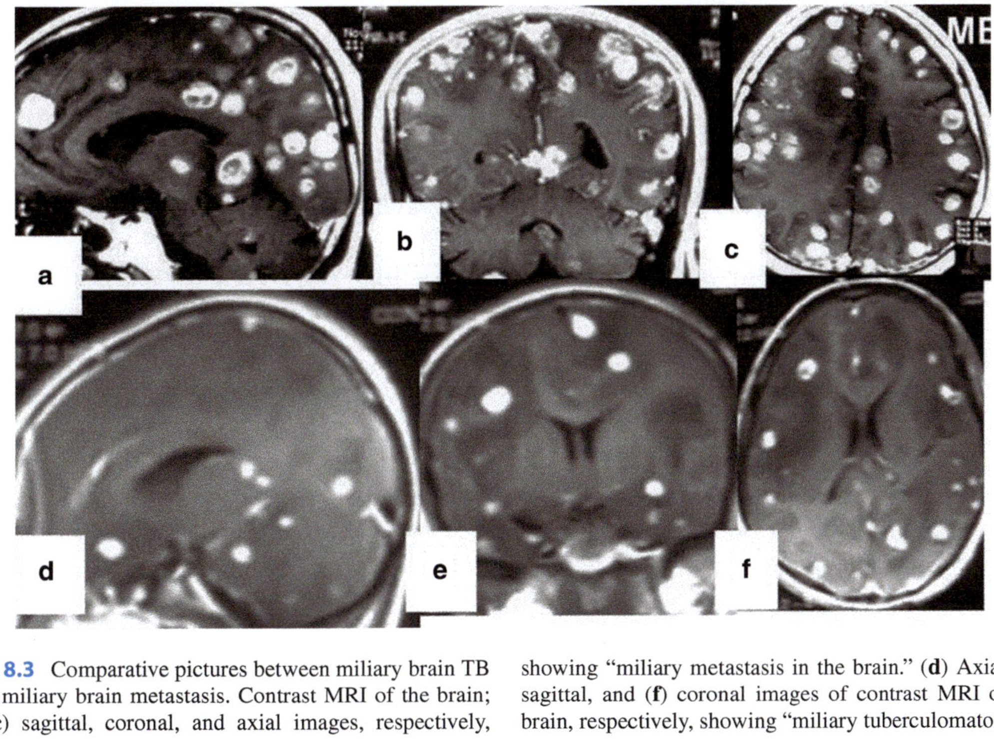

Fig. 8.3 Comparative pictures between miliary brain TB and miliary brain metastasis. Contrast MRI of the brain; (**a**–**c**) sagittal, coronal, and axial images, respectively, showing "miliary metastasis in the brain." (**d**) Axial, (**e**) sagittal, and (**f**) coronal images of contrast MRI of the brain, respectively, showing "miliary tuberculomatosis"

Prevention, and American Thoracic Society guidelines [39], includes an initial 2-month induction therapy regimen including isoniazid (INH), rifampin (RIF), pyrazinamide, and ethambutol, followed by 7–10 additional months of INH and RIF as maintenance therapy for an isolate that is sensitive to these agents. INH, RIF, and the second-line agents, aminoglycosides, capreomycin, and fluoroquinolones, are available in parenteral form if an altered mental status precludes oral intake. The recommended use of this regimen and the duration of therapy are extrapolated from the standard regimen for pulmonary TB, since no randomized control trial has established an optimal treatment course for CNS TB. Recommended duration of anti-TB therapy is at least 9–18 months, depending upon the patient's clinical and radiological response, but may have to be continued for longer or changed to second-line medications [36, 40, 41]. The treatment of multidrug resistance (MDR) and extensive drug resistance (XDR) TB is difficult, and it needs long drug therapy in special combination with first- and second-line drugs. Even in the expert hands, outcome is not good [39, 42–45]. The use of corticosteroids in the treatment of cerebral TB is a controversial issue. It reduces inflammation within the subarachnoid space [46, 47]. So far now, the manner in which dexamethasone affects the neuropathogenesis of CNS TB remains unknown, but the benefit clearly extends to children and adults with CNS TB [17, 39]. Anticonvulsant should be routinely used in cerebral TB due to high incidence of seizure (Fig. 8.4). Commonly used drugs are phenytoin, carbamazepine, oxcarbazepine, and sodium valproate. Phenytoin and INH can produce toxicity due to interaction [48].

Surgical Management (Figs. 8.5, 8.6, 8.7, 8.8, 8.9, 8.10, 8.11, 8.12, 8.13, 8.14, and 8.15) No other CNS infection has seen such a change in management principles as TB [5, 49]. Initial literature is filled with reports of successful treatments with surgical excision of tuberculomas up to mid-1980s, but with the introduction of better medications and with reports of equal or even better results with anti-TB therapy alone, the paradigm shifted toward nonsurgical management [50]. Patients in endemic areas were managed on the basis of clinical suspicion alone without the need for histological diagnosis. Neurosurgical intervention was restricted to stereotactic or CT-guided biopsies of suspect lesions or lesions not responding to medications [51]. Recent reports however suggest that medical therapy may be insufficient for complete cure of these lesions, with 20–46% of the lesions failing to resolve on prolonged (18 months) anti-TB therapy alone [27, 41]. It has been recommended that medical management be initiated for most tuberculomas which can be diagnosed with reasonable confidence based only on their clinical and radiological features [52, 53]. Whenever the diagnosis is suspect, the choice is between an empirical course of antituberculous therapy followed by repeat imaging, or a biopsy of the most superficial lesion in the least eloquent area is recommended [54, 55]. For biopsy, excision of the entire tuberculoma is always preferable if it can be done safely [55]. If lesions near eloquent areas need to be biopsied, stereotactic, neuronavigation, or ultrasound-guided aspirations are useful. For giant tuberculomas, or tuberculomas not responding to therapy, or tuberculomas causing significant mass effect, surgical excision should be considered. When more than one lesion is present, giant tuberculomas are excised [27]. An aggressive attitude toward these giant tuberculomas is due to the fact that these hardly ever resolve with medical therapy alone, require long duration of therapy, have a high risk of reactivation, and may show the paradoxical effect. Debulking of these lesions not only reduces bulk but also improves antibiotic penetration and lowers steroid requirements [27]. Partial excision of tuberculomas carries a higher risk of postoperative hemorrhage. The postoperative course is usually unremarkable. As a policy, biopsy is recommended for all suspected intracranial tuberculomas prior to initiation of chemotherapy [56]. Sometimes despite adequate antimicrobial coverage, the tuberculoma may increase in size, a phenomena referred to as the paradoxical response. This generally occurs over a period of 1–3 months after the commencement of chemotherapy [57]. Under such circumstances, serious thought should

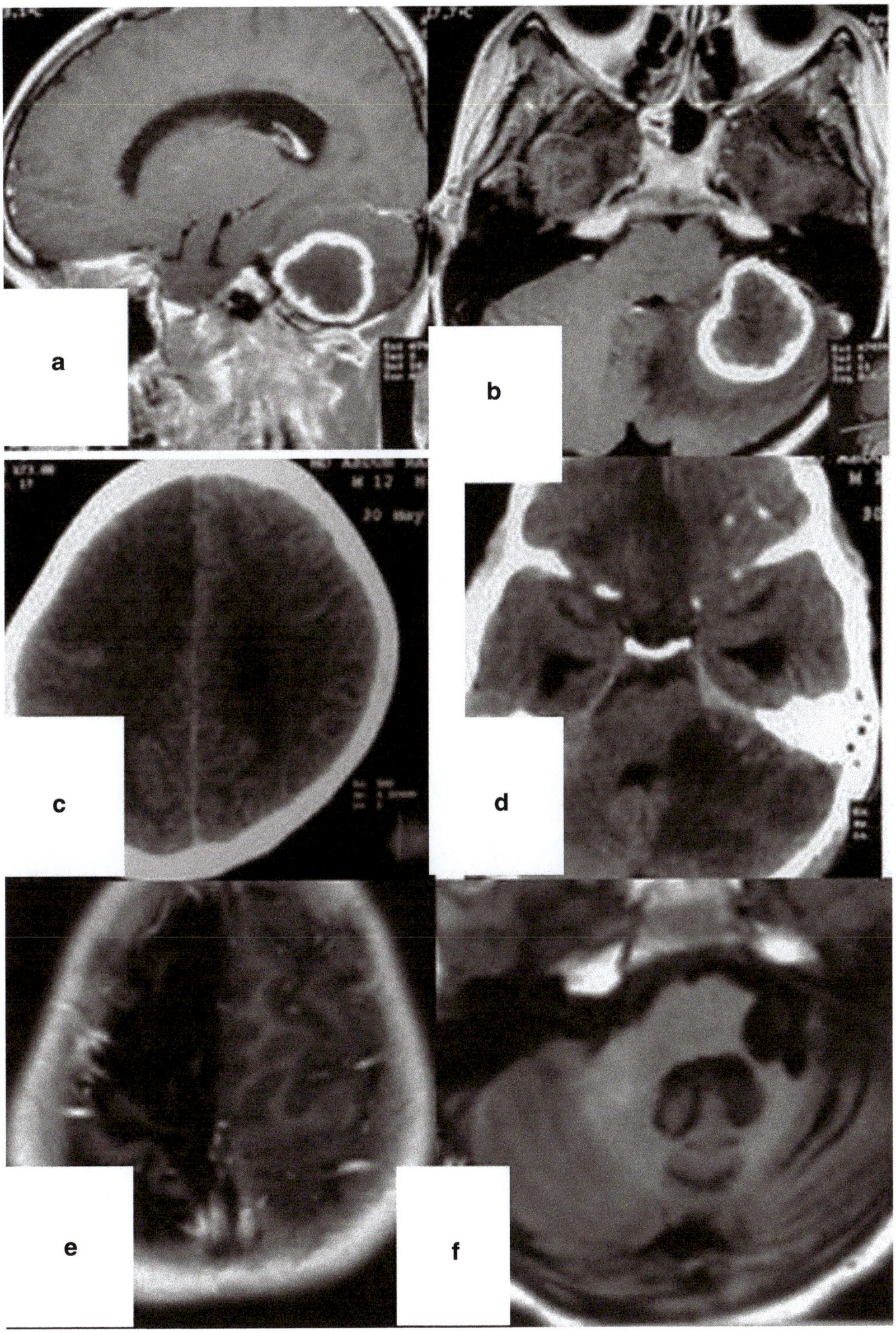

Fig. 8.4 (**a**, **b**) Contrast MRI of the brain in sagittal and axial images showing the large tuberculoma, cerebellum, and middle cerebellar peduncle extending in left cerebellopontine angle (CPA). (**c**, **d**) CT scan of the brain in 16th postoperative day after control of status epilepticus showing edema in the right frontal lobe and left CPA. (**e**) Postoperative contrast MRI axial image (6 months after operation and five and half months after status epilepticus) showing atrophy of the right frontal lobe. (**f**) Postoperative MRI of the brain 6 months after operation showing no residual lesion in the cerebellum and left CPA

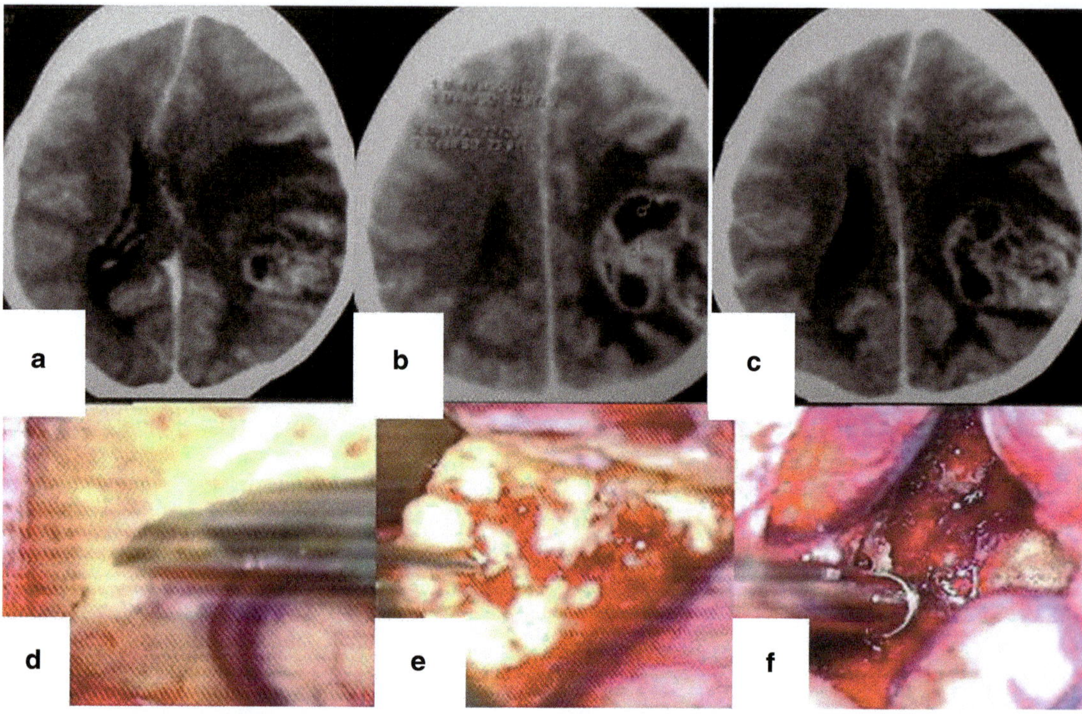

Fig. 8.5 Contrast CT scan of the brain; (**a–c**) axial images showing left frontoparietal TB mass with edema and ventricular effacement. (**d–f**) Per-operative images showing different steps of excision of the TB lesion

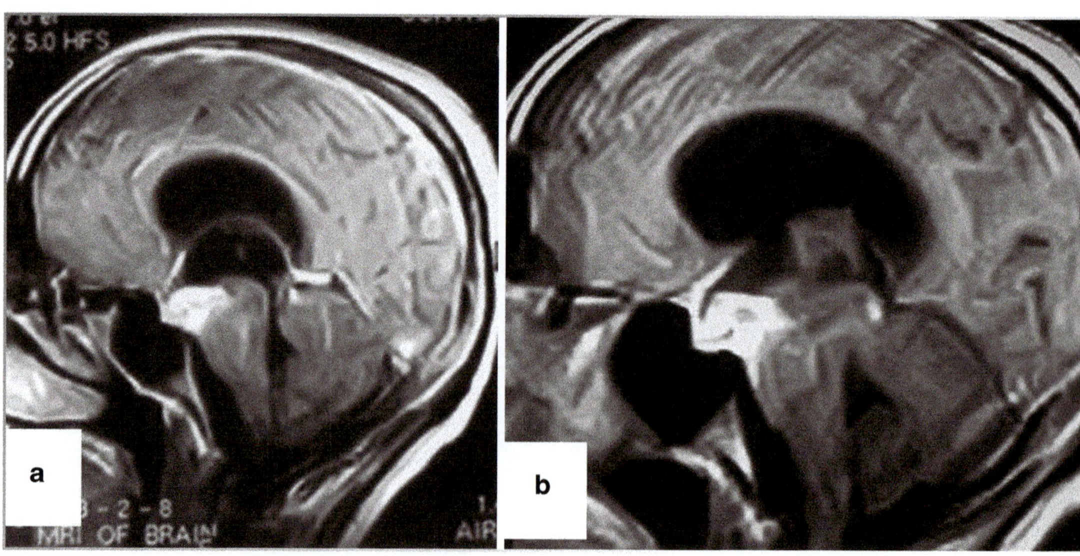

Fig. 8.6 Contrast MRI of the brain; (**a**, **b**) sagittal images and (**c**, **d**) axial images showing TB lesion (abscess was confirmed and drained endoscopically with biopsy. After endoscopic drainage, ETV was successfully done) in the floor of the third ventricle, hypothalamus, infundibulum, and interpeduncular fossa with triventriculomegaly

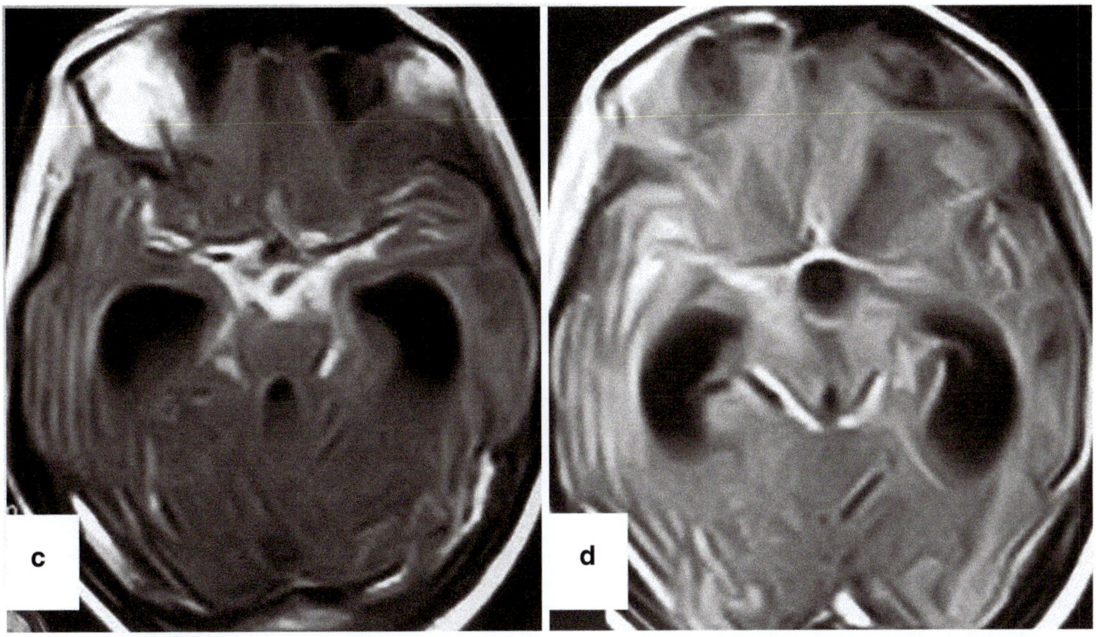

Fig. 8.6 (continued)

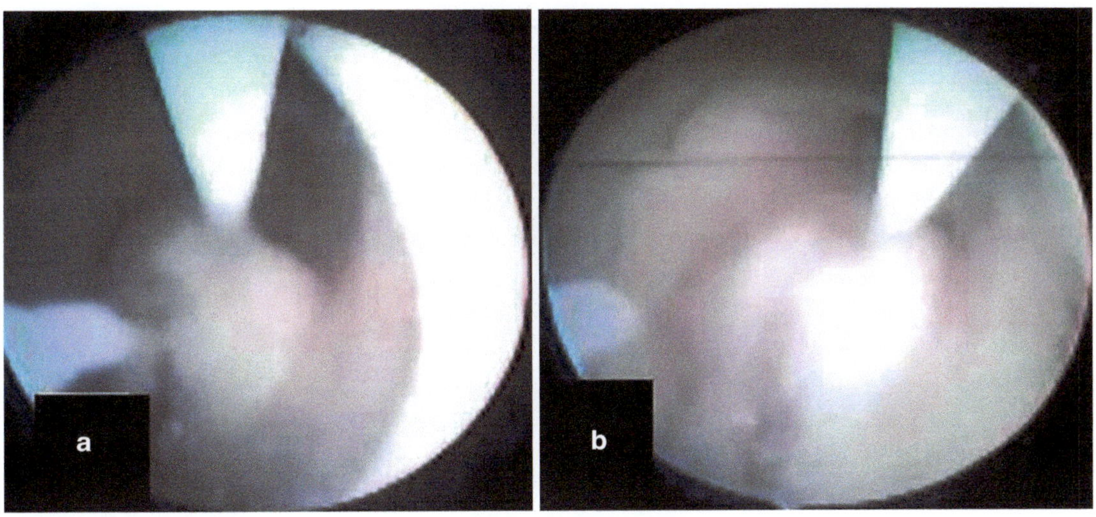

Fig. 8.7 (**a**, **b**) Per-operative pictures of Fig. 8.6 patient during endoscopic third ventricular intervention showing pus coming out from the TBA at the floor of the third ventricle (pus was carefully and slowly aspirated through "cut tip" Fogarty catheter, and finally an endoscopic third ventriculostomy was possible in this case)

be given to reconfirmation of diagnosis and/or excision of tuberculomas. Sequela of disease includes reactivation TB, drug resistance, hydrocephalus, seizures, and paradoxical response to antituberculous therapy [50]. Serial brain imaging is essential to determine the length of therapy. Surgery is indicated for both diagnosis and therapy of tuberculomas [48] or tubercular abscess. A tuberculoma/TBA that severely elevates intracranial pressure (ICP) and threatens life or vision merits emergent surgical excision. In addition, surgical intervention comes into consideration in

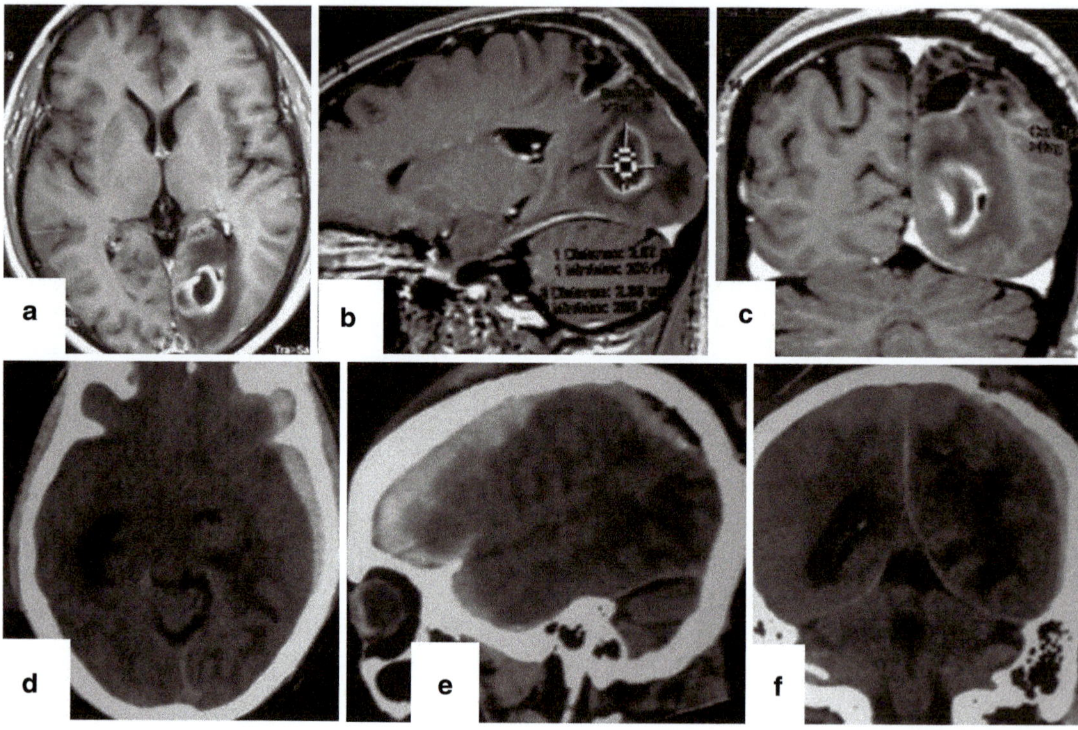

Fig. 8.8 Contrast MRI of the brain; (a) axial images, (b) sagittal images, and (c) coronal images showing left parieto-occipital TBA, recurred after surgical removal of parietal tuberculoma. CT scan of the brain after removal of parieto-occipital TBA; (d) axial images, (e) sagittal images, (f) coronal images showing development of acute subdural hematoma in early postoperative periods

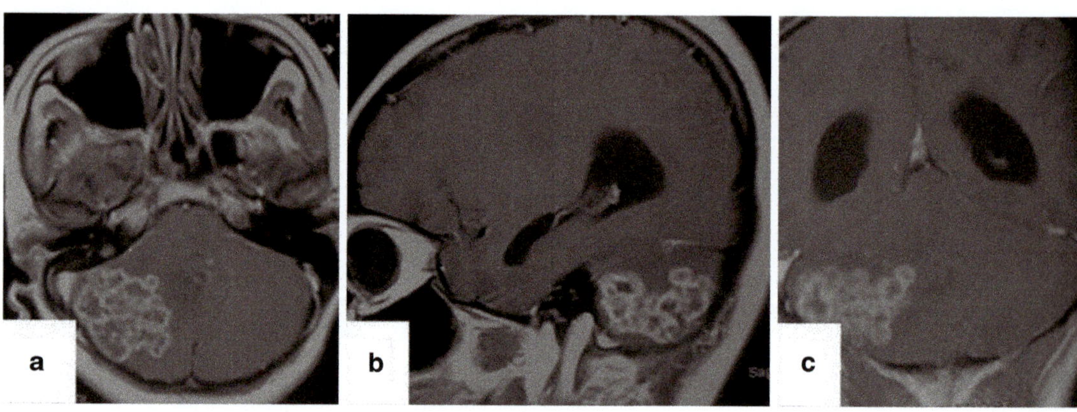

Fig. 8.9 Contrast MRI of the brain; (a) axial, (b) sagittal, and (c) coronal images showing right cerebellar hemispheric large TB lesion (multiple coalescing rings)

(1) patients who do not respond clinically or radiologically to anti-TB therapy; (2) patients whose diagnosis in doubt, such as those with atypical CT or MR images [58]; and (3) patients with obstructive hydrocephalus [48]. An insistence on total excision at the cost of undesirable neurological deficit is to be discouraged [48], though partial excision of tuberculomas carries a

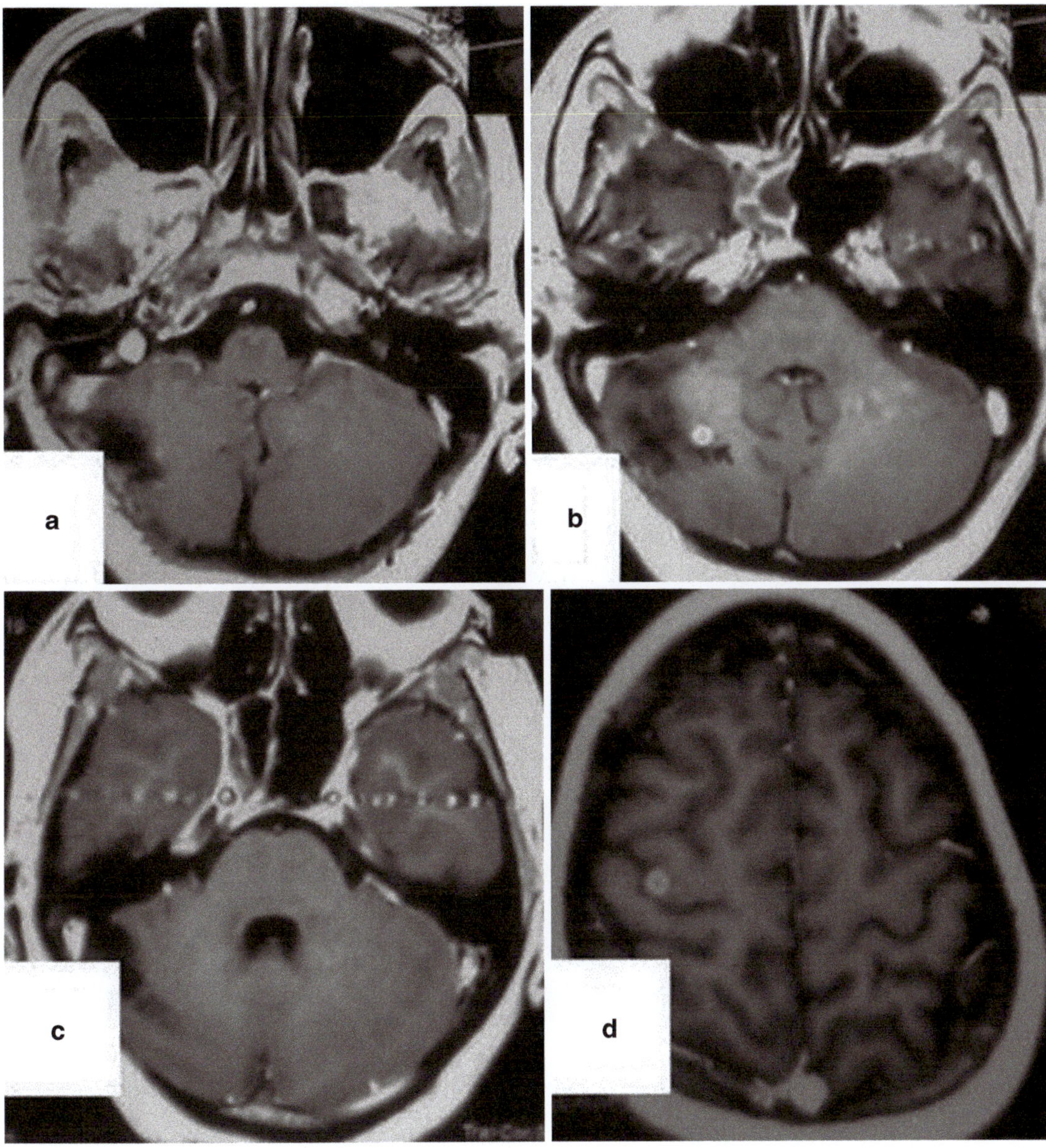

Fig. 8.10 Postoperative contrast MRI of patient of Fig. 8.9; (**a–d**) axial sections showing postoperative state in the right cerebellum and CPA with very small lesion in the right cerebellum and right frontal lobe

higher risk of postoperative hemorrhage [59]. The postoperative course is usually unremarkable [4]. Appropriate surgical treatment options for TBA include simple puncture, continuous drainage, fractional drainage, repeated aspiration through a burr hole, stereotactic aspiration, and total excision of the abscess [23] along with antiTB therapy. From our experiences, when suspected TBA, excision of the abscess gives the best outcome (Figs. 8.1, 8.6, 8.7, and 8.8). Hydrocephalus is an extremely common complication of CNS TB and can be treated with excision of mass lesion (i.e., tuberculomas or abscess), diuretics, osmotic agents, serial lumbar punctures, external ventricular drainage, ventriculoperitoneal shunts (VPS), and ETV [60]. More recently, there are encourag-

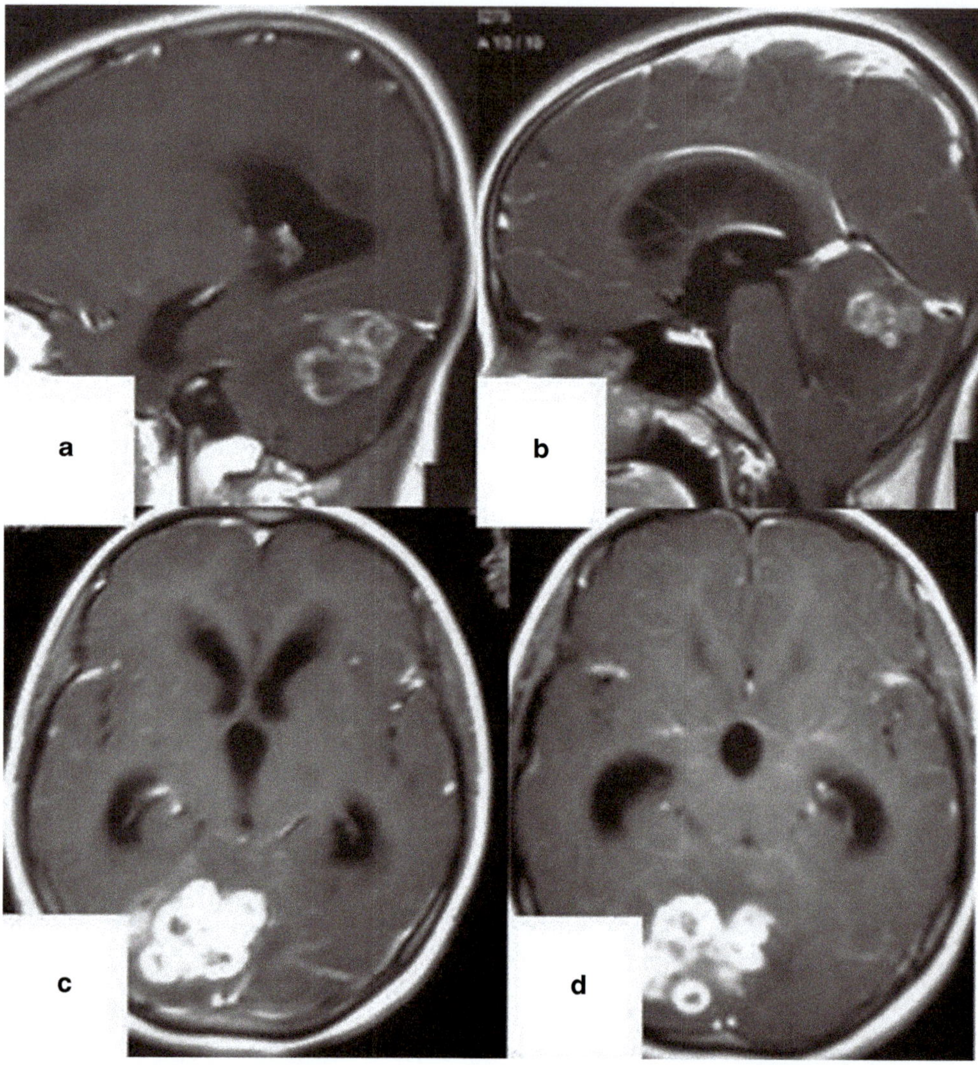

Fig. 8.11 Contrast MRI of the brain; (**a**, **b**) sagittal images and (**c**, **d**) coronal images showing multiple coalescing ring lesions (tuberculomas) in the cerebellum

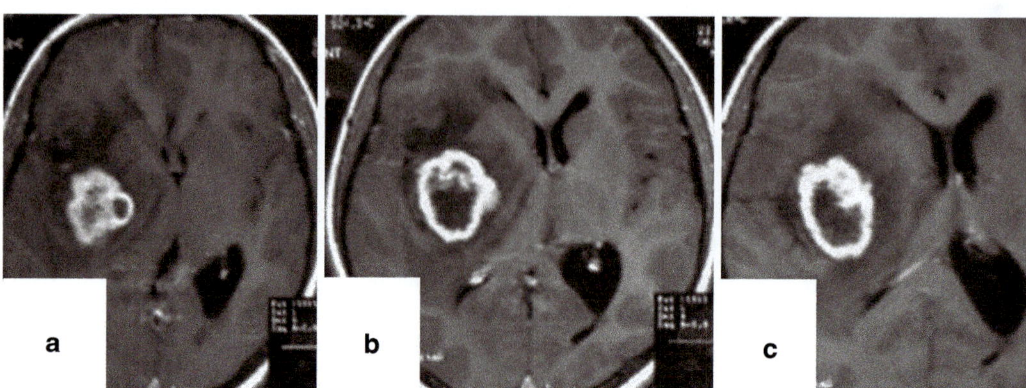

Fig. 8.12 (**a**–**c**) Contrast MRI of the brain showing large tuberculoma in right insulo-putaminal area

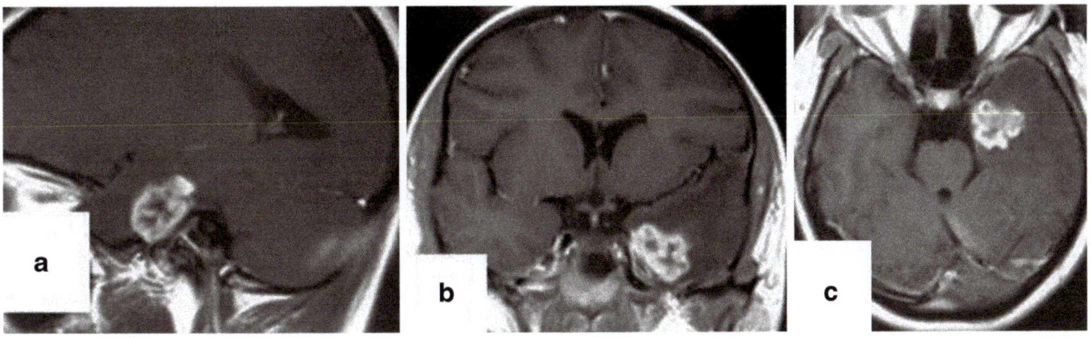

Fig. 8.13 Contrast MRI of the brain; (**a**) sagittal image, (**b**) coronal image, and (**c**) axial image showing left amygdalar tuberculoma (presented with severe form of temporal lobe epilepsy, excised completely with amygdalohippocampectomy)

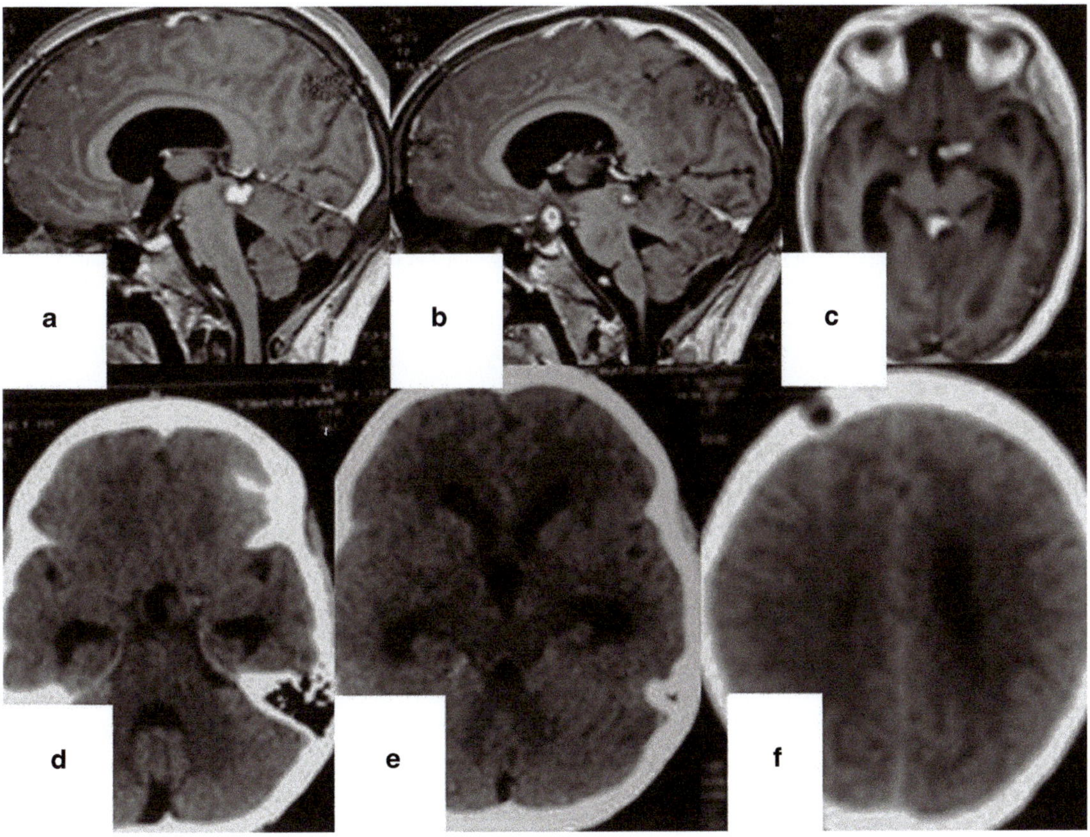

Fig. 8.14 Contrast MRI of the brain; (**a**, **b**) sagittal images and (**c**) axial image showing TB lesion in the infundibulo-hypothalamic region, midbrain tectal area causing triventriculomegaly, and other parts of the brain. (**d–f**) CT scan of the brain's axial sections after endoscopic third ventriculostomy (ETV)

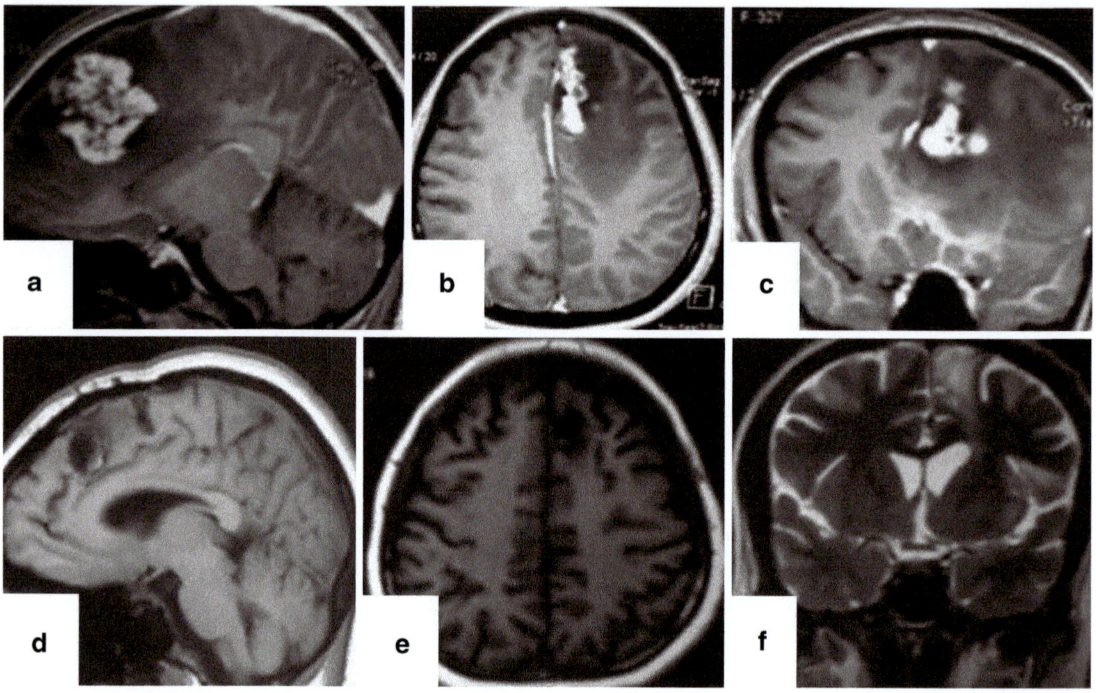

Fig. 8.15 Contrast MRI of the brain; (**a**) sagittal image, (**b**) axial image, and (**c**) coronal image showing large tuberculoma/s in the left medial frontal and superior frontal gyrus. Postoperative (3 months after operation) MRI of the brain; (**d**) sagittal image in T1W, (**e**) axial image in T1W, and (**f**) coronal image in T2W showing postoperative states at the operative field without mass affects and edema

ing data on the safety and efficacy of neuroendoscopy in relieving hydrocephalus in both adults [61] and infants [44] which may negate the need for VPS (Figs. 8.6, 8.7, 8.14, 8.16, 8.17, 8.18, 8.19, and 8.20). In the earlier part of our experiences, we frequently did surgery for cerebral (and cerebellar) tuberculomas, as experiences of increased rate of surgery went down as we learned more conservative way to treat the parenchymal TB lesions by empirical trial/anti-TB therapy. But when surgery is needed, we did radical excision biopsy even in eloquent areas. In this era of microsurgery and modern neurosurgical skill, post-excision neuro-deterioration is unlikely. We did the complete excision of the targeted lesion in almost all cases where surgery was needed or done without any neuro-deterioration.

8.2.6 Cerebral TB and Seizure (Figs. 8.4 and 8.13)

It is considered that tuberculoma in brain parenchyma is relatively less epileptogenic, but patient with CNS TB can present with seizure. But epilepsy the only presenting feature in CNS tuberculoma is rare [62, 63]. Tuberculoma causing seizure can usually manage by antiepileptic drugs. Tuberculoma with only intractable epilepsy is further rare. Tuberculoma in the medial temporal lobe can rarely cause intractable seizure which can respond surgery followed by anti-TB therapy [62]. Chowdhury et al. [64] reported development of postoperative (on 14th postoperative day) status epilepticus in a pediatric patient where large cerebellopontine angle (CPA) tuberculoma (in cer-

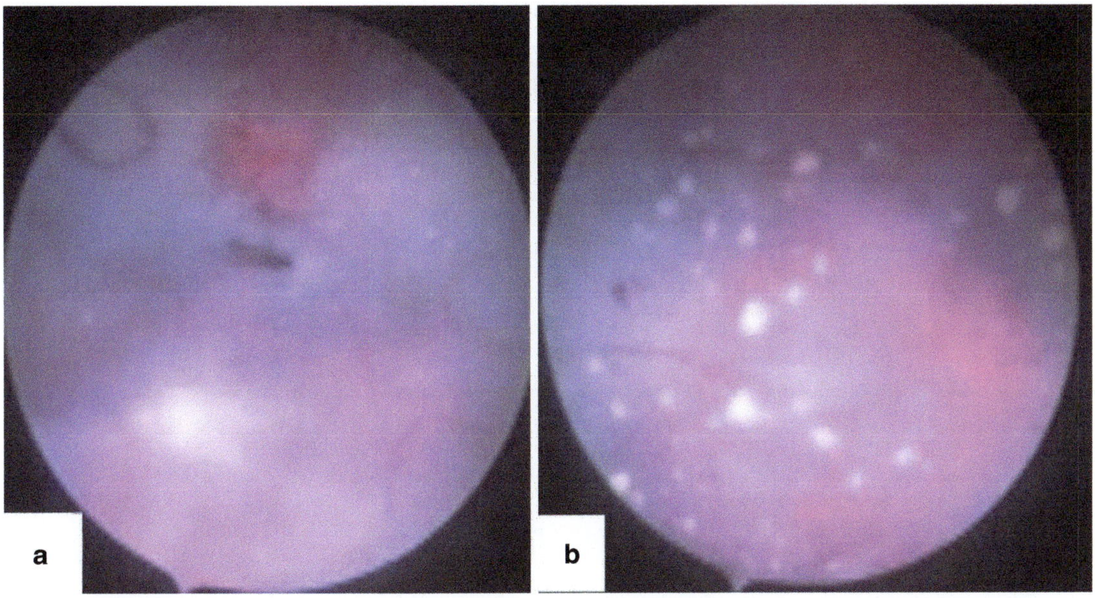

Fig. 8.16 (**a**, **b**) Per-operative pictures during endoscopic ETV and ventriculoscopy showing numerous tuberculomas on the floor of the third ventricle

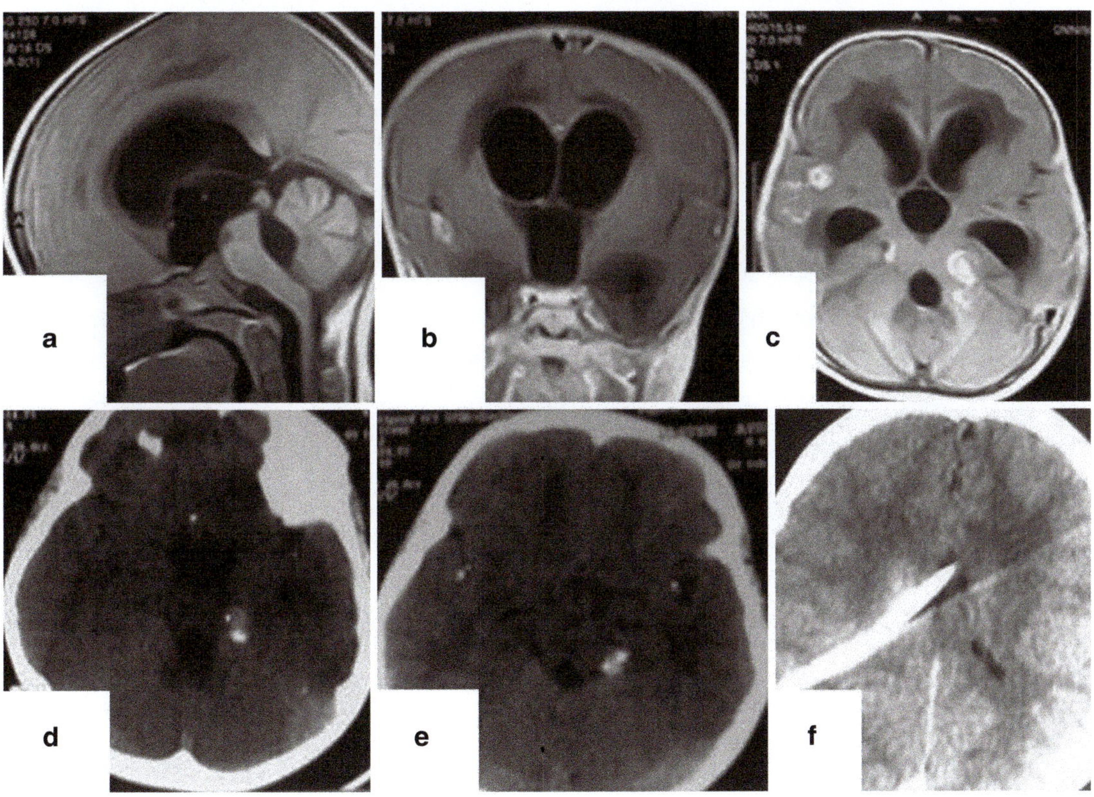

Fig. 8.17 Contrast MRI of the brain; (**a**) sagittal image, (**b**) coronal image, and (**c**) axial image showing post-TBM communicating hydrocephalus with multiple TB lesions in the brain and subarachnoid spaces in patient 18 months of age. (**d–f**) CT scan of the brain at the age of 20 months after ventriculoperitoneal shunt and ongoing anti-TB therapy showing resolution of hydrocephalus, but there is asymptomatic fourth ventricular entrapment

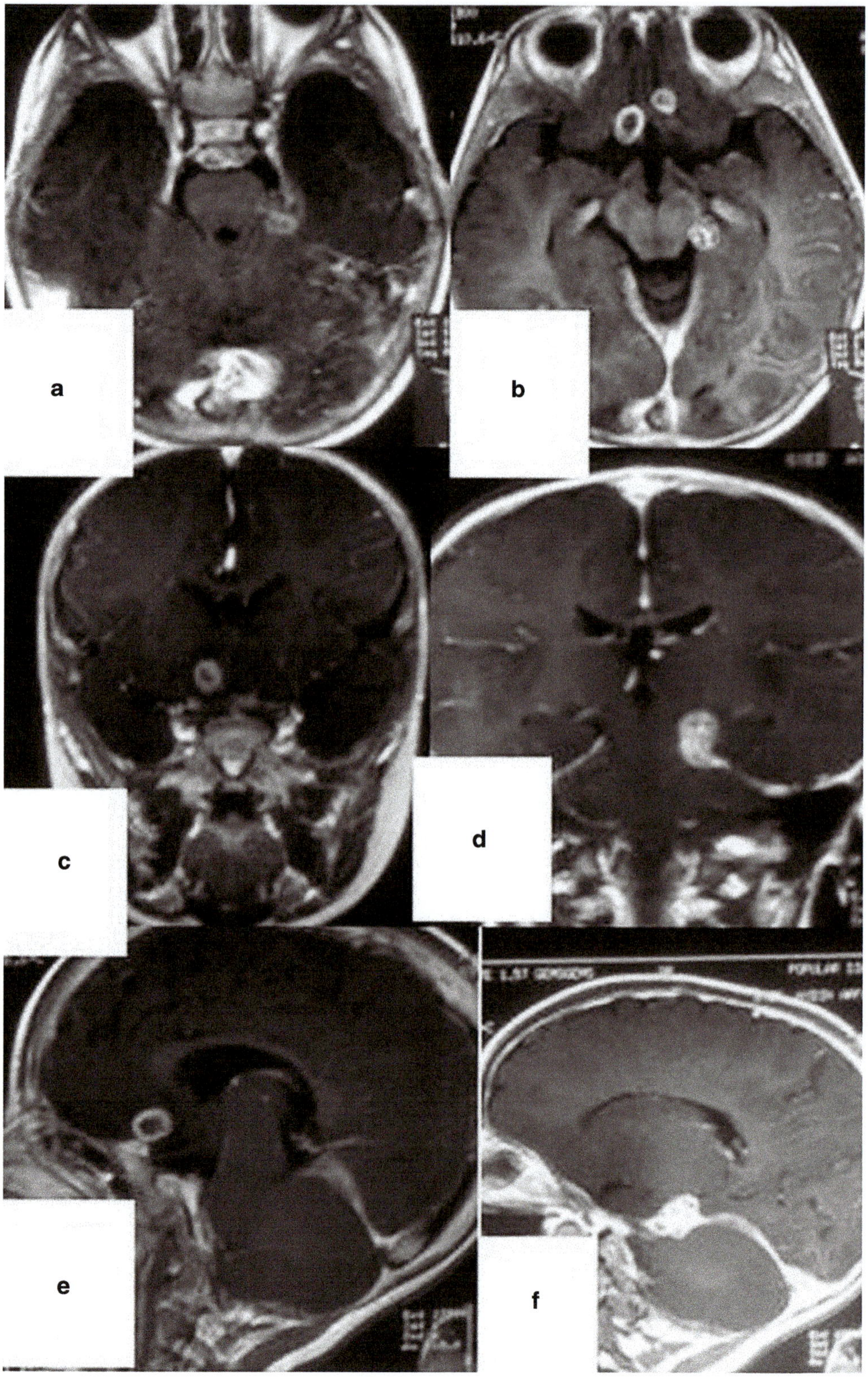

Fig. 8.18 Contrast MRI of the brain at the age of 19 months after VP shunt and ongoing anti-TB therapy; (**a**, **b**) axial images, (**c**, **d**) coronal images, and (**e**, **f**) sagittal images showing resolution of hydrocephalus with persistent tuberculomas in different parts of the brain

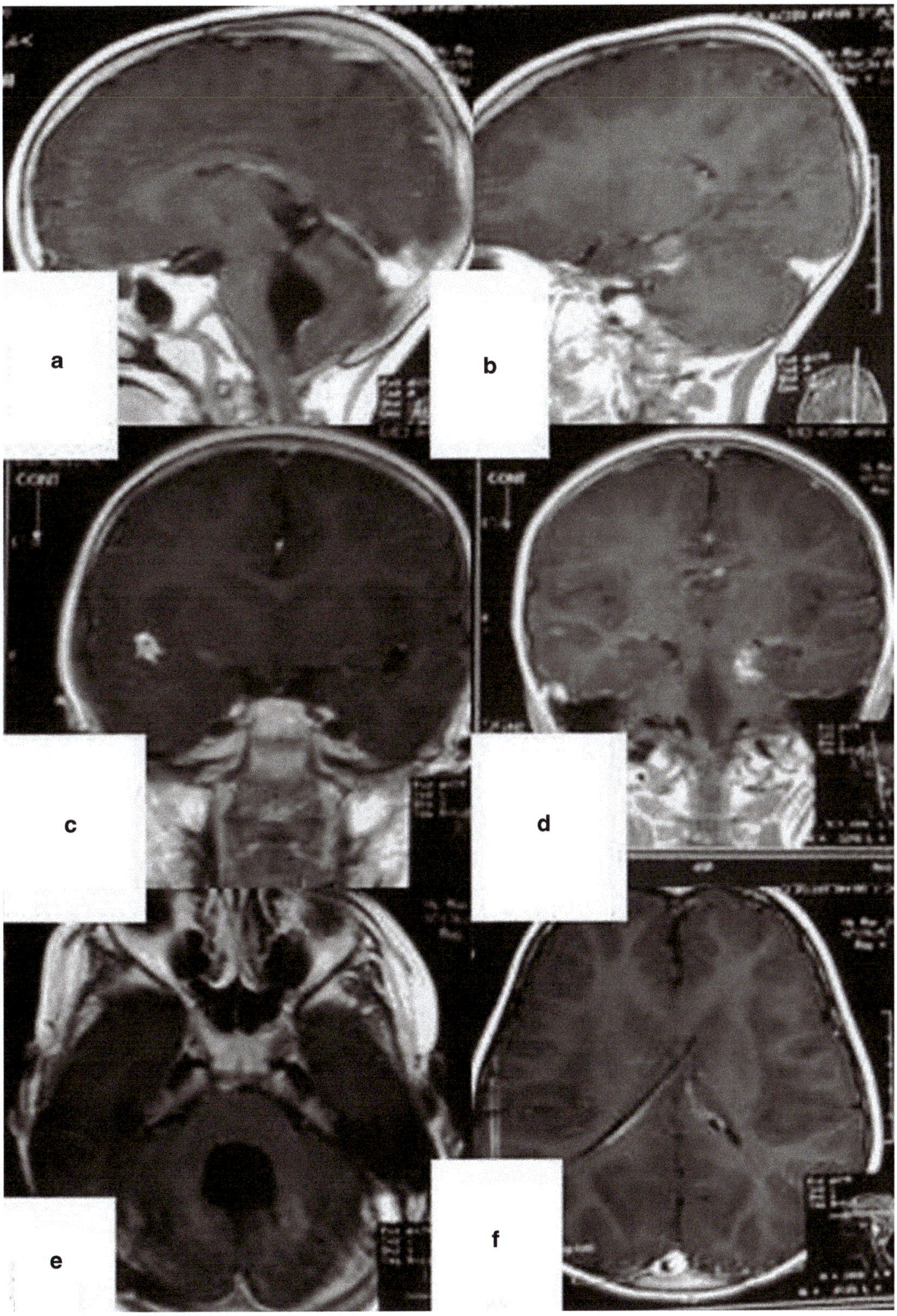

Fig. 8.19 Contrast MRI of the brain at the age of 24 months after VP shunt and ongoing anti-TB therapy; (**a**, **b**) sagittal images, (**c**, **d**) coronal images, and (**e**, **f**) axial images showing resolution of hydrocephalus and resoluting tuberculomas in different parts of the brain

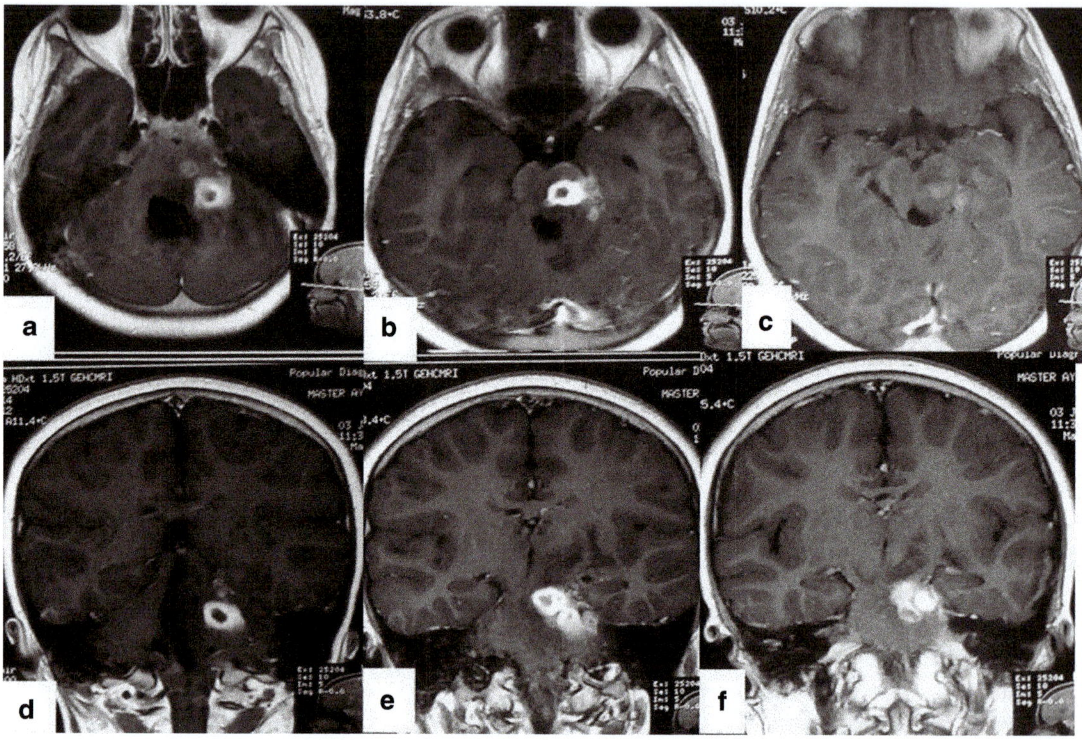

Fig. 8.20 Contrast MRI of the brain at the age of 6 years (the patient developed ataxia and repeated fall); (**a**–**c**) axial images and (**d**–**f**) coronal images showing recurrent tuberculoma in brachium pontis and pons

ebellum) was surgically removed who had a small tuberculoma in the frontal cortex. In this patient, postoperative status epilepticus might be caused by any preexisting cortical lesion, by the ongoing anti-TB drug therapy or by the potentiating effect of both. Anti-TB drugs, especially isoniazid, can cause tonic-clonic seizures by the impairment of pyridoxine metabolism. In the early postoperative period, the patient's status epilepticus was probably due to the combined effect of a frontal lobe lesion and the action of anti-TB drugs that caused severe edema in that lobe and contralateral hemiplegia that recovered slowly and incompletely along with frontal lobe atrophy [64].

8.2.7 Results and Follow-Up

Intracranial tuberculomas usually carry a favorable prognosis, and the predictors of poor outcome include coma at presentation and evidence of miliary TB [65]. Majority of patients make complete recovery although some may have neurological deficits [4]. Initial reports of mortality ranged from 10% to 27%. But the results have dramatically improved in recent years [48]. Early diagnosis and appropriate treatment usually prevent complications such as hydrocephalus, infarct, and paradoxical affect. But the development of sequelae and complications may be delayed, so close monitoring following the initiation of antiTB therapy is essential. Follow-up CT scans at 1 week and 1 month after the initial CT scan have been shown to be particularly important in picking up important diagnostic findings and adverse sequelae in children with CNS TB [66].

8.2.8 Prognosis

The identified predictors of poor outcome in cerebral TB are advanced stage of the disease at presentation, age, and the presence of any infarction other than a purely hemispheric infarction, an HIV coinfection, and the combination of INH and RIF resistance [45, 67].

8.3 TB of Deep Structures of the Brain

8.3.1 TB of the Basal Ganglia

The basal ganglia comprise the lentiform nucleus (putamen and globus pallidus) and caudate nucleus. Isolated lentiform nucleus TB (Fig. 8.12) and isolated caudate nucleus TB are probably very rare and usually involved with other parts of CNS. Lesion in caudate nucleus usually causes chorea. Various types of movement disorders parkinsonism, extrapyramidal syndrome, tremor, chorea, dystonia, myoclonus, hemiballismus can occur in cerebral TB due to involvement of the lentiform nucleus, caudate nucleus, thalamus, subthalamus, and red nucleus [68]. Alarcon et al. [69] studied 180 patients with cerebral TB among whom 30 patients developed various movement disorders. After completion of anti-TB therapy (24 months), seven patients had chorea, three dystonia, and twenty tremor. One of the patients with tremor also had myoclonus, and one with dystonia had tremor. The average age of the patients with chorea was lower than that of the patients with dystonia and tremor. Two patients with chorea, one with dystonia, and three patients with tremor died. The patients with chorea and dystonia had more severe disease. They found little correlation between the types, distribution, or severity of abnormal movements and CT scan or MRI findings. They concluded that tremor is the most common movement disorder. Chorea is more frequently found in young children. Deep vascular lesions are more common among patients with movement disorders [69].

8.3.2 Diencephalic TB

Isolated hypothalamic tuberculoma or TBA is very rare (Figs. 8.6 and 8.7). The hypothalamus can be affected by the tubercular lesion in hypothalamus proper, third ventricle of the suprasellar region. Pathogenesis is the same of cerebral TB as described earlier [17]. Clinical features include general features of TB, headache, vomiting, visual disturbances, altered level of consciousness, behavioral changes, cachexia, memory disturbances, pituitary hypofunctions, precocious puberty in children, diabetes insipidus, seizure, etc. [2, 70]. Diagnosis is mainly based on suspicion, and confirmation is only possible by histological examination tissue specimen from the lesion by microsurgical excision, endoscopic biopsy, or stereotactic cases. Early surgery is useful in visual disturbances caused by the pressure of tubercular mass on optic apparatus and in obstructive hydrocephalus. Management of epilepsy, hypopituitarism, and diabetes insipidus is needed along with anti-TB therapy in indicated cases. Overall management strategy is conservative [17].

The thalamus is usually involved with other parts of CNS in TB (Fig. 8.21). Isolated thalamic TB is very rare [71]. Tuberculoma and TB abscess are the two forms of thalamic TB. Clinical fea-

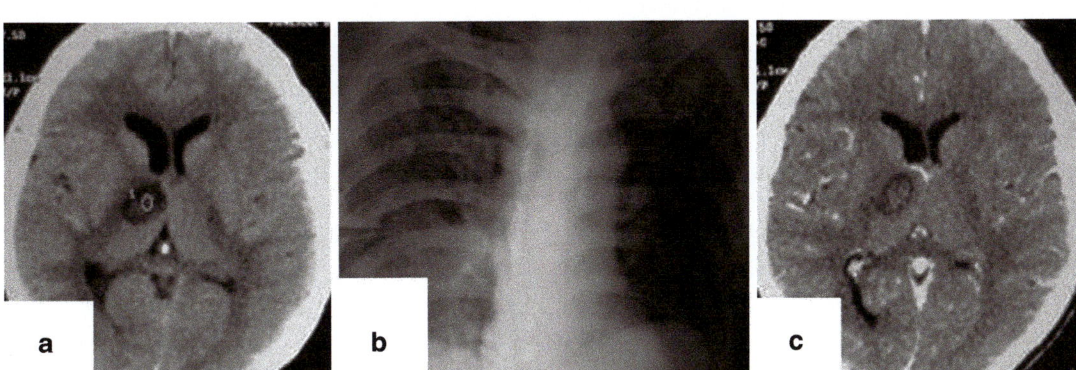

Fig. 8.21 (**a**) CT scan of the brain axial image showing right internal capsular (genu) and anterior thalamic tuberculoma with edema. (**b**) X-ray chest PA view with pulmonary TB. (**c**) CT scan of the brain axial image 6 weeks after anti-TB therapy where edema reduced significantly with clinical improvement of left hemiplegia

tures are like that of thalamic tumor, i.e., features of rised ICP, motor deficit, seizure, behavioral changes, memory disturbances, visual disturbances, etc. [71]. Differential diagnosis of thalamic tuberculoma includes low-grade astrocytoma, glioma, ependymoma, neuroectodermal tumor, lymphoma, metastasis, etc. CT or MRI is the investigation that can show the TB lesion in the thalamus, but no features of CT or MRI are diagnostic. Treatment is usually anti-TB therapy either empirical in suspected cases or after tissue biopsy. Biopsy is obtained by endoscopically or stereotactically or after open surgical excision. Indications of surgery are like that of other parts of CNS. Antiepileptic and steroid are usually prescribed with anti-TB drugs [71]. TB lesion affecting only the subthalamus is very rare, usually affected with other parts of hemisphere and can present with hemiballismus [72]. After diagnosis full-course anti-TB therapy can cure the condition. The subthalamus is usually affected with the thalamus, midbrain, and third ventricle. Isolated epithalamic or metathalamic TB are yet to be reported, and they are usually affected along with other parts of CNS, i.e., the thalamus and third ventricle.

8.4 Cerebellar TB

8.4.1 Introduction

Common site for tuberculoma is cerebellar hemispheres in children, due to the large blood supply to these areas [5]. TB granuloma (tuberculoma) is the most common form of cerebellar parenchymal lesion [58]. Tuberculoma can occur at all age group; however, its incidence is higher in pediatric population [73]. Though solitary tuberculoma is seen occasionally, multiple grape-like tuberculomas are rare which develop as a result of coalescence of multiple small immature tuberculomas and resemble a cluster of neurocysticercosis cyst [74]. Cerebellar involvement in CNS tuberculoma is rare. In a series of 23 CNS tuberculoma cases, Bayindir et al. could detect only two cases of cerebellar involvement [75].

8.4.2 Pathogenesis

These are usually located at the corticomedullary junction and periventricular region, as expected for hematogenous dissemination. They are mostly infratentorial in children. The pathogenesis of cerebellar tuberculoma or tubercular abscess is same as that of supratentorial cerebral tuberculoma or abscess [76, 77]. Isolated TBM in posterior fossa does not occur; posterior fossa meningitis is always part of global meningitis. Types of TB in cerebellum are as follows: (1) meningitis (part of global TBM), (2) tuberculoma, and (3) TBA.

8.4.3 Common Sites (Figs. 8.4, 8.9, 8.10, and 8.11) and Differential Diagnosis (Fig. 8.3)

TB lesion in cerebellum can occur in cerebellar hemispheres, vermis, and subependymal zone near the fourth ventricle and cerebellar peduncle. They can occur in CPA or part of cerebellum near to CPA mimicking CPA tumor [6]. Cerebellar tuberculoma may be associated with supratentorial or spinal tuberculomas [75, 77]. Like supratentorial tuberculoma the differential diagnosis of cerebellar tuberculomas or TBA are metastasis, glioma or lymphoma, pyogenic abscess, toxoplasmosis, neurocysticercosis, sarcoidosis, hydatidosis, and late syphilitic involvement of CNS [77].

8.4.4 Clinical Presentation

Infratentorial tuberculoma is a life-threatening condition. The clinical manifestations of cerebellar TB included various combinations of focal signs and symptoms of subacute onset, similar to those produced by other space-occupying lesions in the brain stem and cerebellum [78]. Like other intracranial mass, cerebellar TB lesion commonly presents with headache, vomiting and visual disturbances, and altered level of consciousness. Infratentorial tuberculomas may present with brain stem syndromes, cerebellar signs, and multiple lower cranial nerve palsies apart from obstructive hydrocephalus [74, 79]. Concomitant extracranial TB is present in 30–50% cases, but tuberculoma is not often associated with TBM.

8.4.5 Diagnosis

Diagnosis can be made by the combination of clinical features, neuroimaging, mycobacterial DNA test, and response to treatment [76]. The gold standard of diagnosis remains on demonstration of hallmark of TB "tubercular granuloma" after histopathological examination of biopsy from tuberculoma/abscess wall or demonstration of innumerable tubercle bacilli in aspirated pus from tubercular abscess [79].

8.4.6 Treatment

Drug therapy Anti-TB drug therapy is like that of cerebral TB therapy as mentioned earlier. In non-resistance cases, the authors practiced initial 3-month four-drug combination therapy followed by RIF and INH therapy for 15–21 months. Antiepileptic therapy is not usually required in isolated cerebellar TB. The principle of steroid therapy is like that of other CNS TB.

Surgical therapy Principles of surgical therapy are like other CNS TB discussed in cerebral TB part of this chapter [4, 17]. But in author's opinion, patient with cerebellar TB where tuberculoma or abscess produced obstructive hydrocephalus, brain stem compression, and altered level of consciousness should be operated on emergency basis: (a) to remove the mass, (b) to relieve brain stem compression, (c) to confirm the diagnosis, and (d) to establish the normal CSF pathway.

8.5 TB of the Cerebellar Peduncle (Fig. 8.22)

Three cerebellar peduncles connect the cerebellum to brain stem. The middle cerebellar peduncle is the largest and connect cerebellum with pons. TB (tuberculoma and TBA) in the cerebellar peduncle usually occurs from the cerebellum or from the brain stem by direct extension. The middle cerebellar peduncle is commonly affected. Rarely the middle cerebellar peduncle can solely be affected by TB [46, 80]. Clinical manifestation of the cerebral peduncle TB is like that of signs and symptoms of cerebellar lesion such as slurred speech, incoordination, progressive difficulty in walking developed, dysarthria with scanning speech, gait ataxia, horizontal nystagmus, dysmetria, etc. [80]. Diagnosis and treatment are same like TB of other parts of CNS.

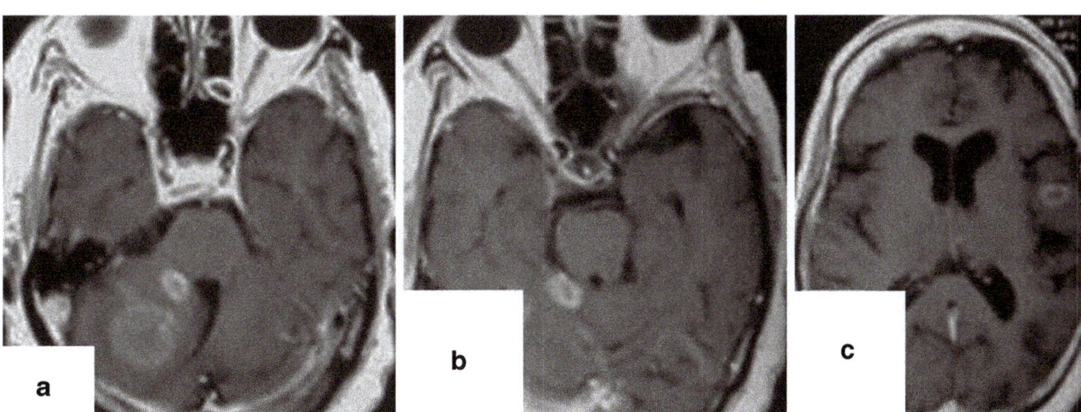

Fig. 8.22 (**a–c**) Contrast MRI of the brain in axial sections showing tuberculomas in the right side of the cerebellum, right superior and middle cerebellar peduncle, and left superior temporal gyrus

8.6 Prevention

Currently, BCG vaccination covers 85% of newborn infants, and it has been estimated that nearly 100 million children are vaccinated with BCG vaccine every year. Several studies have shown that BCG protects against TBM and that its efficacy is around 75–85% [17]. The efficacy of BCG appears to persist through 10 years after infant vaccination [81].

Conclusion

CNS TB specially cerebral or cerebellar TB is a very serious form of TB that can occur in various forms and can cause mortality and morbidity in endemic developing countries and also in developed countries due to emergences of AIDS and other immunocompromised conditions. Even in this modern era of medical sciences, sometimes diagnosis is very challenging. Trial anti-TB therapy has definitive management role in endemic areas of TB. In the treatment of brain TB, though surgery has definitive indications and role, paradigm shifted toward the conservative drug therapy. XDR and MDR TB of brain are extremely difficult conditions to treat and need special attention and special team.

References

1. Sathyanarayana S, Baskaya MK, Fowler M, Roberts R, Nanda A (2003) Solitary tuberculoma of the cerebellopontine angle: a rare presentation. J Clin Neurosci 10:120–122
2. Dutta P, Bhansali A, Singh P (2006) Pituitary Suprasellar tubercular abscess presenting as panhypopituitarism: a common lesion in an uncommon site, a brief review of literature. Pituitary 9:73–77
3. Zuger A (2004) Tubeculosis. In: Scheld WM, Whitley RJ, Mara CM (eds) Infections of central nervous system, 3rd edn. Lippincott-Raven Publishers, New York, pp 441–460
4. Shamim MS, Enam SA, Ali RP, Ali SF, Wasay M (2009) Overview of surgical management of Infectious non-suppurative brain lesions (part 1). Pak J Neurol Sci 4:77–82
5. Arvind C, Korath MP, Raveendranadhan K, Jagadeesan K (1993) A retrospective study of 1247 cases of intracranial tuberculomata diagnosed by computerized tomography. J Assoc Physicians India 41:559–561
6. Bishburg E, Sunderam G, Beichman LB, Kapila R (1986) Central nervous system TB with the acquired immunodeficiency syndrome and its related complex. Ann Med Interne 105:201–213
7. Prabhakar S, Thussu A (1997) Central nervous system TB. Neurol India 45:132–140
8. Grimud-Ayina M, Fari O, Lortholary O, Cruaud P, Kettaneh A, Stirnemann J, Hornstein M, Robineau M, Le Pennec MP, Boudon P, Malbec D, Mechali D, Desrues J, Glowinski J, Guillevin L, Thomas M (2002) Neuromeningeal TB in northeastern suburbs of Paris. Nineteen cases. Ann Med Interne (Paris) 153:75–81
9. Mazodier K, Bernit E, Faure V, Rovery C, Gayet S, Seux V, Donnet A, Bouqui P, Disdier P, Schleinitz N, Kaplanski G, Veit V, Harle JR (2003) Central nervous TB in patients non-HIV: seven case reports. Rev Med Interne 24:78–85
10. Wang JT, Hung CC, Sheng WH, Wang JT, Hung CC, Sheng WH, Wang JY, Chang SC, Luh KT (2002) Prognosis of TB meningitis in adults in the era of modern antituberculous chemotherapy. J Microbiol Immunol Infect 35:215–222
11. de Castro CC, de Barros NG, Campos ZM, Cerre GG (1995) CT scans of cranial TB. Radiol Clin North Am 33:753–769
12. Wallace RC, Brutons EM, Beret FF, Wallace RC, Burton EM, Barrett FF, Laggiadro RJ, Gerald BE, Lasater OE (1991) Intracranial TB in children. CT appearance and clinical outcome. Pediatr Radiol 21:241–246
13. Kaojarern S, Supmonchai K, Phuapradit P, Mokkhavesa C, Krittiyanunt S (1991) Effect of steroids on cerebrospinal fluid penetration of antituberculous drugs in tuberculous meningitis. Clin Pharmacol Ther 49:6–12
14. Bhargava TPN (1980) Intracranial tuberculomas: a CT study. Br J Radiol 53:935–945
15. Welchman JM (1979) CT of intracranial tuberculomata. Clin Radiol 30:567–579
16. Turgut M, Özcan OE, Özgen T, Sağlam S, Bertan V, Erbengi A (1989) Tuberculomas of the craniospinal axis. Turk Neurosurg 1:34–38
17. Rock RB, Olin M, Baker CA, Molitor TW, Piterson PK (2008) Central nervous system TB: pathogenesis and clinical aspects. Clin Microbiol Rev 21:243–261
18. Ulrichs T, Kaufmann SHE (2004) Cell-mediated immune response. In: Rom WN, Garay SM (eds) Tuberculosis, 2nd edn. Lippincott Williams & Wilkins, Philadelphia, pp 251–262
19. Chowdhury FH, Haque MR, Alam MSM (2013) Third ventricular and interpeduncular fossa tubercular abscess with triventriculomegaly – ventriculoscopic surgical management. J Medicine 14:72–73
20. Rich AR, McCordock HA (1933) The pathogenesis of tuberculous meningitis. Bull Johns Hopkins Hosp 52:5–37
21. Khoo JLS, Lau KY, Cheung CM, Tsoi TH (2003) Central nervous system TB. J HK Coll Radiol 6:217–228

22. Shah GV (2000) Central nervous system TB. Neuroimaging Clin N Am 10:355–374
23. Kumar R, Pandey CK, Bose N, Sahay S (2002) Tuberculous brain abscess: clinical presentation, pathophysiology and treatment (in children). Childs Nerv Syst 18:118–123
24. Brooks JB, Daneshvar MI, Haberberger RL, Mikhail IA (1990) Rapid diagnosis of tuberculous meningitis by frequency-pulsed electron-capture gas-liquid chromatography detection of carboxylic acids in cerebrospinal fluid. J Clin Microbiol 28:989–997
25. Sutlas PN, Unal A, Forta H, Senol S, Kirbas D (2003) Tuberculous meningitis in adults: review of 61 cases. Infection 31:387–391
26. Chatterjee S (2011) Brain tuberculomas, tubercular meningitis, and post-tubercular hydrocephalus in children. J Pediatr Neurosci 6(Suppl S1):96–100
27. Poonnoose SI, Rajshekhar V (2003) Rate of resolution of histologically verified intracranial tuberculomas. Neurosurgery 53:873–878
28. Katti MK (2004) Pathogenesis, diagnosis, treatment, and outcome aspects of cerebral TB. Med Sci Monit 10:RA215–RA229
29. Gupta RK, Jena A, Sharma DK, Guha DK, Khushru S, Gupta AK (1988) MR imaging of intracranial tuberculomas. J Comput Assist Tomogr 12:280–285
30. Jinkins JR, Gupta R, Chang KH, Rodriguez-Carbajal J (1995) MR imaging of central nervous system TB. Radiol Clin North Am 33:771–786
31. Bernaerts A, Vanhoenacker FM, Parizel PM, Van Goethem JW, Van Altena R, Laridon A, De Roeck J, Coeman V, De Schepper AM (2003) TB of the central nervous system: overview of neuroradiological findings. Eur Radiol 13:1876–1890
32. Gupta RK, Prakash M, Mishra AM, Husain M, Prasad KN, Husain N (2005) Role of diffusion weighted imaging in differentiation of intracranial tuberculoma and tuberculous abscess from cysticercus granulomas – a report of more than 100 lesions. Eur J Radiol 55:384–392
33. Jayasundar R, Raghunathan P, Banerji AK (1995) Proton MRS similarity between central nervous system non-Hodgkin lymphoma and intracranial tuberculoma. Magn Reson Imaging 13:489–493
34. Jinkins JR (1991) Computed tomography of intracranial TB. Neuroradiology 33:126–135
35. Whitener DR (1978) Tuberculous brain abscess. Report of a case and review of the literature. Arch Neurol 35:148–155
36. Bano S, Chaudhary V, Yadav S (2012) Central nervous system TB, neuroimaging – clinical applications. In: Bright P (ed) InTech, Janeza Trdine 9, 51000 Rijeka, Croatia ISBN: 978-953-51-0200-7, pp 467–498
37. Gee GT, Bazan C III, Jinkins JR (1992) Miliary TB involving the brain: MR findings. AJR Am J Roentgenol 159:1075–1076
38. Yanardag H, Uygun S, Yumuk V, Caner M, Canbaz B (2005) Cerebral TB mimicking intracranial tumour. Singapore Med J 46:731
39. American Thoracic Society, Center for Disease Control and Prevention, and Infectious Diseases Society of America (2003) Treatment of TB. MMWR Recomm Rep 52:1–77
40. Gropper MR, Schulder M, Sharan AD, Cho ES (1995) Central nervous system TB: medical management and surgical indications. Surg Neurol 44:378–384
41. Rajeswari R, Sivasubramanian S, Balambal R, Parthasarathy R, Ranjani R, Santha T, Somasundaram PR, Ganapathy S, Sudarsana K, Sayeed ZA, Kalyanaraman S, Prabhakar R (1995) A controlled clinical trial of short-course chemotherapy for tuberculoma of the brain. Tuber Lung Dis 76:311–317
42. Berning SE, Cherry TA, Iseman MD (2001) Novel treatment of meningitis caused by multidrug-resistant Mycobacterium TB with intrathecal levofloxacin and amikacin: case report. Clin Infect Dis 32:643–646
43. Caws M, Thwaites GE, Duy PM, Tho DQ, Lan NT, Hoa DV, Chau TT, Huyen MN, Anh PT, Chau NV, Chinh TN, Stepniewska K, Farrar J (2007) Molecular analysis of Mycobacterium TB causing multidrug-resistant TB meningitis. Int J Tuberc Lung Dis 11:202–208
44. Padayatchi N, Bamber S, Dawood H, Bobat R (2006) Multidrug-resistant tuberculous meningitis in children in Durban, South Africa. Pediatr Infect Dis J 25:147–150
45. Thwaites GE, Lan NT, Dung NH, Quy HT, Oanh DT, Thoa NT, Hien NQ, Thuc NT, Hai NN, Bang ND, Lan NN, Duc NH, Tuan VN, Hiep CH, Chau TT, Mai PP, Dung NT, Stepniewska K, White NJ, Hien TT, Farrar JJ (2005) Effect of antiTB drug resistance on response to treatment and outcome in adults with tuberculous meningitis. J Infect Dis 192:79–88
46. Kamoto K, Tokiguchi S, Furusawa T, Ishikawa K, Quardery AF, Shinbo S, Sasai K (2003) MR features of diseases involving bilateral middle cerebellar peduncles. AJNR Am J Neuroradiol 24:1946–1954
47. O'Toole RD, Thornton GF, Mukherjee MK, Nath RL (1969) Dexamethasone in tuberculous meningitis. Relationship of cerebrospinal fluid effects to therapeutic efficacy. Ann Intern Med 70:39–48
48. Rosenbulum ML (1985) Chronic granulomatous lesions: TB, leprosy. sarcoidosis. In: Wilkins RH, Rengachary SS (eds) Neurosurgery, 3rd edn. Mc Graw-Hill Book Compo, New York, pp 1980–1983
49. Bass JB Jr, Farer LS, Hopewell PC, O'Brien R, Jacobs RF, Ruben F, Snider DE Jr, Thornton G (1994) Treatment of TB and TB infection in adults and children. American Thoracic Society and The Centers for Disease Control and Prevention. Am J Respir Crit Care Med 149:1359–1374
50. Shamim MS, Enam SA, Ali RP,Ali SF, Wassy M (2009) Overview of surgical management of infectious nonsuppurative brain lesions.Pakistan Journal of Neurological sciences 4(2):77–82
51. Lee WY, Pang KY, Wong CK (2002) Brain tuberculoma in Hong Kong. Hong Kong Med J 8:52–56
52. Tandon PN, Bhargava S (1985) Effect of medical treatment on intracranial tuberculoma–a CT study. Tubercle 66:85–97
53. Tandon PN (1992) Brain biopsy in tuberculoma: the risks and benefits. Neurosurgery 30:301

54. Bouchama A, al-Kawi MZ, Kanaan I, Coates R, Jallu A, Rahm B, Siqueira EB (1991) Brain biopsy in tuberculoma: the risks and benefits. Neurosurgery 28:405–409
55. Selvapandian S, Rajshekhar V, Chandy MJ, Idikula J (1994) Predictive value of computed tomography-based diagnosis of intracranial tuberculomas. Neurosurgery 35:845–850
56. Muthukumar N, Sureshkumar V, Ramesh VG (2007) En plaque intradural extramedullary spinal tuberculoma and concurrent intracranial tuberculomas: paradoxical response to antituberculous therapy. J Neurosurg Spine 6:169–173
57. Bas NS, Guzey FK, Emel E, Alatas I, Sel B (2005) Paradoxical intracranial tuberculoma requiring surgical treatment. Pediatr Neurosurg 41:201–205
58. Vidal JE, Penalva de Oliveira AC, Bonasser Filho F, Schiavon Nogueira R, Dauar RF, Leite AG, Lins DL, Coelho JF (2005) Tuberculous brain abscess in AIDS patients: report of three cases and literature review. Int J Infect Dis 9:201–207
59. Shane SJ, Riley C (1953) Tuberculous meningitis: combined therapy with cortisone and antimicrobial agents. N Engl J Med 249:829–834
60. Schoeman JF, Laubscher JA, Donald PR (2000) Serial lumbar CSF pressure measurements and cranial computed tomographic findings in childhood tuberculous meningitis. Childs Nerv Syst 16:203–208
61. Husain M, Jha DK, Rastogi M, Husain N, Gupta RK (2005) Role of neuroendoscopy in the management of patients with tuberculous meningitis hydrocephalus. Neurosurg Rev 28:278–283
62. Chowdhury FH, Haque MR, Haque AFMM (2012) Intractable temporal lobe epilepsy (TLE) from tuberculoma; microneurosurgical management of by amygdalohippocampectomy with lesionectomy plus standard anterior temporal lobectomy. A case report and short review of literature. J Surg Sci 16:106–109
63. Greenberg MS (2001) Seizures. In: Greenberg MS (ed) Hand book of neurosurgery, 5th edn. Thieme, New York, pp 254–284
64. Chowdhury FH, Haque MR (2012) Large cerebellopontine angle tuberculoma: a case report. Neurol Neurochir Pol 46(2):196–199
65. Wasay M, Moolani MK, Zaheer J, Kheleani BA, Smego RA, Sarwari RA (2004) Prognostic indicators in patients with intracranial tuberculoma: a review of 102 cases. J Pak Med Assoc 54:83–87
66. Andronikou S, Wieselthaler N, Smith B, Douis H, Fieggen AG, Vantoorn R, Wilmshurst J (2005) Value of early follow-up CT in paediatric tuberculous meningitis. Pediatr Radiol 35:1092–1099
67. Andronikou S, Wilmshurst J, Hatherill M, Vantoorn R (2006) Distribution of brain infarction in children with tuberculous meningitis and correlation with outcome score at 6 months. Pediatr Radiol 36:1289–1294
68. Alarcon F, Duenas G, Cevallos N, Lees AJ (2000) Movement disorders in 30 patients with tuberculous meningitis. Mov Disord 15:561–569
69. Alarcón F, Gimenéz-Roldán S (2005) Systemic diseases that cause movement disorders. Parkinsonism Relat Disord 11:1–18
70. Ghanta R, Koti K, Kongara S (2011) Surgical excision of hypothalamic hamartoma in a twenty months old boy with precocious puberty. Indian J Endocrinol Metab 15:255–258
71. Leidl L, Mayanja-Kizza H, Sotgiu G, Baseke J, Ernst M, Hirsch C, Goletti D, Toossi Z, Lange C (2010) Relationship of immunodiagnostic assays for TB and numbers of circulating CD4+ T-cells in HIV infection. Eur Respir J 35:619–626
72. Pai M, Flores LL, Pai N, Hubbard A, Riley LW, Colford JM Jr (2003) Diagnostic accuracy of nucleic acid amplification tests for tuberculous meningitis: a systematic review and meta-analysis. Lancet Infect Dis 3:633–643
73. Jamieson DH (1995) Imaging intracranial TB in childhood. Paediatr Radiol 25:165–170
74. Ahmad FU, Gupta A, Mehta VS (2006) In: Arora VK (ed) Practical approach to TB management, 1st edn. Jaypee brothers, New Delhi, pp 138–148
75. Bayindir C, Mete O, Bilgic B (2006) Retrospectives study of 23 proven cases of central nervous system tuberculomas. Clin Neurol Neurosurg 108:353–357
76. Gupta V, Chhina D, Kaushal RK, Gupta R (2012) Tuberculous brain abscess–Case report. Asian Pac J Trop Dis 2:419–420
77. Wanjari K, Baradkar VP, Nataraj G, Kumar S (2009) A rare case of tubercular cerebellar abscess. Indian J Med Microbiol 27:363–365
78. Guo N, Huang F, Chen X, Zheng M, Zhong D, Feng Y (2013) Infratentorial tuberculoma mimics tumor in immunocompetent adults: an analysis of 11 patients. Open J Mod Neurosurg 3:36–40
79. Agrawal A, Shanthi V, Ramakrishna BA (2015) Tubercular cerebellar abscess in a child. J Mahatma Gandhi Inst Med Sci 20:77–78
80. Avila A, Berrade J (2009) TB involving bilateral middle cerebellar peduncles. Am J Neuroradiol 30(8):E119
81. Colditz GA, Berkey CS, Mosteller F, Brewer TF, Wilson ME, Burdick E, Fineberg HV (1995) The efficacy of bacillus Calmette-Guerin vaccination of newborns and infants in the prevention of TB: meta-analyses of the published literature. Pediatrics 96:29–35

Brainstem Tuberculosis

9

Md Zahed Hossain, Ali Akhaddar,
Ahmet T. Turgut, and Forhad H. Chowdhury

Contents

M.Z. Hossain, FCPS, MS (✉)
F.H. Chowdhury, FCPS, MS
Department of Neurosurgery, National Institute of Neurosciences and Hospital, Sher-e-Bangla Nagar, Dhaka-1207, Bangladesh
e-mail: zaheddr@yahoo.com; forhadchowdhury74@yahoo.com

A. Akhaddar, MD, IFAANS
Department of Neurosurgery, Avicenne Military Hospital of Marrakech, University of Mohammed V, Rabat, Morocco
e-mail: akhaddar@hotmail.fr

A.T. Turgut, MD
Department of Radiology, Hacettepe University School of Medicine, Ankara, Turkey
e-mail: ahmettuncayturgut@yahoo.com

Abbreviations

ADA Adenosine deaminase
AFB Acid-fast bacillus
BCG Bacillus Calmette-Guérin
CNS Central nervous system
CSF Cerebrospinal fluid
CT Computed tomography
EMB Ethambutol
HIV Human immunodeficiency virus
IICP Increased intracranial pressure
INH Isoniazid
MRI Magnetic resonance imaging
MRS Magnetic resonance spectroscopy
NAA Nucleic acid amplification
NHL Non-Hodgkin's lymphoma
PCR Polymerase chain reaction
PZA Pyrazinamide
RIF Rifampicin
SOT Solid organ transplantation
TB Tuberculosis
TBA Tuberculous brain abscess
TBM Tuberculous meningitis

M. Turgut et al. (eds.), *Tuberculosis of the Central Nervous System*,
DOI 10.1007/978-3-319-50712-5_9

9.1 Introduction

Tuberculosis (TB) is caused by the pathogenic microorganism *Mycobacterium tuberculosis.* In spite of the fact that it is a highly prevalent infectious disease in developing countries, it has already become a public health problem in developed countries as well due to increasing human immunodeficiency virus (HIV) epidemics and migration from third world countries [1]. Clinically, one of the most significant manifestations of TB is central nervous system (CNS) involvement, which accounts for 5–10% of extrapulmonary TB and 1% of all TB cases [2]. On the other hand, an even more unusual entity is brainstem tuberculoma, which constitutes approximately 2.5–8% of all intracranial tuberculomas [3, 4]. It is related with a high mortality rate and distressful level of neurological morbidity [2].

Immunosuppression, caused by either HIV infection or solid organ transplantation, is associated with increased susceptibility for acquiring or reactivating TB and also has a negative impact on the proper clinical management of underlying immunosuppression and CNS involvement by TB [5]. In this regard, the effect of HIV infection on TBC involves increased risk for acquisition of TB, rate of progression from latent to active disease, and significant morbidity and mortality associated with TB [5–8]. Importantly, extrapulmonary manifestations occur in approximately in 40% of HIV-infected TB patients [5, 7]. Statistically, HIV-positive individuals with TB are five times more prone to suffer from CNS involvement compared with HIV-negative individuals [5, 6].

The brainstem, occupying the posterior cranial fossa, is a stalklike structure connecting the narrow spinal cord with the expanded cerebrum. It is made up of the medulla, the pons, and the midbrain (Fig. 9.1). The main functions of the brainstem are serving as a channel for the ascending tracts and descending tracts which enables a connection between the spinal cord and higher cerebral centers, controlling the respiratory and cardiovascular system by means of the inherent reflex centers, regulating consciousness, and harboring the important nuclei of cranial nerves III through XII [9].

Unfortunately, the proper diagnosis of CNS TB still remains a challenge because it still relies mainly on insensitive microbiological methods in spite of the fact that promising molecular diagnostic techniques have emerged recently [10]. Although scientific research has focused on clinical manifestations of TB, several aspects of TB of CNS like the pathogenesis, diagnosis, treatment, and management have not been clarified [10].

Brainstem tuberculoma is very unusual and accounting for less than 5% of all intracranial TB

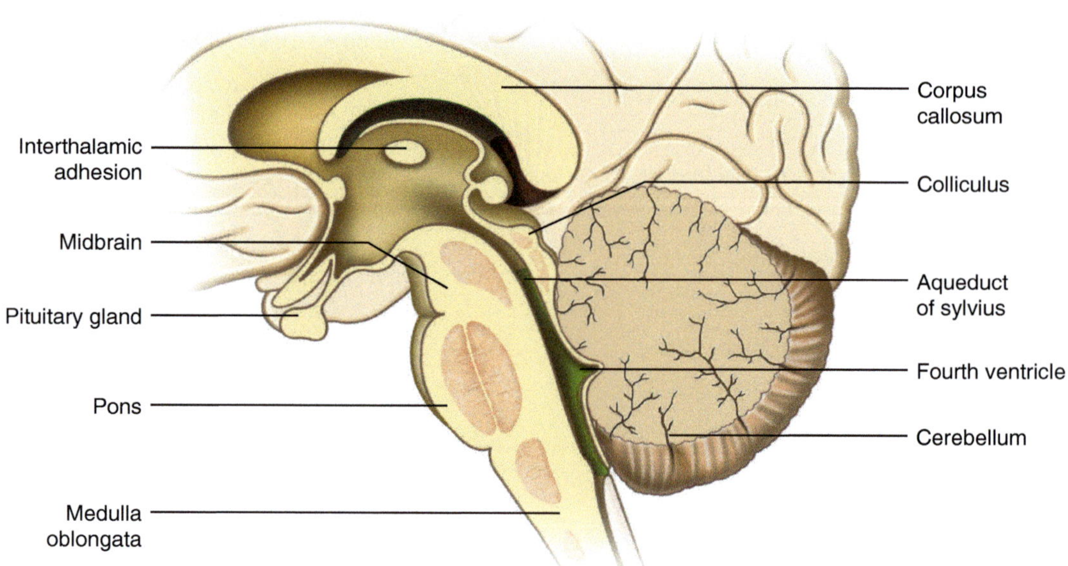

Fig. 9.1 Surgical anatomy of the brainstem

[11, 12]. Radiologically, the diagnosis of the entity may be challenging on conventional magnetic resonance imaging (MRI) as because of the similarity between its appearance and other rim-enhancing lesions such as bacterial abscesses and central tumor necrosis. However, a lesion with a hypointense content on T2-weighted images, a hypointense rim on T1- and T2-weighted images, and marked contrast enhancement is known to be characteristic for caseating tuberculoma which may help differentiation from other rim-enhancing lesions [11–14]. TB of CNS, the most dangerous form of extrapulmonary TB, can present as tubercular meningitis (TBM), intracranial tuberculomas, and abscesses [15]. Intracranial tuberculoma may manifest either with meningitis or without any meningeal involvement. Notably, the vast majority of the tuberculomas are located in the supratentorial compartment in adulthood, and multiple tuberculomas are more common than the solitary form [15, 16].

9.2 Epidemiology

Any organ or tissue can be affected by TB, though the disease mainly involves the lungs. In countries with developed diagnostic and reporting facilities, extrapulmonary TB accounts for 20–25% of reported cases, whereas extrapulmonary disease without concurrent pulmonary involvement is seen in 14% of notified cases in 2007 [17].

TBM and intracranial tuberculomas, with variable incidence in different countries, are the two frequent manifestations of CNS TB. On the other hand, brainstem tuberculomas comprising 2.5–8% of all intracranial tuberculomas are even more rare [3, 4]. According to World Health Organization (WHO) in 2005, the estimated annual number for new cases of active TB was 8 million, with an estimated 1.6 million deaths per year [10, 18]. According to WHO estimates, the number of new TB cases occurring globally was 9.27 million (139/100,000 population) and 9.24 million (140/100,000 population) in 2007 and 2006, respectively [2]. As the overwhelming majority of new active TB cases are detected in underdeveloped and developing countries, the disease remains a worldwide concern [10, 18]. The demographic factors such as poverty, crowding, malnutrition, and a compromised immune system have a substantial role in the worldwide epidemic in 80% of new TB cases, and HIV is related with the disease in the remaining 20% of TB cases in sub-Saharan Africa [10, 18, 19]. As far as the total number of incident cases is concerned, the countries ranking first to fifth are India, China, Indonesia, Nigeria, and South Africa [2].

9.3 Pathogenesis

M. tuberculosis is an aerobic, nonmotile, nonspore-forming, acid-fast bacillus (AFB) that infects primarily humans. Its doubling time is quite long (15–20 h) and requires several weeks to grow on conventional Löwenstein-Jensen medium. There, it has tendency to grow in parallel groups, producing the colonial characteristic of serpentine cording [10]. Brainstem TB is secondary TB as TB of CNS. Pathophysiologically, *M. tuberculosis* infection occurs secondary to the inhalation of droplet nuclei containing the bacilli, which are eventually deposited in the lung alveoli. Once in the alveoli, the bacilli interact with alveolar macrophages through a multitude of different receptors [10, 20–24]. Acquisition can also be occurred through ingestion and direct contact with denuded skin or mucosa. As soon as these innate immune cells are triggered, numerous cytokines and chemokines are released, a type 1 T-helper cell-mediated immune response is activated, and this finally leads to the formation of a granuloma. Earlier, the bacilli are filtered into draining lymph nodes before the actual containment of the infection and *M. tuberculosis* disseminates to distant sites in the body through a low-level bacteremia [10, 25]. This hematogenous seeding involves most frequently highly oxygenated regions of the body such as the brain [10]. TB bacilli are immobilized in end arteries, and this causes the formation of submeningeal TB foci, which may lead to various presentations of TB in turn. In tuberculoma, bacilli get lodged in the brain with rich blood supply. The formation of tuberculoma evokes secondary reaction which leads to the formation of a capsule [26].

The capacity to enter and replicate within macrophages is a distinctive feature of *M. tuberculosis*. The microglial cells, which are the resident macrophages within the CNS, are the main target in the CNS as they are productively infected with *M. tuberculosis* [10, 27, 28]. TB of CNS starts with the development of small TB foci (Rich foci) in the brain, spinal cord, or meninges. The ultimate form of TB in CNS is determined by the location of these foci and the capacity to control them. TB of CNS manifests itself mainly as TBM and less commonly as tubercular encephalitis, intracranial tuberculoma, or a tubercular brain abscess (TBA) [10, 25]. In the brainstem, tuberculoma and TBA are common. Tubercular leptomeningitis can occur as a part of generalized TBM.

9.4 Pathology

Basic pathology of TB is chronic granulomatous inflammation forming caseating granuloma which is a foreign body type of giant cell granuloma

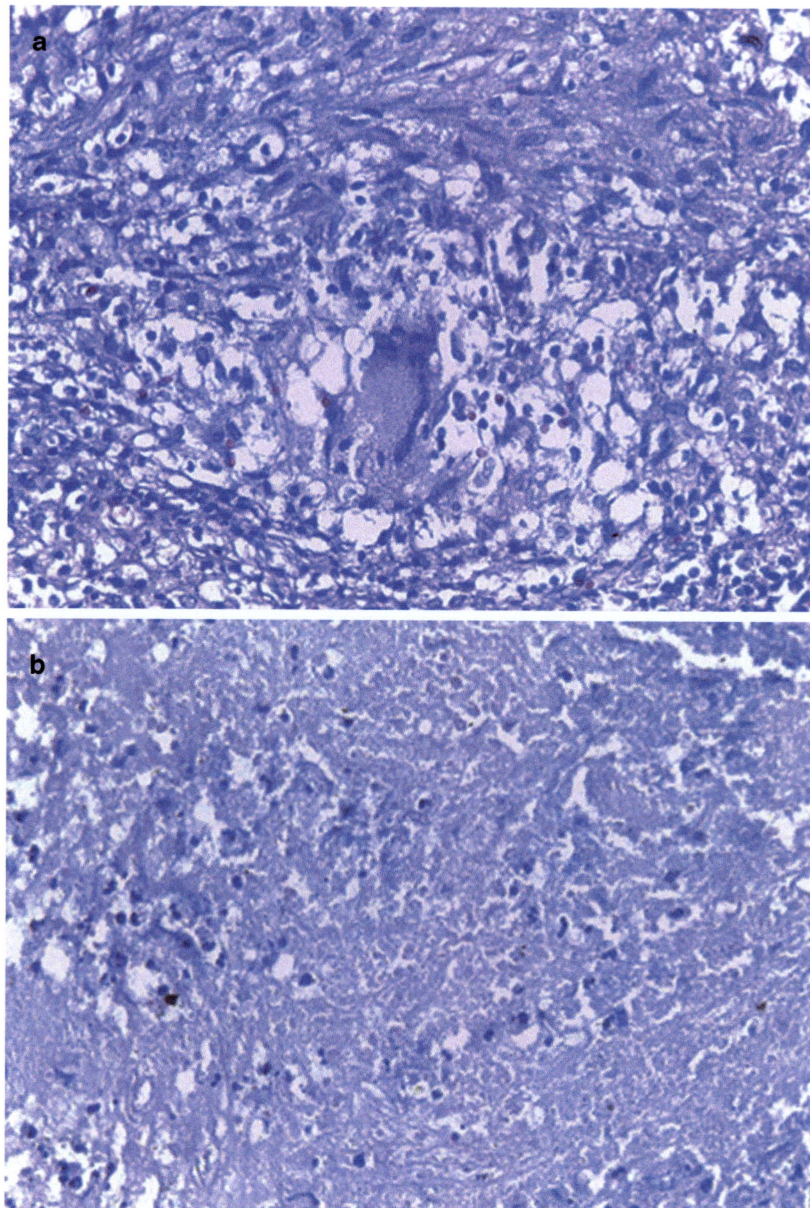

Fig. 9.2 H&E staining of (**a**) TB granuloma and (**b**) caseation necrosis (Courtesy of N. Islam)

(Fig. 9.2). TB of CNS can occur in the form of TBM, tuberculoma in the brain, and TBA. In the brainstem, it can either be tuberculoma or abscess.

9.4.1 Tuberculoma

The formation of tuberculomas is considered to be associated with the enlargement of the tubercles in the brain parenchyma without rupturing into the subarachnoid space. As such, they often occur in the absence of TBM but certainly may occur along with TBM. They more commonly arise as solitary lesions, but multiple tuberculomas are seen. Tuberculomas of the brain show a typical granulomatous reaction consisting of epithelioid cells and giant cells mixed with predominantly lymphocytes around a central area of caseating necrosis. Any liquefaction of the central area of necrosis contains clear or straw-colored fluid, as opposed to pus [10, 29]. According to MRI findings, three types of intracranial tuberculoma have been described: noncaseating, caseating with solid center, and caseating with liquid center (Fig. 9.3) [15]. In children, lesions tend to be infratentorial, whereas in adults they are typically supratentorial [5, 30–33].

Tuberculomas can occur in both supratentorial and infratentorial locations involving the cerebrum, cerebellum, and brainstem (Fig. 9.4). In the brainstem, tuberculomas can occur in any part of it, but more common in pons (Table 9.1).

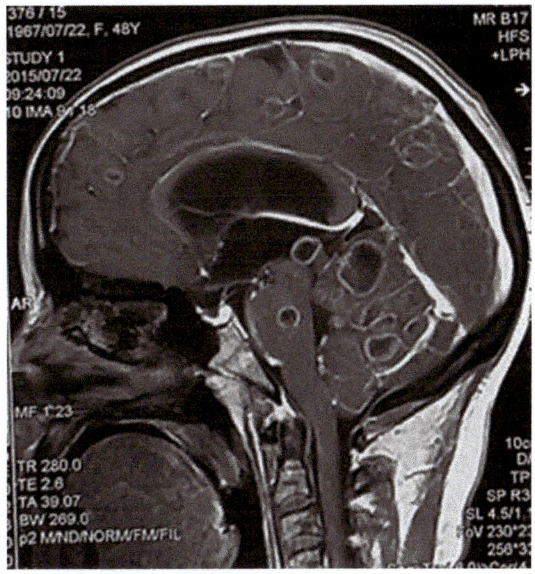

Fig. 9.4 Contrast-enhanced MRI sagittal section shows tuberculoma of pons along with multiple tuberculomas throughout the brain

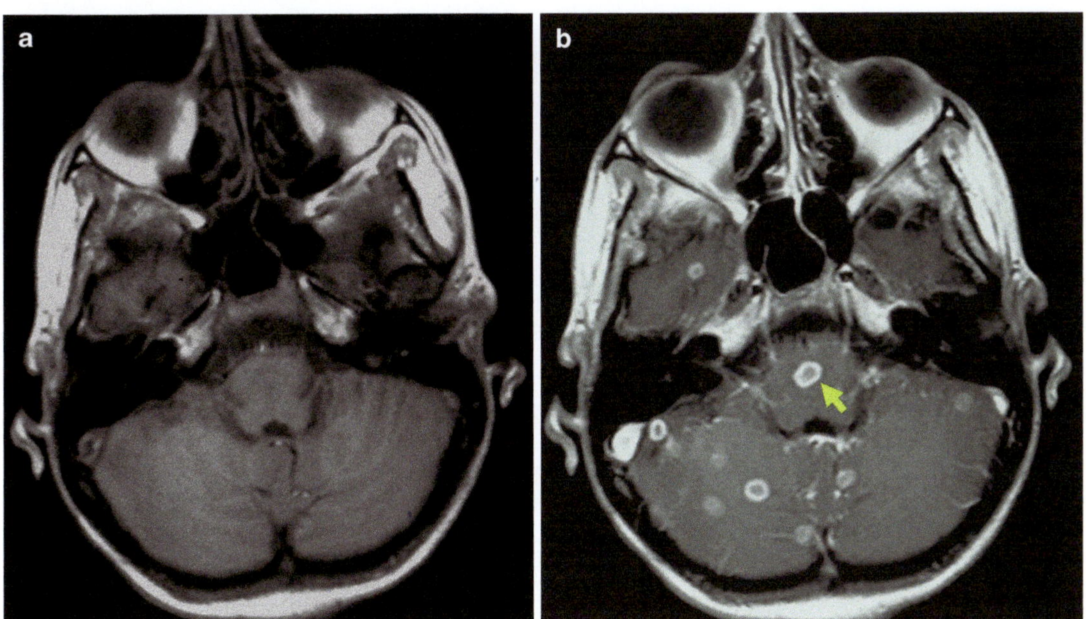

Fig. 9.3 Axial cranial T1-weighted MRI image before (**a**) and after (**b**) gadolinium administration. There is a bulbar tuberculoma (*arrow*) with multiple others

Table 9.1 List of brainstem tuberculosis cases published in world literature to date

Reference and date of publication	No. of cases	Age of patient	Site of involvement	Clinical presentation	Imaging study—diagnosis	Surgical procedure	Outcome
Talamás et al. 1989 [34]	11	20–28 yrs (5 cases) 14 yrs, 34 yrs, 46–53 yrs (4 cases)	Midbrain (4 cases) Pons (4 cases) Midbrain and pons (2 cases) Medulla oblongata and pons (1 case)	CN palsy, long tract sign, gait ataxia, and IICP features in diff. combinations	CT—tuberculoma	Biopsy (1 case) VP shunt (1 case)	Improved (3 cases), Improved with residual deficit (4 cases). No clinical improvement(1 case) Died (3 cases)
Gropper et al. 1994 [3]	2	28 yrs 25 yrs	Pons Pons	Third n palsy, Lt hemiparesis, ataxia Sixth n palsy, ataxia	CT MRI—multiple tuberculomas CT—tuberculoma	VP shunt VP shunt	Improved
Ipekoglu Z 1995 [32]	1	29 yrs	Brainstem	Headache, Lt hemiparesis, multiple CN palsies	CT—tuberculoma	yes	Improved
Lau and Yeun 1996 [35]	1	30 yrs	Midbrain	Headache, numbness	MRI—tuberculoma	No	Improved
Chin-Hua et al. 1999 [36]	1	37 yrs	Brainstem	Headache	CT—tuberculoma	No	Improved
Akhaddar et al. 2000 [37]	2	24 yrs 34 yrs	Pontomesencephalic Pontomesencephalic	Headache, Lt hemiparesis Third CN and sixth CN palsy, dizziness, cerebellar syndrome	CT—tuberculoma CT, MRI—tuberculoma	No No	Improved Improved
Kumar et al. 2000 [4]	6	6 yrs 8 yrs 2 yrs 1 yrs 8 yrs 12 yrs	Brainstem Brainstem Midbrain, pons Brainstem Brainstem Brainstem	Third CN palsy Third CN and sixth CN palsy, noncommunicating hydrocephalus Sixth CN palsy, communicating hydrocephalus Third CN and sixth CN palsy Third CN and seventh CN palsy Sixth CN and seventh CN palsy	CT, MRI—tuberculoma CT—tuberculoma CT—tuberculoma CT—tuberculoma CT—tuberculoma CT—tuberculoma	VP shunt VP shunt	Improved
Minagar et al. 2004 [38]	1	NS	Pons	One-and-a-half syndrome	MRI—tuberculoma	No	Improved

Kumar and Shinghi 2004 [39]	3	1 mo 7 yrs 12 yrs	Pons, medulla oblongata Pons, midbrain Midbrain, pons, medulla oblongata	Hemiparesis, CN palsy Gait disturbance, hoarseness of voice, hemiparesis, CN palsy hoarseness of voice, paraparesis, CN palsy	CT—Abscess CT—Abscess CT and MRI—tuberculoma	Surgical drainage Surgical drainage Surgical excision	Improved Improved Improved
Menon et al. 2004 [40]	1	12 yrs	Midbrain, pons	One-and-a-half syndrome	MRI—tuberculoma	No	Improved
Mushira et al. 2006 [41]	1	73 yrs	Pons	Ptosis, gaze palsy	MRI—tuberculoma	No	improved
Ronald et al. 2006 [42]	1	Child	Pons	Eight-and-a-half syndrome	MRI—tuberculoma		
Akhaddar et al. 2007 [11]	1	34 yrs	Pons and midbrain	Tetraparesis, dizziness double vision, increasing difficulty with speech, hypotonic, headache	MRI—tuberculoma	Stereotactic biopsy but not therapeutic purpose	Improved
Sharma et al. 2008 [43]	1	45 yrs	Pons	Facial numbness	MRI—tuberculoma	No	Improved
Donmez et al. 2009 [44]	1	70 yrs	Medulla oblongata	Stroke-like features	MRI—tuberculoma		
Ertem et al. 2010 [1]	1	17 yrs	Pons	Headache and gaze palsy	MRI—tuberculoma	No	Improved
Demetriou, 2013 [45]	1	38 yrs	Medulla oblongata	Weakness of sixth CN and seventh CN	MRI—cavitating lesion	No	Improved
Gautam VKS et al. 2013 [46]	1	8 yrs	Pons	Weakness and slurring of speech	CT and MRI—tuberculoma	VP shunt	Improved
Chigurupati P and Kumar P 2014 [47]	1	5 yrs	Pons and midbrain	Headache, fever, diplopia, weakness of all four limbs, and gait disturbance	MRI—abscess	Surgical drainage	Improved
Ozan et al. 2014 [48]	1	14 yrs	Pons	Headache, dizziness, vomiting, seizure	CT—abscess	No	Improved
Muin et al. 2015 [49]	1	19 yrs	Midbrain	Rt weakness, Lt CN palsy	MRI—tuberculoma	No	Improved
Agu CC et al. 2015 [50]	1	NS	Pons	Sixth CN palsy	MRI—tuberculoma	No	Improved
Author's cases (unpublished) case 1: Figures 9.5 and 9.6a case 2: Figure 9.4	2	25 yrs 48 yrs	Pons Pons with other parts of the brain	Headache, vomiting, visual blurring Headache, vomiting, seizure, sixth CN palsy	MRI—tuberculoma MRI—multiple tuberculomas in the whole brain	VP- shunt	Died after initial improvement Died

Abbreviations: *CN* cranial nerve, *CT* computed tomography, *IICP* increased intracranial pressure, *Lt* left, *mo* month, *MRI* magnetic resonance imaging, *Rt* right, *VP shunt* ventriculoperitoneal shunt, *yr(s)* year(s)

9.4.2 Tuberculous Brain Abscess

A rare manifestation of TB of CNS is brain abscess. The development of TBA is either from parenchymal TB granulomas or via the spread of TB foci in the meninges. It is characterized by an encapsulated collection of pus with viable bacilli lacking any evidence for the classic TB granuloma and must be differentiated from granuloma with central caseation and liquefaction mimicking pus [10, 29]. TBAs can arise as solitary or multiple lesions [10, 51]. Morphologically, the wall of a TBA is much thicker compared to a pyogenic brain abscess [10, 29]. Histopathologically, the inflammatory reaction in the abscess wall is suggested to be a predominantly vascular granulation tissue where acute and chronic inflammatory cells and bacilli are present in the pus or abscess wall [10, 51].

TBAs, with a diameter frequently greater than 3 cm, tend to be larger than tuberculomas. Clinically, the presentation of TBA which includes fever, headache, and focal neurologic deficits is typically more acute than tuberculoma [5, 52]. The rate of TBAs among HIV-infected persons with TB was reported to be 20% [5, 53], whereas the rate was calculated as 4–7.5% for HIV-negative patients with TB of CNS [5, 54] implying that TBAs may occur more frequently in HIV-infected people. The intracerebral response to TB bacilli may be inhibited by HIV-induced suppression of cell-mediated immunity, increasing the likelihood of an abscess rather than a granuloma formation [5, 53]. In patients with solid organ transplantation (SOT), abscess also seems to be a common manifestation of TB of CNS. In a review by Singh et al., TB abscess was noted to be present in 5 of 18 patients (28%) with TB of CNS after SOT [5, 8].

9.5 Clinical Features

Intracranial tuberculomas, being relatively rarely encountered compared to other types of TB, are morphologically tumorlike masses which are formed by tuberculous granulation tissue. Tuberculomas are frequently multiple, and they may show a mass effect when they are too big in size [1]. Clinically, the patients usually present with headache, seizures, papilledema, or other signs of increased intracranial pressure (IICP), and the clinical manifestations of tuberculoma or TBA depend largely on their location. In patients with tuberculomas, the symptoms develop usually in weeks to months. On the other hand, the onset of TBA with associated findings such as fever, headaches, and focal neurological deficits occurs within a period of 1 week to 3 months and is more acute compared to tuberculoma, whereas the onset is slower than pyogenic brain abscesses [10, 29].

TB is a systemic disease which can present with systemic features of TB as well as with the focal signs depending on the site of involvement. Accordingly, TB involving the brainstem can present with systemic features of TB like fever, malaise, night sweating, anorexia, weight loss, etc.; features of the focal involvement of the midbrain, pons, or medulla in the brainstem; or features of TBM. Also, it can manifest with the features of primary site of involvement like pulmonary or lymph node TB. Additionally, it can present with features of concomitant involvement of other sites of the brain, cerebrum, and cerebellum like seizure, focal sign and gait disturbance, etc.

Clinically, the presenting findings for brainstem tuberculoma or abscess may be features of IICP or signs associated with focal involvement of long tracts such as hemiplegia or hemisensory deficit, involvement of cranial nerve nuclei causing findings related to cranial nerve palsy like diplopia, gaze palsy, facial palsy, dysphagia, etc. The involvement or pressure over the reticular activating system patient may cause depressed level of consciousness. Tuberculoma of the upper brainstem involving mostly the midbrain causes the obstruction to the CSF flow leading to hydrocephalus in turn and presents various findings like headache, nausea and vomiting, visual impairment, papilledema, and impaired consciousness.

A midbrain lesion may also present with different syndromes. In this regard, Weber's syndrome presents with third cranial nerve palsy with contralateral hemiparesis [55]. Benedict's syndrome, on the other hand, presents with third cranial nerve palsy and contralateral hemiparesis without arm involvement where the patient suffers from hyperkinesias, ataxia, and coarse intention tremor when the lesion involves the midbrain tegmentum with red nucleus [56].

A case of tuberculoma of pons presenting with numbness on entire left half of the face, scalp, tongue, and part of auricle and features suggesting trigeminal neuropathy were reported by Sharma et al. (2008) [43]. Later, another case with the involvement of the pons and midbrain by TBA presenting with headache, fever, diplopia, weakness of all four limbs, and gait disturbance with bilateral sixth and seventh cranial nerve paresis (2014) was reported by Pragati and Phani [47]. Vinod et al. (2013), on the other hand, reported a case with brainstem tuberculoma presenting with features suggestive of stroke such as slurring of speech, difficulty in swallowing, and weakness of all four limbs of sudden onset [46].

The clinical presentation of brainstem tuberculoma is variable. In this regard, different types of presentations have been reported in literature including one-and-a-half syndrome, mimicking glaucoma or glioma. Also, it has been reported to present with unilateral paralysis of saccades, Millard-Gubler syndrome, isolated bilateral ptosis, horizontal gaze palsy, myokymia and facial contracture, or Foville's syndrome [46].

Brainstem tuberculomas are usually focal lesions causing focal neurological symptoms associated with the involvement of a cranial nerve nuclei and long tracts. TBM is frequently associated with a TB rhombencephalitis. Hydrocephalus with the presenting findings of headache, vomiting, visual blurring, gait disturbance, up-gaze palsy, and abducens nerve palsy may occur in case it causes obstruction to CSF flow [56].

Clinical presentation of tuberculoma may differ in HIV-infected individuals [5]. Interestingly, CNS tuberculoma after SOT may present up to 11 years following the procedure [5, 57, 58]. In spite of the fact that immunosuppression and comorbidities probably complicate the presentation of posttransplantation CNS tuberculoma, the number of reported cases is too small to allow comment on potential differences in clinical presentation [5].

9.6 Diagnosis

Definitive diagnosis of TB of CNS depends on the detection of the TB bacilli in the CSF or the extraction of tissue from the lesion, either by smear examination or by bacterial culture. Beyond the diagnostic value of these methods, the significance of obtaining a culture is that it allows drug sensitivity testing by means of the growth of *M. tuberculosis* in culture, which can be crucial for appropriate drug selection and prognosis [10].

9.6.1 Microbiology

CSF findings are nonspecific, as smears for AFB are frequently negative in brainstem TB [34]. Unfortunately, traditional staining and culture remain relatively insensitive though it is considered to be important among various diagnostic methods used for TB of CNS, and this is suggested most likely to be due to the typical paucity of AFB in a clinical case with TB of CNS. Standard staining techniques where stains like Ziehl-Neelsen, Kinyoun, or auramine-rhodamine applied to CSF samples have been estimated to allow the detection of approximately 100 AFB/ml of CSF [10, 59]. In several case series, CSF staining sensitivities of <20% have been reported [10, 60–62]. In some techniques, the clot that forms in standing CSF was stained and spinned down the CSF sediment onto a slide for microscopic examination. A sensitivity of 91% was reported with the use of the latter technique in 100 consecutive cases [10, 63]. Long ago, it was reported by Kennedy and Fallon that staining multiple samples of CSF enhanced the sensitivity to 86% [64].

9.6.2 Molecular and Biochemical Analysis

Among currently available molecularly based techniques are commercially available nucleic acid amplification (NAA) methods and other methods based on polymerase chain reaction (PCR), antibody detection, antigen detection, or chemical assays such as adenosine deaminase (ADA) and tuberculostearic acid measurements [2]. All these tests are mostly done from CSF and not very significant for tuberculoma and abscess if not associated with meningitis.

The diagnostic utility of a skin test positive for CNS TB ranges from 10–20% [2, 65] to 50% [2, 66]. The performance of the tuberculin skin test for the diagnosis of TB varies according to age, vaccination with bacillus Calmette-Guérin (BCG), nutritional status, HIV infection, and technique of administration [2, 67].

ADA, being considered to be a marker of cell-mediated immunity, is associated largely with lymphocytic proliferation and differentiation [2, 10, 68]. The reported sensitivity and specificity for ADA in the CSF range from 44 to 100% and 71 to 100%, respectively [2, 10, 69].

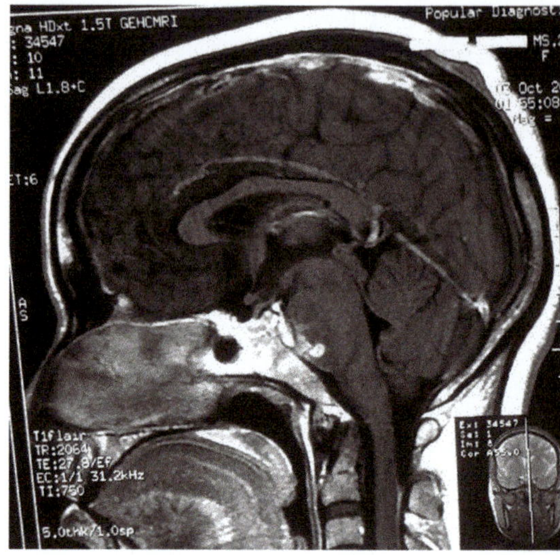

Fig. 9.5 Contrast-enhanced MRI of the brain in sagittal section shows pontine tuberculoma with basal meningeal enhancement

9.6.3 Radiological Evaluation

The diagnostic accuracy for TBM and tuberculomas has been significantly improved with the use of cross-sectional imaging tools such as computed tomography (CT) and MRI in neuroradiology. Contrast-enhanced MRI is accepted to be superior to CT in detecting and assessing TB of CNS [10, 70–72] and is generally considered as the modality of choice. It is particularly useful for the assessment of the location and margins of the lesions as well as ventriculitis, meningitis, and spinal involvement (sensitivity 86%, specificity 90%) [2, 73].

Among the CT criteria for the diagnosis of TB of CNS, basal meningeal enhancement, ventriculomegally, tuberculoma, and infarcts are suggested by Kumar et al. to be characteristics for distinguishing TB of CNS from pyogenic meningitis [10, 74] (Fig. 9.5). On CT, tuberculomas are defined as low- or high-density, round, or lobulated masses with irregular walls and show homogenous or ring enhancement after contrast administration (Fig. 9.6). They occur as solitary or multiple nodules [10, 75]. The "target sign" with a central nidus of calcification surrounded by a ring of enhancement was once considered to be pathognomonic finding for tuberculoma [10, 70], despite being called into question recently [10, 76]. The radiological presentation of tuberculomas depends largely on whether the lesion is noncaseating, caseating with a solid center, or caseating with a liquid center, and the degree of edema surrounding the tuberculoma is considered to be inversely proportional to the age of the lesion [10, 70]. On MRI, tuberculoma is isointense to mildly hyperintense on T1-weighted and hypointense on T2-weighted image [43]. The radiographical response of tuberculoma to treatment can usually be assessed within 4–6 weeks after the diagnosis. While new or enlarging tuberculoma may be detected in some patients on follow-up CT or MRI studies despite undergoing adequate anti-TB chemotherapy, the degree of contrast enhancement may be a clue for the assessment of the activity of the lesion [10, 70]. Late radiographical changes for tuberculomas

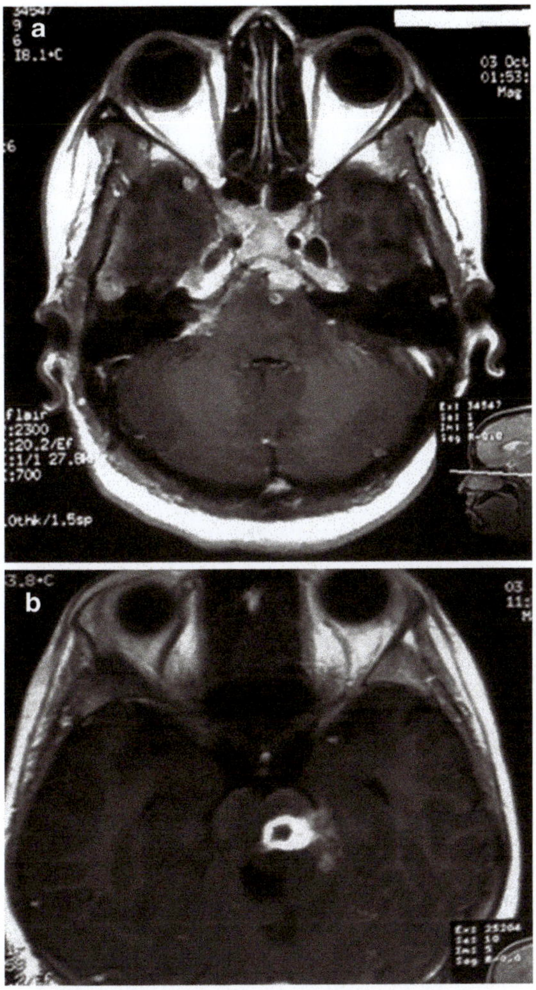

Fig. 9.6 Contrast-enhanced MRI showing homogeneous and ring-enhanced tuberculomas in the brainstem (**a**, **b**) along with basal meningeal enhancement (**a**)

include calcifications and local atrophy though no residual radiological abnormalities may be detected as well [10].

Other radiographic techniques such as magnetic resonance spectroscopy (MRS) have been shown to aid distinguishing tuberculoma from cysticercosis [10, 77], but the technique is of no help for making a distinction from non-Hodgkin's lymphoma (NHL) of the CNS [10, 78]. MRS reveals raised lipid peak with reduced N-acetylaspartate and choline peak tuberculoma [43]. A large lipid, lactate peak has been used to specifically identify tuberculomas by MRS [2, 79] (Fig. 9.7). Owing to the fact that TBAs cannot be reliably differentiated from pyogenic abscesses with the use of radiological tools, they generally require surgical intervention for microbiological diagnosis [10]. All patients should have erythrocyte sedimentation rate and chest X-ray as part of the routine diagnostic assessment and to look for primary focus of TB.

9.7 Differential Diagnosis

Brainstem tuberculoma can be confused with glioma, cysticercosis, lymphoma, metastasis, or nontuberculous pyogenic bacterial abscess. Radiologically, MRI with MRS can differentiate between tuberculoma or TBA and glioma. Any infective foci in the heart or lung or chronic suppurative otitis media or sinus infection hints in favor of pyogenic bacterial abscess. TBA is slower in onset than pyogenic bacterial abscess. Patient's contact history, MRS, and radiological finding (absence of edema) can differentiate cysticercosis from tuberculoma. Lymphoma can be differentiated from tuberculoma by stereotactic biopsy. But sometimes NHL may have peripheral lymphadenopathy which can be biopsied for histopathology to get an indirect evidence.

9.8 Treatment

9.8.1 Antituberculosis Drugs

Treatment of brainstem TB is mostly medical with anti-TB chemotherapy. Depending upon the treatment response and size of the tuberculoma or abscess, however, surgery may be needed.

Recently, WHO-recommended formulations of anti-TB drugs and fixed-dose combinations of drugs appear in the WHO Model List of Essential Medicines [17]. Recommended first-line anti-TB drugs are isoniazid (INH), rifampicin (RIF), pyrazinamide (PZA), ethambutol (EMB), and streptomycin. In general, WHO recommends 6-month treatment regimen for all (pulmonary and extrapulmonary) cases of TB. Nevertheless, some

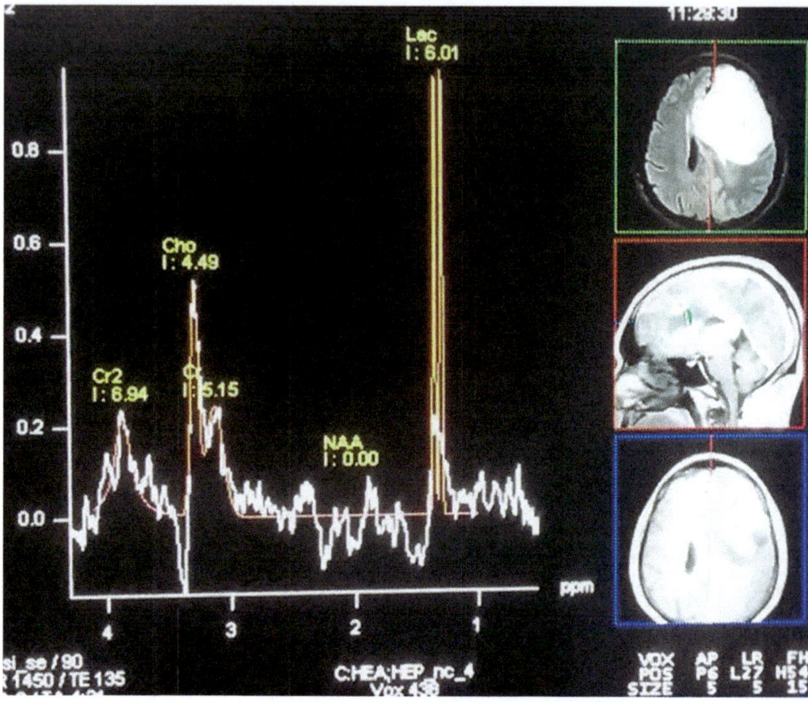

Fig. 9.7 MRS through a tuberculoma reveals raised lipid lactate peak with decreased NAA and choline peak in tuberculoma (Courtesy of Dr. Tariqul Islam, Consultant, Radiology, NINS, Dhaka)

experts recommend 9–12 months of treatment [17]. According to the standard approach endorsed by Infectious Diseases Society of America, Centers for Disease Control and Prevention, and American Thoracic Society guidelines for TB of CNS, an initial 2-month induction therapy regimen including INH, RIF, PZA, and EMB is applied followed by the use of INH and RIF for 7–10 additional months as maintenance therapy for an isolate which is sensitive to these agents. In cases with a mental status precluding oral intake, INH, RIF, and the second-line agents like aminoglycosides, capreomycin, and fluoroquinolones are available in parenteral form [10]. In the literature, most tuberculomas have been reported to resolve with anti-TB chemotherapy (Table 9.1).

9.8.2 Role of Corticosteroids in Tuberculosis of Central Nervous System

Although the use of corticosteroids as adjunctive therapy for the treatment of TB of CNS dates back to the 1950s [10, 80], it still remains a controversial issue. Initially, the main rationale behind the use of steroids was the reduction of inflammation within the subarachnoid space [10, 41]. However, routine use of adjunctive corticosteroids for all patients with tuberculomas without meningitis or with spinal cord TB is arguable, though they may be helpful in the presence of symptoms which cannot be controlled, or are worsening, on anti-TB chemotherapy [2]. The use of dexamethasone at a dose of 4 mg every 6 h for weeks for a presumed paradoxical expansion of the CNS tuberculomas on anti-TB chemotherapy was reported by Mushira et al. (2006), and the therapy was shown to improve the symptoms of ptosis and gaze palsy [41]. Importantly, the use of steroid therapy as an adjunctive therapy coupled with standard anti-TB chemotherapy in cases with TB of CNS has been endorsed by Infectious Diseases Society of America, Centers for Disease Control and Prevention, and American Thoracic Society guidelines [10, 81]. The recommended regimen is an initial dexamethasone dose of 8 mg/day for children weighing less than 25 kg and 12 mg/day for children weighing 25 kg dexamethasone or more and for adults [10, 41]. After an initial dose given for 3 weeks, the dose is decreased gradually during the following 3 weeks [10].

9.8.3 Surgical Treatment

Since the development of effective anti-TB chemotherapy, surgery has been applied to cope with the serious complication of hydrocephalus, reduce the mass effect of tuberculomas, and drain brain abscesses [10]. Hydrocephalus and TBA of the brainstem necessitate urgent neurosurgical intervention though early hydrocephalus, and TBA can be successfully treated by drugs alone [2]. TBA occurs in only 4–8% of patients with TB of CNS who do not have HIV infection, whereas it is seen in 20% of patients having HIV infection. The goal for surgical management of TBA is to reduce the size of the space-occupying lesion, diminish IICP in turn, and eradicate the pathogen [2]. Hydrocephalus is very common in case of brainstem tuberculoma or abscess, and it is mostly obstructive variety. In these situations, urgent ventriculoperitoneal shunt or endoscopic third ventriculostomy is needed. In emergency situation, external ventricular drainage may be given.

Most of the cases of tuberculomas in the brainstem respond to anti-TB chemotherapy and do not need surgery. Moreover surgery on the brainstem is risky. Most of the reported series and case reports show that tuberculomas resolve with anti-TB drugs alone or in combination with dexamethasone (Table 9.1) [1, 3, 4, 11, 32, 34–50]. But very large tuberculoma causing severe mass effect or paradoxical enlargement of tuberculoma or diagnostic dilemma needs surgical intervention. Surgical excision is also recommended as a first-line management when the tuberculoma is superficial and easily accessible [45].

Large abscess and chronic abscess need surgical drainage or excision. Sometimes stereotactic biopsy can also be done for tissue diagnosis in case of smaller and confusing lesions.

9.8.4 Surgical Approaches

Surgical approaches to the brainstem are mostly through midline suboccipital craniotomy/craniectomy followed by transvermian or telovelar approach. The midbrain can also be approached by supracerebellar infratentorial route. If the lesion is laterally placed, it can be approached laterally by lateral suboccipital craniotomy/craniectomy. Anteriorly placed lesions can be approached through fronto-orbito-zygomatic approach. Nowadays minimally invasive surgery is becoming popular. Endonasal endoscopic approach to the brainstem is an alternate approach for anteriorly placed tuberculoma or TBA.

9.9 Outcome and Follow-Up

The morbidity and mortality associated with TB of CNS are highly dependent on the stage of disease at diagnosis, and early diagnosis and treatment are correlated with better outcomes, as expected [82]. In immunocompetent patients, worse outcome of TBM has a correlation with a greater degree of neurologic impairment at presentation [5, 10, 64, 83] and with the presence of hydrocephalus [5, 84, 85]. In most studies, higher mortality rates up to 65% have been reported in HIV-infected patients [5, 83–87]. Among the factors associated with poor prognosis for TBM in HIV-infected patients are severe illness at presentation, CD4 cell count <50 cells/μL, and presence of MDR strains [5, 83, 88]. The mortality rate for tuberculoma is <10% with appropriate anti-TB chemotherapy [5, 52]. However, clinical improvement is usually delayed so as to occur ≥3 months after the onset of treatment [5, 89]. In a small case series of tuberculoma in HIV-infected and HIV-uninfected patients, mortality rates were reported to be similar in both groups [5, 90].

All the patients should be followed up 4–6 weeks after initiation of treatment by CT or MRI and then at regular intervals. The author likes to have an MRI after 4 weeks of treatment and then at 3 months interval and at 6 months interval.

Conclusion

Brainstem TB is a devastating form of TB of CNS, but with rare incidence. Approximately 1% of all TB cases are TB of CNS, among them only 2.5–8% are brainstem TB. Today, BCG vaccine is routinely used against TB in countries where the disease is present. It is difficult to diagnose as clinical features and hematological and CSF findings are not specific for brainstem TB. Radiological findings are also not always specific for brainstem tuberculoma or abscess. Confirmatory diagnosis of TB depends upon the isolation of AFB from the tissue and from the lesion by acid-fast staining or culture, but it is difficult to have the tissue from the brainstem. In most of the cases considering clinical parameters, CSF biochemical and molecular analysis (NAA and PCR), hematological findings, and radiological (contrast-enhanced CT and MRI) features in the brainstem along with contact history, the presence of any other site TB, and social context, diagnosis of brainstem TB is made. Anti-TB chemotherapy is the mainstay of treatment along with corticosteroids in some cases. Most of the cases improve with medical treatment only. Surgical intervention is needed in some cases of large tuberculoma, TBA, acute or chronic hydrocephalus, lesions not responding to medical treatment alone, or neurological deterioration after starting anti-TB chemotherapy.

References

1. Ertem DH, Aslan ND, Ltunkaynak Y, Yıldız DS, Baybaş S (2010) Isolated brain stem tuberculoma: a case report and review of the literature. Düşünen Adam: J Psychiat Neurol Sci 23:288–292
2. Cherian A, Thomas SV (2011) Central nervous system tuberculosis. Afr Health Sci 11:116–127
3. Gropper MR, Schulder M, Duran HL, Wolansky L (1994) Cerebral tuberculosis with expansion into brainstem tuberculoma. Report of two cases. J Neurosurg 81:927–931
4. Kumar R, Jain R, Kaur A, Chhabra DK (2000) Brain stem tuberculosis in children. Br J Neurosurg 14:356–361
5. Snydman DR, Zunt JR, Nelson CA (2011) Tuberculosis of the central nervous system in immunocompromised patients: HIV infection and solid organ transplant recipients. Clin Infect Dis 53:915–926
6. Berenguer J, Moreno S, Laguna F, Vicente T, Adrados M, Ortega AF (1992) Tuberculous meningitis in patients infected with the human immunodeficiency virus. N Engl J Med 326:668–667
7. Kingkaew N, Sangtong B, Amnuaiphon W, Jongpaibulpatana J, Mankatit-tham W, Akksilp S, Sirinak C, Nateniyom S, Burapat C, Kittikraisak W (2009) HIV-associated extrapulmonary tuberculosis in Thailand: epidemiology and risk factors for death. Int J Infect Dis 13:722–729
8. Singh N, Paterson DL (1998) Mycobacterium tuberculosis infection in solid-organ transplant recipients: impact and implications for management. Clin Infect Dis 27:1266–1277
9. Snell RS (2001) The brainstem: clinical neuroanatomy for medical students, 5th edn. Lippincott Williams & Wilkins, Philadelphia, pp 189–224
10. Bryan Rock R, Michael O, Baker CA, Molitor TW, Peterson PK (2008) Central nervous system tuberculosis: pathogenesis and clinical aspects. Clin Microbiol Rev 21:243–261
11. Akhaddar A, Mahi M, Harket A, Elmostarchid B, Belhachemi A, Elasri A, Gazzaz M, Boucetta M (2007) Brainstem tuberculoma in a postpartum patient. J Neuroradiol 34:345–346
12. Akhaddar A, El Hassani MY, Chakir N, Jiddane M (2001) Optochiasmatic tuberculoma: complication of tuberculous meningitis. Report of a case and review of the literature. J Neuroradiol 28:137–142
13. Batra A, Tripathi RP (2004) Diffusion-weighted magnetic resonance imaging and magnetic resonance spectroscopy in the evaluation of focal cerebral tubercular lesions. Acta Radiol 45:679–688
14. Khanna PC, Godinho S, Patkar DP, Pungavkar SA, Lawande MA (2006) MR spectroscopy-aided differentiation: "Giant"extra-axial tuberculoma masquerading as meningioma. Am J Neuroradiol 27:1438–1440
15. Chou PS, Liu CK, Lin RT, Lai CL, Chao AC (2012) Central nervous system tuberculosis-a forgotten diagnosis. Neurologist 18:219–222
16. Bayindir C, Mete O, Bilgic B (2006) Retrospective study of 23 pathologically proven cases of central nervous system tuberculomas. Clin Neurol Neurosurg 108:353–357
17. WHO (2010) Treatment of extrapulmonary TB and of TB in special situations. Treatment of tuberculosis Guidelines, 4th edn. Stop TB Department, World Health Organization, Geneva, Switzerland (WHO/HTM/TB/2009.420) pp 95–99
18. WHO (2007) Global tuberculosis control: surveillance, planning, financing. WHO report, Geneva, World Health Organization (WHO/HTM/TB/2007.376) pp 1–70
19. Waaler HT (2002) Tuberculosis and poverty. Int J Tuberc Lung Dis 6:745–746
20. Bermudez LE, Sangari FJ (2001) Cellular and molecular mechanisms of internalization of mycobacteria by host cells. Microbes Infect 3:37–42
21. El-Etr SH, Cirillo JD (2001) Entry mechanisms of mycobacteria. Front Biosci 6:D737–D747
22. Leemans JC, Florquin S, Heikens M, Pals ST, Van der Neut R, Van Der Poll T (2003) CD44 is a macrophage binding site for Mycobacterium tuberculosis that mediates macrophage recruitment and protective immunity against tuberculosis. J Clin Investig 111:681–689
23. Pieters J (2001) Entry and survival of pathogenic mycobacteria in macrophages. Microbes Infect 3:249–255
24. Velasco-Velazquez MA, Barrera D, Gonzalez-Arenas A, Rosales C, Agramonte-Hevia J (2003) Macrophage-Mycobacterium tuberculosis interactions: role of complement receptor 3. Microb Pathog 35:125–131

25. Rom WN, Garay SM (2004) Tuberculosis, 2nd edn. Lippincott Williams & Wilkins, Philadelphia, pp 773–789
26. Wanjari K, Baradkar VP, Nataraj G, Kumar S (2009) A rare case of tubercular cerebellar abscess. Indian J Med Microbiol 27:363–365
27. Curto M, Reali C, Palmieri G, Scintu F, Schivo ML, Sogos V, Marcialis MA, Ennas MG, Schwarz H, Pozzi G, Gremo F (2004) Inhibition of cytokines expression in human microglia infected by virulent and non-virulent mycobacteria. Neurochem Int 44:381–392
28. Rock RB, Gekker G, Hu S, Sheng WS, Cheeran M, Lokensgard JR, Peterson PK (2004) Role of microglia in central nervous system infections. Clin Microbiol Rev 17:942–964
29. Kumar R, Pandey CK, Bose N, Sahay S (2002) Tuberculous brain abscess: clinical presentation, pathophysiology and treatment (in children). Childs Nerv Syst 18:118–123
30. Nelson CA, Zunt JR (2011) Tuberculosis of the central nervous system in immunocompromised patients: HIV infection and solid organ transplant recipients. Clin Infect Dis 53:915–926
31. Dastur DK, Lalitha VS, Prabhakar V (1968) Pathological analysis of intracranial space-occupying lesions in 1000 cases including children. Part-1. Age, sex and pattern; and the tuberculomas. J Neurol Sci 6:575–592
32. Ipekoglu Z, Aksoy K, Bekar A, Seref Dogan S (1995) Brainstem tuberculoma: case report. Turk Neurosurg 5:65–66
33. Turgut M, Özcan OE, Özgen T, Saglam S, Bertan V, Erbengi A (1989) Tuberculomas of the craniospinal axis. Turk Neurosurg 1:34–38
34. Talamás O, Del Brutto OH, García-Ramos G (1989) Brain-stem tuberculoma. An analysis of 11 patients. Arch Neurol 46:529–535
35. Lau KK, Yeun H (1996) Paradoxical development of brain stem tuberculoma during the treatment for tuberculous meningitis. HKMJ 2:211–212
36. Fu CH, Liu AB, Tsao WL (1999) Disseminated tuberculosis of the brain, brainstem, spinal cord, lung, kidney and retina- a case report. Tzu Chi Med J 11:191–196
37. Akhaddar A, Bourazza B, El Mostarchid B, Rouimi A, Boutaleb N, Ouahabi H, Mosseddaq R (2000) Brain stem tuberculoma- two cases. Rev Neurol (Paris) 156:399–402
38. Minagar A, Schatz NJ, Glaser JS (2004) AIDS Patient Care STDS 14:461–464
39. Kumar R, Singhi V (2004) Tuberculous brain stem abscesses in children. J Pediatr Neurol 2:101–106
40. Menon V, Gogoi M, Saxena R, Singh S, Kumar A (2004) Isolated one and half syndrome in brain stem tuberculoma. Indian J Pediatr 71:469–471
41. Enani M, Al-Nakhli DJ, Bakhsh E (2006) Isolated brain stem tuberculoma presenting with "one and a half syndrome". Saudi Med J 27:1407–1411
42. van Toorn R, Schoeman JF, Donald PR (2006) Brainstem tuberculoma presenting as eight-and-a-half syndrome. Eur J Paediatr Neurol 10:41–44
43. Sharma C, Kumawat B, Tripathi G, Dixit S (2008) Isolated sensory trigeminal neuropathy-a rare clinical presentation of brain stem tuberculoma. Case report. Int J Neurol 11:1
44. Donmez FY, Coskun M, Guven G (2009) Medulla oblongata tuberculoma mimicking metastasis presenting with stroke-like symptoms. Neurol Sci 30:349–352
45. Demetriou GA (2013) Brainstem tuberculosis. BMJ Case Rep 2013(pii):bcr2013010359. doi:10.1136/bcr-2013-010359
46. Gautam VKS, Singh R, Khurana S (2013) Brainstem tuberculoma presenting as stroke. IOSR J Dent Med Sci (IOSR-JDMS) 4:18–19
47. Chigurupati P, Kumar P (2014) Giant tubercular brainstem abscess: a case report. J Mahatma Gandhi Inst Med Sci 19:132–134
48. Kocak O, Bilac B, Harmanci K, Yakut A, Kocak A (2014) Tuberculosis brainstem abscess which is surgically inoperable and treated with medical therapy. J Neuroinfect Dis 5:1–2
49. Muin DA, Wagner K, Burian R, Ghaem Maghami N, Lapaire O (2015) Brainstem tuberculoma in pregnancy. Case Rep Obstet Gynecol 2015:179483. doi:10.1155/2015/179483
50. Agu CC, Aina O, Basunia M, Bhattarai B, Oke V, Schmidt MF, Quist J, Enriquez D, Gayam V (2015) Right gaze palsy and hoarseness: a rare presentation of mediastinal tuberculosis with an isolated prepontine cistern tuberculoma. Case Rep Infect Dis 2015:718289. doi:10.1155/2015/718289
51. Whitener DR (1978) Tuberculous brain abscess. Report of a case and review of the literature. Arch Neurol 35:148–155
52. Garcia-Monco JC (1999) Central nervous system tuberculosis. Neurol Clin 17:737–759
53. Farrar DJ, Flanigan TP, Gordon NM, Gold RL, Rich JD (1997) Tuberculous brain abscess in a patient with HIV infection: case report and review. Am J Med 102:297–301
54. Vidal JE, Penalva de Oliveira AC, Bonasser Filho F, Schiavon Nogueira R, Dauar RF, Leite AG (2005) Tuberculous brain abscess in AIDS patients: report of three cases and literature review. Int J Infect Dis 9:201–207
55. Warenbourg H, Niquet G, Lekieffre J, Thoreux M, Coupin J (1960) Onset of meningeal tuberculosis with Weber's syndrome. Lille Med 1961:3
56. Greenburg MS (2001) Brain stem related syndromes. Handbook of neurosurgery, 5th edn. Thieme medical publishers, New York, p 87
57. Henderson C, Meyers B, Humayun Gultekin S, Liu B, Zhang DY (2003) Intracranial tuberculoma in a liver transplant patient: first reported case and review of the literature. Am J Transplant 3:88–93
58. Vishnubhotla S, Siddhartha B, Sivramakrishna G, Lakshmi AY, Kumaraswamy RM (2009) Proptosis in a post-renal transplant patient with disseminated tuberculosis. Transpl Infect Dis 11:241–242
59. Verdon R, Chevret S, Laissy JP, Wolff M (1996) Tuberculous meningitis in adults: review of 48 cases. Clin Infect Dis 22:982–988
60. Clark WC, Metcalf JC, Muhlbauer MS, Dohan FC, Robertson JH (1986) Mycobacterium tuberculosis meningitis: a report of twelve cases and a literature review. Neurosurgery 18:604–610

61. O'Toole RD, Thornton GF, Mukherjee MK, Nath RL (1969) Dexamethasone in tuberculous meningitis. Relationship of cerebrospinal fluid effects to therapeutic efficacy. Ann Intern Med 70:39–48
62. Sutlas PN, Unal A, Forta H, Senol S, Kirbas D (2003) Tuberculous meningitis in adults: review of 61 cases. Infection 31:387–391
63. Stewart SM (1953) The bacteriological diagnosis of tuberculous meningitis. J Clin Pathol 6:241–242
64. Kennedy DH, Fallon RJ (1979) Tuberculous meningitis. JAMA 241:264–268
65. Kilpatrick ME, Girgis NI, Tribble D, Farid Z (1996) The value of the tuberculin skin test in patients with tuberculous meningitis. J Egypt Public Health Assoc 71:1–8
66. Mahadevan B, Mahadevan S, Serane VT, Narasimhan R (2005) Tuberculin reactivity in tuberculous meningitis. Indian J Pediatr 72:213–215
67. Joos TJ, Miller WC, Murdoch DM (2006) Tuberculin reactivity in bacille Calmette-Guerin vaccinated populations: a compilation of international data. Int J Tuberc Lung Dis 10:883–891
68. Kashyap RS, Kainthla RP, Mudaliar AV, Purohit HJ, Taori GM, Daginawala HF (2006) Cerebrospinal fluid adenosine deaminase activity: a complementary tool in the early diagnosis of tuberculous meningitis. Cerebrospinal Fluid Res 3:5
69. Rock RB, Olin M, Baker CA, Molitor TW, Peterson PK (2008) Central nervous system tuberculosis: pathogenesis and clinical aspects. Clin Microbiol Rev 21:243–261
70. Bernaerts A, Vanhoenacker FM, Parizel PM, Van Goethem JW, Van Altena R, Laridon A, De Roeck J, Coeman V, De Schepper AM (2003) Tuberculosis of the central nervous system: overview of neuroradiological findings. Eur Radiol 13:1876–1890
71. Jinkins JR, Gupta R, Chang KH, Rodriguez-Carbajal J (1995) MR imaging of central nervous system tuberculosis. Radiol Clin North Am 33:771–786
72. Kioumehr F, Dadsetan MR, Rooholamini SA, Au A (1994) Central nervous system tuberculosis: MRI. Neuroradiology 36:93–96
73. Wasay M, Kheleani BA, Moolani MK, Zaheer J, Pui M, Hasan S, Muzaffar S, Bakshi R, Sarawari AR (2003) Brain CT and MRI findings in 100 consecutive patients with intracranial tuberculoma. J Neuroimaging 13:240–247
74. Kumar R, Kohli N, Thavnani H, Kumar A, Sharma B (1996) Value of CT scan in the diagnosis of meningitis. Indian Pediatr 33:465–468
75. Katti MK (2004) Pathogenesis, diagnosis, treatment, and outcome aspects of cerebral tuberculosis. Med Sci Monit 10:RA215–RA229
76. Bargallo J, Berenguer J, Garcia-Barrionuevo UB, Bargallo N, Cardenal C, Mercader JM (1996) The "target sign": is it a specific sign of CNS tuberculoma? Neuroradiology 38:547–550
77. Pretell EJ, Martinot C, Garcia HH, Alvarado M, Bustos JA, Martinot C (2005) Differential diagnosis between cerebral tuberculosis and neurocysticercosis by magnetic resonance spectroscopy. J Comput Assist Tomogr 29:112–114
78. Jayasundar R, Raghunathan P, Banerji AK (1995) Proton MRS similarity between central nervous system non-Hodgkin lymphoma and intracranial tuberculoma. Magn Reson Imaging 13:489–493
79. Kingsley PB, Shah TC, Woldenberg R (2006) Identification of diffuse and focal brain lesions by clinical magnetic resonance spectroscopy. NMR Biomed 19:435–462
80. Shane SJ, Riley C (1953) Tuberculous meningitis: combined therapy with cortisone and antimicrobial agents. N Engl J Med 249:829–834
81. American Thoracic Society, Center for Disease Control and Prevention, and Infectious Diseases Society of America (2003) Treatment of tuberculosis. MMWR Recomm Rep 52:1–77
82. Christie LJ, Loeffler AM, Honarmand S, Flood JM, Baxter J, Jacobson S, Alexander R, Glaser CA (2008) Diagnostic challenges of central nervous system tuberculosis. Emerg Infect Dis 14:1473
83. Thwaites GE, Duc Bang N, Huy Dung N, Thi Quy H, Thi Tuong Oanh D, Thi Cam Thoa N, Quang Hien N, Tri Thuc N, Ngoc Hai N, Thi Ngoc Lan N, Ngoc Lan N, Hong Duc N, Ngoc Tuan V, Huu Hiep C, Thi Hong Chau T, Phuong Mai P, Thi Dung N, Stepniewska K, Simmons CP, White NJ, Tinh Hien T, Farrar JJ (2005) The influence of HIV infection on clinical presentation, response to treatment, and outcome in adults with tuberculous meningitis. J Infect Dis 192:2134–2141
84. El Sahly HM, Teeter LD, Pan X, Musser JM, Graviss EA (2007) Mortality associated with central nervous system tuberculosis. J Infect 55:502–509
85. Misra UK, Kalita J, Srivastava M, Mandal SK (1996) Prognosis of tuberculous meningitis: a multivariate analysis. J Neurol Sci 137:57–61
86. Katrak SM, Shembalkar PK, Bijwe SR, Bhandarkar LD (2000) The clinical, radiological and pathological profile of tuberculous meningitis in patients with and without human immunodeficiency virus infection. J Neurol Sci 181:118–126
87. Vinnard C, Winston CA, Wileyto EP, MacGregor RR, Bisson GP (2010) Isoniazid resistance and death in patients with tuberculous meningitis: retrospective cohort study. BMJ 341:c4451
88. Cecchini D, Ambrosioni J, Brezzo C, Corti M, Rybko A, Perez M (2007) Tuberculous meningitis in HIV-infected patients: drug susceptibility and clinical outcome. AIDS 21:373–374
89. DeAngelis LM (1981) Intracranial tuberculoma: case report and review of the literature. Neurology 31:1133–1136
90. Martinez-Vazquez C, Bordon J, Rodriguez-Gonzalez A, de la Fuente-Aguado J, Sopena B, Gallego-Rivera A (1995) Cerebral tuberculoma: a comparative study in patients with and without HIV infection. Infection 23:149–153

Ventricles

10

Mohammed Benzagmout, Amadou Hassane Ali, and Meryem Himmiche

Contents

M. Benzagmout, MD (✉)
Department of Neurosurgery,
University Hospital Hassan II, Fez, Morocco

Clinical Neurosciences Laboratory, Faculty of Medicine and Pharmacy, University of Fez, BP. 1893; Km 2.200, Sidi Hrazem Road, Fez 30000, Morocco
e-mail: benzagmout@hotmail.fr

A.H. Ali, MD • M. Himmiche, MD
Department of Neurosurgery,
University Hospital Hassan II, Fez, Morocco
e-mail: hassanem8@gmail.com; mariemed.1986@gmail.com

Abbreviations

BBB	Blood-brain barrier
BCSB	Blood-cerebrospinal barrier
CNS	Central nervous system
CSF	Cerebrospinal fluid
CT	Computed tomography
ETH	Ethambutol
IICP	Increased intracranial pressure
INH	Isoniazid
MRI	Magnetic resonance imaging
PCR	Polymerase chain reaction
PZA	Pyrazinamide
QFT	QuantiFERON
RIF	Rifampicin
STR	Streptomycin
TB	Tuberculosis
TBM	Tuberculous meningitis
WHO	World Health Organization

10.1 Introduction

Tuberculosis (TB) still represents one of the main devastating diseases throughout the world, especially in the developing countries [1]. Most commonly it involves the lungs. However, the central nervous system (CNS) involvement is the most severe form of systemic TB due to its high morbidity and mortality rates [2].

Intraventricular tuberculoma represents a rare location of CNS TB. It is usually associated with

M. Turgut et al. (eds.), *Tuberculosis of the Central Nervous System*,
DOI 10.1007/978-3-319-50712-5_10

systemic involvement, multiple cerebral tuberculomas, and/or meningitis [3]. Solitary intraventricular tuberculoma is extremely rare. To date, around 20 cases of intraventricular tuberculomas have been reported in the literature [4–6]. The majority of them were described in the lateral ventricles. Four cases were reported in the third ventricle [6–9], and only one case of fourth ventricular tuberculoma was published in the literature [10]. Table 10.1 summarizes intraventricular tuberculoma cases published in the indexed literature.

Because of the rarity and nonspecific clinical symptoms and imaging features of intraventricular tuberculoma, a preoperative diagnosis of these lesions is challenging, especially in countries where TB is not endemic. Therefore, a high index of suspicion is essential for the diagnosis since it is still a curable disease with a good prognosis if appropriately treated.

10.2 Pathophysiology

The CNS involvement comprises roughly 5–10% of all TB infections and up to 20% of patients with acquired immunodeficiency syndrome-related TB [11–13]. Ventricular involvement in neuro-TB is quite rare, probably due to the specific immune response of cerebrospinal fluid (CSF).

The exact route of entry of tubercle bacilli into the ventricles is controversial. Hematogenous spread through the choroid plexus appears to be the most likely mechanism [3]. Ventricular involvement in the TB process occurs in many forms like choroid plexus inflammation, ependymitis, tubercles (Rich foci), tuberculomas, TB abscess, and asymmetric hydrocephalus secondary to intraventricular adhesions or septa formation [3, 14–18].

Given that about 20% of the systemic blood flow is allocated to the CNS, experimental models have demonstrated that the blood flow allocated to the choroid plexus could be three to six times more than the parenchymal flow. Despite the presence of an efficient and almost impermeable protection system, the ventricular system is vulnerable to chemicals and pathogens especially after long-term contact with the body. In the brain parenchyma, this protection is ensured by the blood-brain barrier (BBB), while at the ventricular level, it is guaranteed by the blood-cerebrospinal barrier (BCSB).

The BCSB is primarily composed of epithelial cells located in the four choroid plexuses (lateral ventricles, third, and fourth ventricles) and endothelial cells forming the subarachnoid veins and venules. In comparison with the BBB, the BCSB has tighter junctions offering better and stricter transcystosis, thus giving the CSF permanent sterility and electrolyte balance. In addition, the choroid plexus offers an important exchange interface between the CSF and the circulatory system which makes it theoretically the ideal site for pathogenic agents to reach the CSF [15, 19, 20].

The mechanism by which *Mycobacterium tuberculosis* passes through the BCSB is unknown but could be largely attributed to the interaction between the host immune response and the virulence of the mycobacterium strains [21]. Theoretically, *M. tuberculosis* can cross the BCSB either as an intracellular microorganism inside an infected macrophage (Trojan horse mechanism) or by a simple phenomenon of transcystosis and/or paracellular traversal (primary infection especially in children) [22].

Study findings of Arnold and Rich Howard McCordock in 1933 coupled with results of Dastur in 1968 showed that autopsy of patients with tuberculous meningitis (TBM) demonstrated granulomatous foci called tubercles or "Rich Foci" [19, 20]. These millimetric lesions would usually rupture into the subarachnoid space and release the pathogen into the CSF causing TBM. Exceptionally, these tubercles may grow and fuse giving rise to intraventricular tuberculomas.

Mature tuberculoma generally consists of a necrotic caseous center surrounded by a capsule comprising fibroblasts, epithelioid cells, Langhans giant cells, and lymphocytes [19, 23]. Ventricular tuberculoma can be located in the choroid plexus, septum pellucidum, or ependymal layer triggering an inflammatory reaction in the surrounding tissue.

Table 10.1 Table summarizing intraventricular tuberculoma cases published in the literature

Authors	Year of publication	Country	Age/sex	Clinical symptoms	Ventricular location	Other cerebral lesions	Pulmonary TB	Anti-TB chemotherapy	Surgery	VP shunt	Outcome
Rucci	1951	Italy	NA	NA	Right lateral ventricle	No	No	Yes	No	No	NA
Berthier	1987	Argentina	04/M	IICP, fever, focal deficit	Left frontal horn	No	Yes	Yes	No	No	Good/3 weeks
Berthier	1987	Argentina	05/F	IICP, fever, weight loss	Left frontal horn	No	No	Yes	No	No	Good
Berthier	1987	Argentina	04/M	IICP, fever, anorexia	Right frontal horn	No	Yes	Yes	No	Yes	Good/1 month
Berthier	1987	Argentina	02/F	IICP	Left occipital horn	Yes	No	Yes	No	No	Partial recovery, psychomotor retardation
Desgeorges	1977	France	15/M	IICP	Left lateral ventricle	No	No	Yes	Total removal	No	Good
Singh JP	1988	India	13/F	IICP, fever	Third ventricle	No	No	Yes/6 months	Partial removal	No	Good/6 months
Okuda	1993	Japan	55/M	IICP, fever, nystagmus	Left lateral ventricle	No	Yes	Yes	Yes/biopsy	No	Good
Vajramani	1999	India	26/F	IICP, fever	Right lateral ventricle	No	No	Yes/14 months	Total removal	Yes	Good
Meshkini	2001	Iran	40/F	IICP, focal deficit	Right temporal horn	No	No	NA	Total removal	No	NA
Desai	2002	India	38/F	IICP, fever	Septum pellucidum	No	No	Yes/24 months	Total removal	No	Good/9 months
Hsu	2004	Taiwan	19/F	IICP	Right frontal horn	No	No	Yes/12 months	Total removal	Yes	Good/10 months
Doglietto	2006	Italy	57/M	IICP, fever, aphasia, ataxia	Left occipital horn	No	Yes	Yes/12 months	Total removal	No	Good/7 years
Sonmez	2008	Turkey	22/M	IICP, fever	Right occipital horn	No	No	NA	Total removal	No	NA
DK Singh	2010	India	43/M	IICP, fever, memory disorders	Right lateral ventricle	No	No	Yes/7 months	Total removal	No	Good/2 months
Mukund	2011	India	04/F	IICP, fever	Fourth ventricle	No	No	Yes/9 months	No	Yes	Good/3 months
Mohindra	2012	India	28/F	IICP, fever, focal deficit	Left frontal horn	No	No	Yes/12 months	No	Yes	Good/12 months
Coulibaly	2013	Morocco	26/M	IICP	Right occipital horn	No	No	Yes/12 months	Total removal	No	Good/3 months
Chowdhury	2013	Bangladesh	18/F	IICP, gait disturbance	Third ventricle	No	No	Yes	Yes/biopsy	No	Good/6 months

(continued)

Table 10.1 (continued)

Authors	Year of publication	Country	Age/sex	Clinical symptoms	Ventricular location	Other cerebral lesions	Pulmonary TB	Anti-TB chemotherapy	Surgery	VP shunt	Outcome
Matsumoto	2013	Japan	70/M	IICP, memory disorders	Right occipital horn	No	No	Yes	Yes/biopsy	No	Good/3 months
N'da	2013	Ivory Coast	10/F	IICP,	Third ventricle	No	No	Yes/6 months	Total removal	No	Good/6 years
Garg	2014	India	16/F	IICP, fever	Third ventricle	Yes	No	Yes	No	Yes	Good/2 months
Singh J	2014	India	13/M	IICP, weight loss	Septum pellucidum	No	Yes	No	Total removal	No	Death

Abbreviations: *TB* tuberculosis, *VP* ventriculoperitoneal, *IICP* increased intracranial pressure, *NA* not available

10.3 Clinical Presentation

There are no specific symptoms for intraventricular tuberculomas [17]. Clinical features may include signs of increased intracranial pressure (IICP) (headache/vomiting/visual symptoms), seizures, and/or focal neurological deficits depending on the number of lesions, their location in the ventricular system, and their relationship with the surrounding affected cerebral regions.

Intraventricular tuberculoma may also be asymptomatic or accidentally discovered in brain imaging upon screening for systemic multivisceral TB. In many cases, the lesions are incidentally picked up in the setting of multiple cerebral parenchymal tuberculoma. Around 30% of cases have evidence of extracranial TB [24].

10.4 Diagnosis

There are no pathognomonic radiological signs for tuberculoma. The confirmation is only made by histopathological study of the lesion. This typically shows a necrotic caseous center surrounded by a capsule composed of fibroblasts, epithelioid cells, Langhans giant cells, and lymphocytes [25].

The radiological characteristics of tuberculoma vary according to their evolutionary stage [20]. The radiological signs are not specific of tuberculoma and can mimic other expansive intraventricular lesions such as plexus choroid tumor, glioma, or metastasis. Nevertheless, the peripheral enhancement of contrast, the central necrosis, the presence of a disproportionate edema, and traction of the septum pellucidum with asymmetrical dilatation of lateral ventricles are all suggestive of intraventricular tuberculomas [3, 6] (Figs. 10.1 and 10.2).

Brain MRI is the tool of choice as it gives the exact location of the lesion, as well as its size, its signal, and the intensity of contrast enhancement. It also searches associated lesions, edema, and hydrocephalus. Radiological findings depend on the maturity of tuberculoma in which we have to distinguish between noncaseating granuloma and caseating lesions with a solid or a liquid center.

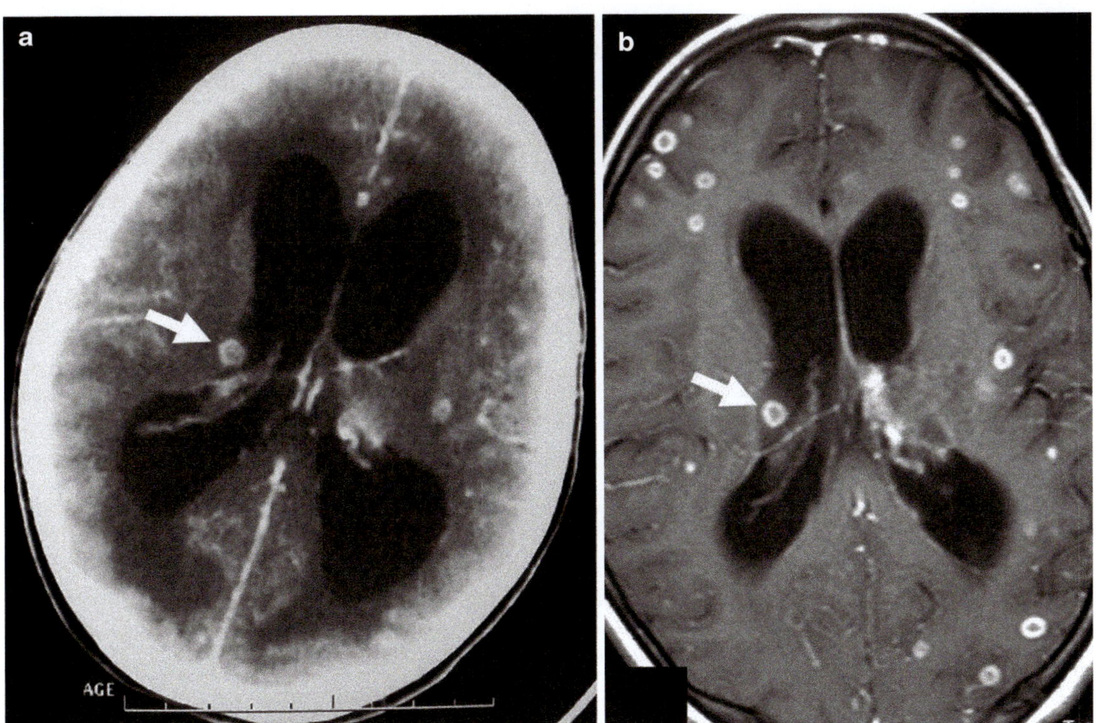

Fig. 10.1 Cerebral axial CT scan (**a**) and T1-enhanced MRI (**b**) demonstrating right intraventricular tuberculoma in a context of multiple cerebral tuberculomas (Courtesy of Ali Akhaddar M.D.)

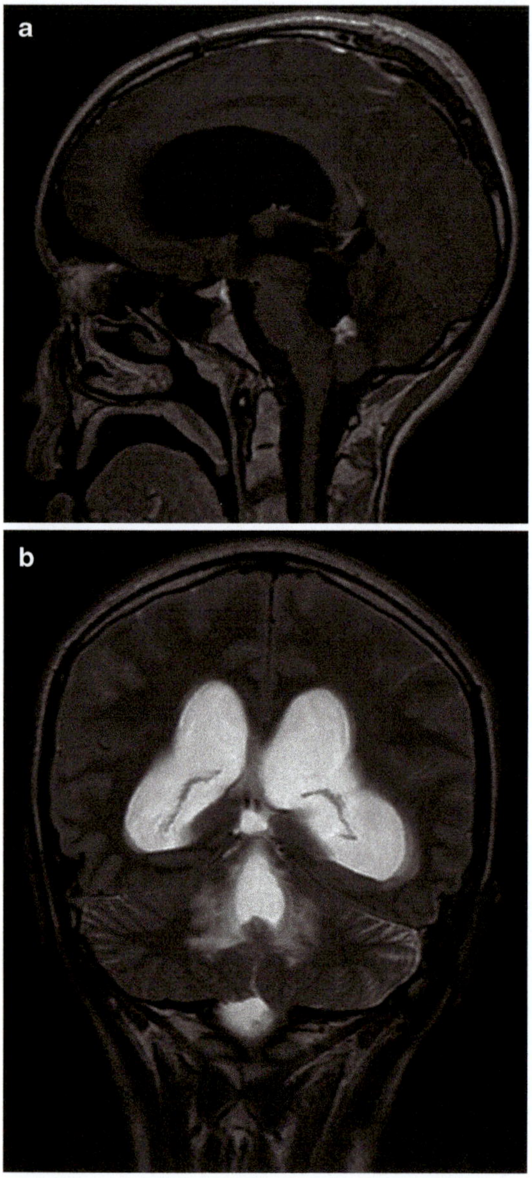

Fig. 10.2 Cerebral MRI in contrast sagittal T1 (**a**) and coronal T2 (**b**) views showing a fourth ventricular tuberculoma with an important perilesional edema

The degree of the surrounding edema is variable and is thought to be inversely proportional to the maturity of the lesion [20, 21]. Moreover, Santy et al. have recommended that magnetic resonance spectroscopy may increase the specificity of tuberculoma diagnosis by identifying lipids within the lesion [26].

Considering the rarity of intraventricular tuberculomas, the preoperative diagnosis of these lesions is very challenging because there are no specific clinical/radiologic symptoms. Nevertheless, various factors should arouse the clinical suspicion of this affection, particularly in countries where TB is endemic. Poor socioeconomic state of the patient, moderate fever, high erythrocyte sedimentation rate, positive Mantoux test, and presence of TB elsewhere in the body are all presumptive indicators of TB.

Some authors suggest also the use of both QuantiFERON test (QFT) and polymerase chain reaction (PCR) to resolve diagnosis difficulties in intracranial tuberculomas. Indeed, QFT does not generate false-positive reactions in patients vaccinated by bacillus Calmette-Guérin and has high sensitivity (86%) and specificity (97.9%) for TB [27]. Additionally, PCR might be useful to detect TB using either CSF or patient sputum samples with variable reported sensitivity and specificity [28].

10.5 Treatment

TB of CNS is a curable disease with appropriate treatment. Its treatment of choice remains conservative and provides a good control of the disease in most cases [5, 29].

Traditionally, anti-TB treatment associates four essential TB drugs of the first class: isoniazid (INH), rifampicin (RIF), pyrazinamide (PZA), and ethambutol (ETH); in some cases streptomycin (STR) can replace ETH. Drugs should be administered orally in the morning on an empty stomach 1 h before meal. STR, a bactericidal antibiotic, was the first effective treatment for TB. As recommended by the WHO, standard treatment of TB consists of a 2-month induction phase with RIF, INH, PZA, and ETH, followed by a consolidation phase using at least INH and RIF [30]. The duration of medical treatment is at least 6 months [31].

Although the medical regimen is the cornerstone of treatment, the surgical treatment is still used in brain tuberculoma management. Shunting procedures such as ventriculoperitoneal shunting or third ventriculostomy could be sometimes required to treat hydrocephalus caused by intraventricular tuberculoma.

Stereotactic or burr-hole biopsy via ventricular endoscopy may be discussed in cases of isolated intraventricular lesions with no associated systemic TB [5]. Besides, surgical intervention has to be considered in cases of uncontrolled IICP induced by the lesion itself or by the associated obstructive hydrocephalus [5]. Surgery is also recommended for a definitive histological diagnosis of the lesion in cases of huge ventricular lesions with unknown history of TB and after 6 weeks of poor response to anti-TB treatment [32–34].

Follow-up radiological examinations (CT scan or MRI) are valuable in monitoring the response to medical treatment. Paradoxical enlargement of a preexisting tuberculoma or the appearance of new CNS tuberculoma lesions in patients receiving anti-TB chemotherapy may be occasionally seen [35]. However, with continuation of adequate treatment, resolution of tuberculoma usually happens [36, 37].

Conclusion

TB remains a major worldwide health problem and a potentially life-threatening disease. Most commonly it involves the lungs. However, CNS location is the most serious form of the disease. The ventricular location of tuberculoma in the brain is extremely rare. Clinical and radiologic manifestations of this affection are miscellaneous and might be misdiagnosed as other infectious or tumoral brain lesions, especially in the absence of other brain or systemic TB lesions. Hence, clinicians should be aware of a potential CNS ventricular involvement in TB. This diagnosis should be kept in mind especially in the presence of atypical solitary lesions in the brain ventricular system in order to reduce the morbidity and mortality of this curable affection.

References

1. Dye C, Scheele S, Dolin P, Pathania V, Raviglione MC (1999) Consensus statement. Global burden of tuberculosis: estimated incidence, prevalence and mortality by country. WHO Global Surveillance and Monitoring Project. JAMA 282:677–686
2. Arvanitakis Z, Long RL, Hershfield ES, Manfreda J, Kabani A, Kunimoto D, Power C (1998) M. tuberculosis molecular variation in CNS infection: evidence for strain-dependent neurovirulence. Neurology 50:1827–1832
3. Berthier M, Sierra J, Leiguarda R (1987) Intraventricular tuberculoma. Report of four cases in children. Neuroradiology 29:163–167
4. Doglietto F, Marchese E, Puca A, Vellone VG, Tirpakova B, Sanguinetti M (2006) Solitary choroid plexus tuberculoma in an adult patient. Case illustration. J Neurosurg 105:933
5. Hsu PW, Lin TK, Chang CN (2004) Solitary intraventricular tuberculoma in adults. Acta Neurochir 146:1151–1154
6. Singh JP, Chandy MJ (1988) Third ventricular tuberculoma: a case report. Br J Neurosurg 2:93–96
7. Chowdhury FH, Haque R, Alam SM (2013) Third ventricular and interpeduncular fossa tubercular abscess with triventriculomegaly – Ventriculoscopic surgical management. J Med 14:72–73
8. Garg K, Gurjar HK, Joseph SG, Shashikant RC, Sharma BS (2014) Third ventricular tuberculoma. Neurol India 62:73–75
9. N'da HA, Haidara A, Drogba L, Derou LK, Yao SK, Ba Zézé V (2013) A rare third ventricle solitary tuberculoma. Pan Afr Med J 16:5
10. Mukund A, Gamanagatti S (2011) Fourth ventricle tuberculoma. Indian Pediatr 48:161–162
11. Berenguer J, Moreno S, Laguna F, Vicente T, Adrados M, Ortega A, González-LaHoz J, Bouza E (1992) Tuberculous meningitis in patients infected with the human immunodeficiency virus. N Engl J Med 326:668–672
12. Bernaerts A, Vanhoenacker FM, Parizel PM, Van Goethem JW, Van Altena R, Laridon A, De Roeck J, Coeman V, De Schepper AM (2003) Tuberculosis of the central nervous system: overview of neuroradiological findings. Eur Radiol 13(8):1876–1890
13. Vidal JE, Penalva de Oliveira AC, Bonasser Filho F, Schiavon Nogueira R, Dauar RF, Leite AG, Lins DL, Coelho JF (2005) Tuberculous brain abscess in AIDS patients: report of three cases and literature review. Int J Infect Dis 9:201–207
14. Bhargava S, Gupta AK, Tandon PN (1982) Tuberculous meningitis-a CT study. Br J Radiol 55:189–196
15. Dastur HM, Desai AD (1965) A comparative study of brain tuberculomas and gliomas based upon 107 case records of each. Brain 88:375–396
16. Dastur DK, Lalitha VS, Prabhakar V (1968) Pathological analysis of intracranial space-occupying lesions in 1000 cases including children. J Neurol Sci 6:575–592
17. Desai K, Nadkarni T, Bhatjiwale M, Goel A (2002) Intraventricular tuberculoma. Neurol Med Chir 42:501–503
18. Vajramani GV, Devi BI, Hegde T, Santosh V, Khanna N, Vasudev MK (1999) Intraventricular tuberculous abscess: a case report. Neurol India 47:327–329
19. Rock RB, Olin M, Baker CA, Molitor TW, Peterson PK (2008) Central nervous system tuberculosis:

pathogenesis and clinical aspects. Clin Microbiol Rev 21:243–261
20. Strazielle N, Mutin M, Ghersi-Egea JF (2005) The choroid plexuses: a dynamic interface between the blood and the cerebrospinal fluid (In French). Morphologie 89:90–101
21. Drevets DA, Leenen PJ, Greenfield RA (2004) Invasion of the central nervous system by intracellular bacteria. Clin Microbiol Rev 17:323–347
22. Kim KS (2008) Mechanisms of microbial traversal of the blood-brain barrier. Nat Rev Microbiol 6:625–634
23. DeLance AR, Safaee M, Oh MC, Clark AJ, Kaur G, Sun MZ, Bollen AW, Phillips JJ, Parsa AT (2013) Tuberculoma of the central nervous system. J Clin Neurosci 20:1333–1341
24. Singh J, Kharosekar H, Vernon Velho MCH (2014) An unusual intraventricular lesion- septum pellucidum tuberculoma. J Spine Neurosurg 3:5
25. Hua SE, Clatterbuck RE, Stern BJ, Sampath P, Rhines LD (2004) Sarcoidosis, tuberculosis, and xanthogranuloma. In: Winn HR (ed) Youmans neurological surgery, vol 1. Saunders, Philadelphia, pp 1435–1447
26. Santy K, Nan P, Chantana Y, Laurent D, Nadal D, Richner B (2011) The diagnosis of brain tuberculoma by (1) H-magnetic resonance spectroscopy. Eur J Pediatr 170:379–387
27. Menzies D, Pai M, Comstock G (2007) Meta-analysis: new tests for the diagnosis of latent tuberculosis infection: areas of uncertainty and recommendations for research. Ann Intern Med 146:340–354
28. Matsumoto Y, Aikawa H, Narita S, Tsutsumi M, Yoshida H, Etou H, Sakamoto K, Inoue R, Nii K, Kazekawa K (2013) Intracranial tuberculoma in non-immunosuppressive state. Neurol Med Chir (Tokyo) 53:259–262
29. Bozbuga M, Boran BO, Bayindir C (2005) Tuberculoma of the cavernous sinus. Int J Neurosurg 2(2)
30. Horsburgh CR Jr, Barry CE 3rd, Lange C (2015) Treatment of tuberculosis. N Engl J Med 373:2149–2160
31. Mitchison DA, Fourie PB (2010) The near future: improving the activity of rifamycins and pyrazinamide. Tuberc (Edinb) 90:177–181
32. Arseni C (1958) Two-hundred- and-one cases of intracranial tuberculoma treated surgically. Neurol Neurosurg Psychiatry 21:308–311
33. Gropper MR, Schulder M, Sharan AD, Eun-Sook Cho BA (1995) Central nervous system tuberculosis: medical management and surgical indications. Surg Neurol 44:378–385
34. Tiel R, Rosenblum ML (1996) Chronic granulomatous lesions: tuberculosis, leprosy, sarcoidosis. In: Wilkins RH, Rengachary SS (eds) Neurosurgery. McGraw-Hill, New York, pp 3341–3350
35. Sanei Taheri M, Karimi MA, Haghighatkhah H, Pourghorban R, Samadian M, Delavar Kasmaei H (2015) Central nervous system tuberculosis: an imaging-focused review of a reemerging disease. Radiol Res Pract 2015:202806
36. Afghani B, Lieberman JM (1994) Paradoxical enlargement or development of intracranial tuberculomas during therapy: case report and review. Clin Infect Dis 19:1092–1099
37. Ku BD, Yoo S (2009) Extensive meningeal and parenchymal calcified tuberculoma as long-term residual sequelae of tuberculous meningitis. Neurol India 57:521–522

11 Sellar-Suprasellar Region

Nayil Khursheed, Rumana Makhdoomi, and Ahmet T. Turgut

Contents

N. Khursheed, MCh (✉)
Department of Neurosurgery, Sheri-Kashmir Institute of Medical Sciences, Srinagar, Kashmir 190011, India
e-mail: nayilkhursh@gmail.com

R. Makhdoomi, MD
Department of Pathology, Sheri-Kashmir Institute of Medical Sciences, Srinagar, Kashmir, India
e-mail: rumanamak@gmail.com

A.T. Turgut, MD
Department of Radiology, Hacettepe University School of Medicine, Ankara, Turkey
e-mail: ahmettuncayturgut@yahoo.com

Abbreviations

CNS	Central nervous system
CSF	Cerebrospinal fluid
INH	Isoniazid
MDR	Multidrug resistance
MRI	Magnetic resonance imaging
RIF	Rifampicin
TB	Tuberculosis
TBM	Tuberculous meningitis

11.1 Introduction

Central nervous system (CNS) tuberculosis (TB) is a serious form of extrapulmonary TB, occurring among approximately 10% of all patients with TB. Intracranial tuberculomas account for 0.15–4% of intracranial space-occupying lesions [1, 2]. In developing countries, tuberculomas constituted up to 30% of space-occupying intracranial lesions until recently. However, the incidence has dramatically decreased after the advent of anti-TB chemotherapy.

11.2 Pathogenesis

The pathway for spread of *Mycobacterium tuberculosis* to this region is unclear; either hematogenous spread or continuous extension from a local TB infection of the paranasal sinuses has been

M. Turgut et al. (eds.), *Tuberculosis of the Central Nervous System*,
DOI 10.1007/978-3-319-50712-5_11

proposed [3]. In some patients, the primary focus cannot be demonstrated. It has been reported that intracranial tuberculomas can develop or enlarge during anti-TB therapy where exaggerated host reaction to TB protein is thought to play a role [4]. Pituitary involvement in TB infection may be secondary to tuberculous meningitis (TBM) [5]. Sharma et al. reported that history or existing TB infection elsewhere in the body was present only in 30% of patients. This observation was based in a review on 18 cases of sellar tuberculomas [6].

11.3 Clinical Features

TB of CNS can present as meningitis, arachnoiditis, or spinal or intracranial tuberculomas [7]. Tuberculoma of CNS might occur at any site and in any age group; however, sellar and suprasellar regions are not the usual sites of tuberculomas. The first reported case of a sellar tuberculoma was by Coleman in 1940 [8]. Most of the literature data on sellar tuberculomas unsurprisingly largely arises from the Indian subcontinent and other developing countries. Tuberculomas of the sellar and suprasellar regions comprise 1% of all intracranial tuberculomas; a review of literature reveals 77 cases [2, 9–11], which includes two cases reported by us [10]. Most of the reported patients are females with headache and visual symptoms as the most frequent complaints [6, 12]. Headache is present in more than 90% patients and visual symptoms in more than 46%. Headache is reported as throbbing and severe in most patients. Visual disturbances in the form of visual field cuts, diminution of visual acuity, diplopia, mydriasis, and blurred vision are common [9].

Specific cause of headache in pituitary tuberculomas is attributed to the associated meningitic process or infarction caused by inflammatory vasculitis or secondary to the dural stretch [13]. Fever is present in patients who are usually less than 12 years of age while as it is much less frequent in adult patients [4]. More than 80% of affected individuals are less than 45 years of age, mean age of 32 years (range of 5–68 years) with a female-to-male ratio of 2.2:1 (53 females, 24 males) (Table 11.1). Retrosellar extension of sellar tuberculomas can cause cranial nerve palsies, hemiparesis, and cerebellar signs resulting from brainstem and peduncular compression [13].

Patients may present with anterior pituitary hormone deficiencies, central diabetes insipidus at onset, and hypogonadism secondary to low levels of GH, FSH/LH, TSH, and ACTH deficiencies. About 60% of patients have complete anterior panhypopituitarism, and 28% had central diabetes insipidus as initial presentation [21]. Another frequent finding is raised prolactin levels due to pituitary stalk effect [20].

Hemorrhage in a sellar tuberculoma is extremely rare, with only three case reports in the literature. Such patients present with the classical features of pituitary apoplexy. They report with acute onset headache, vomiting, and sometimes with altered sensorium. Oculomotor nerve palsy may also be a feature. Besides, acute visual diminution is almost invariably noticed. The mechanism is supposed to be secondary to vasculitis. All these symptoms may have a subacute onset also which could be secondary to repeated small hemorrhages within the granuloma [22].

Interestingly, moyamoya phenomenon also has been described in association with suprasellar tuberculoma [11] recently in an 8-year-old boy who presented with headache and visual diminution. In this patient digital subtraction angiography showed complete occlusion of the left internal carotid artery distal to posterior communicating artery and formation of some moyamoya collaterals. Bilateral anterior cerebral arteries were filling from the right A2. On external carotid artery injection, the entire cerebral circulation was supplied by multiple dural collaterals, mainly from the middle meningeal artery.

11.4 Imaging

Tuberculomas appear on imaging as round or oval nodules varying in size from 2 to 12 mm. Sometimes the central necrosis may result in ring-enhancing appearance on contrast imaging. On magnetic resonance imaging (MRI), tuberculomas are usually hypointense on T1-weighted images and iso- to hyperintense on T2-weighted

Table 11.1 Published cases of pituitary tuberculoma in the literature to date

No. of cases	Reference	Age/sex	Presentation	Tuberculosis elsewhere	Endocrinology before treatment	Endocrinological profile after treatment
1	Coleman et al. (1940) [8]	57, F	Headache, bitemporal hemianopsia	No	NM	NM
2	Glass and Davis (1944) [9]	54, M	Fever	No	Hypopituitarism	NM
3	Brooks et al. (1973) [1]	33, F	Headache, amenorrhea, mild bitemporal field cut	Lung	Hypopituitarism	Improved
4	Esposito et al. (1987) [2]	54, F	Headache	Lung	Normal	Normal
5	Eckland et al. (1987) [2]	37, F	Headache, VI nerve palsy, temporal hemianopia	Cervical lymph nodes	Hypopituitarism	Improved
6	Delsedime et al. (1988) [2]	45, F	Headache, amenorrhea, deafness	Sinusitis	Hyperprolactinemia	Same
7	Kamiya et al. (1991) [9]	41,M	Headache	Pulmonary TB	Hypopituitarism	Improved
8	Taparia et al. (1992) [2]	40, M	Headache, constricted visual fields	No	Normal	Normal
9	Ghosh et al. (1992) [2]	35, F	Headache, amenorrhea, bitemporal field cut	No	Hypopituitarism, hyperprolactinemia	Improved
10	Ranjan et al. (1994) [12]	32, F	Headache, nausea	–	Hypopituitarism	Worse
11	-do-	40, M	Headache, lethargy	–	Hypopituitarism	Improved
12	-do-	18, F	Headache, vomiting	–	Normal	Worse
13	-do-	27, M	Headache, lethargy, headache, galactorrhoea	–	Hypopituitarism	Improved
14	-do-	35, F	Amenorrhea, bitemporal field cut	–	Hypopituitarism	Improved
15	Pereira et al. (1995) [2]	55, F	Headache, VI nerve palsy	No	Hypopituitarism	Improved
16	Ashkan et al. (1997) [14]	33, F	Headache, amenorrhea, fatigue, weight loss, headache galactorrhoea	Bilateral lymph adenopathy	Hypopituitarism	Improved
17	-do-	31, F	Amenorrhea, bitemporal upper quadrantanopia	No	Panhypopituitarism	Improved
18	Gazioglu et al. (1998) [2]	34, F	Acromegaly, oligomenorrhea	No	GH level raised	Improved
19	Kim et al. (1998) [2]	47, F	Headache	No	–	Improved
20	-do-	36, F	Headache	No	–	Improved
21	Petrossians et al. (1998) [9]	54, F	Headache, vomiting			
22	Basaria et al. (2000) [9]	NA, F	Headache	No	NM	NM
23	Sharma et al. (2000) [6]	35, F	Headache, vomiting, decrease of vision	No	Normal	–
24	-do-	17, F	Headache, blindness	No	Normal	–

(continued)

Table 11.1 (continued)

No. of cases	Reference	Age/sex	Presentation	Tuberculosis elsewhere	Endocrinology before treatment	Endocrinological profile after treatment
25	-do-	14, F	Headache, decrease of vision, III nerve palsy	No	Normal	–
26	-do-	36, M	Headache, decrease of vision	No	Normal	–
27	-do-	8, F	Fever, headache, blindness	Dorsal spine TB	Normal	–
28	-do-	21, F	Headache, vomiting, loss of vision	No	Normal	–
29	-do-	40, M	Headache, diminution of vision	No	Hypopituitarism	–
30	-do-	43, M	Headache, vomiting	No	Hypopituitarism	–
31	-do-	16, M	Weight gain, generalized weakness	No	Hypogonadism	–
32	-do-	22, F	Headache, vomiting, fever, galactorrhoea	Tuberculous meningitis	Proactin raised	–
33	-do-	20, M	Headache, vomiting, fever	Pulmonary TB	Hypopituitarism	–
34	-do-	35, F	Headache, vomiting, loss of vision	No	Hypopituitarism	–
35	-do-	14, F	Headache, diplopia, sixth nerve palsy, fever	No	Normal	–
36	-do-	14, F	Headache, third nerve palsy	No	Normal	–
37	-do-	25, F	Headache, galactorrhea	No	Prolactin raised	–
38	-do-	22, F	Headache, amenorrhea, hoarseness	No	GH level raised	–
39	-do-	32, F	Headache, amenorrhea, loss of vision	Pulmonary TB	Prolactin raised	–
40	-do-	13, F	Headache, blindness	Pulmonary TB	Normal	–
41	Jain et al. (2001) [15]	5, M	Irritability of 10-month duration, decreased visual field	No	Hypothyroidism, diabetes insipidus	Improved
42	Paramo et al. (2001) [5]	32, F	Headache, asthenia, amenorrhea, polydipsia, polyuria	No	Normal	Hypopituitarism
43	Arunkumar et al. (2001) [16]	27, M	Headache with giddiness	No	Normal	Improved
44	Manghani et al. (2001) [17]	24, M	Headache, loss of libido	No	Prolactin, ACTH level minimally raised	Improved
45	Domingues et al. (2002) [9]	46/F	Confusion	No	Hypopituitarism	Improved
46	Stalldecker et al. (2002) [9]	16, F	Headache, polyuria, polydipsia, amenorrhea	No	Hypopituitarism	Improved
47	-do-	15, F	Hemianopia	Pulmonary TB	Hypopituitarism	Improved
48	-do-	19, F	Headache, amenorrhea	No	Hypopituitarism	Improved
49	Desai et al. (2003) [13]	22, F	Headache, amenorrhea, decreased vision	Yes	Hypopituitarism	Hypopituitarism
50	-do-	30, F	Headache	No	Hypopituitarism	Improved

51	-do-	47, M	Headache, oligomenorrhea, galactorrhea	No	Raised prolactin	Improved
52	Satyarthee et al. (2003) [9]	32, F	Polyuria, polydipsia, amenorrhea,	No	Raised prolactin	Improved
53	Kim et al. (2003) [2]	29, F	Headache, decreased vision	No	Hypopituitarism	Improved
54	Harzallah et al. (2004) [9]	52, F	Headache, vomiting, oculomotor nerve palsy	No	Hypopituitarism	Improved
55	-do-	62, M	Fever, seizures, confusion	No	Hypopituitarism	Improved
56	Ahmad et al. (2005) [18]	22, F	Headache, decrease in vision	No	Normal	Normal
57	Trabelsi et al. (2005) [9]	42, F	Polyuria, polydipsia amenorrhea, galactorrhea	No	Raised prolactin	Improved
58	Deogaonkar et al. (2006) [9]	27, F	Headache, vomiting, oculomotor nerve palsy	No	Normal	Normal
59	Sunil et al. (2007) [4]	42, M	Polyuria, polydipsia, polyphagia, decreased libido	No	Raised prolactin	Improved
60	Yilmazlar et al. (2007) [9]	37, F	Galactorrhea and menstrual irregularity	No	Raised prolactin	Improved
61	Hussain et al. (2008) [9]	40, F	Headache, fatigue	No	Hypothyroidism and hypocortisolism	Improved
62	Rao et al. (2008) [9]	47, F	Headache, vomiting, galactorrhea	No	Raised prolactin	Improved
63–70	Behari et al. (2009) [19]	Eight cases, mean age of 25 years, range 15–40 years, M:F = 5:3	Headache and vomiting were main symptoms	In some patients	Most had hypopituitarism	Improved
71	Mittal et al. (2010) [9]	40, F	Headache, blurred vision	No	Hypopituitarism	Improved
72	Domiciano et al. (2010) [9]	33, F	Polyuria, polydipsia	No	Anterior pituitary hormones were normal	Normal
73	Shukla et al. (2010) [9]	68/M	Left temporal field cut	No	Normal	Normal
74	Furtado et al. (2011) [20]	31, F	Headache, lethargy	No	Hypopituitarism	Normal
75	Nayil et al. (2011) [10]	8, M	Known case of tubercular meningitis on treatment developed headache and vomiting	No	Hypothyroidism and hypocortisolism	Improved
76	Nayil et al (2011) [10]	6, F	Polyuria and polydipsia	No	Normal	Remained normal
77	Nupur et al. (2014) [11]	8, M	Headache, vomiting	No	Not mentioned	Not mentioned

Case numbers 4–6, 8, 9, 15, and 18–20 have been cited from by Kim SH et al. [2], and case numbers 2, 7, 21, 22, 45–48, 52, 54, 55, 57, 58, 60–62, and 71–73 have been cited from Bonifacio-Delgadillo et al. [9]

Abbreviations: *NM* not mentioned

images with perilesional edema. The enhancement in intracranial tuberculomas may reveal solid-enhancing lesions, ring-enhancing lesions, or/and mixed-enhancing lesions [15, 16, 23]. MRI may also depict thickening of pituitary stalk in pituitary tuberculomas which is a nonspecific sign seen in other non-TB conditions, such as sarcoidosis, Wegner's granulomatosis, and lymphocytic hypophysitis [10, 24–26].

There are five major radiological types of sellar/suprasellar tuberculomas:

Type A – sellar/suprasellar tuberculomas with hydrocephalus due to obstruction at the level of the third ventricle. Such patients usually present with signs of increased intracranial pressure (IICP) and visual diminution.

Type B – multiple coalescing sellar-suprasellar ring-enhancing tuberculomas with mild perilesional edema which may involve the hypothalamus. There usually is no hydrocephalus.

Type C – intrasellar abscess.

Type D – pachymeningitis with suprasellar extension. MRI reveals markedly enhancing tissue layering the supra- and infratentorial surfaces of the tentorium. There also may be extension of the granulation tissue into the brain stem and upper cervical cord.

Type E – enhancing granulation tissue eroding into the clivus with extension into the sphenoidal and ethmoidal sinuses and the sella [19].

The sellar mass lesions must be differentiated from inflammatory lesions such as lymphocytic or granulomatous hypophysitis, sarcoidosis, and Langerhans cell histiocytosis and from neoplasms such as astrocytoma, lymphoma, metastasis, germ cell tumor, and meningioma. The ring-enhancing lesions must be especially distinguished from neurocysticercosis and abscess. The differential diagnosis also includes several clinical entities with a clinicoradiological picture of pachymeningitis such as lymphoma, leukemia, sarcoidosis, and idiopathic pachymeningitis. Skull base tuberculoma may have similar appearance with clival chordomas, chondromas, giant cell tumors of the sphenoid, adenoid cystic carcinoma, and fungal granuloma [10, 16]. Magnetic resonance spectroscopy of a tuberculoma shows prominent lipid peaks at 0.9, 1.3, 2.0, and 2.8 ppm and for phosphoserine at 3.7 ppm. An increase in the normalized choline/creatinine ratio is also found. The lipid resonances occur due to the presence of methylene and terminal methyl groups on fatty acids found in the caseous material in the center of tuberculomas; however a similar pattern may, however, also be observed in patients with toxoplasmosis and primary CNS lymphoma [27].

11.5 Management Options

There has been no agreement on the duration of treatment for TB of CNS, which is partly because of the numerous variables that may have an impact on therapeutic response. The American Thoracic Society and the Centers for Disease Control and Prevention recommend that treatment for TBM, intracranial tuberculomas, or tuberculomas with meningitis should be administered for 12 months when the bacterial strain is sensitive to the antibiotics. They also recommend that treatment should be extended to 18 months for patients who do not receive pyrazinamide during the first 2 months of therapy, whereas the therapy should be extended to 24 months for patients with multidrug resistance (MDR)-TB of the CNS [28].

In case of residual lesion, anti-TB therapy is to be continued beyond this initial period. Steroid administration during the first 2 weeks is used to decrease inflammation and adhesions around the optic nerve in patients presenting with rapid visual deterioration [10]. Patients presenting with definite systemic manifestations of TB such as chronic cough, weight loss, malaise, evening fever or night sweats, and residing in endemic areas, with a positive history of TB or with prolonged contact with a patient suffering from TB, can undergo anti-TB chemotherapy without any histopathological confirmation for the diagnosis. Also, a raised erythrocyte sedimentation rate, fluorescein microscopy, mycobacterial DNA amplification, and enzyme-linked immunosorbent assay for immunoglobulins against TB may be considered as further evidence to diagnose a TB infection [6]. Mantoux positivity in an endemic area such as the Indian subcontinent is not accepted to be diagnostic because of the high rate of false positivity. The significant clinical response to anti-TB chemotherapy within the time frame of 6 to 12 weeks establishes the diagnosis [7, 19].

Tuberculomas in the sellar-suprasellar region may be resistant to anti-TB therapy which can be challenging to the treating physician. Two cases of MDR-tuberculomas in the sellar/suprasellar region have been reported by us previously. Both the cases were of pediatric age group who developed the tuberculomas, while being treated for TBM [10] (Fig. 11.1). MDR-TB has been defined by the World Health Organization as resistant to isoniazid (INH) and rifampicin (RIF) [29]. About 50% of cases with MDR-TB are encountered in China and India [10]. It has been noted by Farnial et al. that drug-resistant strains of *M. tuberculosis* have asymmetric Y- and V-branching-type cell types on atomic force microscopy, whereas drug-sensitive strains have more symmetric cell types [30]. The genetic basis of drug resistance has been linked to catalase-peroxidase gene (kat G) and inhA gene for INH resistance, the rpoB gene, which encodes the RNA polymerase beta subunit in RIF resistance. In a similar fashion, mutation in the rrs gene causes resistance to second-line anti-TB therapy drugs such as amikacin, kanamycin, and capreomycin [10].

In case of treated cases of tuberculomas, we can follow up the patients radiologically. The histopathological evaluation may be the only means for verifying the true nature of the residual contrast-enhancing lesions. This approach is clinically impractical, because such patients are asymptomatic, and it would be inappropriate to suggest an invasive procedure such as a biopsy. Therefore, the issue of whether to continue anti-TB chemotherapy for patients with contrast-enhancing residual lesions is difficult to resolve. However, the presence of clinical features consistent with an active lesion, such as headaches, progressive focal deficits, and possibly seizures, and the presence of perilesional edema or the appearance of new lesions on computed tomography scans imply active disease and the need for continuing medication [31]. Therefore, total surgical excision should be considered for tuberculomas in noneloquent and accessible regions of the brain, especially if they are solitary or persist after the application of anti-TB therapy for a reasonable period. However, total excision should not be considered in cases where it is likely to result in additional neurological morbidity. The preferred prophylactic anticonvulsants following transcranial surgery is carbamazepine or phenobarbitone, which are less hepatotoxic than other anticonvulsants drugs and therefore do not worsen the hepatotoxic effect of the first-line anti-TB chemotherapy [19].

The main challenge for the management of sellar/suprasellar tuberculomas is the lack of any single specific imaging sign which may preclude a preoperative diagnosis. Most patients require surgery which offers immediate decompression of the optic apparatus and provides tissue samples for histopathologic examination as well. Technically, the transsphenoidal corridor is the approach of choice as it is the least-invasive approach for sellar lesions. This route obviates the chance of cerebrospinal fluid (CSF) contamination, which is a risk with the transcranial approach. Nevertheless, suprasellar extension of the lesion warrants a transcranial approach [14, 17, 32]. The lesion is usually yellowish or grayish, firm, avascular to moderately vascular, and relatively non-suckable [18].

In patients with a significant suprasellar component, a transylvian, subfrontal approach is a good option. The infiltrative spread of the TB granulation usually prevents enlargement of the sella though sellar and suprasellar component is significant. Thus, accessing the suprasellar component in order to attain adequate optic nerve decompression in patients with rapidly decreasing vision may be challenging with the transsphenoidal approach. Not infrequently, stereotactic or an endoscopic endonasal transsphenoidal biopsy of the lesion may be essential to confirm the diagnosis of tuberculoma. An endoscopic third ventriculostomy may be difficult in patients with associated hydrocephalus because of the opalescent ventricular CSF, the thickened third ventricular floor related to ventricular ependymitis, and the obstruction of CSF pathway at the

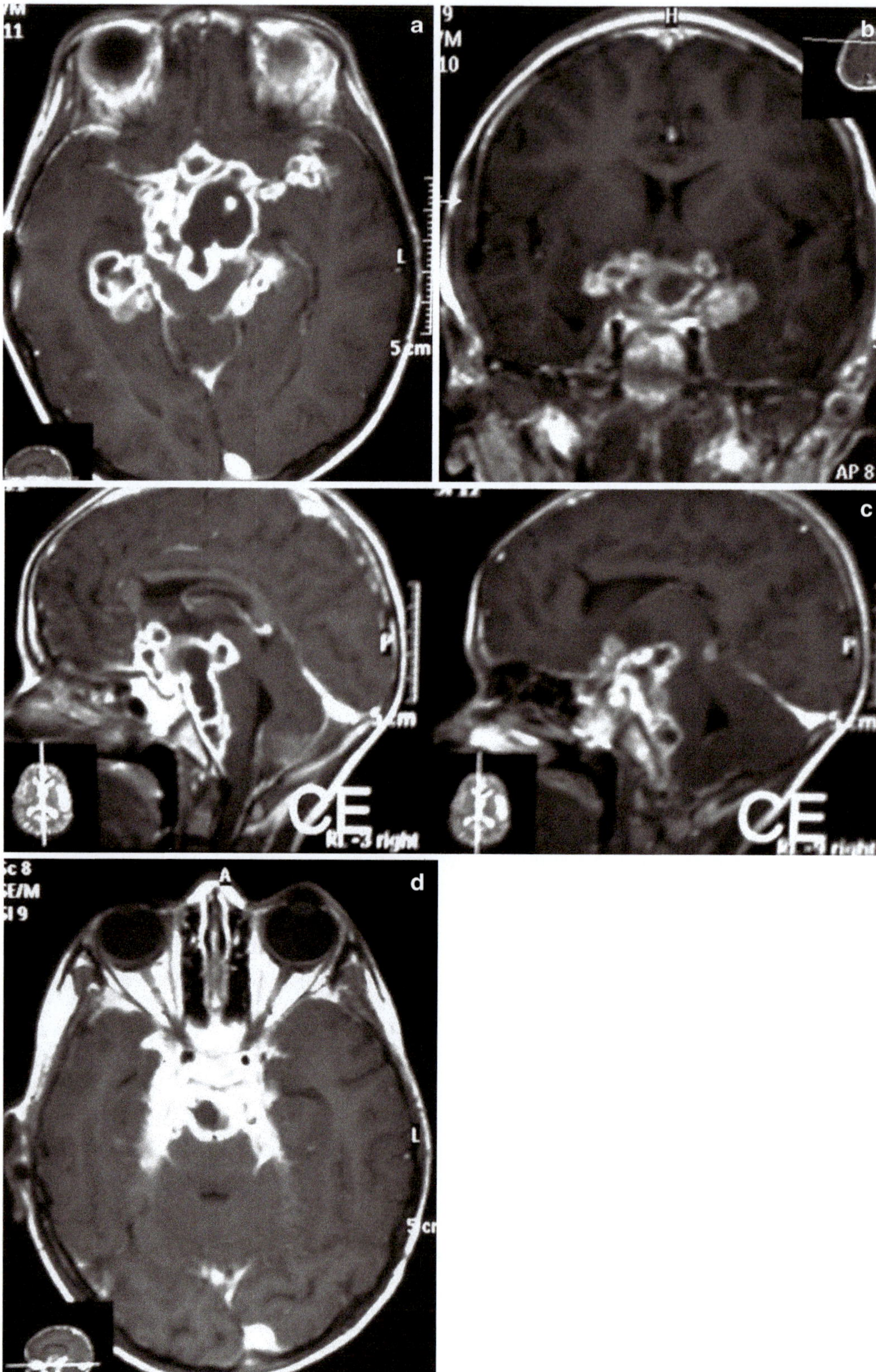

Fig. 11.1 MRI brain demonstrates enhancing tuberculoma in sellar-suprasellar area with extension medially along the temporal lobes, axial (**a**), coronal (**b**), and retroclival area (**c**) and evidence of severe pachymeningitis (**d**)

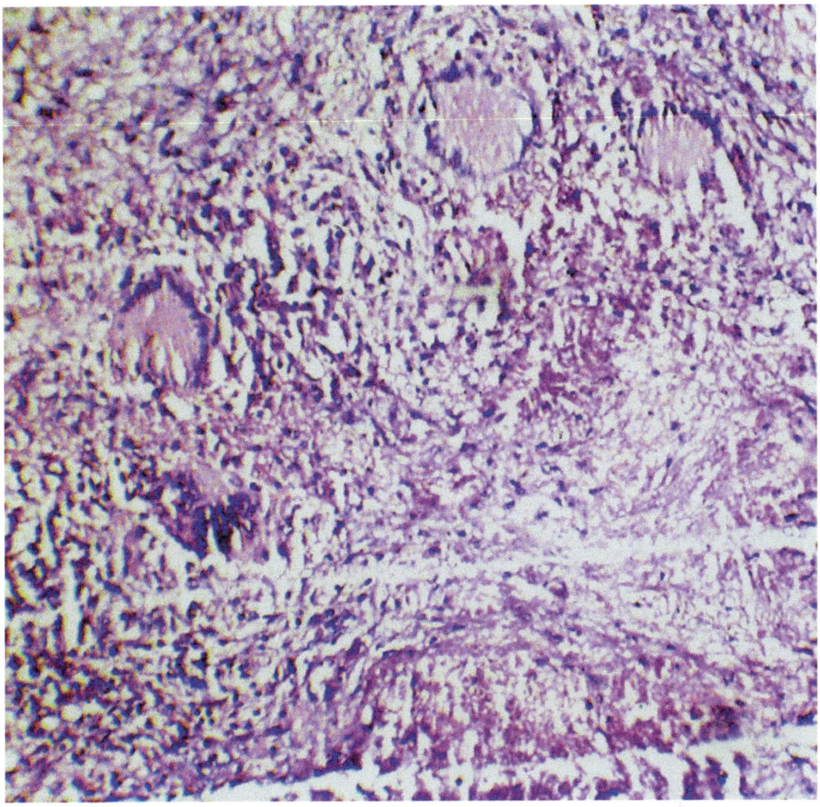

Fig. 11.2 Hematoxylin and eosin (HE ×20) photomicrograph showing Langhans-type giant cells with epithelioid cell granulomas

subarachnoid cisternal and arachnoid granulation at the superior sagittal sinus level [19].

11.6 Histopathological Features

The histopathological features of a central caseating necrosis surrounded by lymphocytes, plasma cells, and Langerhans giant cells suggest the diagnosis of TB. Histologically, TB, sarcoidosis, mycotic infection, hypophysitis secondary to ruptured intrasellar Rathke's cleft cyst, and idiopathic causes should be considered in the differential diagnosis of granulomatous hypophysitis. Also, the infiltration of hypophysis with histiocytes may be seen in histiocytosis X, if the pituitary parenchyma is involved by the disease. A central area of caseous necrosis with surrounding epithelioid cells, macrophages, lymphocytes, and plasma cells is a characteristic for granulomas in TB. Caseation is diagnostic of TB. The presence of acid-fast bacilli has also been reported though in very few cases [33] (Fig. 11.2).

Conclusion

The differential diagnosis of sellar lesions should include TB, especially if contrast enhancement and thickening of sphenoid sinus mucosa or pituitary stalk is encountered in patients from TB endemic areas. Most of these patients are negative for workup for systemic TB. There may be five radiological manifestations of sellar-suprasellar tuberculomas which include a mass lesion, multiple coalescing ring lesions, intrasellar abscess, skull base lesion, or pachymeningitis with extension to the sellar-suprasellar region. Surgery is useful in establishing the histological diagnosis of TB after which anti-TB chemotherapy may be instituted. Short-term steroid therapy under cover of anti-TB therapy may aid in decreasing edema and adhesions around the optic nerve in patients with rapidly deteriorating vision and for lessening the symptoms related to IICP in patients with intracerebral tuberculomas. Overall prognosis is excellent. MDR-tuberculomas also have been reported in the literature involving the sellar/suprasellar region. Surgically, a decompression for biopsy alone should be performed after an intraoperative frozen section biopsy is reported to be consistent with inflammatory pathology. We do not advise radical decompression of these lesions as anti-TB treatment is sufficient for cure.

References

1. Brooks MH, Dumbao JS, Bronsky D, Waldestein SS (1973) Hypophysial tuberculoma with hypopituitarism. Am J Med 54:777–781
2. Kim SH, Kim DG (2003) Sellar tuberculoma mimicking pituitary adenoma. J Korean Neurosurg Soc 34:245–248
3. Rich AR (1933) The pathogenesis of tuberculous meningitis. Bull Johns Hopkins Hosp 52:5–37
4. Sunil K, Menon R, Goel N, Sanghvi D, Bandgar T, Joshi SR, Menon P, Shah N, Goel A (2007) Pituitary tuberculosis. J Assoc Physicians India 55:453–456
5. Paramo C, Fuente de L, Nodar A, Miramontes S, Quinlela JL, Garcia-Mayor RV (2002) Intrasellar tuberculoma: a difficult diagnosis. Infection 30:35–37
6. Sharma MC, Arora R, Mahapatra AR, Sarat Chandra P, Gaikwad SD, Sarkar C (2000) Intrasellar tuberculoma: an enigmatic pituitary infection: a series of 18 cases. Clin Neurol Neurosurg 102:72–77
7. Ramzan A, Nayil K, Asimi R, Wani A, Makhdoomi R, Jain A (2013) Childhood tubercular meningitis: an institutional experience and analysis of predictors of outcome. Pediatr Neurol 48:30–35
8. Coleman CC, Meredith JM (1940) Diffuse tuberculosis of the pituitary gland simulating tumor with postoperative recovery. Arch Neurol Psychiatry 44:1076–1085
9. Bonifacio-Delgadillo D, Aburto-Murrieta Y, Salinas-Lara C, Sotelo J, Montes-Mojarro I, Garcia-Marquez A (2014) Clinical presentation and magnetic resonance findings in sellar tuberculomas. Case Rep Med 2014:961913
10. Nayil K, Singh S, Makhdoomi R, Ramzan A, Wani A (2011) Sellar-suprasellar tuberculomas in children: 2 cases and literature review. Pediatr Neurol 44:463–466
11. Nupur P, Karanth S, Nagarjun MN, Pandey P (2014) Suprasellar tuberculoma associated with unilateral moyamoya phenomenon: case report. Neurol India 62:453–455
12. Ranjan A, Chandy MJ (1994) Intrasellar tuberculoma. Br J Neurosurg 8:179–185
13. Desai KJ, Nadkarni TD, Goel A (2003) Tuberculomas of the hypophysis cerebri: report of five cases. J Clin Neurosci 10:526–526
14. Ashkan K, Papadopoulos MC, Casey AT, Thompson DN, Jarvis S, Powell M, Thomas DG (1997) Sellar tuberculoma: report of two cases. Acta Neurochir (Wein) 139:523–525
15. Jain R, Kumar R (2001) Suprasellar tuberculoma presenting with diabetes insipidus and hypothyroidism. A case report. Neurol India 49:314–316
16. Arun Kumar MJ, Rajshekhar V (2001) Intrasellar tuberculoma presenting as pituitary apoplexy. Neurol India 49:407–410
17. Mahghani DK, Gaitonde PS, Dastur DK (2001) Pituitary tuberculoma: a case report. Neurol India 49:299–301
18. Ahmad FU, Sarat Chandra P, Sanyal S, Garg A, Mehta VS (2005) Sellar tuberculoma. an unusual infection. Indian J Tuberc 52:215–217
19. Behari S, Singhal U, Jain M, Jaiswal AK, Wadwekar V, Das KB (2009) Clinicoradiological presentation, management options and a review of sellar and suprasellar tuberculomas. J Clin Neurosci 16:1560–1566
20. Furtado SV, Venkatesh PK, Ghosal N, Hegde AS (2011) Isolated sellar tuberculoma presenting with panhypopituitarism: clinical diagnostic considerations and literature view. Neurol Sci 32:301–304
21. Dalan R, Leow MK (2008) Pituitary abscess: our experience with a case and a review of literature. Pituitary 11:299–306
22. Mittal P, Dua S, Saggar K, Gupta K (2010) Magnetic resonance findings in sellar and suprasellar tuberculoma with hemorrhage. Surg Neurol Int 1:73
23. Salgado P, Del Brutto OH, Talamas O (1989) Intracranial tuberculomas: MR imaging. Neuroradiology 31:299–302
24. Czarnecki E, Spickler E (1995) MR demonstration of Wegner granulomatosis of the infundibulum: a cause of diabetes insipidus. AJNR Am J Neuroradiol 16:968–970
25. Rosete A, Carbal AR, Krans A, Alarcan-Segona D (1991) Diabetes insipidus secondary for Wegner granulomatosis: report and review of the literature. J Rheumatol 18:761–765
26. Rumana M, Kirmani A, Khursheed N, Besina S, Khalil MB (2010) Lymphocytic hypophysitis with normal pituitary function mimicking a pituitary adenoma: a case report and review of literature. Clin Neuropathol 29:26–31
27. Saini KS, Patel AL, Shaikh WA, Magar LN, Pungaonkar SA (2007) Magnetic resonance spectroscopy in pituitary tuberculoma. Singapore Med J 48:783–786
28. Bass JB Jr, Farer LS, Hopewell PC, O'Brien R, Jacobs RF, Ruben F, Snider DE Jr, Thornton G (1994) Treatment of tuberculosis and tuberculosis infection in adults and children. American Thoracic Society and

the Centers for Disease Control and Prevention. Am J Respir Crit Care Med 149:1359–7134
29. Aziz MA, Wright A, Laszlo A, De Muynck A, Portaels F, Van Deun A, Wells C, Nunn P, Blanc L, Raviglione M (2006) Epidemiology of antituberculosis drug resistance (the global project on anti-tuberculosis drug resistance surveillance): an update analysis. Lancet 368:2142–2154
30. Farnial P, Masjedi MR, Merza MA, Tabarsi P, Zhavnerko GK, Ibrahim TA, Kuan HO, Ghanavei J, Farnia P, Ranjbar R, Poleschuyk NN, Titov LP, Owlia P, Kazampour M, Setareh M, Sheikolslami M, Migliori GB, Velayati AA (2010) Growth and cell-division in extensive (XDR) and extremely drug resistant (XXDR) tuberculosis strains: transmission and atomic force observation. Int J Clin Exp Med 3:308–314
31. Poonnoose SI, Rajshekhar V (2003) Rate of resolution of histologically verified intracranial tuberculomas. Neurosurgery 53:873–878
32. Ghosh S, Chandy MJ (1992) Intrasellar tuberculoma. Clin Neurol Neurosurg 94:251–252
33. Dastur DK, Lalitha VS, Prabhkar V (1968) Pathological analysis of intracranial space occupying lesions in 1000 cases including children. J Neurol Sci 6:575–182

12 Vascular Complications of Tuberculous Meningitis

Hardeep Singh Malhotra and Ravindra K. Garg

Contents

H.S. Malhotra, MD, DM • R.K. Garg, MD, DM (✉)
Department of Neurology, King George's Medical University, Lucknow, UP, India
e-mail: drhsmalhotra@gmail.com; garg50@yahoo.com

Abbreviations

CNS	Central nervous system
ACA	Anterior cerebral artery
CSF	Cerebrospinal fluid
CT	Computed tomography
ICA	Internal carotid artery
MCA	Middle cerebral artery
MMP	Matrix metalloproteinase
MRA	Magnetic resonance angiography
MRI	Magnetic resonance imaging
MRV	Magnetic resonance venography
PCA	Posterior cerebral artery
SPECT	Single photon emission computed tomography
TB	Tuberculosis
TBM	Tuberculous meningitis
TCD	Transcranial Doppler
WHO	World Health Organization

12.1 Introduction

Tuberculosis (TB) may be regarded as a true ancient disease with its root as deep as the known civilizations. In one of the earliest molecular documentations, it has been traced back to at least 9000 years from the bone samples at the Atlit Yam site in the eastern Mediterranean [1]. TB is such a public health problem that World Health Organization has decided to revise its policy from the earlier "Stop TB" strategy to an "End TB"

M. Turgut et al. (eds.), *Tuberculosis of the Central Nervous System*,
DOI 10.1007/978-3-319-50712-5_12

strategy [2]. Among different types of extrapulmonary TB, tuberculous meningitis (TBM) is the most deadly form, whose vascular complications are responsible, for most part, for the morbidity and mortality observed in patients.

12.2 Historical Aspects

The credit of the earliest description of vascular pathology in patients showing miliary tubercles in the pia mater goes to Dr. Eduard Rindfleisch who in 1862 described the affliction and the possible pathophysiology [3]. Another publication in German by Baumgarten in 1881 supported the involvement of vessels of the pia mater in such patients [4]. In the English literature, Hektoen in 1896 gave an excellent description of vascular changes, focusing on the endarteritis, in patients with TBM [5]. In a series of four patients, Greitz gave the initial description of carotid and vertebral angiographic changes in patients with TBM [6]. He demonstrated that constrictions were most often evident at the level of intradural carotid siphon, followed by the proximal parts of anterior cerebral arteries (ACAs) and middle cerebral arteries (MCAs) [6].

12.3 Epidemiology

Among the vascular complications of TBM, ischemic lesions (infarcts) have been observed more commonly than hemorrhagic lesions. Moyamoya-like pathology and the presence of subarachnoid hemorrhages are uncommon, while the co-occurrence of aneurysm, causal or incidental, is rare; this information, thus, exists either in isolation or in small case series. It is imperative to understand that the frequency of radiological detection of vascular lesions would always lie on the higher side in comparison to clinical features since not all vascular lesions would have a clinical correlate.

12.3.1 Clinical

Approximately 14–19% patients with TBM present with a stroke at baseline [7, 8]. During the course of the illness, the time of development of which may vary, the number increases owing either to delay in treatment, lack of appropriate treatment, drug-resistant disease, or secondary to development of a paradoxical reaction. Not less than 15% patients develop a focal neurological deficit as a result of these processes [9, 10].

Interestingly, not only does TBM but non-central nervous system (CNS)/meningeal TB, per se, also increases the risk of development of stroke in afflicted patients. A three-year follow-up of patients suggests that the risk of sustaining a stroke is 1.5 times when compared to their healthy counterparts, having adjusted for common predisposing factors of stroke [11].

12.3.2 Imaging

MRI is superior to CT in detecting as well as correctly identifying stroke in patients with TBM. In an earlier CT study conducted in 60 patients with TBM, infarcts could be demonstrated in approximately 28% of them [12]. Twenty-five to 74% patients may exhibit an infarct on the MRI [13–19]. Angiographic abnormalities have been reported variably between 20.8% and 100% depending upon the sample and modality used [12, 14, 18, 20–23]. Mycotic aneurysms are rare; they usually occur either with exudates or in close proximity with TB granulomas [14, 24–27].

12.3.3 Autopsy

Approximately 25% patients of TBM ($n = 44$) had infarcts at postmortem examinations in a study from Uganda [28]. Evidence of arteritis was noted in 35 of 39 patients with TBM in an autopsy series. Associated changes in the hypothalamus were observed in 37 of 39 patients and pituitary involvement in 4 of 21 patients examined [29]. In a recent Indian study, specifically looking at vasculature in patients with TBM, it was shown that more than two-thirds had evidence of an infarct; arterial aneurysms were observed in two patients [30]. The presence of multiple aneurysms in an infant with TBM and subarachnoid hemorrhage has also been described [27].

12.4 Clinical Features

Development of a focal neurological deficit is the most common manifestation in a patient with TBM having involvement of the cerebral vasculature. The deficits most often correlate with their structural analogue, but not all structural lesions may manifest clinically [31]. This may occur secondary to several reasons, viz., a very small infarct, infarct not involving the motor area or its pathway, altered state of consciousness limiting meaningful examination, or the presence of additional lesions (besides vascular) with or without perilesional edema preventing segregation of the etiology.

Focal neurological deficit, defined at onset or during the course of CNS TB, may be seen in 42% of children ($n = 500$) among whom nearly 20% each may present with hemiparesis and quadriparesis, 2.6% with monoparesis, and 0.6% with cerebral paraparesis [31]. Tuberculomas may be a common accompaniment of TBM and can be demonstrated in approximately 28% patients with TBM [32]. In a mixed population (children and adults, $n = 232$) with TBM, the frequency of paralysis was found to be 16.5% [7]. On an average, focal neurological deficits may be seen in approximately one-fourth of patients (18–27%) at baseline taking into consideration all the three affected populations, viz., children, adults, and elderly [15, 17, 33, 34]. A study has specifically centered on brainstem ischemic lesions in children with TBM and states that, of those with brainstem involvement, 43% present with quadriparesis and 21.5% each with either right or left hemiparesis [35]. At follow-up, paradoxical development of lesions referable to vascular involvement may be seen in 15% patients in the brain and in 13.8% patients in the spinal cord [10]. Manifestations suggestive of involvement of the venous system (venous sinus thrombosis or thrombophlebitis alone) may be there which may lead to a lot of confusion in the presence of hydrocephalus and lateral rectus involvement. Such an involvement has been proven on autopsy too [36, 37].

Besides focal (motor) neurological deficits, which have an organic vascular correlate, other clinical manifestations in patients with TBM have not been studied in detail to delineate the underlying process. The symptoms such as altered sensorium, seizures, involuntary movements, endocrinological complaints, etc. might not relate to vascular impairment on one-on-one basis. The presence of intracerebral and subarachnoid hemorrhage, secondary either to a pure TB process (vasculitis) or as a result of a mycotic extravascular aneurysm, may in addition complicate the clinical picture [24, 26, 27, 38–41]. It may be noted that subarachnoid hemorrhage in a patient with TBM might not axiomatically imply that an aneurysm is present. Such a hemorrhage may either be a non-aneurysmal subarachnoid hemorrhage [39–41] or a mycotic aneurysmal hemorrhage [26, 27] which would depend on how and in which form the vessel is involved. Thus, such a presentation must be interpreted with caution and attributed to vascular involvement only in light of appropriate clinicoradiological features.

For the sake of clarity, only movement disorders, syringomyelia, and involvement of the hypothalamo-pituitary axis shall be discussed further.

Movement disorders have been noted in 6.46–18.2% of patients with TBM [7, 31, 42]. The most commonly reported movement disorder is tremor, followed by chorea and dystonia. The presence of chorea and dystonia may be associated with a more severe disease. Although direct correlation does not exist, the frequency of deep vascular lesions is said to be more in patients with movement disorders [42].

Syringomyelia or syringobulbia has been shown to occur both as an early as well as a delayed complication of TBM [43–45]. It has been proposed that vascular involvement occurs in the majority of patients, either primarily or secondarily. This seems to occur over and above the association with exudates/arachnoiditis and hydrocephalus.

Involvement of the hypothalamus or hypothalamo-pituitary axis resulting into symptoms suggestive of an endocrinological disorder has been recorded to lie between 1.6% and 20% in patients with TBM [31, 46, 47]. In a recent evaluation, probably the largest (n = 75, adults), almost a half of patients with TBM were detected to have hormonal dysfunction. The most common abnormality noted was hyperprolactinemia; next in line were cortisol deficiency and central hypothyroidism [48]. However, an explicit vascular involvement was not observed in any patient in this study. In other series, and case report with reviews, children have been found to be affected more commonly and with more sequelae [46, 47, 49–51]. Almost all types of endocrine abnormalities have been described such as hyperprolactinemia, growth hormone deficiency, gonadotropin deficiency, diabetes insipidus, precocious puberty and associated behavioral or personality changes, corticotropin deficiency, and cortisol deficiency. Associated changes in electrolytes and metabolites have also been noted.

12.5 Imaging

It is important to appreciate the superiority of MRI over CT. Not only does it help in better detection of vascular complications (good sensitivity), it also separates certain commonly encountered situations mimicking stroke (good specificity). For example, infarcts occurring in the region of basal ganglia are commonly missed on CT. Similarly, tuberculomas, with accompanying perilesional edema, developing during the course of TBM might not be definable on CT.

12.5.1 Computed Tomography

In possibly the first description of infarcts in TBM, 17 of 60 (28.3%) patients demonstrated the finding as a hypodense lesion in the basal ganglia or the perisylvian area [12].

In a serial CT-based evaluation of 25 patients with TBM, it was shown that two-thirds of children developed an infarct, while just one out of 13 adults (aged 50 years) developed the same. Infarcts in these children were found to be more common at higher MRC stages. It was, thus, suggested that infarcts were commoner in children [46]. In another evaluation, 25 of 65 children (38.5%) were found to have infarcts; all but two patients had anterior circulation infarcts, most of which conformed to the MCA territory [25].

12.5.2 Magnetic Resonance Imaging

MRI of the brain is considered to be superior than CT in demonstrating abnormalities associated with TBM, particularly infarcts. The frequency of detection of infarction may actually vary depending on the age, time to presentation, time to diagnosis, time to treatment, the presence of comorbidities, adherence to treatment, etc. at baseline as well as during follow-up.

In a study on 27 children in stage II (n = 10) and stage III (n = 17) TBM, 20 (74%) had parenchymal ischemic lesions. The lesions were found to be distributed in the basal ganglia-diencephalon region (n = 20) and brainstem-parahippocampal gyri-hypothalamus region (n = 10, also had supratentorial lesions). This study demonstrated the superiority of MRI over CT especially in detecting the brainstem lesions [13].

MRI may show infarcts in 54–60% patients which may be hemorrhagic or bland [14, 16, 18, 52]. Specifically using a diffusion-weighted imaging protocol, infarcts were observed in 17 of 30 (56.7%) patients with TBM [15]. In a series of 100 patients, stroke was detected in 30% [17]. In a retrospective chart review of adult population with tuberculosis of the CNS (n = 404), it was found that approximately 25% of patients (n = 99) had an evidence of an infarct; concomitant occurrence of a tuberculoma was noted in 10% of patients (n = 39) [19].

The distribution of infarcts in patients with TBM generally follows the location as defined by the "TB zone." "TB zone" is constituted by head of the caudate, anteromedial part of the thalamus, and anterior plus genu of the internal capsule [53] (Fig. 12.1). In terms of the arterial territories, MCA is most commonly involved. A majority of series published till date have demon-

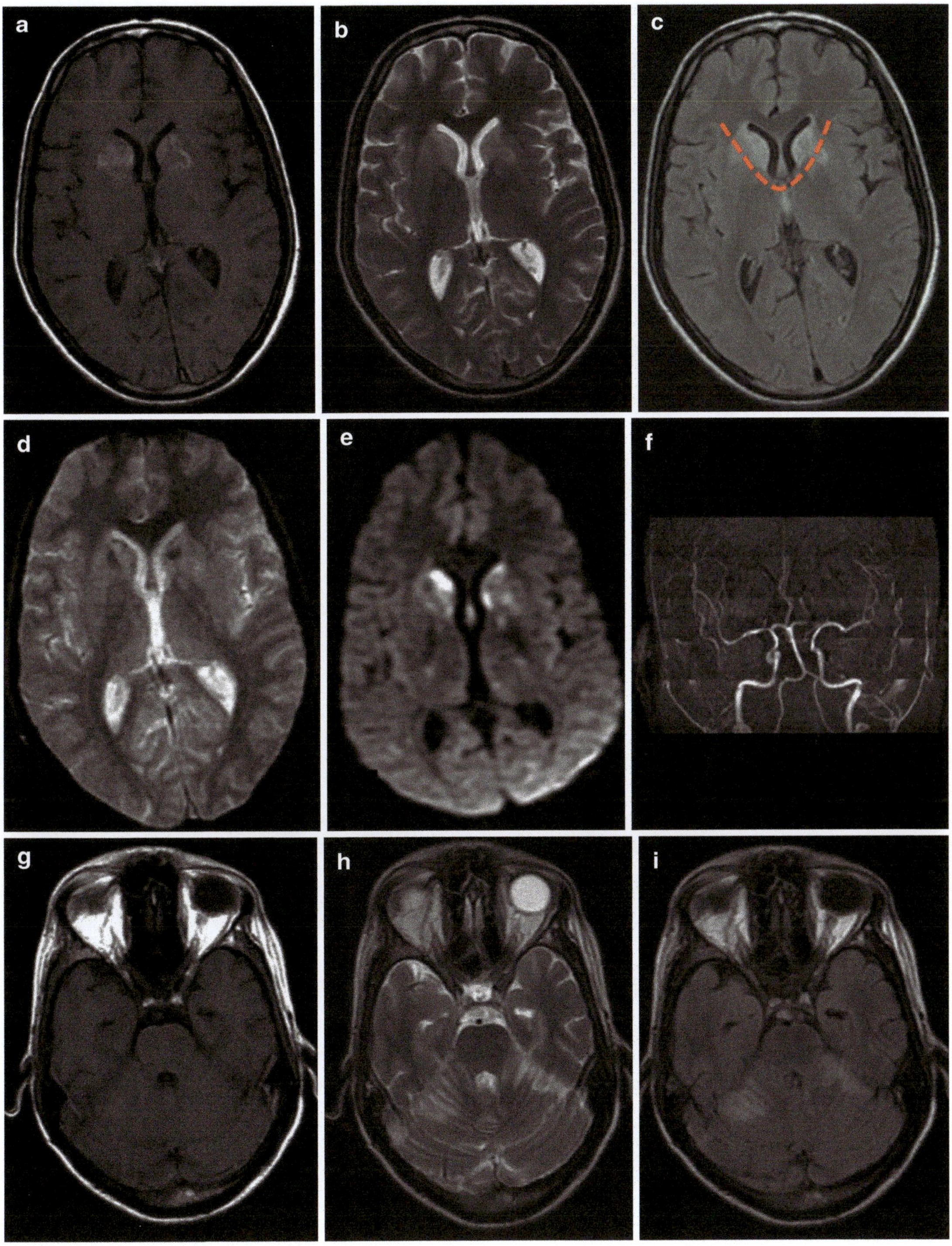

Fig. 12.1 MRI of the brain in a patient with TBM depicts a typical (TB zone, *red dotted line*) bi-basal ganglia infarct (**a–c**, **e**) with suggestion of hemorrhage (**d**, gradient recalled echo sequence). MRA is suggestive of right distal internal carotid artery (ICA) stenosis with segments of narrowing of right middle cerebral artery (MCA) (**f**). More foci of nonhemorrhagic infarction are evident involving the superior parts of the cerebellum (**g–k**). MRV of the same patient is suggestive of non-visualization of the right-sided transverse, sigmoid, and jugular sinus flow with multiple collateral drainages (**l**)

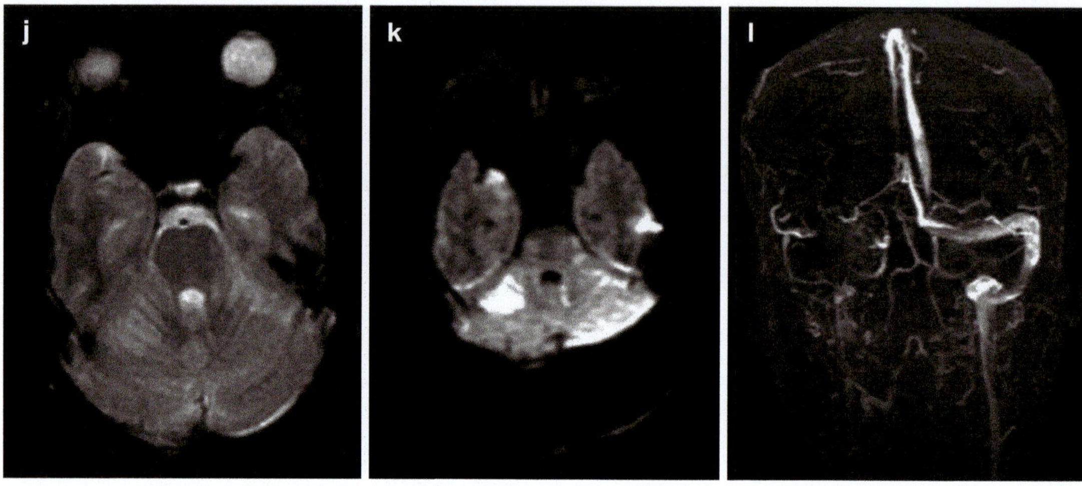

Fig. 12.1 (continued)

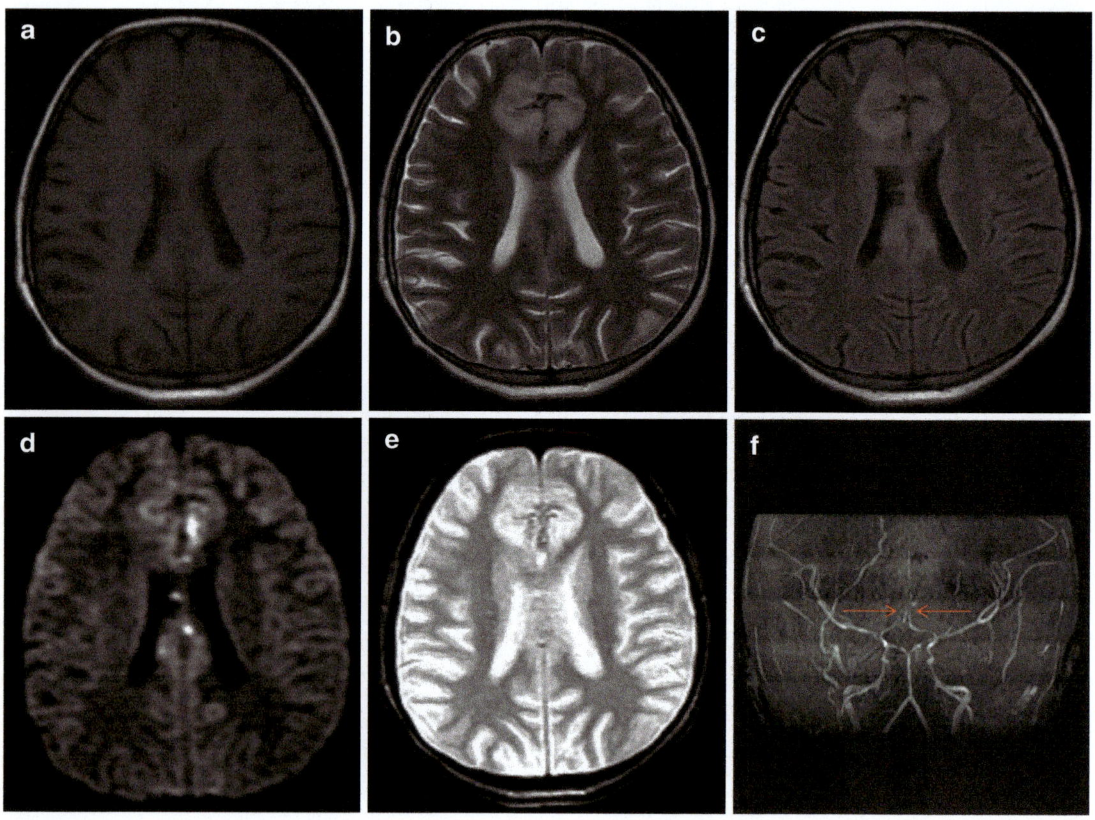

Fig. 12.2 MRI of the brain depicts an infarction in a patient with TBM in the territory of anterior cerebral artery (ACA) (**a–d**) with no suggestion of hemorrhage (**e**, gradient recalled echo sequence). MRA is suggestive of involvement of both ACA (*arrows*, **f**)

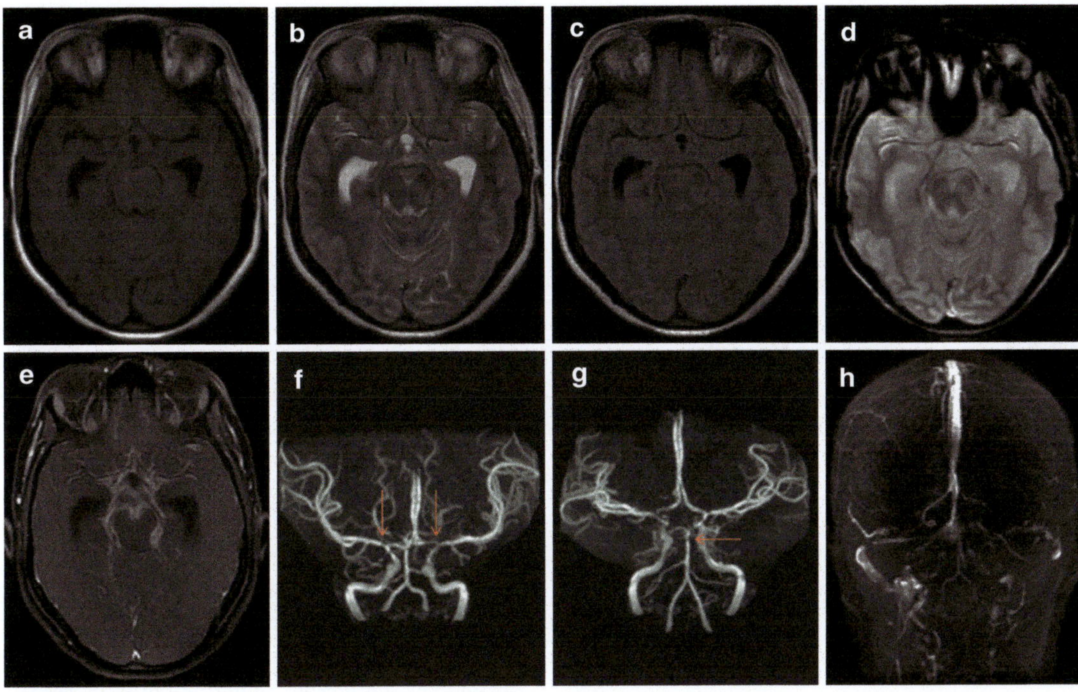

Fig. 12.3 MRI of the brain of a patient with TBM presenting with hydrocephalus at onset (**a–d**) and extensive exudates lining the basal cisterns and fissures (**e**, gadolinium contrast). Non-infarct-related vascular involvement (smooth plus segmental involvement) can be seen involving the distal ICA (**f**, *arrows*) and basilar artery (**g**). MRV of the same patient shows poor visualization of the left-sided transverse, sigmoid, and jugular flow with multiple collateral drainage (**h**)

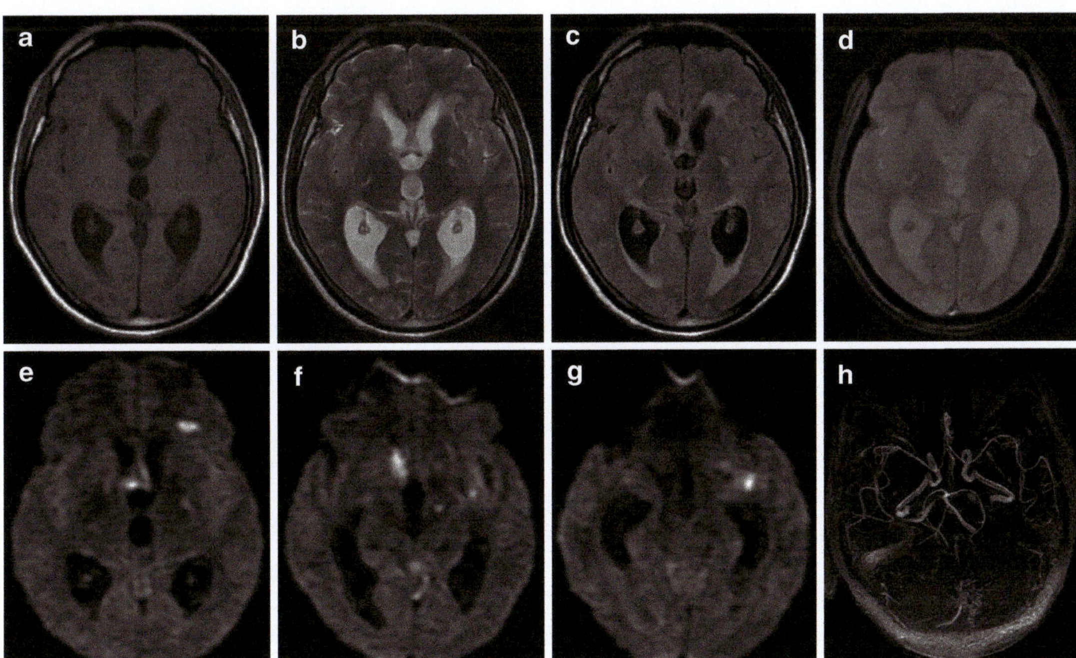

Fig. 12.4 MRI of the brain in a patient with TBM presenting with hydrocephalus (**a–d**) with multiple small infarcts (**e–g**) and thinning of the distal vasculature (**h**)

strated this conformity in most patients (75% or more). In contrast to stroke unrelated to infections, infarcts observed in patients with TBM may be bilateral in almost 50% patients and defy the territorial restrictions of anterior and posterior circulation (Figs. 12.2, 12.3, and 12.4). Large territory infarctions, anterior or posterior, are less often seen [14, 16–18, 54].

12.5.3 Imaging of the Vessels

Needless to say, assessment of the vasculature of the central nervous system is incomplete without a dedicated imaging of the arterial as well as the venous system. Conventional cerebral angiography had been the modality of choice to image the vessels till a couple of decades back; with advances in imaging, MRI- or CT-based evaluation is considered more appropriate.

12.5.3.1 Angiography

Conventional and Digital Subtraction Angiography

The performance of conventional cerebral angiography was initiated in patients with TBM to rule out the possibility of a space-occupying lesion, abscess, aneurysm, or malignancy and not primarily to assess the status of cerebral vasculature during the course of TB process. In his seminal paper on "Angiography in tuberculous meningitis," published five decades back, Greitz gave an excellent précis of vascular changes in TBM derived from four female patients [6]. Constriction or narrowing of the intradural carotid siphon, with or without involvement of the proximal MCA/proximal ACA, was demonstrated in three patients, while the posterior cerebral artery (PCA) was shown to be involved in the fourth one. He highlighted the concept of functional versus organic stenosis and summarized the speculated causative factors as a localized basal cisternal or generalized intracranial pressure rise, spasm of the arteries similar to that observed in subarachnoid hemorrhage, and tuberculous vasculitis. He concluded that the vascular involvement in TBM was secondary to inflammatory changes in vessels [6]. Lehrer formulated a "radiopathologic triad," based on his observations in eight patients with TBM who underwent conventional cerebral angiography, to suggest or substantiate the diagnosis of TBM. This triad consisted of ventricular dilatation (depending on the course of ACA or thalamostriate vein), narrowing of vessels in the basal region (tuberculous arteritis versus spasm), and occlusive TB vasculitis involving small-to-medium-sized vessels [55].

Subsequent studies directed their objective toward delineation of site and type of vascular involvement in patients with TBM, besides ruling out a space-occupying lesion. In a large series (48 cerebral angiographic evaluations), an abnormal angiography was observed in ten (20.8%) patients. "Moyamoya-like" appearance was also observed by this group [20]. In an evaluation of five patients, three patients had involvement of vessels both at the base and the periphery, while two had involvement of vessels only at the base [21]. Serial CT ($n = 60$) with conventional angiography ($n = 14$) in patients with TBM revealed angiographic abnormalities in 11 (78.6%) of them. It was attributed to arteritis in eight (those "with" enhancing exudates) and vasospasm in three (those "without" enhancing exudates) patients. The MCA territory alone was affected most commonly (82.35%) followed by the combined territories of MCA and ACA; involvement of PCA territory was observed in one patient [12].

In probably the solitary study directed at assessing adult population with TBM ($n = 24$) by digital subtraction angiography, it was shown that the positive and the negative predictive values of the technique were 0.82 and 0.46, respectively. The sensitivity was low while the specificity was moderate in terms of infarcts. Interestingly, 1 of 11 patients with an abnormal angiogram had superior sagittal sinus thrombosis [22].

CT Angiography

The value of CT angiography has not been evaluated in as much detail as MR Angiography. In a prospective study to demonstrate the vascular abnormalities in TBM, 33 of 47 (70.2%) patients were found to have an abnormal angiogram; of note, only 32% patients had hemiparesis.

At follow-up, in the normal angiogram group ($n = 9$), new abnormalities were seen in two patients, while in the abnormal angiogram group ($n = 17$), angiogram normalized in three patients. The presence of basal exudates was found to be a significant predictor of angiographic abnormalities on multivariate analysis; those which were significant only on univariate analysis were impaired vision, hemiparesis, hydrocephalus, meningeal enhancement, and infarcts [23]. In our experience, delineation of vessels is better with CT angiography, but it occurs at the cost of loss of good parenchymal details; we prefer a combination of MRI of the brain with contrast plus four-vessel CT angiography to evaluate a patient with TBM (Figs. 12.5 and 12.6).

MR Angiography

Not many dedicated studies have evaluated the role of MR angiography (MRA); the vascular assessment in these cases has neither been uniform nor on absolute basis. In a nutshell, the available data replicates the existent findings in the form of narrowing of the terminal ICA and proximal parts of MCA and ACA (Figs. 12.1, 12.2, 12.3, and 12.4). Detection of an occasional aneurysm might be incidental in these patients [14, 18]. It is important to understand that not all patients with an abnormality on MRA will have an infarct; not more than two-thirds may have a corresponding infarct [18].

12.5.3.2 Venography

Despite of an ample amount of histopathological evidence suggesting involvement of the venous system in patients with TBM, no formal evaluation of this aspect has been done so far. Few individual case reports in the literature have predicted an association between TB and venous sinus thrombosis, but this cannot be substantiated at the present time [22, 37, 52, 56, 57]. It may be noted that a systematic evaluation of the venous system might reveal more than expected changes on venography (Figs. 12.1 and 12.3).

12.5.3.3 Transcranial Doppler

Transcranial Doppler (TCD) is an encouraging modality to evaluate the cerebral vasculature in view of its portability, ease of use and access, safe application, and real-time functional assessments. Its ability to insonate corroborates with commonly involved vessels in TBM, viz., distal internal carotid artery, proximal MCA, proximal ACA, and PCA [58]. The use of TCD in TBM appeared after the demonstration of its utility in performing ventriculoperitoneal shunt as a diversion procedure in patients with hydrocephalus [59]. In the first of its kind evaluation, 15 children with TBM were evaluated in terms of pre- and postoperative pulsatility index (PI) determination against 15 children with congenital hydrocephalus. This study demonstrated that the difference (essentially fall) in PI was statistically significant in the two groups. It was also shown that statistically significant difference existed in the TBM group between those who had and those who did not have an infarct. It was proposed that the reason for vascular changes in TBM is arteritis, with or without a contribution from exudates, and not vasospasm [60].

Blood flow velocity and PI measurements are used to aid in the diagnosis and prognosis of patients with TBM. In a study on patients with TBM (20 patients, mean age of 9 years), they were divided to fall in either phase I, II, or III, in terms of increasing severity of disease. Serial correlative assessments in these patients showed that an increase in mean velocity and a decrease in PI occurred through phases I to II. In phase III, there was absence of blood flow and was associated with poor outcome. It was suggested that TCD is especially good for patients presenting with a focal neurological deficit (phase II) [61]. Another study done in 20 children with TBM has shown that a correlation exists between large infarcts and three estimated parameters on TCD, complete MCA blockage, subnormal mean MCA velocities (<40 cm/s), and PI of <0.4 [62].

12.5.4 Other Imaging Modalities

Single-photon emission computed tomography has been used to study the areas of hypoperfusion in patients with TBM. Seventeen patients (3 in stage I, 3 in stage II, 11 in stage III) were evaluated using SPECT; cortical hypoperfusion ($n = 10$) was observed along with hypoperfusion in basal ganglia ($n = 14$) and midbrain ($n = 1$).

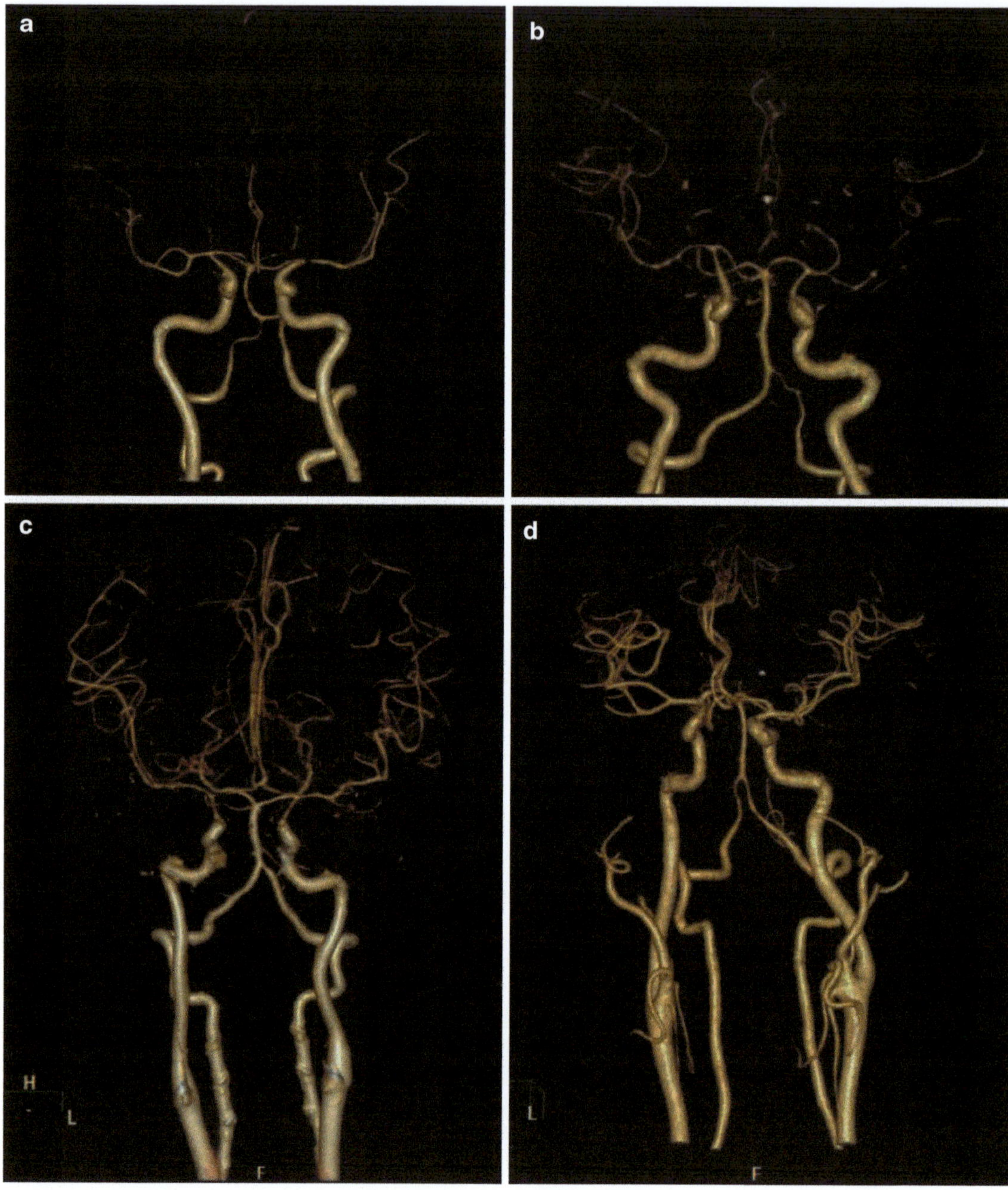

Fig. 12.5 CT angiography of the brain (different patients with TBM) depicts classical narrowing of the supraclinoid segment of the ICA along with proximal segments of the MCA and the ICA; segments of narrowing can also be seen in the basilar artery (**a**). Multiple areas of narrowing with markedly reduced perfusion can be seen beyond the stenosed distal ICA (**b**). Multiple areas of narrowing with relatively preserved perfusion can be seen beyond the stenosed distal ICA (**c**). Stenosis of distal vertebral arteries just before the formation of basilar artery (**d**)

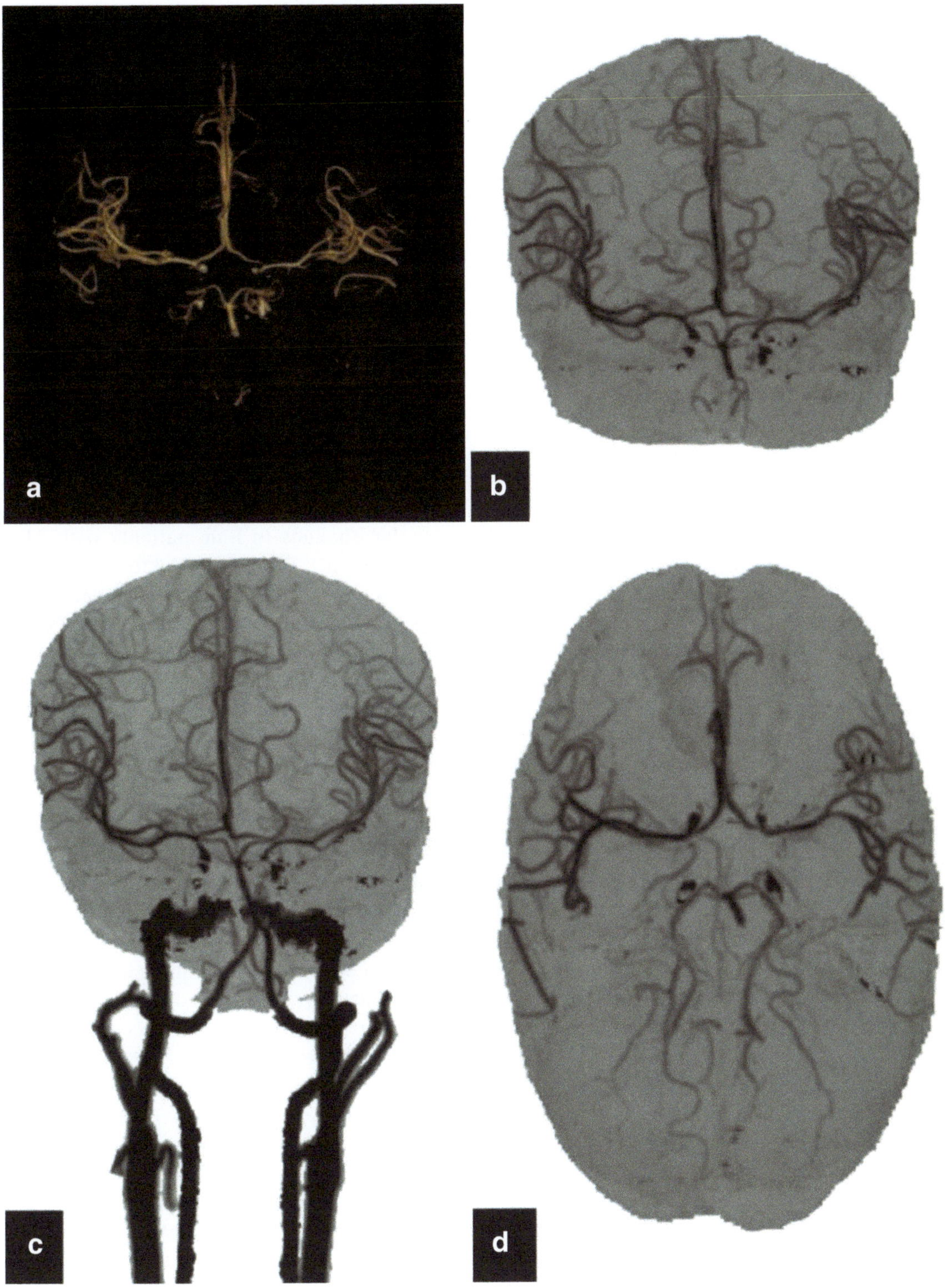

Fig. 12.6 CT angiography of the brain in a patient with TBM depicts severe stenosis of distal ICA leading to its non-visualization; the anterior and the posterior circulation are seemingly independent (**a**–**d**)

These hypoperfusion abnormalities, however, did not correlate either with the stage or the outcome of the patient [63].

12.6 Pathology and Pathophysiological Processes

12.6.1 Structural Pathology

The gross pathology of the brain reveals thick exudate at the base of the brain, with or without involvement of the superolateral surfaces, in which the vessels forming the circle of Willis bathe. These exudates extend anteriorly into the optochiasmatic area, laterally into the sylvian fissures, and posteriorly into the interpeduncular, ambient, and prepontine cisterns [64]. It is this distribution of exudates that is responsible for the corresponding changes observed in the affected vessels traversing this region. Thus, it is not surprising that involvement of the supraclinoid (intradural) part of the ICA and proximal parts of ACA and MCA are most commonly affected in patients with TBM. The small-caliber perforating arteries bear the brunt of the injury, whereby the basal ganglia, structurally, is the commonest involved area. The substance of the brain may show capillary hemorrhages involving the gray matter. Areas of "yellow softening" may be observed in the territory of the involved/stenosed arteries, e.g., MCA. Miliary tubercles may be seen lining the vessels in the subarachnoid space and may additionally contribute to compression and infiltration of vessels [65]. In an autopsy series of 39 patients, 37 patients demonstrated presence of exudates; in this series arteritis was observed in 35 cases, and the histopathology was based on the presence of infarcts and border-zone reaction. Out of 35 patients with arteritis, corresponding infarcts were not observed in nine cases, and border-zone reaction was observed in 29 cases in totality [29].

The presence of intracerebral hemorrhage or subarachnoid hemorrhage, though uncommon, has been studied pathologically in the past [66]. The aneurysms detected in patients with TBM have been described as "mycotic aneurysm of extravascular origin" suggesting an effect of nearby focus of tuberculous infection, either in the form of exudates or a tuberculoma [24]. In a large autopsy series, where subarachnoid hemorrhage was not observed in TBM, it was suggested that despite of a necrotizing process, vessels may maintain their integrity strong enough to resist a leak [30].

The earliest description of the microscopic pathology, with special reference to meningeal vessels, in patients with TBM is available in the German literature where Rindfleisch and Baumgarten, respectively, have described vascular changes [3, 4]. In the English literature, an excellent description of vascular changes in nine patients with TBM has been provided by Hektoen [5]. The changes described in these early years have not changed much in their basic form in the past one-and-a-half century; what has actually evolved during this period is the insight into the actual pathophysiology defined by the march of events from seeding of the bacilli to full-blown meningitis.

One of the most controversial issues regarding the vascular involvement in TBM is the aspect of "what initiated the process?"—i.e., what was the primary event? The opinion carried forward by most researchers is that the *Mycobacterium tuberculosis* bacillemia gets co-localized in the adventitia of arteries, subsequent to which invasion of other two layers, media and intima, may take place. Simple as this may seem, the actual processes are very complex.

It seems intuitive to accept that the involvement of vessel occurs from without [67] but descriptions of arteritis (endarteritis) have existed from the very beginning [4, 5, 64]. Adventitial as well as intimal lesions have also been described where the progression has been depicted toward the intima [68]. Since the media of the vessels in these patients have been found to be relatively intact and considered resistant to infection, how does infection actually travel through the vessel wall? [64, 68]. Thus, the process of seeding through the blood (bacillemia) and by way of involvement of adventitia may occur in tandem or in unison instead of behaving in pure individuality.

Similarly, the description of various forms of vascular involvement described in the literature need to be viewed collectively rather than being separate processes [69]. The types of involvement, viz., infiltrative/inflammatory/vasculitic, proliferative/obliterative/stenosing/occlusive, and necrotizing, are not mutually exclusive and may be viewed from the perspective of mild to moderate to severe disease, respectively. Such a classification will help in simplifying the seemingly complex classifications and will help in characterizing the patients better via histopathology. We need to ease down on the issue of thrombosis too because the evidence is again conflicting where thrombosis of arteries is present [49, 68, 70, 71] or not present/minimal [55, 64, 72]. Thrombosis cannot occur independently, and a lot of factors may contribute to its occurrence right from vascular flow abnormalities to abnormal expression of cytokines and growth factors. Thus, it may be regarded both as a precipitating event as well as a complication of the disease process.

As far as the pathology with respect to pial veins is concerned, intense phlebitis has been shown in veins moving through the exudate. It has been stated that at places, viz., borderland zone, phlebitis may actually precede arteritis [64]. Thrombosis may be observed in these patients as part of the disease process [68, 73].

12.6.2 Molecular Pathology

Our knowledge of molecular processes occurring in tuberculosis, especially with respect to cerebrovascular complications, is limited. As is true for most inflammatory-infective disorders, interaction of a multitude of factors leads to the expression of a specific disease. Most research translating into TBM has risen from those done in other inflammatory disorders, especially bacterial meningitis and fungal meningitis. In a first, 29 patients with TBM were assessed for vascular endothelial growth factor (VEGF), a marker of angiogenesis, along with 31 infectious non-TBM patients. It was shown that the titers of VEGF, both in serum and CSF, were significantly higher in patients with TBM than their counterparts; corresponding decrease in CSF titers was noted, in addition, in those who were improving [74]. The role of VEGF, as a vascular permeability factor, was assessed in 26 children with TBM in a later study which found that it correlates with blood-brain-barrier breach in patients with TBM and that its inhibition might be responsible for the role of corticosteroids in TBM [75]. As far as the clinical translation is concerned, significant correlation with intracranial pressure or infarcts was not observed.

Matrix metalloproteinase 2 and matrix metalloproteinase 9 (MMP-2, MMP-9), enzymes of the larger group of calcium-dependent zinc-containing endopeptidases, have been evaluated in patients with meningitis ($n = 21$, including seven with TBM). It was suggested that MMP-9 might be a good marker of "encephalitogenecity" when measured against MMP-2 [76]. In a combined in vitro and in vivo analysis, besides highlighting the utility of MMP-9 in TBM, it was shown to correlate significantly with signs of damage to the cerebral parenchyma [77].

High CSF concentrations of lactate, interleukin-8 (IL-8), and interferon-γ have been observed in drug-naïve adult patients with TBM, which decrease on follow-up with anti-tuberculosis treatment [78]. High IL-8 and IL-10 levels have been found to correlate significantly with infarcts in adult patients ($n = 11$ with infarct, $n = 16$ without infarct) with TBM [34]. However, in a later study no correlation was observed between cytokine levels and stage of meningitis or clinical and radiological outcome [79].

12.7 Management

Management of vascular complications in patients with TBM is yet to see a major breakthrough. The use of corticosteroids is recommended in HIV-negative patients with TBM to prevent death and disability; its use in HIV-positive patients does not have sufficient evidence to push a recommendation [80]. A serial MRI study, to assess the effect of dexamethasone in adult patients with TBM (n = 43, HIV-positive = 1), has shown that infarcts are almost halved in those receiving dexamethasone (27% versus 58%). But this effect was nonsignificant; it was also stated that the use of dexamethasone does not affect the location of the commonly affected area, i.e., basal ganglia of the brain [34]. A study, done earlier, in 141 children with TBM had revealed similar results both in terms of frequency and location of infarcts [81]. An important diagnostic issue may arise with the use of adjunctive corticosteroids where endocrinological abnormalities may be masked [29].

The use of aspirin (150 mg/day) has been evaluated in patients with TBM in an open-label placebo controlled trial (n = 59 in each group, also included six children). It was shown that aspirin resulted in insignificantly lesser strokes but a significant reduction in mortality at 3 months [82]. The results of this study, however, need further validation owing to certain critical issues such as lack of uniformity in administration of adjunctive corticosteroids, significant lost to follow-up, and small subgroup size. In another evaluation, done specifically in children (n = 146), different dose groups of aspirin were made; no significant benefit in terms of morbidity or mortality was observed [83].

Thalidomide has been used to improve the outcome in a rabbit model simulating mycobacterial infection of the nervous system [84, 85]. This may be a potential clinical target in patient suffering from TBM, provided the issue of teratogenicity is adequately taken care of.

Regulation of cerebral tissue oxygenation has been looked at in two patients with severe TBM. It was suggested that delayed cerebral ischemia (infarct) can be prevented by maintaining adequate oxygenation of the cerebral tissue guided by appropriate estimation of the same [86].

A group has also looked into the role of hypervolemia-hypertension-hemodilution (HHH) regime in patients with TBM similar to its usage in subarachnoid hemorrhage. Against five patients on conservative management, seven patients were offered HHH therapy. It was concluded that HHH therapy might be a safe and beneficial option in patients with TBM [87].

12.8 Prognosis

The presence of infarcts has been considered as a predictor of poor outcome, morbidity, or mortality in patients with TBM [17, 19]. Ischemic lesions of the brainstem have also been shown to be associated with poor outcome in children [35].

12.9 Future Research

Future research should target the pathophysiology of vascular involvement which to our understanding is the largest gray zone limiting our advances toward adoption of better preventive modalities and development of better treatment modalities. Newer molecules, antithrombotic or anti-inflammatory, may be studied in patients with TBM to look for a positive effect.

Conclusion

Vascular complications are commonly observed in patients with TBM, either at baseline or during the course of the disease. Angiographic abnormalities outnumber clinical as well as radiological manifestations and portend a poor outcome in those with the ischemic lesions. Early and prompt treatment of TBM is essential as vascular abnormalities are related with the duration of TBM, and no specific treatment is available to reverse the sequelae.

References

1. Hershkovitz I, Donoghue HD, Minnikin DE, May H, Lee OY, Feldman M, Galili E, Spigelman M, Rothschild BM, Bar-Gal GK (2015) Tuberculosis origin: the neolithic scenario. Tuberculosis (Edinb) 95:122–126
2. World Health Organization (2015) Global tuberculosis report. http://apps.who.int/iris/handle/10665/191102. Accessed 07 Apr 2016

3. Rindfleisch E (1862) Der Miliare Tuberkel. Virchows Arch 24:571–578
4. Baumgarten P (1881) Gamose arteritis und entsprechende tuberculose veranderungen. Virchows Archiv fur Pathologische Anatomie 86:179–221
5. Hektoen L (1896) The vascular changes in tuberculous meningitis especially in tuberculous endarteritis. J Exp Med 1:112–163
6. Greitz T (1964) Angiography in tuberculous meningitis. Acta Radiol (Sweden) 2:369–378
7. Thomas MD, Chopra JS, Walia BNS (1977) Tuberculous meningitis (TBM)-(a clinical study of 232 cases). J Assoc Physicians India 25:633–639
8. Thwaites GE, Nguyen DB, Nguyen HD, Hoang TQ, Do TT, Nguyen TC, Nguyen QH, Nguyen TT, Nguyen NH, Nguyen TN, Nguyen NL, Nguyen HD, Vu NT, Cao HH, Tran TH, Pham PM, Nguyen TD, Stepniewska K, White NJ, Tran TH, Farrar JJ (2004) Dexamethasone for the treatment of tuberculous meningitis in adolescents and adults. N Engl J Med 351:1741–1751
9. Garg RK, Jain A, Malhotra HS, Agrawal A, Garg R (2013) Drug-resistant tuberculous meningitis. Expert Rev Anti Infect Ther 11:605–621
10. Garg RK, Malhotra HS, Kumar N (2014) Paradoxical reaction in HIV negative tuberculous meningitis. J Neurol Sci 340:26–36
11. Sheu JJ, Chiou HY, Kang JH, Chen YH, Lin HC (2010) Tuberculosis and the risk of ischemic stroke: a 3-year follow-up study. Stroke 41:244–249
12. Bhargava S, Gupta AK, Tandon PN (1982) Tuberculous meningitis-a CT study. Br J Radiol 55:189–196
13. Schoeman J, Hewlett R, Donald P (1988) MR of childhood tuberculous meningitis. Neuroradiology 30:473–477
14. Gupta RK, Gupta S, Singh D, Sharma B, Kohli A, Gurjal RB (1994) MR imaging and angiography in tuberculous meningitis. Neuroradiology 36:87–92
15. Shukla R, Abbas A, Kumar P, Gupta RK, Jha S, Prasad KN (2008) Evaluation of cerebral infarction in tuberculous meningitis by diffusion weighted imaging. J Infect 57:298–306
16. Kalita J, Misra UK, Nair PP (2009) Predictors of stroke and its significance in the outcome of tuberculous meningitis. J Stroke Cerebrovasc Dis 18:251–258
17. Anuradha HK, Garg RK, Agarwal A, Sinha MK, Verma R, Singh MK, Shukla R (2010) Predictors of stroke in patients of tuberculous meningitis and its effect on the outcome. QJM 103:671–678
18. Kalita J, Prasad S, Maurya PK, Kumar S, Misra UK (2012) MR angiography in tuberculous meningitis. Acta Radiol 53:324–329
19. Wasay M, Farooq S, Khowaja ZA, Bawa ZA, Ali SM, Awan S, Beg MA, Mehndiratta MM (2014) Cerebral infarction and tuberculoma in central nervous system tuberculosis: frequency and prognostic implications. J Neurol Neurosurg Psychiatry 85:1260–1264
20. Mathew NT, Abraham J, Chandy J (1970) Cerebral angiographic features in tuberculous meningitis. Neurology 20:1015–1023
21. Leeds NE, Goldberg HI (1971) Angiographic manifestations in cerebral inflammatory disease. Radiology 98:595–604
22. Rojas-Echeverri LA, Soto-Hernández JL, Garza S, Martínez-Zubieta R, Miranda LI, García-Ramos G, Zenteno M (1996) Predictive value of digital subtraction angiography in patients with tuberculous meningitis. Neuroradiology 38:20–24
23. Singh B, Garg RK, Singh MK, Verma R, Malhotra HS, Jain A, Singh R, Kohli N, Phadke RV, Shukla R, Parihar A (2012) Computed tomography angiography in patients with tuberculous meningitis. J Infect 64:565–572
24. Suwanwela C, Suwanwela N, Charuchinda S, Hongsaprabhas C (1972) Intracranial mycotic aneurysms of extravascular origin. J Neurosurg 36:552–559
25. Leiguarda R, Berthier M, Starkstein S, Nogues M, Lylyk P (1988) Ischemic infarction in 25 children with tuberculous meningitis. Stroke 19:200–204
26. Griffiths SJ, Sgouros S, James G, John P (2000) Intraventricular haemorrhage due to ruptured posterior inferior cerebellar artery aneurysm in tuberculous meningitis. Childs Nerv Syst 16:872–874
27. Gupta K, Radotra BD, Suri D, Sharma K, Saxena AK, Singhi P (2012) Mycotic aneurysm and subarachnoid hemorrhage following tubercular meningitis in an infant with congenital tuberculosis and cytomegalovirus disease. J Child Neurol 27:1320–1325
28. Poltera AA, Templeton AC (1973) Intracranial tuberculosis in Uganda: a post-mortem survey. Afr J Med Sci 4:343–349
29. Vani KR, Shankar SK, Das S, Asha T, Rao TV (1991) Involvement of hypothalamus in tuberculous meningitis: pathological changes at autopsy. Indian J Tuberc 38:149–153
30. Chatterjee D, Radotra BD, Vasishta RK, Sharma K (2015) Vascular complications of tuberculous meningitis: an autopsy study. Neurol India 63:926–932
31. Udani PM, Parekh UC, Dastur DK (1971) Neurological and related syndromes in CNS tuberculosis. Clinical features and pathogenesis. J Neurol Sci 14:341–357
32. Dastur DK, Lalitha VS, Udani P, Parekh U (1970) The brain and meninges in tuberculous meningitis: gross pathology in 100 cases and pathogenesis. Neurol India 18:86–94
33. Srikanth SG, Taly AB, Nagarajan K, Jayakumar PN, Patil S (2007) Clinicoradiological features of tuberculous meningitis in patients over 50 years of age. J Neurol Neurosurg Psychiatry 78:536–538
34. Thwaites GE, Macmullen-Price J, Chau TT, Mai PP, Dung NT, Simmons CP, White NJ, Hien TT, Summers D, Farrar JJ (2007) Serial MRI to determine the effect of dexamethasone on the cerebral pathology of tuberculous meningitis: an observational study. Lancet Neurol 6:230–236
35. van der Merwe DJ, Andronikou S, Van Toorn R, Pienaar M (2009) Brainstem ischemic lesions on MRI in children with tuberculous meningitis: with diffusion weighted confirmation. Childs Nerv Syst 25:949–954

36. Mangalore S, Desai S, Mahadevan A, Kovoor JM, Vasudev LM, Tally AB, Shankar SK (2014) Cerebral tubercular thrombophlebitis presenting as venous infarct: magnetic resonance imaging and pathologic correlation. Ann Indian Acad Neurol 17:130–134
37. Natarajan V, George S, Eapen G, Arulneyam J (2015) An unusual association: tuberculous meningitis causing cerebral venous thrombosis. J Case Reports 5:343–346
38. Hu CH (1986) Tuberculous meningitis complicated by massive intracerebral hemorrhage: report of 2 cases. Zhonghua Shen Jing Jing Shen Ke Za Zhi 19:119–121
39. Mohapatra AK, Sharma SN, Sethi PK, Ahuja IM (1988) Subarachnoid haemorrhage in tubercular meningitis. J Assoc Physicians India 36:237
40. Yeh STY, Lee WJ, Lin HJ, Chen CY, Te AL, Lin HJ (2003) Nonaneurysmal subarachnoid hemorrhage secondary to tuberculous meningitis: report of two cases. J Emerg Med 25:265–270
41. Kim SM, Lee E, Kim BJ, Kim JH, Khang SK, Kim JS, Kang JK (2009) Tuberculous meningoencephalitis complicated by subarachnoid hemorrhage. J Korean Neurol Assoc 27:409–412
42. Alarcón F, Dueñas G, Cevallos N, Lees AJ (2000) Movement disorders in 30 patients with tuberculous meningitis. Mov Disord 15:561–569
43. Schon F, Bowler JV (1990) Syringomyelia and syringobulbia following tuberculous meningitis. J Neurol 237:122–123
44. Fehlings MG, Bernstein M (1992) Syringomyelia as a complication of tuberculous meningitis. Can J Neurol Sci 19:84–87
45. Moghtaderi A, Alavi-Naini R, Rahimi-Movaghar V (2006) Syringomyelia: an early complication of tuberculous meningitis. Trop Doct 36:254–255
46. Kingsley DPE, Hendrickse WA, Kendall BE, Swash M, Singh V (1987) Tuberculous meningitis: role of CT in management and prognosis. J Neurol Neurosurg Psychiatry 50:30–36
47. Lam KS, Sham MMK, Tam SCF, Ng MMT, Ma HT (1993) Hypopituitarism after tuberculous meningitis in childhood. Ann Intern Med 118:701–716
48. Dhanwal DK, Kumar S, Vyas A, Saxena A (2011) Hypothalamic pituitary dysfunction in acute non mycobacterial infections of central nervous system. Indian J Endocrinol Metab 15:233–237
49. Smith HV, Vollum RL, Cairns H (1948) Treatment of tuberculous meningitis with streptomycin. Lancet 251:627–636
50. Lorber J (1958) Diabetes insipidus following tuberculous meningitis. Arch Dis Child 33:315–319
51. Haslam RHA, Winternitz WW, Howieson J, Ky L (1969) Selective hypopituitarism following tuberculous meningitis. Am J Dis Child 118:903–908
52. Uesugi T, Takizawa S, Morita Y, Takahashi H, Takagi S (2006) Hemorrhagic infarction in tuberculous meningitis. Intern Med 45:1193–1194
53. Hsieh FY, Chia LG, Shen WC (1992) Locations of cerebral infarctions in tuberculous meningitis. Neuroradiology 34:197–199
54. Nair PP, Kalita J, Kumar S, Misra UK (2009) MRI pattern of infarcts in basal ganglia region in patients with tuberculous meningitis. Neuroradiology 51:221–225
55. Lehrer H (1966) The angiographic triad of tuberculous meningitis: a radiographic and clinicopathologic correlation. Radiology 87:829–835
56. Finsterer J, Kladosek A, Nagelmeier IE, Becherer A, Matula C, Stradal KH, Wolf K, Czech T, Stanek G (2000) Chronic granulomatous meningitis with multiple cranial nerve lesions hydrocephalus, stroke, sinus thrombosis, and epilepsy. South Med J 93:1108–1111
57. Fiorot Júnior JA, Felício AC, Fukujima MM, Rodrigues CA, Morelli VM, Lourenço DM, Prado GF (2005) Tuberculosis: an uncommon cause of cerebral venous thrombosis? Arq Neuropsiquiatr 63:852–854
58. Aaslid R, Markwalder TM, Nornes H (1982) Noninvasive transcranial Doppler ultrasound recording of flow velocity in basal cerebral arteries. J Neurosurg 57:769–774
59. Chadduck WM, Seibert JJ, Adametz J, Glasier CM, Crabtree M, Stansell CA (1989) Cranial Doppler ultrasonography correlates with criteria for ventriculoperitoneal shunting. Surg Neurol 31:122–128
60. Nadvi SS, Van Dellen JR, Gouws E (1995) Transcranial Doppler ultrasonography in hydrocephalic children with tuberculous meningitis. Br J Neurosurg 9:519–526
61. Kilic T, Elmaci I, Ozek MM, Pamir NM (2002) Utility of transcranial Doppler ultrasonography in the diagnosis and follow-up of tuberculous meningitis-related vasculopathy. Childs Nerv Syst 18:142–146
62. van Toorn R, Schaaf HS, Solomons R, Laubscher JA, Schoeman JF (2014) The value of transcranial Doppler imaging in children with tuberculous meningitis. Childs Nerv Syst 30:1711–1716
63. Misra UK, Kalita J, Das BK (2000) Single photon emission computed tomography in tuberculous meningitis. Postgrad Med J 76:642–645
64. Doniach I (1949) Changes in meningeal vessels in acute and chronic (streptomycin-treated) tuberculous meningitis. J Pathol Bacteriol 61:253–259
65. Barlow T (1910) Tuberculous meningitis. In: Albutt C, Rolleston HD (eds) A system of medicine. Macmillan & Co., London, pp 201–228
66. Smith HV, Daniel P (1947) Some clinical and pathological aspects of tuberculosis of the central nervous system. Tubercle 28:64–80
67. Rich AR, McCordock HA (1933) The pathogenesis of tuberculous meningitis. Bull Johns Hopkins Hosp 52:2–37
68. Goldzieher JW, Lisa JR (1947) Gross cerebral haemorrhages and vascular lesions in acute tuberculous meningitis and meningo-encephalitis. Am J Pathol 23:133–145
69. Lammie GA, Hewlett RH, Schoeman JF, Donald PR (2009) Tuberculous cerebrovascular disease: a review. J Infect 59:156–166
70. Rigdon RH, Lefeber EJ (1950) Thrombosis of cerebral vessels with necrosis of the basal nuclei; a complication of tuberculous meningitis and streptomycin therapy. Am Rev Tuberc 61:247–256

71. Poltera AA (1977) Thrombogenic intracranial vasculitis in tuberculous meningitis. A 20 year "post mortem" survey. Acta Neurol Belg 77:12–24
72. Winkleman NW, Moore T (1940) Meningeal blood vessels in tuberculous meningitis. Arch Neurol Psychiatry 42:315–333
73. Dastur DK, Lalitha VS (1973) The many facets of neurotuberculosis: An epitome of neuropathology. In: Progress in Neuropathology, Vol 2. Edited by HM Zimmerman. New York, Grune & Stratton, pp 351–408
74. Matsuyama W, Hashiguchi T, Umehara F, Matsuura E, Kawabata M, Arimura K, Maruyama I, Osame M (2001) Expression of vascular endothelial growth factor in tuberculous meningitis. J Neurol Sci 186:75–79
75. van der Flier M, Hoppenreijs S, van Rensburg AJ, Ruyken M, Kolk AH, Springer P, Hoepelman AI, Geelen SP, Kimpen JL, Schoeman JF (2004) Vascular endothelial growth factor and blood-brain barrier disruption in tuberculous meningitis. Pediatr Infect Dis J 23:608–613
76. Matsuura E, Umehara F, Hashiguchi T, Fujimoto N, Okada Y, Osame M (2000) Marked increase of matrix metalloproteinase 9 in cerebrospinal fluid of patients with fungal or tuberculous meningoencephalitis. J Neurol Sci 173:45–52
77. Price NM, Farrar J, Chau TTH, Mai NTH, Hien TT, Friedland JS (2001) Identification of a matrix-degrading phenotype in human tuberculosis in vitro and in vivo. J Immunol 166:4223–4230
78. Thwaites GE, Simmons CP, Quyen NT, Chau TT, Mai PP, Dung NT, Phu NH, White NP, Hien TT, Farrar JJ (2003) Pathophysiology and prognosis in Vietnamese adults with tuberculous meningitis. J Infect Dis 188:1105–1115
79. Misra UK, Kalita J, Srivastava R, Nair PP, Mishra MK, Basu A (2010) A study of cytokines in tuberculous meningitis: clinical and MRI correlation. Neurosci Lett 483:6–10
80. Prasad K, Singh MB (2008) Corticosteroids for managing tuberculous meningitis. Cochrane Database Syst Rev 1:CD002244
81. Schoeman JF, Van Zyl LE, Laubscher JA, Donald PR (1997) Effect of corticosteroids on intracranial pressure, computed tomographic findings, and clinical outcome in young children with tuberculous meningitis. Pediatrics 99:226–231
82. Misra UK, Kalita J, Nair PP (2010) Role of aspirin in tuberculous meningitis: a randomized open label placebo controlled trial. J Neurol Sci 293:12–17
83. Schoeman JF, Janse van Rensburg A, Laubscher JA, Springer P (2011) The role of aspirin in childhood tuberculous meningitis. J Child Neurol 26:956–962
84. Tsenova L, Sokol K, Freedman VH, Kaplan G (1998) A combination of thalidomide plus antibiotics protects rabbits from mycobacterial meningitis-associated death. J Infect Dis 177:1563–1572
85. Tsenova L, Bergtold A, Freedman VH, Young RA, Kaplan G (1999) Tumour necrosis factor a is a determinant of pathogenesis and disease progression in mycobacterial infection in the central nervous system. Proc Natl Acad Sci USA 96:5657–5662
86. Figaji AA, Sandler SI, Fieggen AG, Le Roux PD, Peter JC, Argent AC (2008) Continuous monitoring and intervention for cerebral ischemia in tuberculous meningitis. Pediatr Crit Care Med 9:E25–E30
87. Gujjar AR, Srikanth SG, Umamaheshwara Rao GS (2009) HHH regime for arteritis secondary to TB meningitis: a prospective randomized study. Neurocrit Care 10:313–317

Imaging Findings of Tuberculosis of the Brain and Its Coverings

13

Mohammad Ali Karimi, Morteza Sanei Taheri, and Ahmet T. Turgut

Contents

M.A. Karimi, MD (✉) • M.S. Taheri, MD
Department of Radiology, Shohada-e-Tajrish Hospital, Shahid Beheshti University of Medical Sciences, Tehran, Iran
e-mail: mkarimidr@yahoo.com; saneim@gmail.com

A.T. Turgut, MD
Department of Radiology, Hacettepe University School of Medicine, Ankara, Turkey
e-mail: ahmettuncayturgut@yahoo.com

Abbreviations

AIDS	Acquired immunodeficiency syndrome
CNS	Central nervous system
CSF	Cerebrospinal fluid
CT	Computed tomography
FLAIR	Fluid attenuation inversion recovery
MRA	Magnetic resonance angiography
MRI	Magnetic resonance imaging
MT	Magnetization transfer
TB	Tuberculosis
TBA	Tuberculous brain abscess
TBM	Tuberculous meningitis

13.1 Introduction

Tuberculosis (TB) is a historical disease which has reemerged and considered as a major worldwide health problem due to increasing frequency of immunocompromising conditions such as diabetes, alcoholism, cancer, and acquired immunodeficiency syndrome (AIDS) in recent decades. *Mycobacterium tuberculosis* may involve any organ, and the lungs are the most common location; however, central nervous system (CNS) TB is the most tremendous form of this disease. CNS TB consists about 5–10% of all patients with TB and up to 20% of patients with AIDS-related TB [1–3].

CNS TB usually has a distant origin, e.g., the lung, and the organism reaches to the brain or meninges via hematogenous spread. Sometimes, it

M. Turgut et al. (eds.), *Tuberculosis of the Central Nervous System*,
DOI 10.1007/978-3-319-50712-5_13

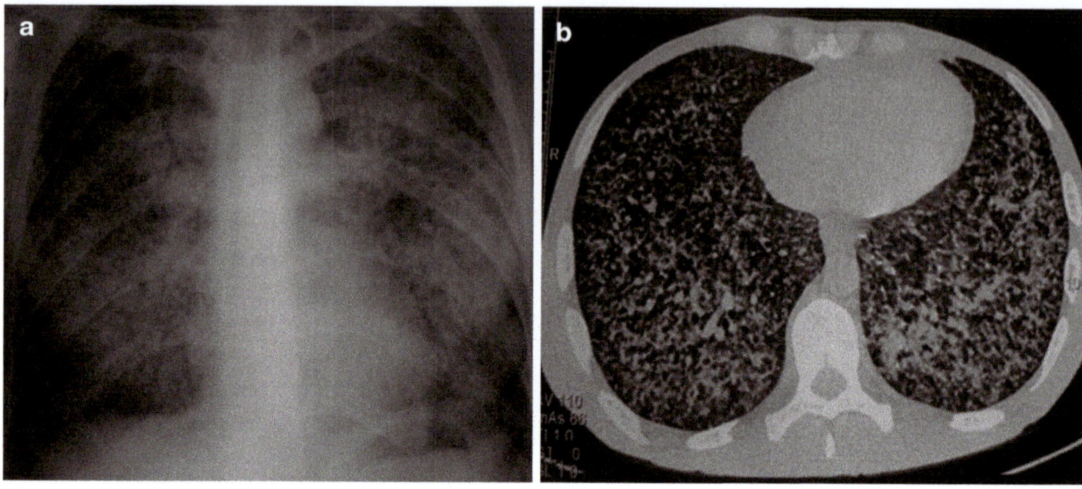

Fig. 13.1 Miliary tuberculosis (TB). Frontal chest radiograph (**a**) shows bilateral diffuse fine tiny nodules. Axial high-resolution chest CT scan (**b**) demonstrates innumerable randomly distributed fine discrete nodules bilaterally.

may result from direct spread from intra- or extracranial foci [4]. Clinical and imaging manifestations of CNS TB may simulate other neurological diseases such as tumors and other infectious and noninfectious conditions [5]. Since CNS TB has no unique characteristics on neuroimaging and clinical manifestation, diagnosis of this disease remains a challenging issue. Therefore, familiarity with the radiological manifestations of CNS TB has a key role in timely and precise diagnosis of this disease. CNS TB may present as tuberculous meningitis (TBM), cerebritis, ventriculitis, cerebral abscesses, tuberculomas, miliary TB, and spinal and calvarial involvement [6–8]. In this chapter, we describe imaging findings of TB of the brain and its coverings.

13.2 Pulmonary Tuberculosis as a Diagnostic Clue

Most of patients with CNS TB have a diagnostic clue in their lung imaging, and sometimes a plain radiograph can help us to make a correct diagnosis. Therefore, we first briefly describe the imaging manifestations of pulmonary TB. Pulmonary TB may be primary or postprimary (reactivation). Primary form is common in children, and postprimary infection usually presents in adults.

Primary TB characteristically presents as hilar (and/or mediastinal) lymphadenopathy which is typically unilateral but may be asymmetrically bilateral. Other findings are pleural effusion (typically unilateral), miliary nodules, and consolidation (Fig. 13.1). In primary infection, the parenchymal disease and adenopathy may completely resolve, or there may be a residual focus of scarring or calcification [9, 10].

Postprimary TB typically involves apical and posterior segments of upper lobes and to a lesser degree superior segment of lower lobes. The main manifestations include cavitations, nodular infiltrations, typically as tree-in-bud appearance, multifocal patchy opacities, lymphadenopathies, and pleural effusion. Cavitations usually indicate active and transmissible disease (Fig. 13.2) [9, 10].

When we encounter patients with CNS TB, lung radiograph or computed tomography (CT) may show the sequels of old pulmonary TB, including parenchymal fibrosis, architectural distortion, bronchiectasis, and volume loss in the upper lobes.

13.3 Tuberculous Meningitis

Tuberculous Meningitis (TBM) is the most common type of CNS TB. It is most frequent in children or immunocompromised individuals [11, 12].

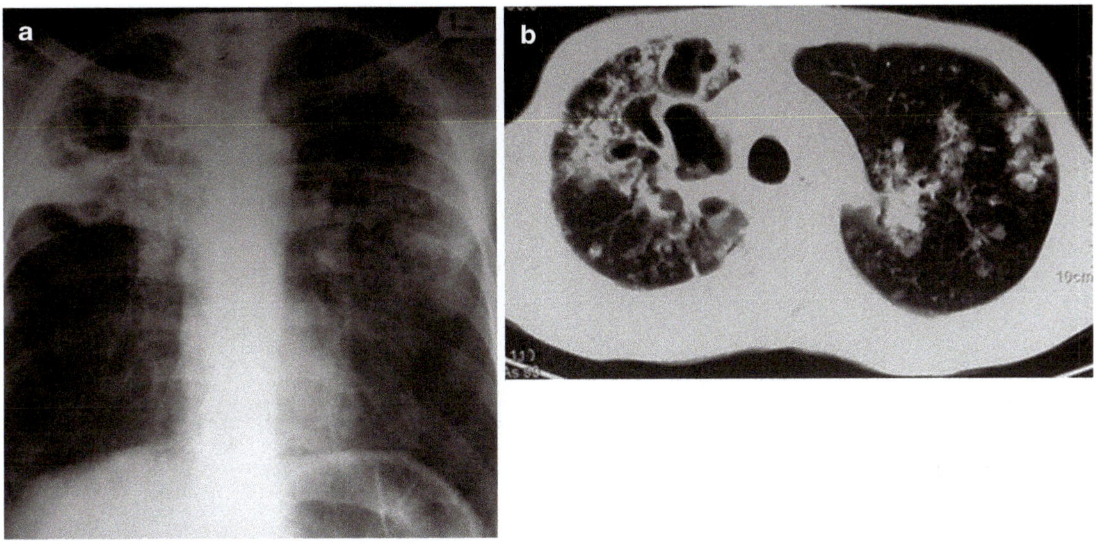

Fig. 13.2 Reactivated pulmonary TB. (**a**) Frontal chest radiograph shows typical location of TB involvement in *right* upper lobe with cavitary consolidation and volume loss. There are also some nodular opacities in *left* upper lobe. (**b**) Axial chest CT scan of another HIV-positive patient demonstrates multiple cavities in *right* upper lobe associated with clumped nodular and some linear opacities in both upper lobes

TBM results from hematogenous spread of *M. tuberculosis*; however, it may also result from spread of adjacent focus (Rich focus) in cortical subpial or subependymal into the subarachnoid spaces or into the ventricular system [13]. Insidious course of TBM along with its nonspecific manifestations may result from misdiagnosis or delayed diagnosis of TBM. Hence, high index of suspicion and early imaging play important role in the timely detection of TBM and thereby reducing its morbidity and mortality rate.

Radiologically, the most common finding is enhancing exudate in the basal cisterns. This is a relatively specific neuroimaging finding of leptomeningeal TB on CT and magnetic resonance images (MRIs) [14]; however, sometimes this feature may also be seen in meningitis due to other infectious including fungal ones and granulomatous (sarcoidosis) and neoplastic (lymphoma; carcinomatosis) diseases [1]. The tuberculous exudate is composed of bacilli and the host immune cells.

The most sensitive imaging finding of tubercular meningitis is meningeal enhancement that has been reported in up to 90% of patients [7, 14, 15]. The subpial exudate is commonly located in the lateral cerebral fossa and the sylvian fissure, inferomedial surface of the frontal lobes, the anteromedial surface of the temporal lobes, the superior aspect of the cerebellum, and the floor of the third ventricle [16]. Sometimes, extension to adjacent areas such as suprasellar, pontomesencephalic, or interpeduncular cisterns may also occur [17]. Meningeal enhancement over the cerebral convexities and the sylvian fissures is another common finding. Involvement of ependymal surfaces of the ventricles usually occurs in the later stages of the TBM [1, 17, 18]. In later stages, also there may be widening of subarachnoid spaces.

CT images of TBM usually demonstrate obliteration of basal cisterns by exudates of iso- to mild hyperattenuation [1, 6, 16, 19]. MRI is more sensitive than CT for detection of the findings, especially post-contrast MRIs which will demonstrate the leptomeningeal enhancement and enhancing cisternal exudates (Figs. 13.3, 13.4, and 13.5) [6].

Some studies reported that in comparison to contrast-enhanced T1-weighted images, post-contrast fluid attenuation inversion recovery (FLAIR) images show a higher specificity for discovery of leptomeningeal enhancement [20]. Also, contrast-enhanced magnetization transfer

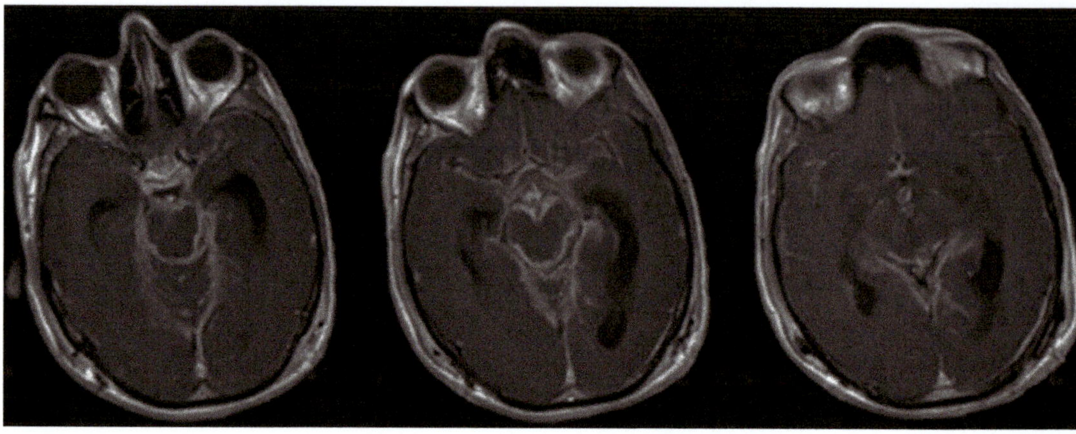

Fig. 13.3 Meningeal TB. Axial post-contrast T1-weighted MRIs demonstrate enhancing basilar exudates and leptomeningeal enhancement

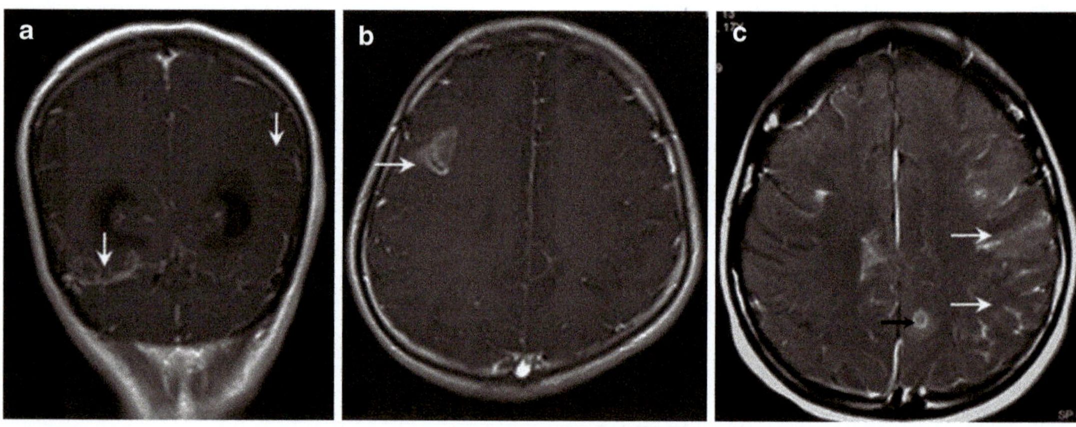

Fig. 13.4 Meningeal TB. Coronal (**a**) and axial (**b**, **c**) post-contrast T1-weighted MRIs show leptomeningeal enhancement (*white arrows*). A small tuberculoma in *left* parasagittal parietal region (*black arrow* in **c**) is also evident

(MT) imaging is superior to the conventional post-contrast imaging in detecting meningeal involvement [11]. As mentioned above, TBM imaging findings may overlap with other conditions; this form of meningeal enhancement may be seen in carcinomatous meningitis, other infective meningitis, and inflammatory diseases such as rheumatoid arthritis or sarcoidosis [11].

Progressive hydrocephalus, cranial neuropathies, infarction, and vasculitis with their own imaging features are the complications of TBM which may alter the face of the disease [8, 12]. Obstruction of cerebrospinal fluid (CSF) flow in the basal cisterns results to the most common complication of TBM, communicating hydrocephalus (Fig. 13.6) [1, 4, 8, 11]. Noncommunicating hydrocephalus may be seen in some cases which is due to obstruction by tuberculoma or TB abscess.

Ischemic infarct (Fig. 13.6) secondary to vascular compression and obstruction of perforating vessels (necrotizing arteritis) [17, 21, 22], especially the lenticulostriate and thalamoperforating arteries, is also a common complication with detection rate of 20–40% of patients. This event is seen mostly in the basal ganglia or internal capsule which is enriched by vessels that perfuse the so-called medial TB zone [19]. Dural venous sinus thrombosis and secondary hemorrhagic infarct may be seen in patients with TBM. We encountered a patient with CNS TB in our institute in which the only finding was dural venous sinus thrombosis (Fig. 13.7).

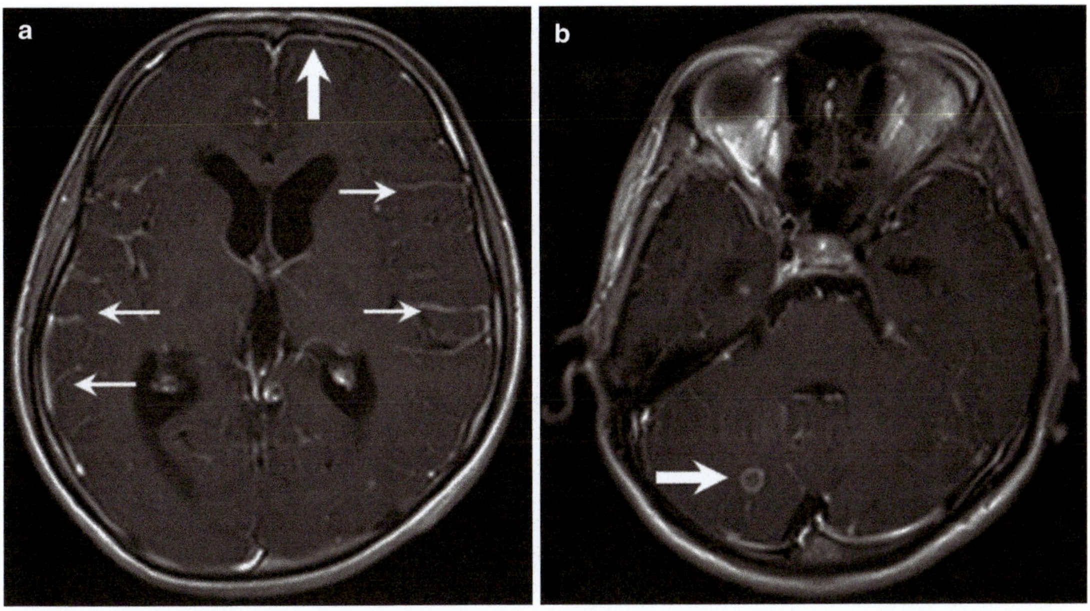

Fig. 13.5 Meningeal TB. (**a**) Leptomeningeal (*small arrows*) and dural pachymeningeal (*large arrow*) enhancements are seen in this axial post-contrast T1-weighted MRIs. (**b**) A small tuberculoma is seen in *right* cerebellar hemisphere (*arrow*)

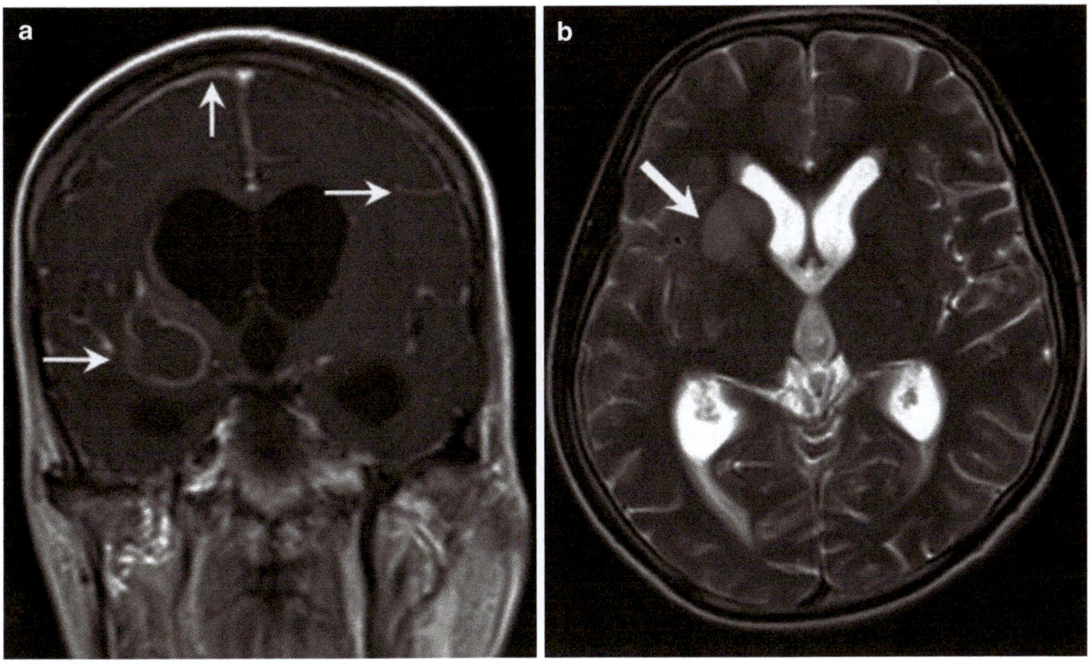

Fig. 13.6 Complications of meningeal TB. (**a**) Coronal post-contrast T1-weighted MRI demonstrates leptomeningeal and pachymeningeal enhancement (*arrows*). Hydrocephalus is also seen which is secondary to the obstruction of cerebrospinal fluid (CSF) flow in the basal cisterns. (**b**) Axial T2-weighted MRI of another patient with TBM shows a lesion in *right* basal ganglia due to ischemic infarct

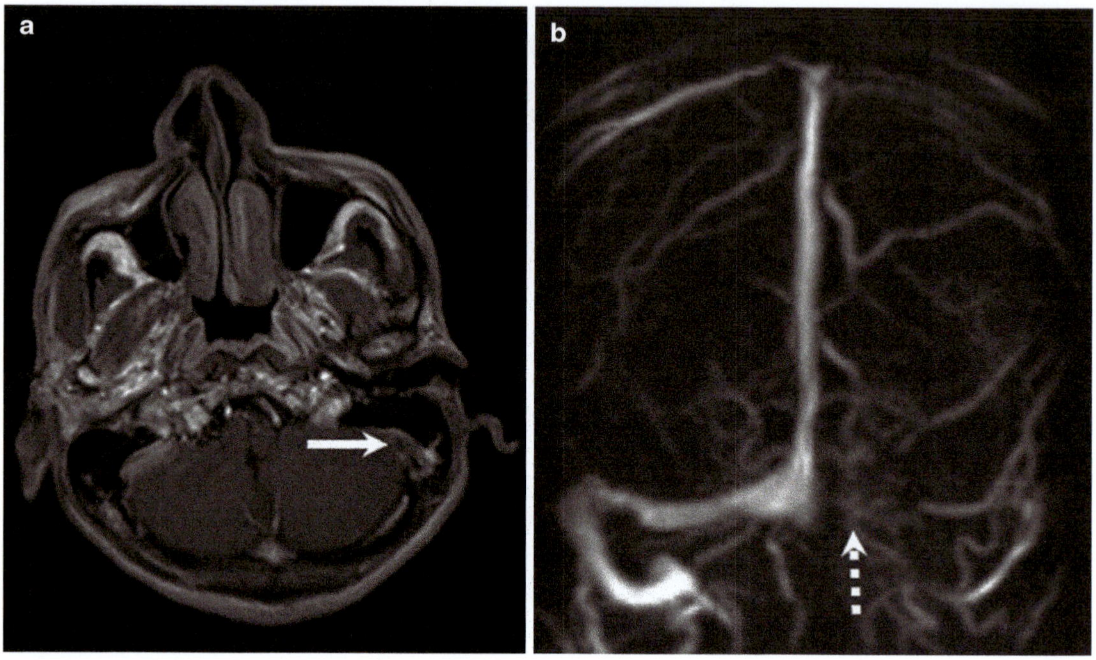

Fig. 13.7 Dural venous sinus thrombosis. (**a**) Axial post-contrast T1-weighted MRI demonstrates a filling defect within *left* sigmoid sinus (*white arrow*). (**b**) MRA reveals nonvisualization of transverse and sigmoid sinuses in *left* side (*white arrow*). This was the only imaging evidence of TBM in a man presented with headache. Because the patient was an immigrant from an endemic area for TB, we assessed CSF PCR for *M. tuberculosis* which revealed a positive result

TBM may also complicate by cranial nerve involvement which occurs in 17–40% of cases. It occurs secondary to ischemia, vascular compromise, or nerve entrapment within basal exudates. Second, third, fourth, and seventh cranial nerves are the most commonly involved nerves [16, 18]. MRI is the preferred imaging for evaluation of the affected cranial nerves; they usually appear as thickened enhanced nerves, particularly in proximal segments. These thickened nerves have high signal intensity on T2-weighted images.

13.4 Brain Parenchymal Tuberculosis

The most common form of brain parenchymal TB disease is tuberculoma. Other forms include cerebritis, cerebral abscess, miliary TB, or TB encephalopathy. Parenchymal disease may occur with or without TBM.

13.4.1 Cerebritis and Cerebral Abscess

Some parenchymal TB is associated with concomitant TBM, and sometimes it occurs without accompanying meningitis. Cerebritis refers to pyogenic inflammation of the brain parenchyma and may lead to abscess formation in the setting of inadequate or incorrect treatment. TB cerebritis or abscess may mimic pyogenic bacterial infection on CT or MRI.

TB cerebritis is infrequent and usually appears as a single or multiple focal ill-defined hypoattenuated lesion(s) on CT images. These lesions appear hyposignal on T1-weighted and hypersignal on T2-weighted images. On post-contrast MRI, areas of patchy enhancement may be seen (Fig. 13.8) [6, 23].

Tuberculous brain abscess (TBA) (Fig. 13.9) is also infrequent and consists of a central zone of pus and liquefied material. The abscess may be single or multiple and often has multilocu-

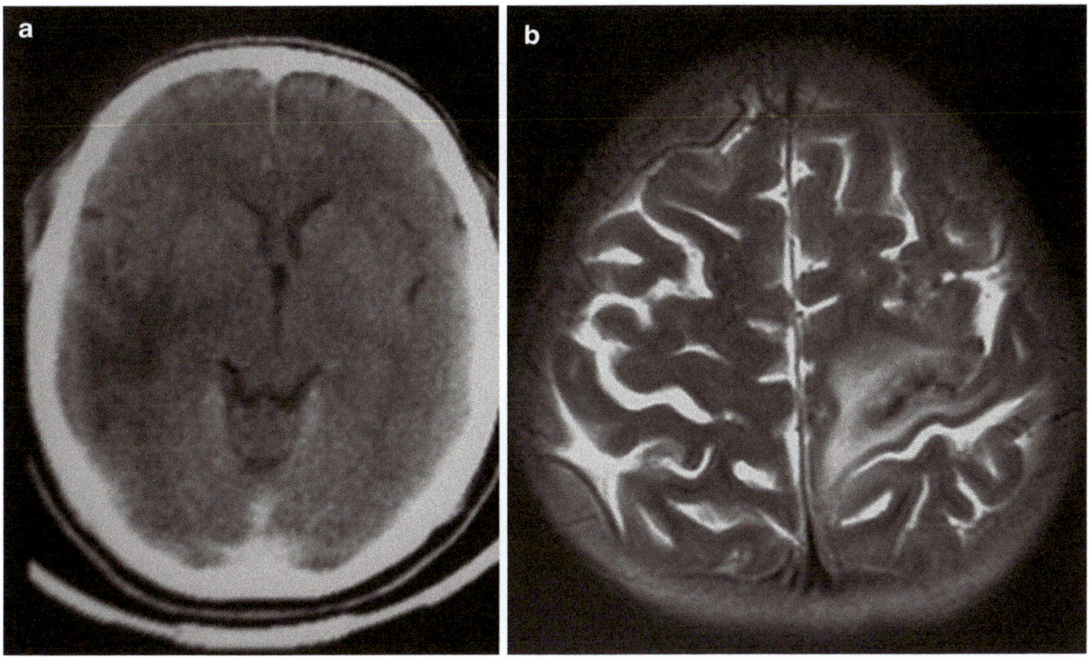

Fig. 13.8 TB cerebritis. (**a**) Axial post-contrast CT image demonstrates an irregular hypodensity in *right* temporal region with faint peripheral enhancement in anterior part. (**b**) Axial T2-weighted MRI in another patient shows nonspecific hypersignality in *left* frontoparietal region

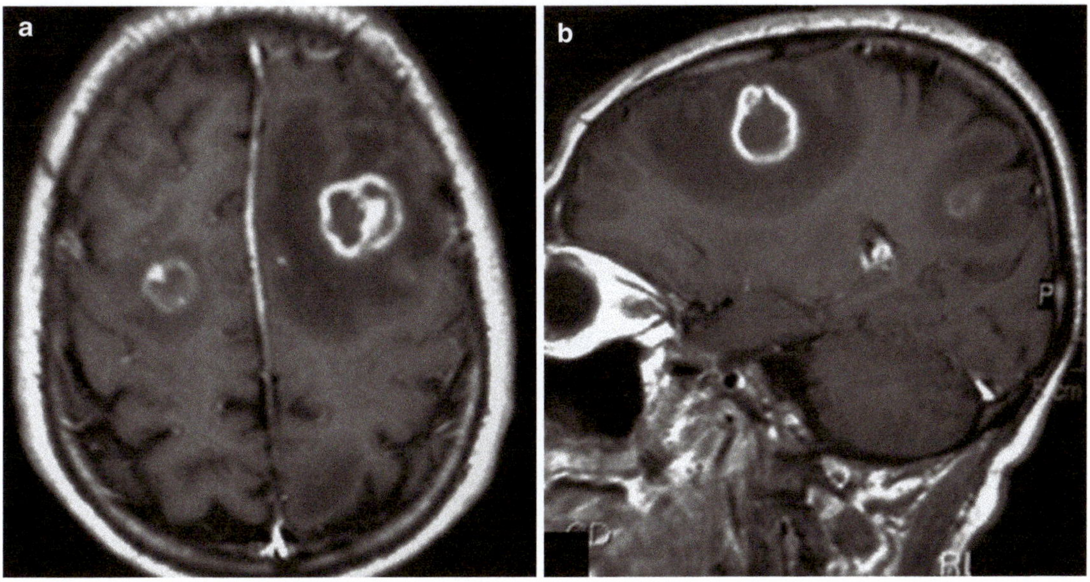

Fig. 13.9 Tuberculous brain abscess (TBA). Axial (**a**) and sagittal (**b**) post-contrast T1-weighted MRIs show multiple TBAs as irregular thick ringlike enhancing lesions in both frontal lobes and *left* parietal region with peripheral edema

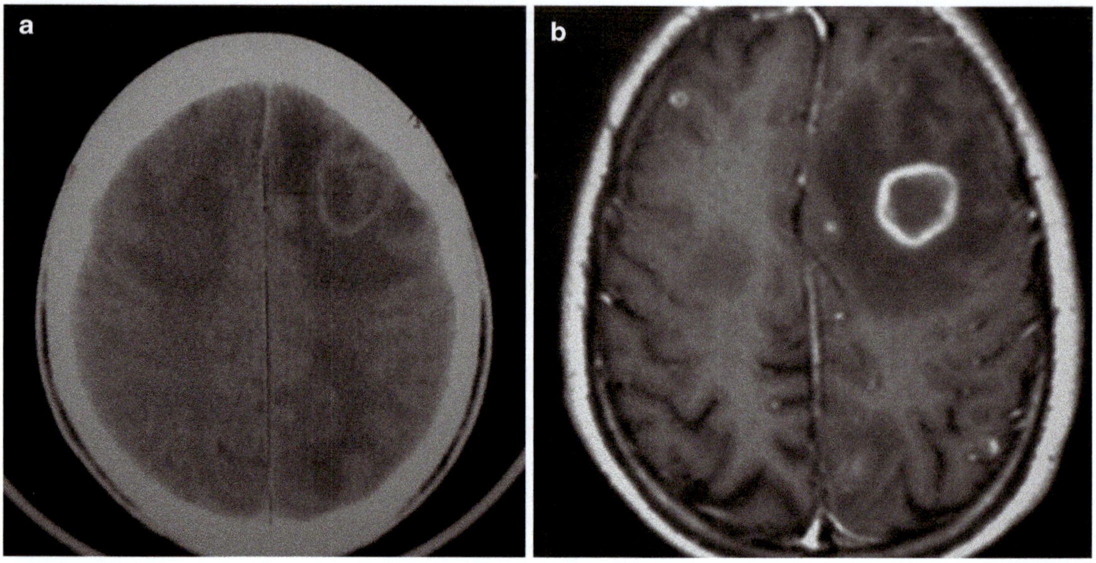

Fig. 13.10 TBA. (**a**) Axial post-contrast CT image shows ring-enhancing lesions in *left* frontal lobe with marked peripheral edema. (**b**) Axial post-contrast T1-weighted MRI in another patient also reveals a lesion in *left* frontal lobe with thick ring enhancement and marked peripheral edema and mass effect leading to midline shift

lar appearance [15]. On CT images the TBA presents as hypodense round or multiloculated lesion(s) accompanied with peripheral edema. It may show some mass effect. Since the abscess contains a central necrotic and liquefied zone, it shows an increased signal intensity on T2-weighted images. Ring enhancement is a dominant feature in post-contrast CT or MRIs (Fig. 13.10). This enhancement is often thin and uniform. However, it may be irregular and thick, particularly in immunodeficient patients [1, 3, 7, 8, 24, 25].

Some studies have shown that application of MT spine echo images make the CNS TB lesions more obvious [26–31]. By increasing the detectability of the lesions, MT images improve the assessment of extent of CNS TB. MT ratio measurements on MRI help to distinguish CNS TB from other infectious brain lesions; MT ratios in TB are lower than those in pyogenic infections and higher than those in viral infections, with the difference related to variations in protein content [5]. Furthermore, on MR spectroscopy, unlike the pyogenic abscess, the peak of amino acids is not a usual finding in TBA [26, 31].

13.4.2 Tuberculoma

Tuberculoma is the most common form of parenchymal involvement in CNS TB. The lesion may be single or multiple and may be seen in any part of the intracranial space. Tuberculoma and TBM may occur concomitantly (Fig. 13.11).

Unlike the TBA which contains central area of pus, tuberculoma has a necrotic caseous center. Its peripheral capsule contains Langerhans cells, epithelioid cells, fibroblasts, and lymphocytes [32]. Tuberculoma in nonenhanced CT images may be isodense, hyperdense, or of mixed density. On contrast-enhanced CT, tuberculoma shows a ringlike enhancement. It may also exhibit irregular or nodular nonhomogeneous enhancement. Some studies have shown that presence of a central calcification within a ringlike enhancement (target sign) is suggestive of tuberculoma [22]. T2-weighted or FLAIR images show a mixed intensity lesion (mainly low signal) which contains a central zone of high signal intensity [33]. The central caseating necrosis makes high signal intensity zone, and peripheral collagenous capsule presents as low signal intensity rim. The capsule is a layer with low water content and high protein content [33].

Surrounding edema may be seen as high signal intensity edema. Post-contrast MRIs often show a ring enhancement (Figs. 13.12 and 13.13).

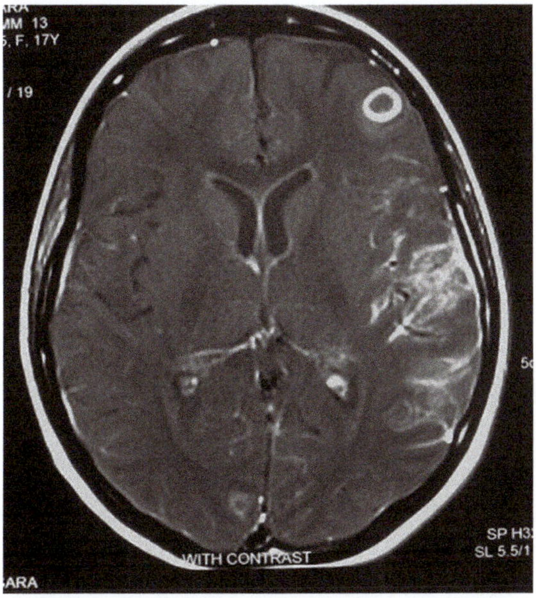

Fig. 13.11 Tuberculoma with TBM. Axial post-contrast T1-weighted image through the lateral ventricles shows a tuberculoma as a cortical ring-enhancing lesion in *left* frontal lobe. There is also another small tuberculoma in *right* occipital lobe. Dural and leptomeningeal enhancements in *left* frontoparietal region indicate associated TBM

Caseating solid granulomas are hypointense on T1-weighted images and strikingly hypointense on T2-weighted images. This hypointensity is due to the granulation tissue and a compact cellularity which is higher than that of brain parenchyma. These typical imaging findings are not seen in noncaseating granulomas; they usually are hypointense to isointense on T1-weighted and hyperintense on T2-weighted images. On post-contrast images homogeneous enhancement is typical [8].

Evaluation of response to medical treatment can be performed by follow-up CT or MRI studies. Regression of the lesions is not a role, and some patients who receive suitable treatment may show paradoxical enlargement of a tuberculoma. Sometimes, a new intracranial and spinal tuberculoma may be seen. Nevertheless, with continuation of anti-TB treatment, the lesions often eventually resolve [33, 34].

Occasionally, healed tuberculomas appear as calcified points on noncontrast CT (Fig. 13.14). Also, several years after healed TBM, calcifications within basal cisterns or brain sulci may be seen [35]. On MR spectroscopy tuberculomas demonstrate lipid level peaks at 0.9 ppm, 1.3 ppm, 2.0 ppm, and 2.8 ppm; these peaks are due to presence of the high lipid content of the mycolic

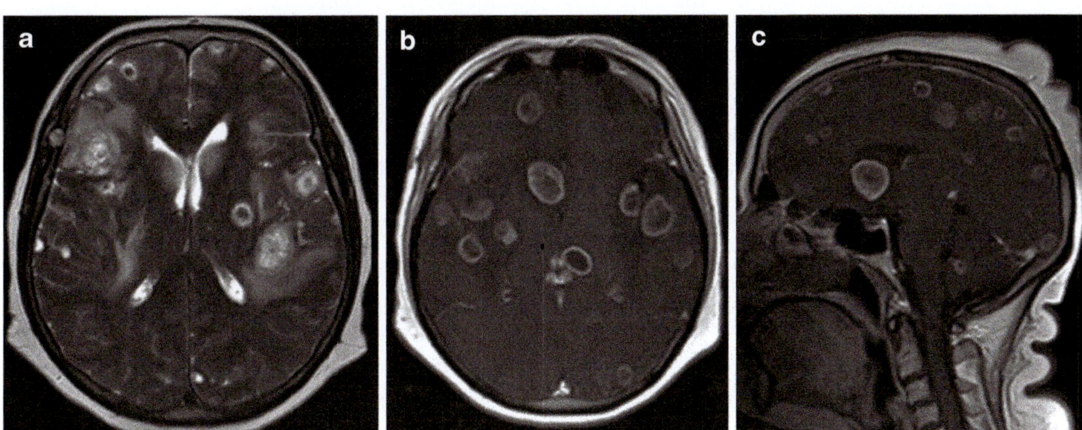

Fig. 13.12 Multiple tuberculomas. (**a**) T2-weighted image through the lateral ventricles shows lesions with hypointense core and peripheral hyperintensity in bilateral frontotemporal regions. Axial (**b**) and sagittal (**c**) post-contrast T1-weighted images show scattered bilateral cerebral tuberculomas as ring-enhancing lesions without peripheral edema. A cerebellar tuberculoma is also seen (**c**)

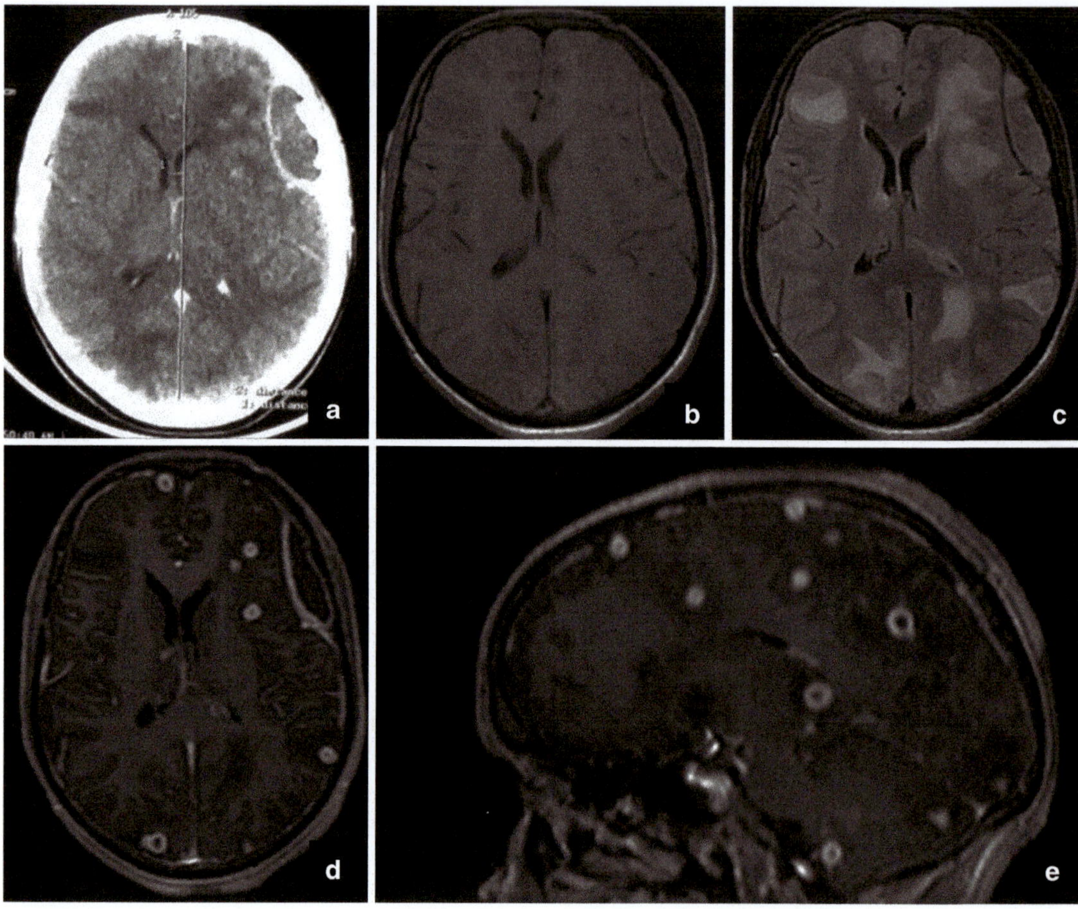

Fig. 13.13 Contrast-enhanced CT of the head showing multiple enhancing lesions with perilesional edema and an extra-axial collection in *left* frontal region, with suggestion of midline shift to the *right* (**a**). The extra-axial collection is iso- to hypointense on T1 W (**b**) and T2-FLAIR (**c**). SPGR-contrast images (axial, **d**; sagittal, **e**) show multiple ring lesions (tuberculomas) with an extra-axial enhancing collection (en plaque tuberculoma) (Courtesy of R. K. Garg, M.D.)

acid in the mycobacterial cell wall. In contrast to pyogenic abscesses which show amino acid resonances at 0.9 ppm at MR spectroscopy, this feature is not seen in TBAs [5].

13.4.3 Miliary Tuberculosis

Brain miliary TB is a very rare form of TB which is seen mainly in severely immunodeficient patients. It is often accompanied with meningitis or an extracranial primary TB infection [36]. The dissemination is always hematogenous, and therefore the military lesions often lodge at the corticomedullary junctions.

Miliary tuberculomas are usually tiny (2–3 mm) dispersed lesions. The lesions usually are not seen on CT images and may be also invisible on noncontrast MRIs. In visible lesions, MRI shows small lesions that are hypointense on T2-weighted sequences. These lesions occasionally can be hardly seen as small hypodense foci on CT images [16]. Post-contrast MRIs usually demonstrate innumerable homogeneously enhancing small round lesions (usually ring enhancing) (Fig. 13.15) [26]. MT spin echo

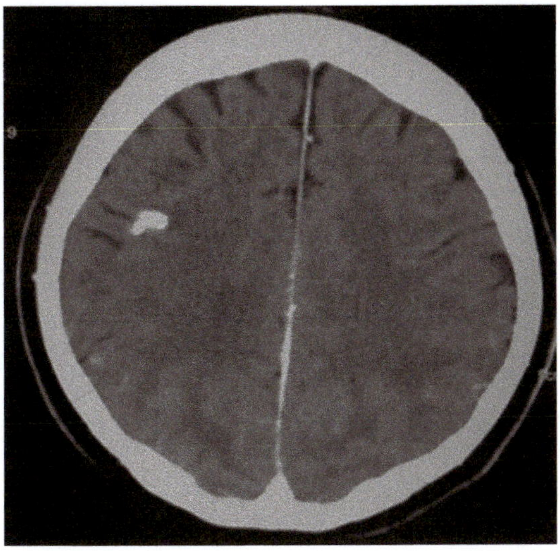

Fig. 13.14 Treated tuberculoma. Axial CT image in a patient with history of treated TB shows a calcified lesion in *right* frontal lobe without edema or mass effect

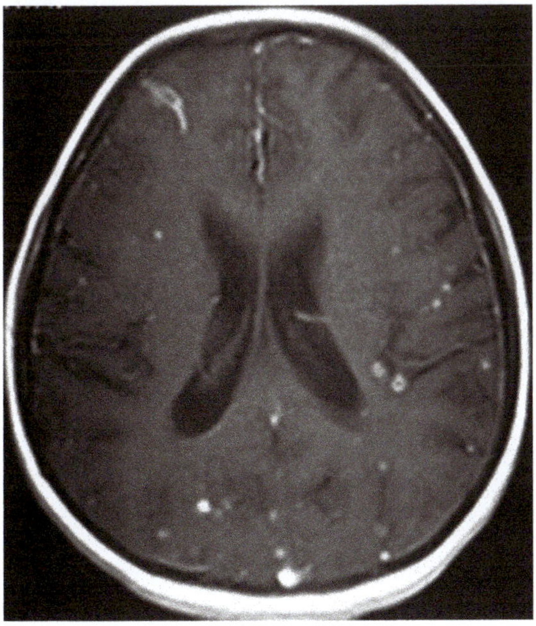

Fig. 13.15 Miliary brain TB. Axial post-contrast T1-weighted image shows numerous bilateral tiny enhancing nodules. This young female patient presented with chronic cough, headache, dizziness, nausea, and vomiting

T1-weighted images (with or without contrast) can detect invisible lesions on routine MRIs even those without enhancement [27].

13.4.4 Tuberculous Encephalopathy

This type of CNS TB characteristically involves the young children. These patients may present with neurologic signs such as convulsion, stupor, and coma. There may be no signs of focal neurological deficit or meningeal irritation. Severe cerebral edema, which may be unilateral or bilateral, is the main neuroimaging finding. Sometimes, hypoattenuating areas on CT images and hyperintensity areas on T2-weighted MRIs may be seen due to myelin loss in the white matter [8, 13, 37].

13.5 Tuberculous Ventriculitis

In addition to the subarachnoid space and brain parenchyma, *M. tuberculosis* can infect the ventricles called "ventriculitis." Despite high incidence of TBM in endemic areas, there are a few reports of TB ventriculitis [38, 39], and it seems to be underestimated [38]. Main CT and MRI findings include intraventricular debris (mostly in occipital horns), ventricular dilatation, periventricular edema, subependymal (or choroidal) enhancement, and restricted diffusion (Fig. 13.16). Singh et al. [38] reported five patients of TB ventriculitis. Enhancement of ependymal wall of lateral ventricle or fourth ventricle was seen on MRIs of these patients along with restricted diffusion and hydrocephalus. Intraventricular septations, sequestered ventricles, and ventricular sludge were also seen in some patients. They concluded that sequestered ventricles (intraventricular septations) and enhanced or hyperintense ependymal wall on MT images are suggestive for TB ventriculitis.

13.6 Miscellaneous Forms of CNS Tuberculosis

Beside the abovementioned presentations, CNS TB may present as other forms such as subdural or epidural abscess, spinal or spinal cord

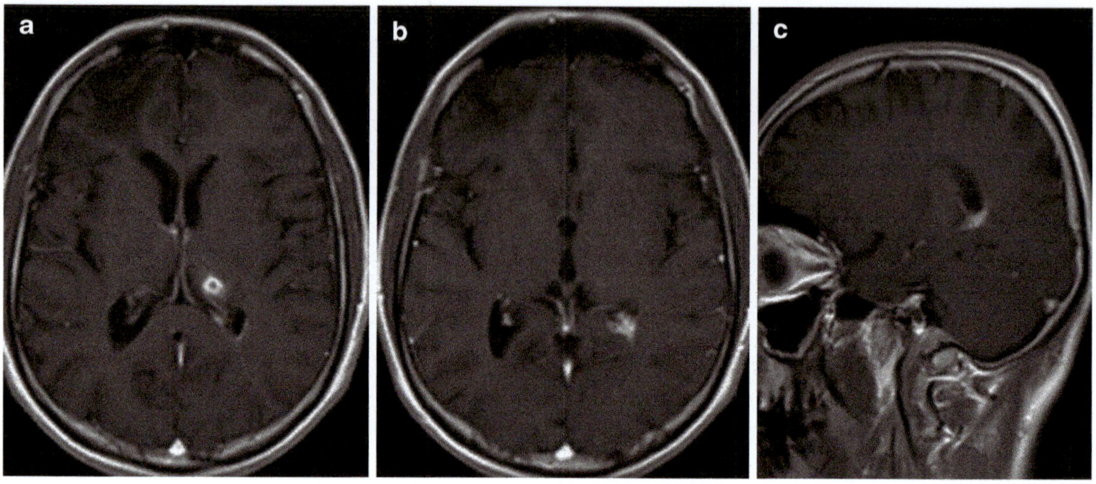

Fig. 13.16 Axial (**a**, **b**) and sagittal (**c**) post-contrast T1-weighted MRIs demonstrate marked enhancement in posterior horn of *left* lateral ventricle and adjacent subtle ventricular wall enhancement. There is also a ring-enhancing tuberculoma in *left* thalamus

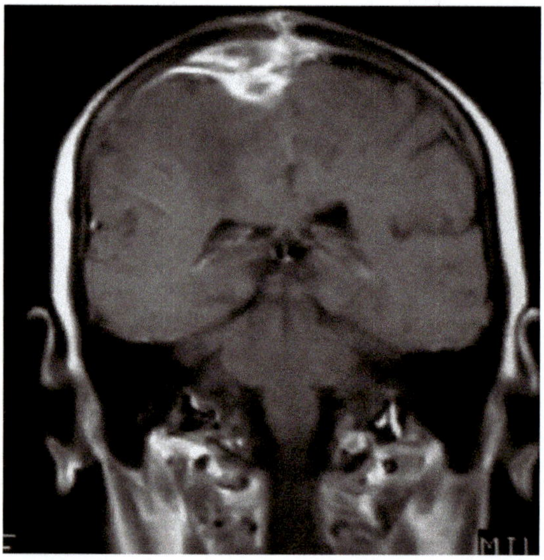

Fig. 13.17 TB epidural and subdural empyema. Coronal post-contrast T1-weighted MRI demonstrates dural enhancement and epidural and subdural collections with thick enhancing walls in *right* frontal region. The epidural component extended to the *left* side. Involvement of diploe indicates calvarial involvement

TB, and calvarial TB. Intracranial subdural or epidural abscess may be seen with or without a primary CNS TB. Imaging features of the abscess are similar to that of other pyogenic abscesses, i.e., isosignal to hyposignal intensity on T1-weighted images and hypersignal or mixed signal intensity on T2-weighted images. These lesions typically show rim enhancement on post-contrast MRI or CT images (Fig. 13.17) [33]. Atypical imaging presentation of CNS TB is not infrequent, and brain TB sometimes mimics a mass lesion leading to unnecessary surgery (Fig. 13.18).

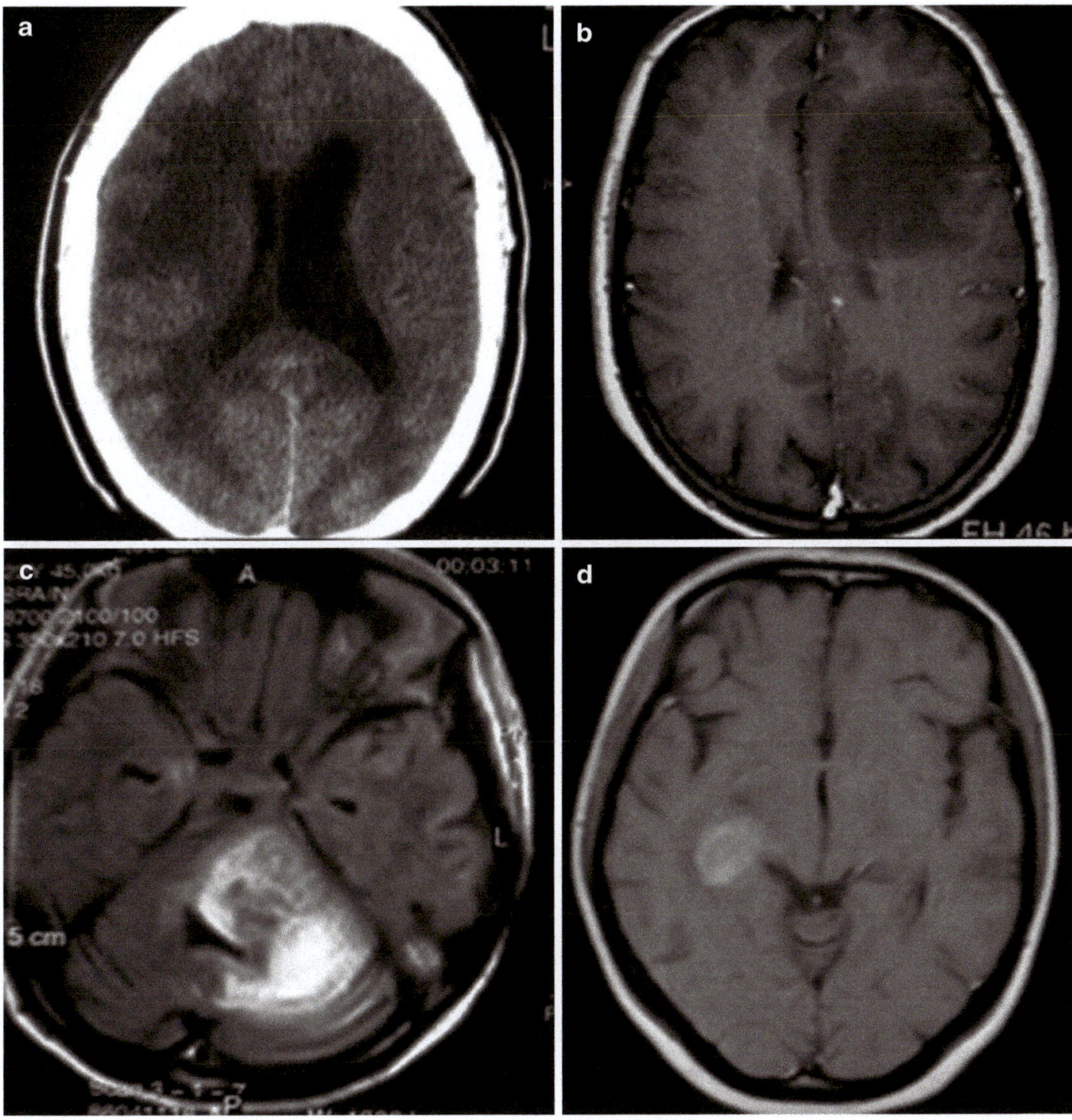

Fig. 13.18 Atypical presentations of CNS TB. (**a–d**) These are four different patients with CNS TB mimicking cerebral or cerebellar mass lesions. In case of (**c**) the diagnosis of TB was made after a complicated surgery

Conclusion

TBM is the most common form of CNS TB, followed by tuberculoma. Enhancing exudate in the basal cisterns is the hallmark of TBM. Tuberculoma often presents as single or multiple ring-enhancing lesion(s) with or without evidence of TBM. Diagnosis of CNS TB is a challenging issue because of its insidious course and nonspecific clinical presentations and also sometimes atypical imaging presentations such as a mass-like lesion. Therefore, the neuroimaging plays a key role in early diagnosis of this curable disease and reducing its morbidity and mortality rates.

References

1. Bernaerts A, Vanhoenacker FM, Parizel PM, Van Goethem JW, Van Altena R, Laridon A, De Roeck J, Coeman V, De Schepper AM (2003) Tuberculosis of the central nervous system: overview of neuroradiological findings. Eur Radiol 13:1876–1890
2. Berenguer J, Moreno S, Laguna F, Vicente T, Adrados M, Ortega A, González-LaHoz J, Bouza E (1992) Tuberculous meningitis in patients infected with the human immunodeficiency virus. N Engl J Med 326:668–672
3. Vidal JE, Penalva de Oliveira AC, Bonasser Filho F, Schiavon Nogueira R, Dauar RF, Leite AG, Lins DL, Coelho JF (2005) Tuberculous brain abscess in AIDS patients: report of three cases and literature review. Int J Infect Dis 9:201–207
4. Rock RB, Olin M, Baker CA, Molitor TW, Peterson PK (2008) Central nervous system tuberculosis: pathogenesis and clinical aspects. Clin Microbiol Rev 21:243–261
5. Shih RY, Koeller KK (2015) Bacterial, fungal, and parasitic infections of the central nervous system: radiologic-pathologic correlation and historical perspectives. Radiographics 35:0000–0000
6. Burrill J, Williams CJ, Bain G, Conder G, Hine AL, Misra RR (2007) Tuberculosis: a radiologic review. Radiographics 27:1255–1273
7. Bathla G, Khandelwal G, Maller VG, Gupta A (2001) Manifestations of cerebral tuberculosis. Singapore Med J 52:124–130
8. Ahluwalia VV, Sagar GD, Singh TP, Arora N, Narayan S, Singh M (2013) MRI spectrum of CNS tuberculosis. JIACM 14:83–90
9. Harisinghani MG, McLoud TC, Shepard JA, Ko JP, Shroff MM, Mueller PR (2000) Tuberculosis from head to toe. Radiographics 20:449–470
10. Bhalla AS, Goyal A, Guleria R, Gupta AK (2015) Chest tuberculosis: Radiological review and imaging recommendations. Indian J Radiol Imaging 25:213–225
11. Raviglioni MC, Snider DE, Kochi A (1995) Global epidemiology of tuberculosis: morbidity and mortality of a worldwide epidemic. JAMA 273:220–226
12. Andronikou S, Wilmshurst J, Hatherill M, VanToorn R (2006) Distribution of brain infarction in children with tuberculous meningitis and correlation with outcome score at 6 months. Pediatr Radiol 36:1289–1294
13. Dastur D, Manghani D, Udani PM (1995) Pathology and pathogenetic mechanisms in neurotuberculosis. Radiol Clin North Am 33:733–750
14. Andronikou S, Smith B, Hatherhill M, Douis H, Wilmshurst J (2004) Definitive neuroradiological diagnostic features of tuberculous meningitis in children. Pediatr Radiol 34:876–885
15. Uysal G, Köse G, Güven A, Diren B (2001) Magnetic resonance imaging in diagnosis of childhood central nervous system tuberculosis. Infection 29:148–153
16. Arbeláez A, Medina E, Restrepo F, Castillo M (2004) Cerebral tuberculosis. Semin Roentgenol 39:474–481
17. Jinkins JR, Gupta R, Chang KH, Rodriguez-Carbajal J (1995) MR imaging of central nervous system tuberculosis. Radiol Clin North Am 33:771–786
18. Morgado C, Ruivo N (2005) Imaging meningo-encephalic tuberculosis. Eur J Radiol 55:188–192
19. Shah GV (2000) Central nervous system tuberculosis: imaging manifestations. Neuroimaging Clin N Am 10:355–374
20. Parmar H, Sitoh YY, Anand P, Chua V, Hui F (2006) Contrast-enhanced FLAIR imaging in the evaluation of infectious leptomeningeal diseases. Eur J Radiol 58:89–95
21. Dastur DK, Lalitha VS, Udani PM, Parekh U (1970) The brain and meninges in tuberculous meningitis - gross pathology in 100 cases and pathogenesis. Neurology 18:86–100
22. Whiteman ML (1997) Neuroimaging of central nervous system tuberculosis in HIV-infected patients. Neuroimaging Clin N Am 7:199–214
23. Rath TJ, Hughes M, Arabi M, Shah GV (2012) Imaging of cerebritis, encephalitis, and brain abscess. Neuroimaging Clin N Am 22:585–607
24. Sharma P, Garg RK, Verma R, Singh MK, Shukla R (2011) Incidence, predictors and prognostic value of cranial nerve involvement in patients with tuberculous meningitis: a retrospective evaluation. Eur J Intern Med 22:289–295
25. Garg RK (1999) Tuberculosis of central nervous system. Postgrad Med J 75:133–140
26. Trivedi R, Saksena S, Gupta RK (2009) Magnetic resonance imaging in central nervous system tuberculosis. Indian J Radiol Imaging 19:256–265
27. Gupta RK, Husain N, Kathuria MK, Datta S, Rathore RK, Husain M (2001) Magnetization transfer MR imaging correlation with histopathology in intracranial tuberculomas. Clin Radiol 56:656–663
28. Saxena S, Prakash M, Kumar S, Gupta RK (2005) Comparative evaluation of magnetization transfer contrast and fluid attenuated inversion recovery sequences in brain tuberculoma. Clin Radiol 60:787–793
29. Gupta RK, Kathuria MK, Pradhan S (1999) Magnetization transfer MR imaging in CNS tuberculosis. AJNR Am J Neuroradiol 20:867–875
30. Gupta R (2002) Magnetization transfer MR imaging in central nervous system infections. Indian J Radiol Imaging 12:51–58
31. Gupta RK, Vatsal DK, Husain N, Chawla S, Prasad KN, Roy R, Kumar R, Jha D, Husain M (2001) Differentiation of tuberculous from pyogenic brain abscesses with in vivo proton MR spectroscopy and magnetization transfer MR imaging. AJNR Am J Neuroradiol 22:1503–1509
32. Kim TK, Chang KH, Kim CJ, Goo JM, Kook MC, Han MH (1995) Intracranial tuberculoma: comparison of MR with pathologic findings. AJNR Am J Neuroradiol 16:1903–1908
33. Ku BD, Yoo SD (2009) Extensive meningeal and prenchymal calcified tuberculoma as long-term residual sequelae of tuberculous meningitis. Neurol India 57:521–522

34. Afghani B, Lieberman JM (1994) Paradoxical enlargement or development of intracranial tuberculomas during therapy: case report and review. Clin Infect Dis 19:1092–1099
35. Neumann R, Pohanka P, Prunyi E (1963) Intracranial calcification following tuberculous meningitis in children. Acta Radiol 18:487–492
36. Krishnan N, Robertson BD, Thwaites G (2010) The mechanisms and consequences of the extrapulmonary dissemination of *Mycobacterium tuberculosis*. Tuberculosis 90:361–366
37. Udani PM, Dastur DK (1970) Tuberculous encephalopathy with and without meningitis clinical features and pathological correlations. J Neurol Sci 10:541–561
38. Singh P, Paliwal VK, Neyaz Z, Srivastava AK, Verma R, Mohan S (2014) Clinical and magnetic resonance imaging characteristics of tubercular ventriculitis: an under-recognized complication of tubercular meningitis. J Neurol Sci 342:137–140
39. Kumar S, Kumar R, Radotra BD, Singh M (2014) Tubercular ventriculitis: an uncommon entity. Indian J Pediatr 81:608–610

14 Surgical Therapy

Ali Akhaddar

Contents

A. Akhaddar, MD, IFAANS
Department of Neurosurgery, Avicenne Military Hospital of Marrakech, Mohammed V University in Rabat, Rabat, Morocco
e-mail: akhaddar@hotmail.fr

Abbreviations

AFB	Acid-fast bacilli
Anti-TB	Antituberculous
CNS	Central nervous system
CSF	Cerebrospinal fluid
CT	Computed tomography
HIV	Human immunodeficiency virus
IICP	Increased intracranial pressure
MRI	Magnetic resonance imaging
Neuro-TB	Neurotuberculosis
SAH	Subarachnoid hemorrhage
TB	Tuberculosis
TBA	Tuberculous brain abscess
TBM	Tuberculous meningitis

14.1 Introduction

Tuberculosis (TB) is one of the few infectious diseases that have resisted eradication despite the improvement of valuable anti-TB drugs. Prior to any successful treatment, initial diagnosis of craniocerebral TB should be suspected and confirmed early. The correct diagnosis can generally be recognized based on the patient's comorbidities, the neurologic status, the duration of disease before diagnosis was established, the potential primary source of infection, biologic and imaging results, and more pertinent the microbiologic or histologic confirmation. While the main tools in the treatment of central nervous system (CNS)

M. Turgut et al. (eds.), *Tuberculosis of the Central Nervous System*,
DOI 10.1007/978-3-319-50712-5_14

TB are chemotherapeutic drugs, their correct selection and dosage, the indication for adjunctive surgical therapy, and the radiological follow-up monitoring may go over the scope of a single specialist. So, the need for interdisciplinary and cooperative management of patients with neurotuberculosis (neuro-TB) has been recognized. The part of surgery in the treatment of craniocerebral TB has declined clearly with the advent of successful anti-TB chemotherapy. However, neurosurgeons are still applied in the management of many presentations with this complex and potentially devastating disease.

The indications and performance of surgery for different varieties of cranial and intracranial TB are presented in this chapter. It deals comprehensively with the modern techniques concerned in the surgical strategy of brain parenchymal lesions. A part of the chapter is dedicated to the indications and procedures of surgical treatment of cranial bone TB. At the end of this chapter, there is a presentation of surgical management of TB of CNS with cerebrovascular involvement.

14.2 Surgical Therapy for Brain Tuberculoma

Tuberculoma is the second most common complications of neuro-TB [1–3]. The presentations of intracranial tuberculomas are highly variable, including brain tuberculomas, miliary tuberculomas, and tuberculoma en plaque among others. Different pathological changes probably depend on the type and virulence of *Mycobacterium tuberculosis* and on the host immune response to the infection. Brain tuberculomas can be single or multiple, with or without coexisting meningitis. They can occur in any part of the brain, mainly in the posterior fossa in children and supratentorial compartment in adults. Miliary tuberculomas may be a component of generalized pathological process, with primary focus located in the lung or elsewhere in the body [1, 2] (Fig. 14.1). These lesions are small (less than 5 mm), located at cortico-subcortical junction of the brain parenchyma in the distribution of perforating vessels [4] (Fig. 14.2). Tuberculomas may mimic "en plaque meningiomas" with dural-based, mass-forming localized meningeal process. They are usually found along the frontal convexity, interhemispheric fissures, tentorium, and in the posterior fossa [5–7] (Fig. 14.3).

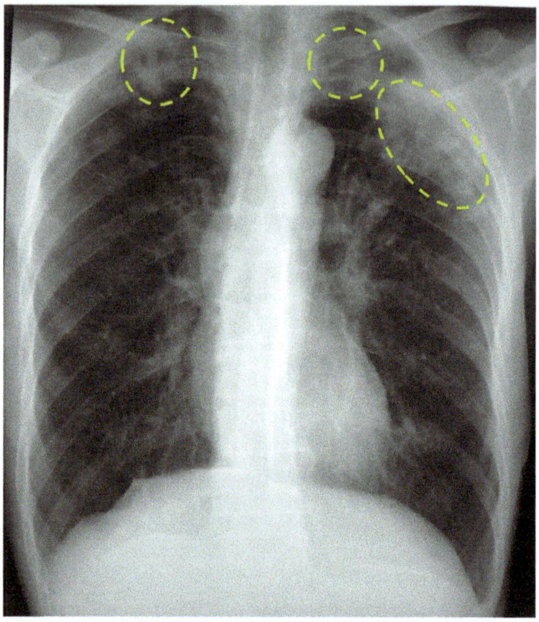

Fig. 14.1 Chest radiography findings of pulmonary tuberculosis (TB) in a patient with brain tuberculoma (bilateral *upper* lobe TB lesions)

Treatment of TB of CNS is primarily medical: all confirmed intracranial tuberculomas should be treated with anti-TB drugs. Neurosurgical intervention may be required for treatment of mass lesions, no success of medical therapy, management of increased intracranial pressure (IICP), and for CSF diversion in cases of hydrocephalus.

For many authors, each patient's care should be individualized and adapted to the particular characteristics of the patient and the brain tuberculomas [1–3, 8–10]. Undoubtedly the location, the size of tuberculoma, and the confirmation of TB through other diagnostic studies have to be taken into consideration when planning therapy for presumed intracranial tuberculoma. Single brain tuberculomas causing midline shift and IICP, and do not succeed to respond to anti-TB therapy, must

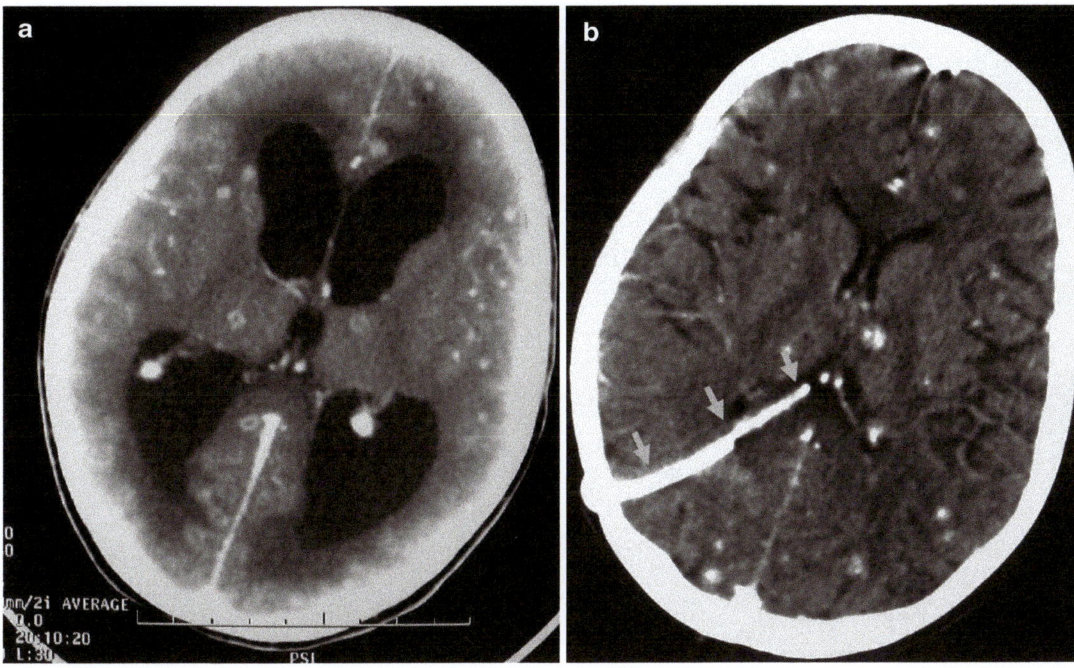

Fig. 14.2 Axial cranial CT scan with contrast administration before (**a**) and after (**b**) ventricular shunting for a communicating hydrocephalus with miliary brain tuberculoma and meningitis (Note the shunt placement inside the *right* brain's lateral ventricle (*arrows*))

be removed surgically. In this optic, tuberculoma requires complete excision. Sometimes the lesions are relatively hard and it is usually not easy to cut them. Open surgical resection has some inconvenience, especially when located in critical structures, since surgery itself may cause unexpected extensive damage to the contiguous viable parenchyma in an already edematous tissue [3].

Occasionally, surgical excision is performed for a brain mass which on imaging is diagnosed as a different tumoral or infectious entity, and an unsuspected tuberculoma is encountered (Figs. 14.4, 14.5, and 14.6). Indeed, many patients were misdiagnosed as a brain parenchyma tumor and underwent a surgical biopsy, with or without total removal of the lesions. The diagnosis of "tuberculoma" was made after surgery on histopathologic studies [11–17]. Neuro-TB should be considered in the differential diagnosis of cerebral tumors and other granulomatous lesions, especially in endemic regions, and mainly if the patient has a history of previous TB.

Rarely, decompressive craniectomy may be proposed to save life in some patients with multiple tuberculomas, important brain edema, or potentially uncontrollable IICPs. This surgical technique involves the removal of a large portion of the cranium (unilateral, bifrontal, or suboccipital) [3, 18]. Large cerebellar tuberculoma may cause sudden complete occlusion of cerebrospinal fluid pathways early. So, it should be completely excised via a suboccipital craniectomy or more rarely through a craniotomy (Figs. 14.7 and 14.8). For some authors, patients with optochiasmatic tuberculoma may require urgent surgical decompression when vision deteriorated rapidly even under anti-TB chemotherapy [11, 19, 20].

Surgery is not just a therapeutic choice but also allows confirmation of the diagnosis and the sampling of material for bacteriological and histopathological diagnosis. Neuroradiology-guided stereotactic surgery has established itself

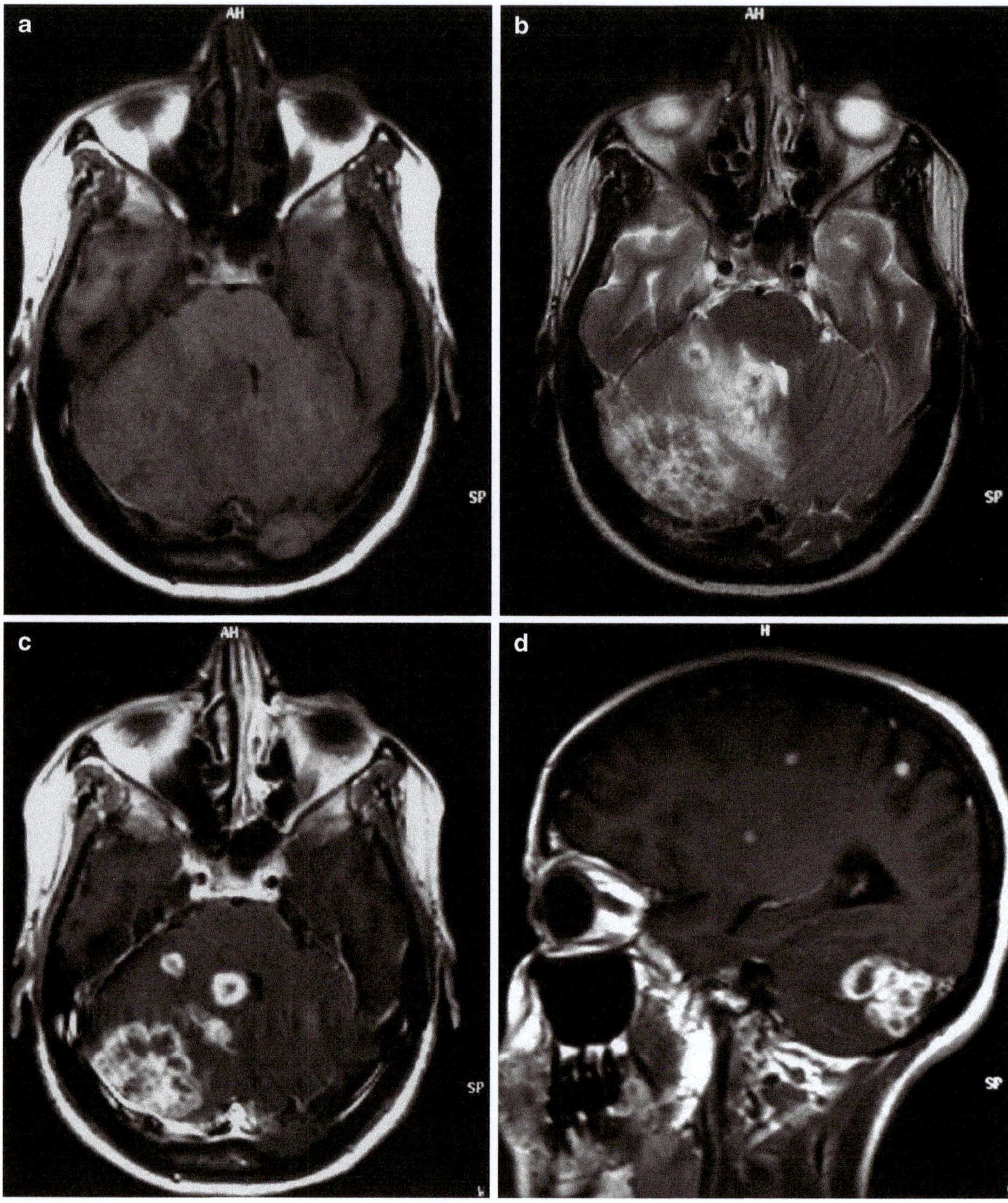

Fig. 14.3 Brain miliary tuberculoma with "tuberculomas en plaque" appearance in the posterior fossa. Axial cranial MRI on T1- (**a**) and T2-weighted image (**b**). Axial (**c**) and sagittal (**d**) MRI on T1-weighted images after gadolinium injection

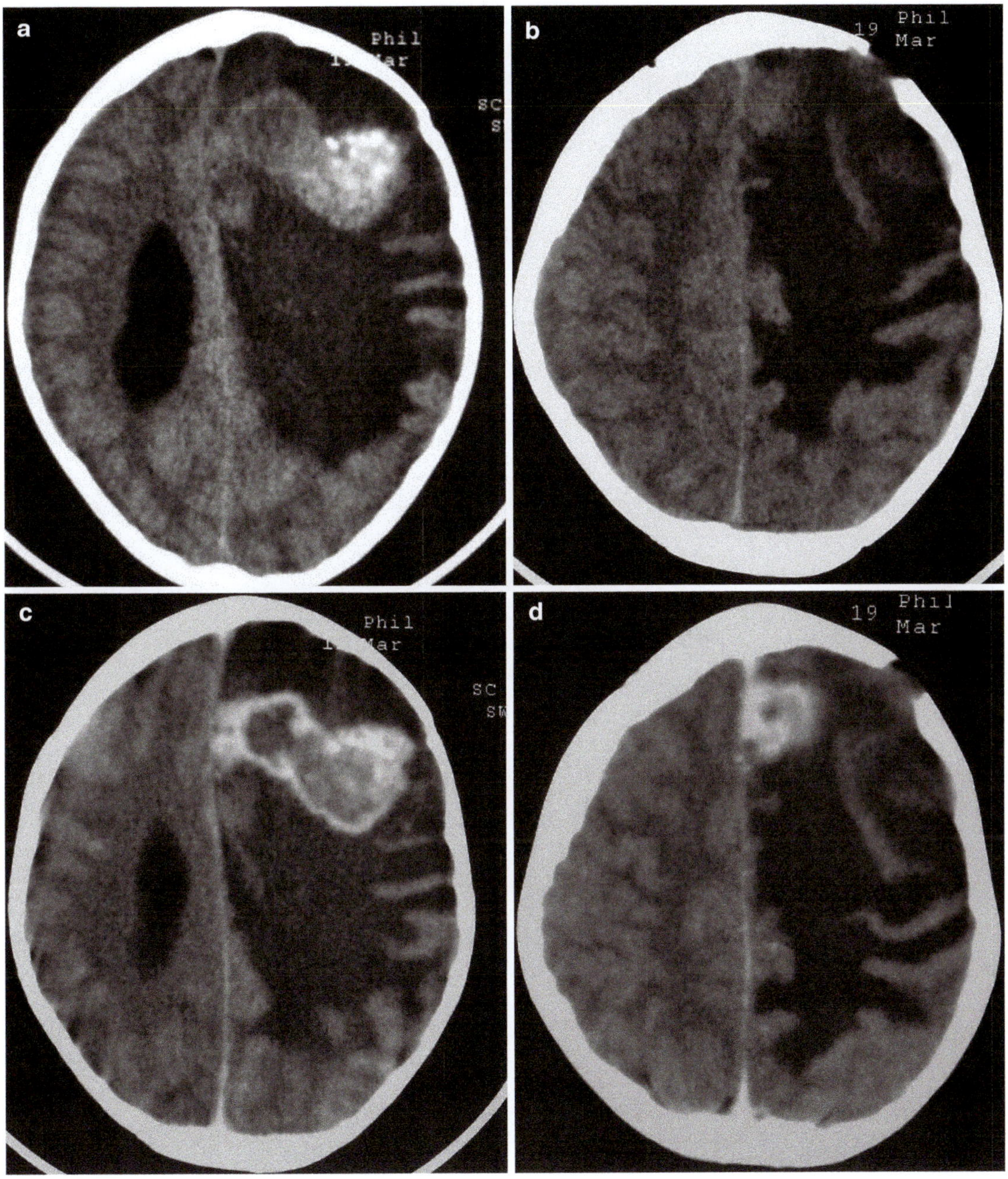

Fig. 14.4 Large calcified brain tuberculoma in the *left* frontoparietal area with important perilesional edema and significant mass effect (case n°1). Axial cranial CT scan before (**a**, **b**) and after contrast injection (**c**, **d**)

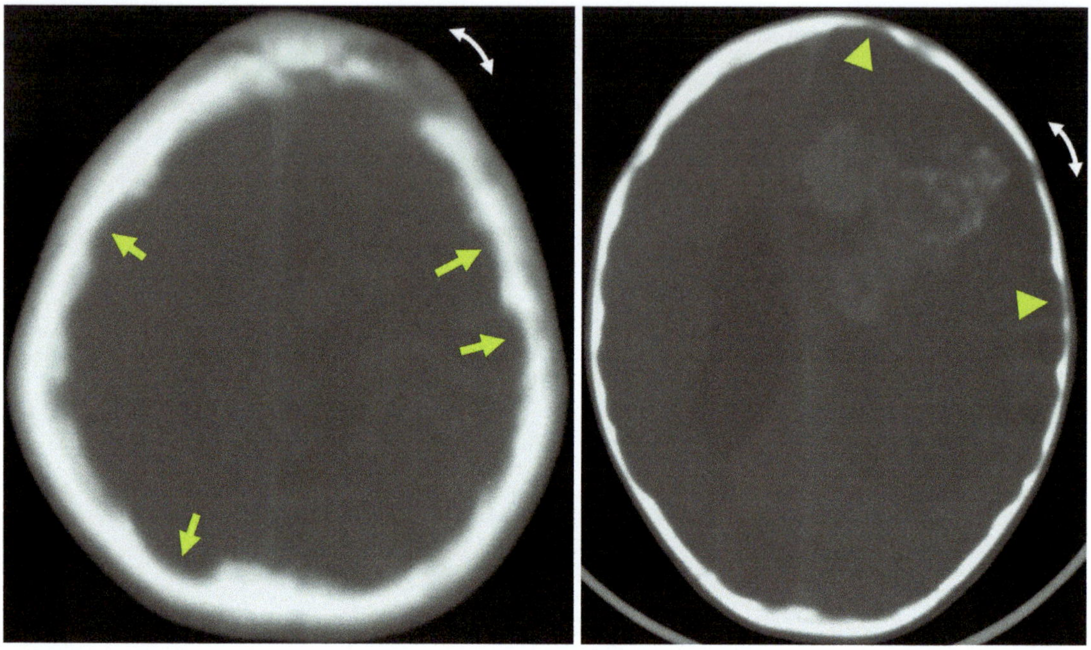

Fig. 14.5 Axial cranial CT scan on bone windows with signs of increased intracranial pressure: prominent impressions on the inner table of the skull (beaten copper appearance) (*arrows*) associated with disjunction of the coronal suture (*double arrows*) (case n°1)

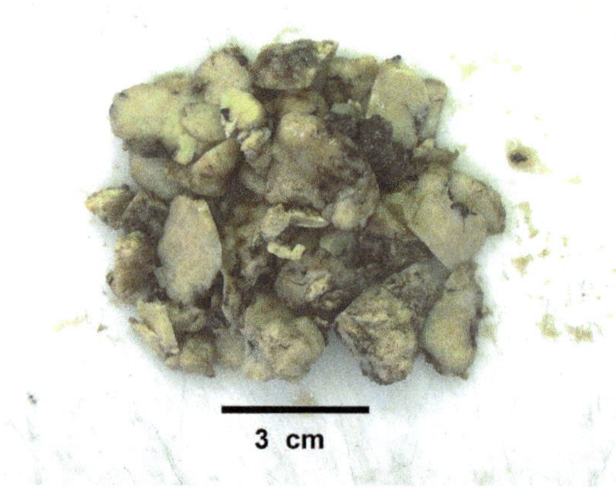

Fig. 14.6 Macroscopic appearance of the brain tuberculoma: *yellowish*, firm, and relatively avascular mass (case n°1)

as a safe and consistent technique in obtaining histological diagnosis of intracranial lesions under local anesthesia [8, 21, 22] (Figs. 14.9, 14.10, and 14.11). Also stereotactic procedure may be performed for surgical localization (pre-planning), especially when brain tuberculomas are deep seated, small, and situated in the eloquent areas of the brain [9]. Small, superficial lesions are best excised because of stereotactic biopsy being technically difficult and potentially hemorrhagic due to bleeding from superficial cortical vessels. Transsphenoidal biopsy may be used with a suspected sellar tuberculoma; however, CSF fistula should be avoided [10].

Proof of TB origin is by either a positive culture of the specimen for *M. tuberculosis*, demonstration of acid-fast bacilli (AFB), or histopathologic evidence of TB granulomas. Newer genomic techniques like polymerase chain reaction (PCR) for *M. tuberculosis* can provide valuable tool for diagnosis of TB particularly from paucibacillary specimens as tuberculoma [23].

Hydrocephalus in patients with TB of CNS is most frequently "communicating" rather than "obstructive" [24, 25]. Classical features of

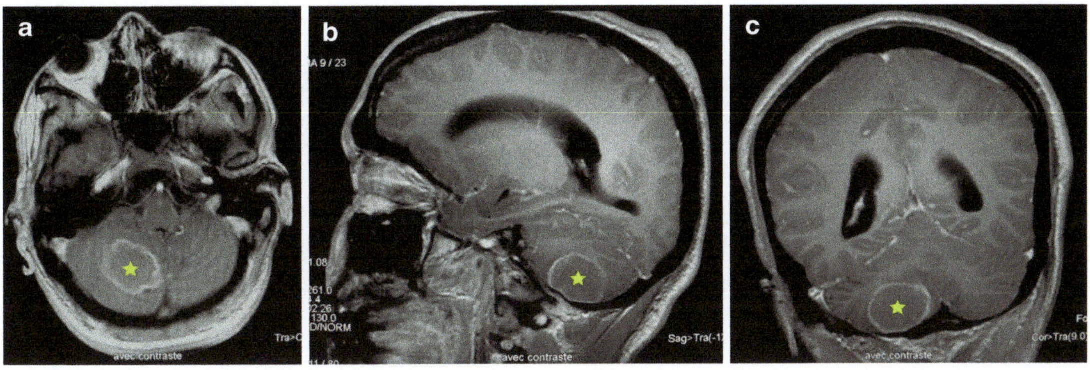

Fig. 14.7 Axial (**a**), sagittal (**b**), and coronal (**c**) T1-weighted MRI after gadolinium injection revealing a cerebellar tuberculoma (*star*) in the right side (case n°2)

tuberculous meningitis (TBM) are thick enhancing basal exudates, associated tuberculomas, and infarcts in addition to the presence of hydrocephalus (Figs. 14.2 and 14.12). For patients with acute obstructive hydrocephalus or with large cerebellar tuberculoma, urgent CSF diversion with an external ventricular drain is mandatory in life-threatening conditions or as a salvage method. The CSF drainage will be either progressively withdrawn over time and removed or changed by a definitive shunt afterward. Persistent hydrocephalus is treated with an internal shunting system (Fig. 14.13). Shunts may need replacement due to obstruction by high proteinorrachia. Although there was an initial apprehension of propagating the disease via a ventriculoperitoneal shunt with the risk of a TB peritonitis, this has not been described to date in any patient under anti-TB therapy [3]. In cases of communicating hydrocephalus, the surgical plan is more complex: please refer to Chaps. 29 and 30 about shunt surgery and endoscopic third ventriculostomy in TBM with hydrocephalus. Unfortunately, complications of shunt surgery are higher in patients with TBM than in patients with other conditions. Common complications include shunt obstruction, shunt infections, abdominal pseudocysts, and erosion of the skin over the shunt components [26, 27]. Relating to the operating theater, no special measures are needed when patients with neuro-TB are operated on [3].

Although prescription of corticosteroids in brain tuberculomas is controversial, steroids may be useful in patients with IICP, significant brain edema with mass effect/midline shift, compromised mental or neurological condition, and potentially life-threatening situations such as brain herniation [2]. Besides surgical procedures, anti-TB drugs, and corticosteroids, many other adjunctive therapies may be required. These concomitant therapies differ with site and severity of the disease and may include:

- Intubation and mechanical ventilation.
- Corrections of electrolyte imbalances.
- Proper nutrition against anorexia and malnutrition.
- Management of comorbidities and other underlying medical problems.
- Identification and treatment of any other source of infection.
- Anticonvulsants, anticoagulations, analgesics, and antipyretics.
- Functional rehabilitation may be needed in the aftercare of the patient.

Immunocompetent patients with single noncomplicated brain tuberculoma have a good outcome [2]. Seizures most often resolve after successful treatment of the underlying TB of CNS [28]. Residual deficits are not rare. Patients with poor general health, those with drug

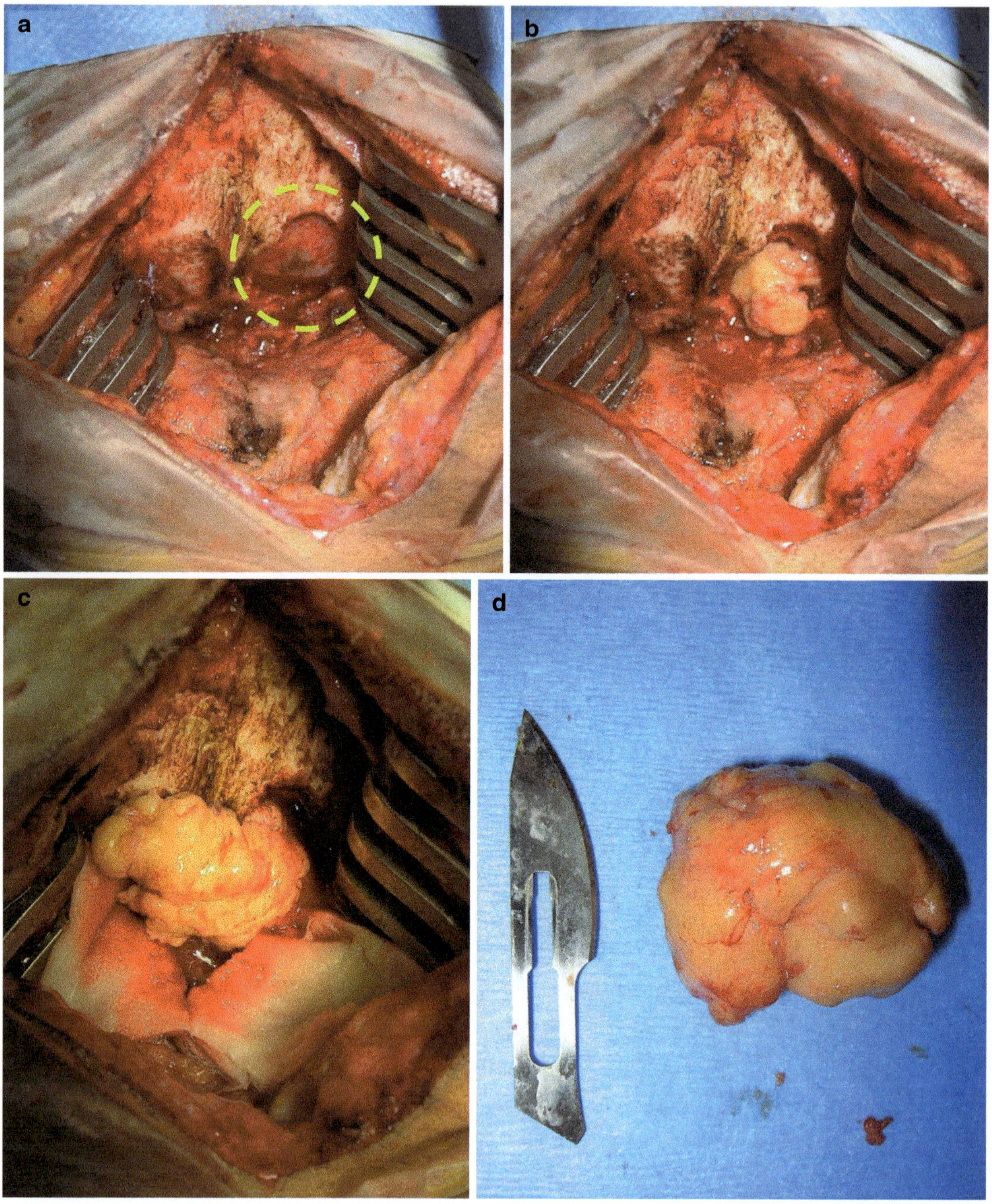

Fig. 14.8 Operative views in the same patient (case n°2). *Right* side, suboccipital craniectomy (**a**) and total excision of the cerebellar tuberculoma (**b**, **c**). Macroscopic appearance of the completely removed granulomatous mass (**d**)

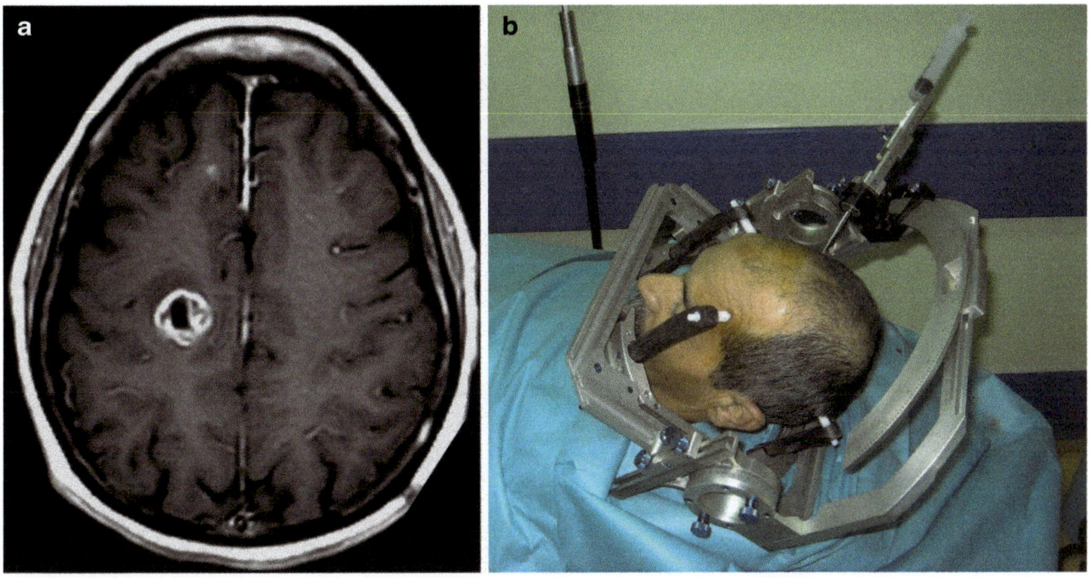

Fig. 14.9 Axial cranial T1-weighted MRI following gadolinium administration revealing a Rolandic tuberculoma in the *right* side (**a**). Stereotacic-guided brain biopsy of the lesion in the same patient (Radionics* CRW* frame) (**b**)

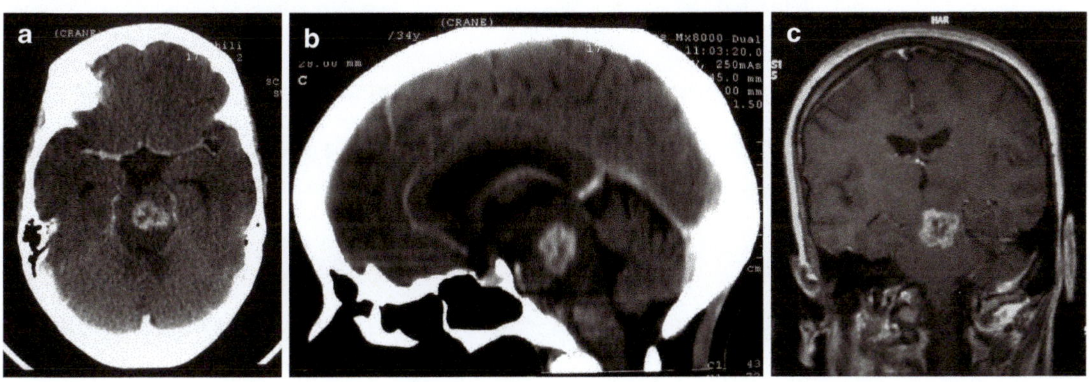

Fig. 14.10 Brainstem (pontomesencephalic) tuberculoma (case n°3). Axial (**a**) and sagittal reconstructions (**b**) CT scan after contrast administration and coronal cranial T1-weighted MRI after gadolinium injection (**c**)

resistance TB, and those with immunodeficiency disorders have a poor prognosis [2, 3, 29].

14.3 Surgical Therapy for Tuberculous Brain Abscess

Tuberculous brain abscess (TBA) is a rare form of TB of CNS distinct from tuberculoma [30, 31]. According to Whitener's criteria of 1978 [32], TBA is characterized by verification of pus formation within brain parenchyma, vascular granulation tissue containing acute and chronic inflammatory cells without epitheloid granuloma, or the presence of AFB or *M. tuberculosis* growth on culture. Liquefied tuberculoma can lead to the formation of central purulent material without evidence of AFB. These also mimic a tuberculous abscess on CT scan and MRI studies but can only be distinguished at histopathologic study [33]. Abscesses are usually single and larger, have greater mass effect and edema, and grow more rapidly than the tuberculomas. Before the

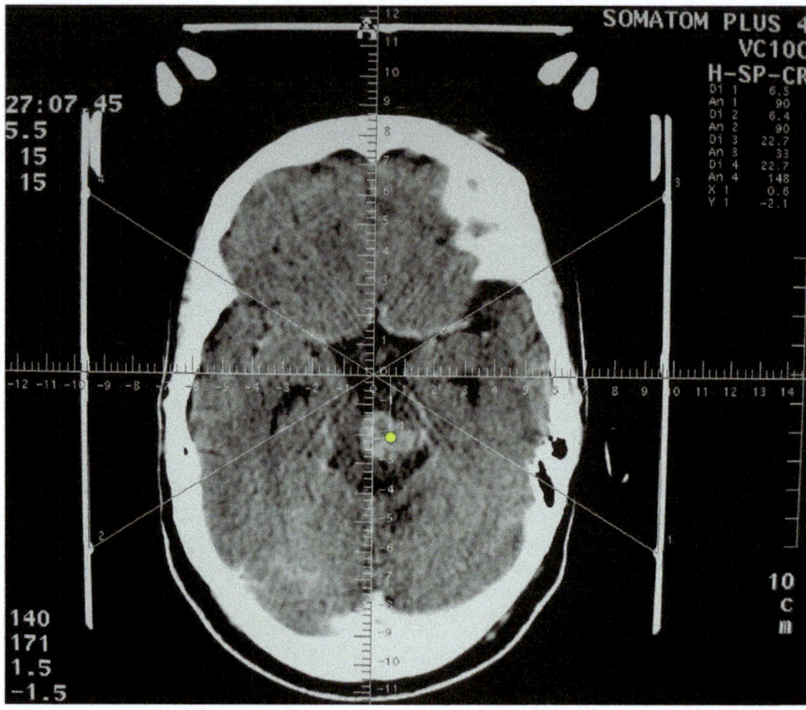

Fig. 14.11 Axial cranial CT scan with contrast injection during preplanning procedure of stereotactic-guided brainstem biopsy in the same patient (Leksell* frame) (case n°3)

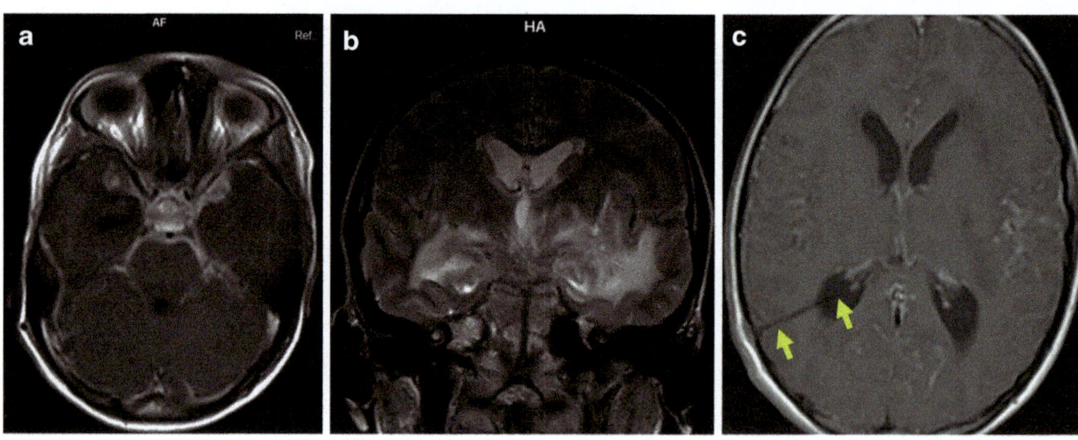

Fig. 14.12 Brain MRI on axial enhanced- T1-weighted image (**a**) and coronal T2-weighted image (**b**) of a patient with meningoencephalitis (Note the prominent exudates involving the basal meninges and the extensive brain edema). He was also operated on for a communicating hydrocephalus. Axial T1-weighted image (**c**) showing a *right* lateral ventricular shunting [*arrows*]

introduction of antibiotics, most TBAs were found at autopsy in patients who died of meningitis, TB, or generalized sepsis [32]. Today, TBA is still a diagnostic challenge especially in the absence of concomitant extracranial disease. Epidemiologically, more than two-thirds of patients with TBAs had a previous history of tuberculosis, and many are receiving anti-TB therapy when the abscess is diagnosed [34, 35]. Indeed, TBAs will occur or paradoxically increase during continuation of anti-TB chemotherapy for pulmonary or TB of CNS [30, 36–38]. On neuroimaging studies, TBA is often indistinguishable from other infectious, parasitic, neoplastic, or

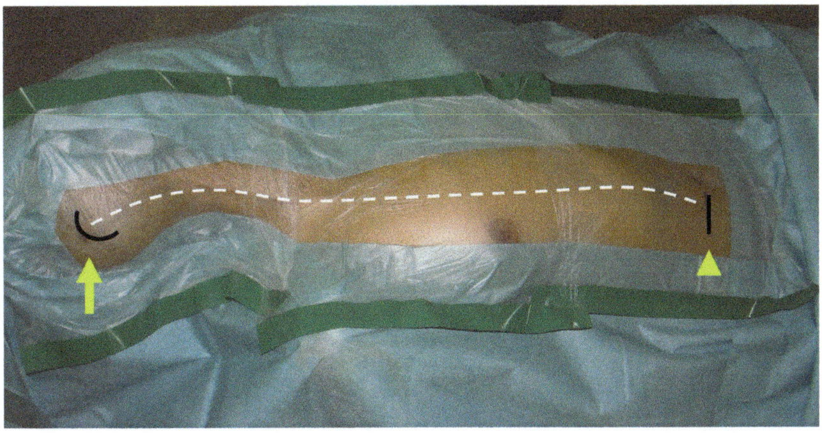

Fig. 14.13 View of the operative field for a ventriculoperitoneal shunting procedure. The surgeon will make a small incision behind the *right* ear [*arrow*] and drill a small hole in the skull. One catheter is threaded into the brain through this opening, and another is placed under the skin behind the ear. This tube is snaked down to the chest and abdomen; this allows excess CSF to drain away into the abdominal cavity (via a small paraumbilical incision [*arrowhead*]) where the body absorbs it

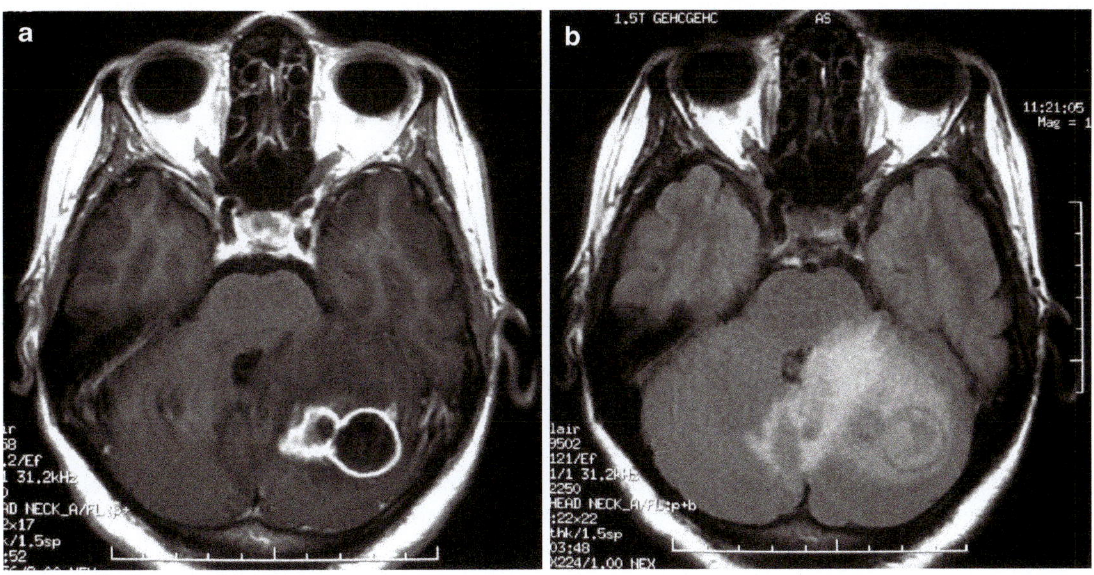

Fig. 14.14 TB cerebellar abscess in the *left* side with surrounded edema. Axial T1-weighted MRI following gadolinium injection (**a**) and on FLAIR sequence (**b**)

cystic lesions [39, 40] (Fig. 14.14). Unlike pyogenic bacterial infections, microbiologic sensitivity testing for TBA is difficult, as the mycobacterial cultures may take weeks to become positive. Although it is benign and curable, a delayed diagnosis and treatment may lead to considerable morbidity and mortality especially in immunocompromised hosts [38, 41–43].

The most important indications for surgery in a patient with a TBA on imaging explorations are (a) to reduce intracranial pressure, (b) to obtain a definitive diagnosis, (c) to diminish the size of the abscess collection, and (d) to eradicate the pathogen agent if possible. Anyway, anti-TB therapy remains the mainstay of treatment.

Clinical status of the patient, neuroimaging appearance of the abscess, and the effectiveness of medical therapy help in the surgical treatment planning. In general, neurosurgical indications for TBA do not differ significantly from those of other infectious pathogens. All intraparenchymatous brain abscesses bigger than 2 cm must be aspired [44, 45]. Urgent surgical procedure should be performed with considerable mass effect, obstructive hydrocephalus, edema, IICP, progressive focal neurological deficit, or clinical worsening during conservative management. Posterior fossa abscesses often necessitate urgent surgery due to the important possibility of brain herniation [46, 47] (Fig. 15.4). In addition, juxtaventricular abscess presents the risk of intraventricular rupture.

The main methods for surgical management of brain abscesses are freehand or endoscope-assisted aspiration of the purulent material with or without stereotactic neuroimaging guidance, drainage by craniotomy or craniectomy with/without intraoperative ultrasound guidance, or complete removal of the abscess collection [21, 22, 45, 48]. The choice of the best procedure is not easy. Each surgical method has its distinct advantages and indications. Although craniotomy with surgical excision was the main treatment used for many years, needle aspiration has gradually substituted this technique, thinning the aggressiveness of surgical approaches. As mentioned above, this enhanced management has been possible, thanks to the advances of neuroimaging technology and stereotactic techniques which allow the accurate puncture of these lesions through burr holes with minimum brain damage.

Stereotactic-guided approaches optimize the selection of the trajectory and needle placement for pus aspiration. This technique is preferred in eloquent or deep-seated location (thalamus, basal ganglia, or brainstem areas) [8, 22]. This is also the ideal procedure in patients with poor clinical status as the biopsy can be done under local anesthesia. The introduction and improvement of frameless stereotactic systems have partly simplified this procedure. Now, neuronavigation is widely used for brain abscess drainage. The most disadvantage of stereotactic aspiration is the need for repeated procedures (because incomplete evacuation of thick purulent material), surgical bleeding into the abscess cavity [21], and CSF leakage.

Whereas open surgical excision is an appropriate alternative for large, multiloculated, cerebellar abscesses and in those that do not respond to aspiration or to medical anti-TB therapy alone [44]. Worsening of neurological deficits, cognitive and learning impairment in children, and seizures have been described in some cases following surgical excision. However, for many authors, craniotomy and surgical excision (when possible) still have better results for TBAs because they have a lower frequency of recurrence, shorter hospitalization, and overall lesser cost of treatment [34, 37]. In this context, monobloc removal (in one piece) of the abscess is the ideal method to avoid the spillage of purulent content in the operative field and the reinfection of injury surrounding brain parenchyma.

Great care should be taken at the time of surgery not to inoculate the ventricular system with purulent material. Regarding bone flap, it may be replaced at the end of operative time if not grossly infected [45]. For some authors, early anti-TB chemotherapy should be well respected in all cases of suspected TBAs even before surgery, in order to reduce the risk of postoperative TBM [34, 49].

All pus sample should be sent for bacteriologic (both aerobic and anaerobic, specific and non-specific), mycologic, parasitologic, and histopathologic studies. Surgically excised and pathologically evaluated specimens remain the gold standard for diagnosing TBAs [37]; however a second concomitant pathogen may be associated and should always be taken into consideration [47, 50, 51]. As mentioned previously, CSF diversion is mandatory in the presence of obstructive or persistent hydrocephalus. Supportive therapy measures should also be taken into consideration.

There is still some controversy regarding the best surgical approach for other intracranial purulent collections. Surgical management is indicated in almost all cases of subdural empyema for cerebral decompression, drainage of purulent content, and identification of the causative pathogens. Interventions include burr hole drainage, stereotactic drainage for deep-seated parafalcine or tentorial empyemas, and large craniotomy for irrigation, debridement, and drainage. Although good results have been reported via burr hole drainage, many authors prefer to achieve a generous craniotomy covering as much as the affected brain surface as possible, crossing the midline when interhemispheric collections are present [52–54]. The dura matter may be not easy to open because of its friability and thickness. While observable, the pus is softly aspirated by moderate suction. Subdural collections under the craniotomy edge should be able to be drained by passing a flat dissector into the subdural space and gently depressing the brain surface by a few millimeters. The dura should be closed following draining the empyema to avoid a CSF leak. Repeat surgical procedures may be necessary if needed. Burr hole craniotomy for decompression with irrigation, debridement, and drainage is required in a majority of patients with epidural abscess [55]. However, in some cases with more solid organized granulomatous collection with/without cranial vault osteomyelitis, a large bone flap is needed [56]. A delay in surgical treatment has been related with important morbidity and mortality rates.

Finally, combination of surgical treatment with standard anti-TB regimen appears to decrease morbidity and mortality of intracranial suppurations due to TB.

14.4 Surgical Therapy for Cranial Osteomyelitis Due to Tuberculosis

Management of tuberculous cranial osteomyelitis is a challenge due to the intimate anatomical relationship of the brain and its coverings with the cranial bone and the scalp. Because tuberculous cranial osteomyelitis is somewhat unusual, it may not be widely recognized. It should be suspected in disseminated TB or in any draining lesion of the skull that is sterile or fails to respond to usual antibiotic therapy (Fig. 14.15). As mentioned above, some presentations may occur in the setting of human immunodeficiency virus (HIV) infection [57]. The part of surgery in the treatment of cranial bone TB has declined clearly with the advent of effective anti-TB drugs. For numerous authors, surgery is indicated only for diagnosis purposes, for removal of epidural collections and/or large sequestra, and for patients with discharging sinuses, intracranial

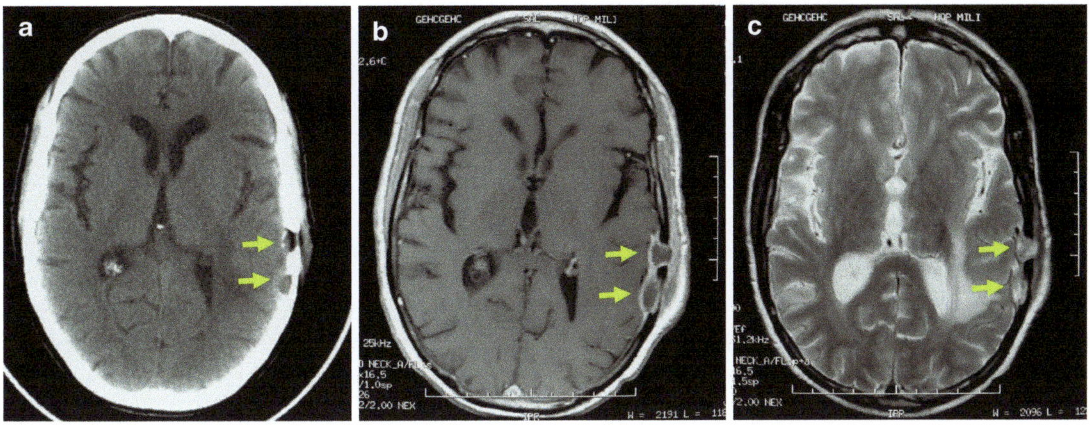

Fig. 14.15 Chronic temporoparietal tuberculous osteomyelitis. Axial cranial CT scan (**a**), T1-weighted MRI after gadolinium injection (**b**), and on T2-weighted image (**c**) showing bifocal (*arrows*) cranial bone defect (*arrows*) with mild extracranial and epidural extensions

extensions, or large collections of caseating material causing mass effect or IICP [56, 58–61]. For others, debridement of bone lesion not only offers tissue for microbiological and histopathological examinations but also facilitates in accelerated healing by allowing chemotherapeutic drugs to penetrate the infected regions [58, 62, 63].

When performed, extradural granulation tissue and osteolytic lesion should be removed till normal bone is encountered, but dura matter should be left intact to avoid CSF fluid contamination. It is important to collect as much material as possible from fluid, granulomatous lesions, purulent substance, and tissue specimens [64]. The possibility of polymicrobial infections with a mixture of mycobacteria and pyogenic bacteria or fungi must be always taken in consideration [58, 60, 65]. One of our patients had a temporal cranial vault osteitis with brain extension involving *Serratia liquefaciens* and *M. tuberculosis* at the same time [50]. Discharging sinuses should also be excised and the scalp closed [66]. The quality and integrity of extracranial soft tissue must be evaluated for postoperative wound closure and the necessity of flap coverage [60]. If necessary, cranial bone defect (cranioplasty) may be closed following a minimum of 6 months after the healing of the infectious process [64]. It is also important to consider TB in post-craniotomy bone flap osteomyelitis (surgical site infections). Two cases were previously described: following craniotomy for a glioma [67] and secondary to evacuation of an acute subdural hemorrhage [68]. Although unusual, attention should be paid to the possible occurrence of TB cranial osteomyelitis following a traumatic head injury [69–71].

Superficial extracranial infection with mild osteomyelitis of the skull can be treated with anti-TB drugs alone. However, all patients should be followed vigilantly and reevaluated if there is evidence of clinical and/or paraclinical worsening, and if necessary surgical intervention must be performed. Sometimes, simple percutaneous drainage and limited scalp incision are sufficient to drain small superficial abscess and to collect specimens for bacteriologic and histopathologic examinations. In some superficial limited infection, fine needle aspiration cytology was able to diagnose TB infection without using surgical debridement [60].

In the skull base, surgical debridement is often not suggested because of the elevated risk of complication [64, 72]. The danger of incontrollable bleeding and injury to the brainstem or important cranial nerves is important. However, surgery can be limited to biopsy, drainage of large abscesses, debridement of extracranial soft tissue, and removal of osseous sequestrum if possible [58, 73, 74].

Prognosis of TB cranial osteomyelitis depends on the general health status, the extension of local lesion, the early confirmation of diagnosis, and the response to treatment. Regular follow-up (clinical, biological, and on neuroimaging study) is necessary for an entire cure. When infection remains or progresses even with anti-TB regimen or when it recurs, reoperation may be indispensable [58]. Overall, the prognosis is usually favorable.

14.5 Surgical Therapy for Cerebrovascular Manifestations of Tuberculosis

Cerebrovascular manifestations of neuro-TB are common in the medical literature and may represent its most serious complication with significant morbidity and mortality [75–83]. These conditions may cause cerebral infarcts and rarely hemorrhages [84–93]. From the neuropathologic point of view, vascular damages are related to variable lesions such as infiltrative, necrotizing (small branches), and proliferative changes (larger branches) [12, 94]. More rarely, venous thrombosis and mycotic aneurysms with or without rupture may occur [70, 95–100]. In some patients, the severity of the neurological presentation makes impossible to recognize a specific stroke syndrome, and cerebrovascular complications are only identified on autopsy [77, 101, 102]. Surgical intervention may be discussed in some situations.

Intracranial aneurysms related to TB of CNS are rare, representing about 1% of all infectious intracranial aneurysms [103]. In reviewing the literature, we found reports of only six cases since 2000 [77, 92, 96, 97, 99, 104]. Three recognized sources of tubercular intracranial aneurysmal formation were previously suggested [92]: endovascular spread or intravascular source [78], hematogenous extension with autoimmune response to TB [87], and direct extravascular infection [87, 92, 97]. Classically, patient who presents a mycotic aneurysm must be placed on appropriate antibiotics that realize therapeutic levels in the CNS, inspite of whether the patient is to undergo surgical therapy. Patients with ruptured infectious aneurysm and intracranial bleeding should be considered for surgical removal if they have a peripheral aneurysm without important anesthetic risk. A more conservative approach was suggested in patients with proximal aneurysms, because these aneurysms are not easy to clip in the acute period. For unruptured lesions, surgery must be performed only if the aneurysm enlarges. We must take in mind that because of the friable nature of mycotic aneurysms, clip ligation cannot always be achievable. In this case wrapping the aneurysm dome is a surgical alternative, as is trapping the parent artery [103]. Delayed surgical therapy may reduce the danger of perioperative rupture and permit the aneurysm to mature from a friable acute lesion to a more fibrotic chronic lesion [105].

Although these recommendations are relatively reasonable, one cannot be dogmatic about managing patients with this rare complication. In 2000, a 9-year-old boy presented with an intraventricular bleeding due to a ruptured posterior inferior cerebellar artery infectious aneurysm. He had been diagnosed as having miliary TB and TBM and had been treated with chemotherapy and ventriculoperitoneal shunting 7 months previously. The aneurysm was successfully treated by craniotomy and clipping [96]. Manka et al. presented a young woman with acute intracerebral hemorrhage secondary to a ruptured septic arteria cerebri media aneurysm. She had also miliary lung TB. Surgery was not performed, and the patient was treated only by anti-TB regimen with acceptable minor neurologic symptoms after cessation of the treatment [104]. Roh et al. reported the case of a 76-year-old woman who had two saccular aneurysms arising from the right distal internal carotid artery and proximal middle cerebral artery complicated by subarachnoid hemorrhage (SAH) with concomitant TBM [92]. The aneurysms were treated conservatively and the patient's condition was last reported to be stable [92]. Another young woman presented with a subcortical tuberculoma of the left parietal lobe with adjacent multiple small inflammatory unruptured aneurysms in the distal middle cerebral arteries. The tuberculoma was totally removed, and the aneurysms were secured by wrapping and fibrin tissue adhesive with a good outcome [97]. The sophistication and usefulness of endovascular options for aneurysm treatment have increased in the past three decades. Saraf and Limaye presented an atypical case of intracranial tuberculomas complicated by intralesional bleeding secondary to a mycotic TB aneurysm managed successfully by endovascular treatment [99].

In some cases, surgery may also be performed to prevent cerebral ischemia after TBM [76, 106]. Misch et al. presented a 5-year-old girl with recurring ischemic episodes in the left middle cerebral artery territory that were refractory to repetitive endovascular procedures [106]. For this patient an extracranial-intracranial bypass surgical procedure was successfully performed with a favorable outcome [106].

In patients who develop clinical and radiological signs of impending brain herniation including hemispheric infarction, ischemic swelling, SAH, and spontaneous intracerebral hemorrhage, early neurosurgical consultation is recommended. In some selected cases, decompressive craniectomy may be proposed. As seen above, this surgical technique involves the resection of a large portion of the cranium in the setting of life-threatening brain swelling or potentially unmanageable intracranial pressures.

Conclusion

Craniocerebral TB is a complex and potentially devastating infection. Since early diagnosis and initiation of medical treatment are very important in preventing morbidity and mortality, the possibility of surgery is required in some patients such as treatment of mass lesions, failure of medical therapy, management of IICP, and for CSF diversion in cases of hydrocephalus. Surgical interventions can be also diagnostic by collecting specimens of material for microbiological and histopathological studies. Close harmonization of care between infectious disease specialists and neurosurgeons is extremely important. Each patient's care must be individualized and adapted to the particular characteristics of the patient and the craniocerebral lesions. Undoubtedly the location, the type, the number, and the size of lesions, as well as the confirmation of TB through other diagnostic studies, have to be taken into consideration when planning therapy. Neuroradiology-guided stereotactic surgery has established itself as a safe and consistent technique for aspiration, localization, and biopsy of intracranial lesions under local anesthesia.

References

1. DeLance AR, Safaee M, Oh MC, Clark AJ, Kaur G, Sun MZ, Bollen AW, Phillips JJ, Parsa AT (2013) Tuberculoma of the central nervous system. J Clin Neurosci 20:1333–1341
2. Li H, Liu W, You C (2012) Central nervous system tuberculoma. J Clin Neurosci 19:691–695
3. Rajshekhar V (2015) Surgery for brain tuberculosis: a review. Acta Neurochir 157:1665–1678
4. Akhaddar A, Boucetta M (2011) Images in clinical medicine. Multiple intracranial tuberculomas. N Engl J Med 365:1527
5. Adachi K, Yoshida K, Tomita H, Niimi M, Kawase T (2004) Tuberculoma mimicking falx meningioma-case report. Neurol Med Chir (Tokyo) 44:489–492
6. Aggarwal A, Patra DP, Gupta K, Sodhi HB (2016) Dural tuberculoma mimicking meningioma: a clinicoradiologic review of dural en-plaque lesions. World Neurosurg 88:e1–e7
7. Raheja A, Kedia S, Sinha S, Nambirajan A, Sharma MC (2014) Giant extra-axial en-plaque tuberculoma with gyriform enhancement: unusual presentation of a common disease. Neurol India 62:697–699
8. Akhaddar A, Mahi M, Harket A, Elmostarchid B, Belhachemi A, Elasri A, Gazzaz M, Boucetta M (2007) Brainstem tuberculoma in a postpartum patient. J Neuroradiol 34:345–346
9. Ersahin M, Hakan T, Ayan E, Berkman Z, Ekinci O, Ceran N, Aker FV (2010) Diagnostic and therapeutic role of CT-guided stereotactic surgery in the management of intracranial tuberculomas. Turk Neurosurg 20:295–302
10. Ranjan A, Chandy MJ (1994) Intrasellar tuberculoma. Br J Neurosurg 8:179–185
11. Aversa do Souto A, Fonseca AL, Gadelha M, Donangelo I, Chimelli L, Domingues FS (2003) Optic pathways tuberculoma mimicking glioma: case report. Surg Neurol 60:349–353
12. Chatterjee S, Saini J, Kesavadas C, Arvinda HR, Jolappara M, Gupta AK (2010) Differentiation of tubercular infection and metastasis presenting as ring enhancing lesion by diffusion and perfusion magnetic resonance imaging. J Neuroradiol 37:167–171
13. Doraiswamy V, Vaswani RK, Lahiri KR, Kondekar SS (2010) Neurotoxoplasmosis mimicking intracranial tuberculoma. J Postgrad Med 56:31–34
14. Peng J, Ouyang Y, Fang WD, Luo TY, Li YM, Lv FJ, Zhang ZW, Li XY (2012) Differentiation of intracranial tuberculomas and high grade gliomas using proton MR spectroscopy and diffusion MR imaging. Eur J Radiol 81:4057–4063
15. Raheja A, Sinha S, Sable MN, Sharma MC, Sharma BS (2015) A case of giant intracranial tuberculoma in an infant: clinical and radiologic pitfalls. J Child Neurol 30:364–367
16. Shih RY, Koeller KK (2015) Bacterial, fungal, and parasitic infections of the central nervous system: radiologic-pathologic correlation and historical perspectives. Radiographics 35:1141–1169
17. Sumer S, Koktekir E, Demir NA, Akdemir G (2015) Intracranial giant tuberculoma mimicking brain tumor: a case report. Turk Neurosurg 25:337–339
18. Yamashita K, Suzuki Y, Yoshizumi H, Takahashi JB, Nogawa T (1994) Tuberculous hypertrophic pachymeningitis involving the posterior fossa and high cervical region-case report. Neurol Med Chir (Tokyo) 34:100–103
19. Akhaddar A, El Hassani MY, Chakir N, Jiddane M (2011) Optochiasmatic tuberculoma: complication of tuberculous meningitis. Report of a case and review of the literature (in French). J Neuroradiol 28:137–142
20. Teoh R, Poon W, Humphries MJ, O'Mahony G (1988) Suprasellar tuberculoma developing during treatment of tuberculous meningitis requiring urgent surgical decompression. J Neurol 235:321–322
21. Barlas O, Sencer A, Erkan K, Eraksoy H, Sencer S, Bayindir C (1999) Stereotactic surgery in the management of brain abscess. Surg Neurol 52:404–410
22. Mohanty A, Venkatarama SK, Vasudev MK, Khanna N, Anandh B (1999) Role of stereotactic aspiration in the management of tuberculous brain abscess. Surg Neurol 51:443–446

23. Akhaddar A, Bourazza A, El Mostarchid B, Rouimi A, Boutaleb N, Ouahabi H, Mosseddaq R (2000) Brainstem tuberculomas: two cases (in French). Rev Neurol (Paris) 156:399–402
24. Nadvi SS, Van Dellen JR, Gouws E (1995) Transcranial Doppler ultrasonography in hydrocephalic children with tuberculous meningitis. Br J Neurosurg 9:519–526
25. Raut T, Garg RK, Jain A, Verma R, Singh MK, Malhotra HS, Kohli N, Parihar A (2013) Hydrocephalus in tuberculous meningitis: Incidence, its predictive factors and impact on the prognosis. J Infect 66:330–337
26. Akhaddar A (2015) Infective complications. In: Di Rocco C, Turgut M, Jallo G, Martinez-Lage DJF (eds) Complications of CSF shunting in Hydrocephalus. Springer International Publishing, Cham, pp 141–148
27. Mohindra S (2012) Symptomatic, paradoxical intracranial tuberculomas along non-functional ventricular catheter necessitating its removal. Br J Neurosurg 26:909–911
28. AlSemari A, Baz S, Alrabiah F, Al-Khairallah T, Qadi N, Kareem A, Alrajhi AA (2012) Natural course of epilepsy concomitant with CNS tuberculomas. Epilepsy Res 99:107–111
29. Cheng VC, Ho PL, Lee RA, Chan KS, Chan KK, Woo PC, Lau SK, Yuen KY (2002) Clinical spectrum of paradoxical deterioration during antituberculosis therapy in non-HIV-infected patients. Eur J Clin Microbiol Infect Dis 21:803–809
30. Menon S, Bharadwaj R, Chowdhary A, Kaundinya D, Palande D (2011) Tuberculous brain abscesses: case series and review of literature. J Neurosci Rural Pract 2:153–157
31. Naama O, Boulahroud O, Elouennass M, Akhaddar A, Gazzaz M, Elmoustarchid B, Boucetta M (2010) Primary tuberculous cerebellar abscess in an immunocompetent adult. Intern Med 49:875–876
32. Whitener DR (1978) Tuberculous brain abscess. Report of a case and review of the literature. Arch Neurol 35:148–155
33. Chakraborti S, Mahadevan A, Govindan A, Nagarathna S, Santosh V, Yasha TC, Devi BI, Chandramouli BA, Kovoor JM, Chandramuki A, Shankar SK (2009) Clinicopathological study of tuberculous brain abscess. Pathol Res Pract 205:815–822
34. Cárdenas G, Soto-Hernández JL, Orozco RV, Silva EG, Revuelta R, Amador JL (2010) Tuberculous brain abscesses in immunocompetent patients: management and outcome. Neurosurgery 67:1081–1087
35. Narang M, Gomber S, Upreti L, Dua S (2010) Multiple intracranial tubercular abscesses in a child. Kathmandu Univ Med J (KUMJ) 8:244–246
36. Joshi V, Germano I, Meenakshi R, Doshi A (2014) Paradoxical evolution of a cerebellar tuberculosis abscess after surgical drainage and antibiotic therapy. Surg Neurol Int 5:143
37. Mohindra S, Savardekar A, Gupta R, Tripathi M, Rane S (2016) Tuberculous brain abscesses in immunocompetent patients: a decade long experience with nine patients. Neurol India 64:66–74
38. Pandit V, Valsalan R, Seshadri S, Bahuleyan S (2009) Disseminated tuberculosis presenting as mesenteric and cerebral abscess in HIV infection: case report. Braz J Infect Dis 13:383–386
39. du Plessis J, Andronikou S, Wieselthaler N, Theron S, George R, Mapukata A (2007) CT features of tuberculous intracranial abscesses in children. Pediatr Radiol 37:167–172
40. Gupta RK, Vatsal DK, Husain N, Chawla S, Prasad KN, Roy R, Kumar R, Jha D, Husain M (2001) Differentiation of tuberculous from pyogenic brain abscesses with in vivo proton MR spectroscopy and magnetization transfer MR imaging. AJNR Am J Neuroradiol 22:1503–1509
41. Gump WC, Summers LE, Walsh JW (2006) Tuberculosis infection presenting as brain abscess in an immunocompromised host. J La State Med Soc 158:292–295
42. Megarbane B, Lebrun L, Marchal P, Axler O, Brivet FG (2000) Fatal *Mycobacterium tuberculosis* brain abscess in an immunocompetent patient. Scand J Infect Dis 32:702–703
43. Vidal JE, Penalva de Oliveira AC, Bonasser Filho F, Schiavon Nogueira R, Dauar RF, Lins DL, Coelho JF (2005) Tuberculous brain abscess in AIDS patients: report of three cases and literature review. Int J Infect Dis 9:201–207
44. Akhaddar A, Elouennass M, Baallal H, Boucetta M (2010) Focal intracranial infections due to *Actinomyces species* in immunocompetent patients: diagnostic and therapeutic challenges. World Neurosurg 74:346–350
45. Kim PD, Hall WA (2014) Bacterial brain abscess. In: Hall WA, Kim PD (eds) Neurosurgical infectious disease: surgical and nonsurgical management. Thieme, New York, pp 95–103
46. Akhaddar A, El Mostarchid B, Gazzaz M, Boucetta M (2002) Cerebellar abscess due to *Lactococcus lactis*. A new pathogen. Acta Neurochir (Wien) 144:305–306
47. Simsek H, Kutlay M, Colak A, Haholu A, Kaya H, Ozyurt M, Demircan MN (2013) Concomitant tubercular and fungal cerebellar abscess in an immunocompromised girl. Turk Neurosurg 23:88–94
48. Muzumdar D, Jhawar S, Goel A (2011) Brain abscess: an overview. Int J Surg 9:136–144
49. Barber PA, Sieradzan KS, Schady W (1999) Superior sagittal sinus obstruction and tuberculous abscess. Acta Neurol Scand 99:202–203
50. Akhaddar A, Baallal H, Elouennass M, Elgharbaoui H, Mahi M, Boucetta M (2011) Combined *Serratia liquefaciens* and *Mycobacterium tuberculosis* in temporal osteitis with brain extension. Surg Infect (Larchmt) 12:329–331
51. Siddiqui AA, Sarwari AR, Chishti KN (2001) Concomitant tuberculous and pyogenic brain abscess. Int J Tuberc Lung Dis 5:100–101
52. Banerjee AD, Pandey P, Ambekar S, Chandramouli BA (2010) Pediatric intracranial subdural empyema

caused by *Mycobacterium tuberculosis* – a case report and review of literature. Childs Nerv Syst 26:1117–1120
53. Nathoo N, Nadvi SS, Gouws E, van Dellen JR (2001) Craniotomy improves outcomes for cranial subdural empyemas: computed tomography-era experience with 699 patients. Neurosurgery 49:872–877
54. Turel MK, Moorthy RK, Rajshekhar V (2012) Multidrug-resistant tuberculous subdural empyema with secondary methicillin-resistant *Staphylococcus aureus* infection: an unusual presentation of cranial tuberculosis in an infant. Neurol India 60:231–234
55. Gettler JF, El-Sadr W (1993) Cranial epidural abscess due to *Mycobacterium tuberculosis* in a patient infected with the human immunodeficiency virus. Clin Infect Dis 17:289–290
56. Jacques C, Boukobza M, Polivka M, Ferrario A, George B, Merland JJ (2000) Cranial epidural tuberculoma. A case report. Acta Radiol 41:367–370
57. Tripathi AK, Gupta N, Khanna M, Ahmad R, Tripathi P (2007) Tuberculosis presenting as osteolytic soft tissue swellings of skull in HIV positive patient: a case report. Indian J Tuberc 54:193–195
58. Akhaddar A (2016) Unusual pathogens. In: Akhaddar A (ed) Cranial osteomyelitis. Diagnosis and treatment. Springer International Publishing, Cham, pp 259–283
59. Gupta PK, Kolluri VR, Chandramouli BA, Venkataramana NK, Das BS (1989) Calvarial tuberculosis: a report of two cases. Neurosurgery 25:830–833
60. Mukherjee KK, Kaushik R, Nada R, Khosla VK, Khandelwal N, Kak VK (2002) Calvarial tuberculosis. Surg Neurol 57:195–202
61. Tyagi AK, Kirollos RW, Kang NV (1996) Tuberculous osteitis of the skull: a case report and review of the literature. Br J Neurosurg 10:399–401
62. Mohanty S, Rao CJ, Mukherjee KC (1981) Tuberculosis of the skull. Int Surg 66:81–83
63. Ramdurg SR, Gupta DK, Suri A, Sharma BS, Mahapatra AK (2010) Calvarial tuberculosis: uncommon manifestation of common disease – a series of 21 cases. Br J Neurosurg 24:572–577
64. Akhaddar A (2016) General considerations and surgical therapy. In: Akhaddar A (ed) Cranial osteomyelitis. Diagnosis and treatment. Springer International Publishing, Cham, pp 191–223
65. Sethi A, Sethi D, Mrig S, Passey JC, Srivastav N (2006) Coexistent acute pyogenic and tubercular petrous apicitis: a diagnostic dilemma. J Laryngol Otol 120:875–878
66. Jadhav RN, Palande DA (1999) Calvarial tuberculosis. Neurosurgery 45:1345–1349
67. Biniwale SN, Rajshekhar V (2000) Tuberculous osteomyelitis of bone flap following craniotomy for a glioma. Neurol India 48:91–92
68. Pandey AS, Surana A (2011) Tuberculous osteomyelitis of the bone flap following craniotomy. Indian J Tuberc 58:129–131
69. Sundar VI, Shekhawat J, Gupta A, Sinha VD (2013) Post traumatic tubercular osteomyelitis of skull vault. J Neurosci Rural Pract 4(Suppl 1):138–141
70. Sundaram PK, Sayed F (2007) Superior sagittal sinus thrombosis caused by calvarial tuberculosis: case report. Neurosurgery 60:E776
71. Zettel H (1961) Post-traumatic tuberculosis of the skull (in German). Monatsschr Unfallheilkd Versicherungsmed 64:299–307
72. Indira Devi B, Tyagi AK, Bhat DI, Santosh V (2003) Tuberculous osteitis of clivus. Neurol India 51:69–70
73. Clark MP, Pretorius PM, Byren I, Milford CA (2009) Central or atypical skull base osteomyelitis: diagnosis and treatment. Skull Base 19:247–254
74. Farshchi S, Hasibi M, Ashtiani MT, Yazdani N, Mokhtari Z, Farshchi A (2013) A misdiagnosis led to an extensive skull base surgery: infratemporal tuberculosis mimicking giant cell tumor. Indian J Otolaryngol Head Neck Surg 65:83–85
75. Chen CH, Chang YJ, Sy HN, Chen WL, Yen HC (2014) Risk assessment of the outcome for cerebral infarction in tuberculous meningitis. Rev Neurol (Paris) 170:512–519
76. Figaji AA, Sandler SI, Fieggen AG, Le Roux PD, Peter JC, Argent AC (2008) Continuous monitoring and intervention for cerebral ischemia in tuberculous meningitis. Pediatr Crit Care Med 9:e25–e30
77. Gupta K, Radotra BD, Suri D, Sharma K, Saxena AK, Singhi P (2012) Mycotic aneurysm and subarachnoid hemorrhage following tubercular meningitis in an infant with congenital tuberculosis and cytomegalovirus disease. J Child Neurol 27:1320–1325
78. Leiguarda R, Berthier M, Starkstein S, Nogués M, Lylyk P (1988) Ischemic infarction in 25 children with tuberculous meningitis. Stroke 19:200–204
79. Rotta NT, Silva AR, Firpo-Freire C, Sebben G, Rd S-R, Ohlweiler L (2004) Cerebrovascular disease as an initial finding in childhood tuberculosis meningoencephalitis (in Spanish). Rev Neurol 39:1034–1037
80. Sahin S, Cansu A, Kamaşak T, Eyüboğlu İ, Esenülkü G, Ökten A (2014) Lumbar puncture requirement in acute hemiparesis: diagnosis of tuberculous meningitis after hemiparesis in a child. Childs Nerv Syst 30:2139–2142
81. Schoeman JF, Van Zyl LE, Laubscher JA, Donald PR (1995) Serial CT scanning in childhood tuberculous meningitis: prognostic features in 198 cases. J Child Neurol 10:320–329
82. Sheu JJ, Hsu CY, Yuan RY, Yang CC (2012) Clinical characteristics and treatment delay of cerebral infarction in tuberculous meningitis. Intern Med J 42:294–300
83. Wen LS, Noble JA (2011) A case of a young girl with fever and seizure. Acad Emerg Med 18:e86–e92
84. Clemente Morgado T, Kinsky M, Carrara H, Rothemeyer S, Semple P (2013) Prognostic value of computed tomography-evident cerebral infarcts in adult patients with tuberculous meningitis and

hydrocephalus treated with an external ventricular drain. World Neurosurg 80:e255–e260
85. Hendin AS, Margolis MT, Glickman MG (1973) Occlusion of the basilar artery in tuberculous meningitis. Neuroradiology 6:193–195
86. Kashiwagi S, Abiko S, Harada K, Yamashita K, Ito H (1990) Ischemic cerebrovascular complication in tuberculous meningitis; a case of Fröhlich syndrome and hemiparesis (in Japanese). No Shinkei Geka 18:1141–1145
87. Lammie GA, Hewlett RH, Schoeman JF, Donald PR (2009) Tuberculous cerebrovascular disease: a review. J Infect 59:156–166
88. Lu CH, Chang WN, Chang HW, Chung KJ, Tsai NW, Lui CC, Wang HC (2007) Clinical relevance of intracranial arterial stenoses in tuberculous and cryptococcal meningitis. Infection 35:359–363
89. Pathare AV, Patil RR, Chikhalikar AA, Dalvi SG (1988) Association of tuberculoma with arterio-venous malformation (a case report). J Postgrad Med 34:190–192
90. Radmanesh F, Nejat F, El Khashab M (2010) Cerebral infarction as the first presentation of tuberculosis in an infant: a case report. J Microbiol Immunol Infect 43:249–252
91. Ramdasi R, Mahore A, Kawale J, Thorve S (2015) Cerebral venous thrombosis associated with tuberculous meningitis: a rare complication of a common disease. Acta Neurochir 157:1679–1680
92. Roh JK, Kang DW (1998) A case of tuberculosis meningitis complicated by intracerebral hemorrhage. Eur Neurol 40:50–52
93. Uesugi T, Takizawa S, Morita Y, Takahashi H, Takagi S (2006) Hemorrhagic infarction in tuberculous meningitis. Intern Med 45:1193–1194
94. Podlecka A, Dziewulska D, Rafałowska J (1998) Vascular changes in tuberculous meningoencephalitis. Folia Neuropathol 36:235–237
95. de Almedia GM, Lee KC, Ciappetta P (1997) Middle cerebral artery aneurysm complicated by tuberculosis. Surg Neurol 48:448–450
96. Griffiths SJ, Sgouros S, James G, John P (2000) Intraventricular haemorrhage due to ruptured posterior inferior cerebellar artery aneurysm in tuberculous meningitis. Childs Nerv Syst 16:872–874
97. Kim IY, Jung S, Jung TY, Kang SS, Moon KS, Joo SP (2008) Intracranial tuberculoma with adjacent inflammatory aneurysms. J Clin Neurosci 15:1174–1176
98. Madhusudan HV, Krishnamoorthy N, Suresh PK, Subramaniam V (2015) Superficial temporal artery pseudoaneurysm presenting as extradural hematoma: a case report and review of literature. Asian J Neurosurg 10:63–65
99. Saraf R, Limaye U (2013) Ruptured intracranial tubercular infectious aneurysm secondary to a tuberculoma and its endovascular management. Br J Neurosurg 27:243–245
100. Vitali AM (2008) Acquired encephalocele attributable to tuberculous osteitis: case report. Neurosurgery 62:E976
101. Chatterjee D, Radotra BD, Vasishta RK, Sharma K (2015) Vascular complications of tuberculous meningitis: an autopsy study. Neurol India 63:926–932
102. Shuangshoti S, Phisitbutr M (1979) Fatal hemorrhage in tuberculosis of the brain. J Med Assoc Thai 62:639–645
103. Choi H, Hall WA, Deshaies EM (2014) Infectious intracranial aneurysms. In: Hall WA, Kim PD (eds) Neurosurgical infectious disease: surgical and nonsurgical management. Thieme, New York, pp 133–146
104. Manka R, Lentini S, Manka C, Lüderitz B, Tasci S (2005) A case of arteria cerebri aneurysm, sepsis, and miliary lung infiltrates in a 32-year-old woman (in German). Med Klin (Munich) 100:740–743
105. Chun JY, Smith W, Halbach VV, Higashida RT, Wilson CB, Lawton MT (2001) Current multimodality management of infectious intracranial aneurysms. Neurosurgery 48:1203–1213
106. Misch M, Thomale UW, Keitzer R, Vajkoczy P (2010) Prevention of secondary ischemic events by superficial temporal artery-middle cerebral artery bypass surgery after tuberculosis-induced vasculopathy in a 5-year-old child. J Neurosurg Pediatr 6:69–72

Part III

Tuberculosis of the Spine and Its Coverings

Pott's Disease

15

Mehmet Turgut, Ahmet T. Turgut,
and Ali Akhaddar

Contents

M. Turgut, MD, PhD (✉)
Department of Neurosurgery, Adnan Menderes University School of Medicine, Aydın, Turkey
e-mail: drmturgut@yahoo.com

A.T. Turgut, MD
Department of Radiology, Hacettepe University School of Medicine, Ankara, Turkey
e-mail: ahmettuncayturgut@yahoo.com

A. Akhaddar, MD, IFAANS
Department of Neurosurgery, Avicenne Military Hospital of Marrakech. Mohammed V University in Rabat, Rabat, Morocco
e-mail: akhaddar@hotmail.fr

Abbreviations

AIDS	Acquired immunodeficiency syndrome
ALL	Anterior longitudinal ligament
BCG	Bacillus Calmette–Guerin
CT	Computed tomography
EMB	Ethambutol
INH	Isoniazid
IVD	Intervertebral disc
MRI	Magnetic resonance imaging
PLL	Posterior longitudinal ligament
PZA	Pyrazinamide
RIF	Rifampicin
TB	Tuberculosis
TST	Tuberculin skin test
WHO	World Health Organization

15.1 Introduction

Tuberculosis (TB) of the bones remains rare, accounting for only about 1% of all cases of TB [1–4]. Based on findings reported by over 200 countries that account for almost all of TB cases in the world, the latest report from the World Health Organization (WHO) on TB control indicates a global decrease on its prevalence and

M. Turgut et al. (eds.), *Tuberculosis of the Central Nervous System*,
DOI 10.1007/978-3-319-50712-5_15

mortality rates since 1990, suggesting existence of major progress [5]. Nevertheless, spinal TB, known as "Pott's disease", as an important cause of vertebral infection is still frequent in underdeveloped countries, and the most common extrapulmonary location of TB is the spine, accounting for over 50% of the cases of osseous involvement [3, 4, 6]. As a result of haematogenous dissemination, vertebral involvement develops and then infection spreads to the intervertebral disc (IVD) tissue, the adjacent vertebrae and/or paraspinal area. TB predominantly involves the thoracic spine and then cervical and lumbar regions of the spine with late sequelae including severe kyphosis and paraplegia. This chapter focuses on certain aspects of Pott's disease with emphasis on pathogenesis, imaging modalities and current surgical techniques.

15.2 History

In 1782, the English surgeon Sir Percivall Pott (1714–1788) firstly described the clinical presentation and pathologic findings of spinal TB infection [7]. In 1905, the German microbiologist Robert Koch isolated the causative organism, *Mycobacterium tuberculosis* [8]. However, TB disease has been known for many centuries, and scientists found that humans were infected with the disease in Africa approximately 5000 years ago [9], while other researchers suggested that the TB bacteria typical vertebral lesions are older than 6000 years in Peru, called the Peruvian pre-Columbian era [9]. The Ebers Papyrus which was found between the legs of a mummy in Egypt from around 1550 BC, called the Egyptian predynastic era, described involvement of TB disease [10, 11]. Then, Greek physician Hippocrates described the characteristics of the disease as "phthisis" and "consumption" and stated the illness as nearly always fatal [12].

The incidence of TB grew gradually during the Middle Ages and Renaissance period [12]. Historically, the first evidence for TB in humans relies on lesions compatible with bone TB in a 500,000-year-old skull in Turkey [13]. Recently, however, a morphological and molecular evidence of TB infection was detected in humans in the eastern Mediterranean from the Neolithic period dating from 9000 years ago [14]. To the best of our knowledge, this finding is the oldest scientific evidence of TB infection in humankind to date.

15.3 Epidemiology

In 2013, Dara et al. [15] reported that TB-related deaths decreased by 40% between 1990 and 2010 [15]. In recent years, however, there are increased inflation, poverty, unemployment, human immunodeficiency virus/acquired immunodeficiency syndrome (AIDS) infections, resistance to anti-TB chemotherapeutic agents and immigration from endemic areas to non-endemic regions of the world, albeit extensive efforts for control of TB infection [16, 17]. As a result, in many countries of the world like Turkey, the revival in TB has been associated with an associated increase in TB of central nervous system including in Pott's disease [3, 4, 18–20]. Today, it is accepted that about one-third of the world's population harbour TB caused by the bacillus, *M. tuberculosis*, which is rarely seen in organs other than the lung [17].

15.4 Pathogenesis

Vertebral involvement originates from dissemination patterns of the TB infection in a distant focus or as a result of latent reactivation [17]. Due to differences in the normal vascular anatomy of the spine, anatomical localization of involvement of the vertebral body may be (a) peridiscal region, within metaphyseal bone and beneath the anterior longitudinal ligament (ALL) or posterior longitudinal ligament (PLL) with involvement of adjacent areas; (b) central region, the centre of the vertebral body, or adjacent regions to the cartilage end plate; and (c) anterior subperiosteal region, the anterior part of the vertebral body near the cortex. Classically, TB infection generally starts in the anterior vertebral body and propagates along the ALL or PLL, while the IVD

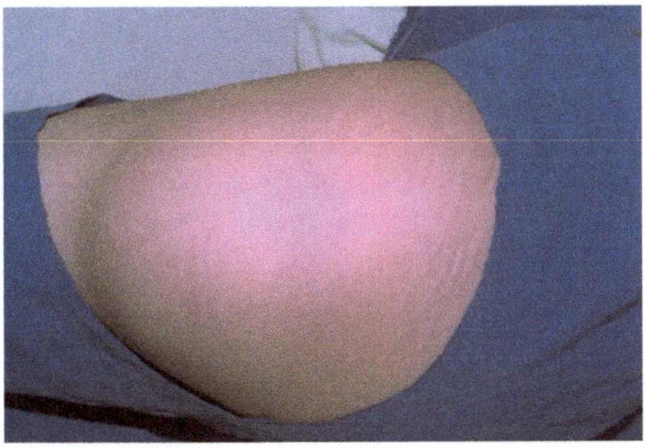

Fig. 15.1 Cold abscess in the *left* thigh in case of thoracolumbar Pott's disease (Courtesy of M. Benzagmout, M.D.)

is spared until very late stages of the disease. As a result of disease progression, kyphotic angulation and gibbus deformity due to anterior vertebral body collapse and then a paraspinal abscess develop. In some cases, it may cause destruction in adjacent segments called "contiguous lesions," or it may result in "skip lesions" or typical cold abscess formations (Fig. 15.1), by spread from the primary focus by way of the Batson vertebral venous system [3, 4, 21]. In some patients with Pott's disease, infection produces an extradural abscess without bony involvement, possibly via the internal vertebral venous plexus in the extradural space [22]. Typically, the lower thoracic and upper lumbar regions of the spine are the most common sites of involvement (50% of patients), and cervical spine and lumbar spine are each involved in 25% of patients with Pott's disease [3, 4, 23]. On the other hand, atypical Pott's disease with involvement of the posterior vertebral elements alone is an uncommon entity [24].

15.5 Clinical Features

Most common presenting symptom manifestation of Pott's disease is low back pain, but systemic signs, such as fever, anorexia, fatigue, night sweats and weight loss, are frequent. Pain is the most common presenting manifestation and neurologic deficit is uncommon. The incidence of neurologic deficit in Pott's disease ranges from 5% to 100% in various clinical series, possibly due to varying incidence of advanced stage of the disease [1–4, 25, 26]. Pathophysiologically, spinal cord involvement may result from direct pressure from abscess formation and/or bony sequestrum as a complication of osteomyelitis in Pott's disease. In clinical practice, the limited symptoms and absence of specific radiological changes early in the course of the infection often result in diagnostic delays.

15.6 Diagnostic Studies

All over the world, an elevated erythrocyte sedimentation rate and a positive intradermal tuberculin skin test (TST) are still used for the diagnosis of extrapulmonary latent TB including Pott's disease. It is important to remember that TST will occur as false negative in malnourished patients and AIDS patients, while they will give false-positive results for those who had been given the bacillus Calmette–Guerin (BCG) vaccine, as did many countries of the world including Turkey and Morocco. Therefore, these patients should be tested using measurement of the interferon gamma released into venous blood by infected T cells [17]. In patients with a strong suspicion of clinical TB, molecular biology techniques such as DNA amplification techniques (polymerase chain reaction) may be used as an alternative, although both specificity and sensitivity of these techniques are lower than to those of TB cultures [17, 27].

Accurate diagnosis can be obtained by the bacteriological isolation of *M. tuberculosis* in the materials of computed tomography (CT)-guided needle biopsy or open surgical intervention. Histological examination of formalin-fixed and paraffin-embedded tissue specimen blocks usually provides granulomatous pattern with caseating necrosis and giant-cell granuloma, but it is difficult to show typical acid-fast bacilli on staining with haematoxylin–eosin in cases receiving anti-TB chemotherapy in the preoperative period, and results of TB cultures are generally negative in such cases [3, 4, 28]. In these cases, however, every attempt should be done to obtain an adequate tissue sample because of the high occurrence of false-negative results with only aspiration.

15.7 Imaging Modalities

15.7.1 Radiography

In cases of Pott's disease, spinal lesions suggesting TB infection may be evaluated on standing conventional lateral radiographs as first-step diagnostic methods, and they are usually osteolysis involving contiguous body of the vertebra with diffuse osteopenia, destruction and kyphosis caused by bone destruction and ultimately bony briding, sparing the posterior elements (Figs. 15.2 and 15.3). Typically, Pott's disease results in destruction of anterior parts of two adjacent vertebrae and destruction of the intervening IVD.

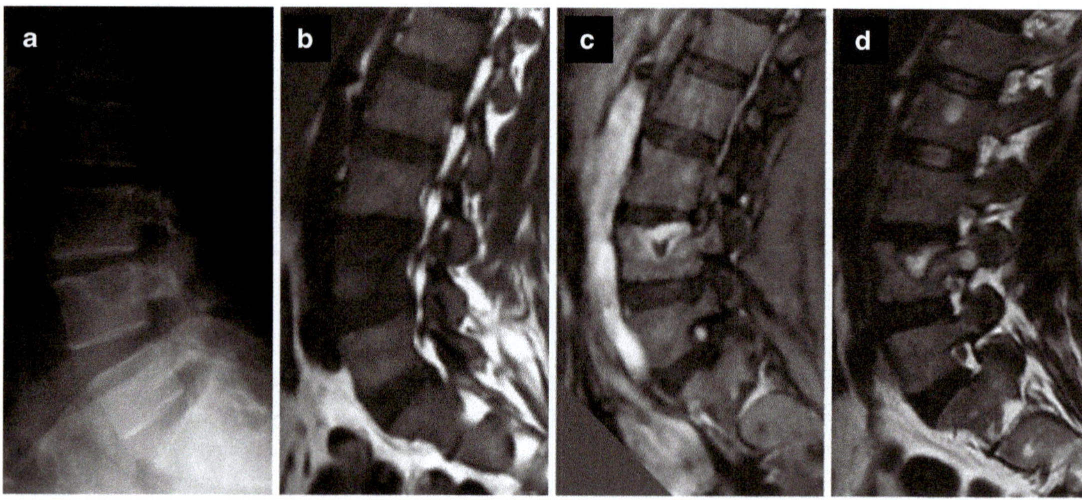

Fig. 15.2 L4 spondylitis with centro-somatic and superior cartilage end plate invasion due to TB. Plain radiography (**a**), sagittal MRI on T1-weighted image before (**b**) and after gadolinium injection (**c**) and on T2-weighted image (**d**)

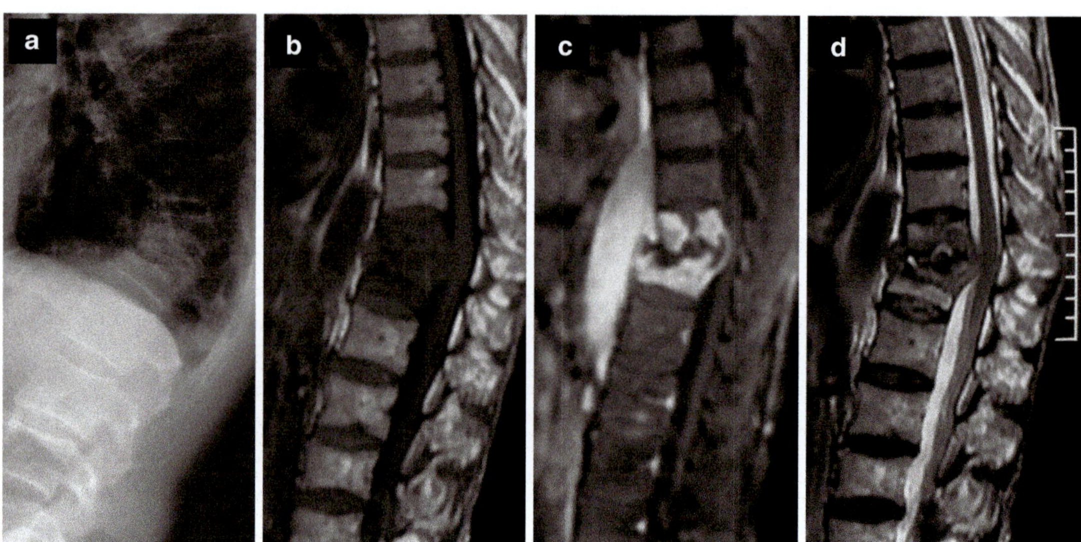

Fig. 15.3 Thoracolumbar Pott's disease. Plain radiography (**a**), sagittal MRI on T1-weighted image before (**b**) and after gadolinium injection (**c**) and on T2-weighted image (**d**) (Note the conus medullaris compression)

15.7.2 CT Scan

CT, a valuable diagnostic tool, clearly demonstrates the extension of soft tissue involvement, called paraspinal TB abscess, in addition to osseous destruction in cases with Pott's disease (Figs. 15.4, 15.5, 15.6 and 15.7). Specifically, soft tissue calcification will provide differential diagnosis of spinal TB from other conditions on 3-D CT scans, thus strongly suggesting diagnosis of Pott's disease [29].

15.7.3 MRI

Magnetic resonance imaging (MRI) is a very useful noninvasive diagnostic tool among currently available techniques for spinal lesions earlier than the other ones (Figs. 15.2, 15.3, 15.7, 15.8, 15.9, 15.10, 15.11, 15.12 and 15.13), although the definitive diagnosis of Pott's disease cannot be established based on imaging finding alone [17, 29–31]. As a general rule, histopathological diagnosis remains essential in cases with Pott's disease [27]. In cases with cold abscesses, MRI reveals the locations and numbers of these lesions and also demonstrates the lesions causing the spinal cord compression (Figs. 15.3, 15.7 and 15.13), allowing their relationship with the clinical manifestations of the patients and a guide for biopsy procedure for identification of *M. tuberculosis* and the best treatment strategy [17]. Recently, it has been reported that T2 STIR images can ensure the early detection of inflammatory oedema [17]. Moreover, it is important to note that TB osteomyelitis is encountered in 25% of cases of spinal extradural abscess [24–26, 29].

15.8 Anti-TB Chemotherapy

Nowadays, the recommended anti-TB chemotherapy protocol composed of 2 months of pyrazinamide (PZA) (30–40 mg/kg), isoniazid (INH) (5–15 mg/kg), ethambutol (EMB) (15–25 mg/kg) and rifampicin (RIF) (10–20 mg/kg), followed by the next 4 months of INH and RIF [17]. Nevertheless, a long treatment of 9 months is used if the clinical, laboratory and imaging findings show the presence of persistent inflammation [32]. At present, treatment of cases with Pott's disease consists of anti-TB chemotherapy and immobilization with bracing, when observed early before collapse of more than one vertebral body and mild kyphosis without any neurologic deficit. With the use of adequate anti-TB chemotherapy under the control of dispensaries for fighting TB infection and/or internal medicine clinics in hospitals, a regression of neurologic symptoms and angle of

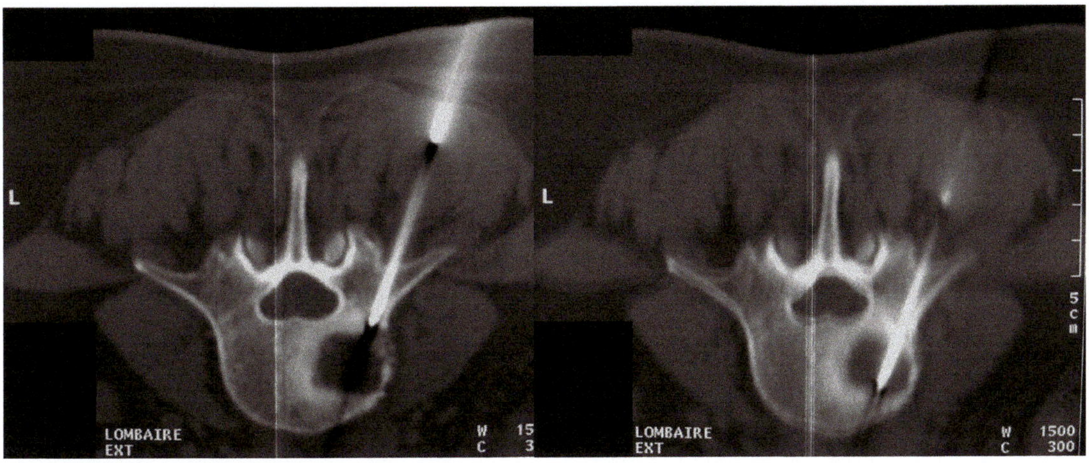

Fig. 15.4 Axial spinal lumbar CT scan when performing CT-guided needle biopsies in the same patient as in Fig. 15.2

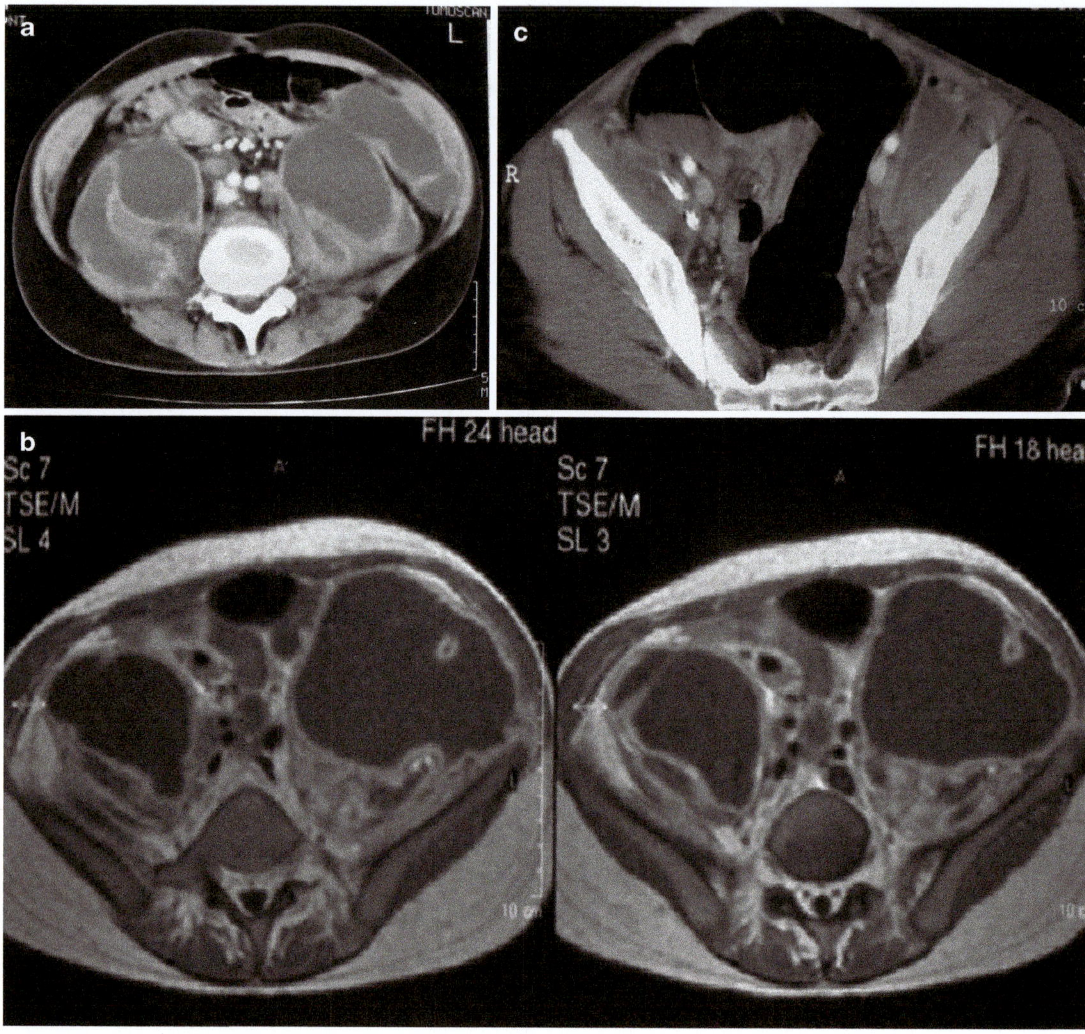

Fig. 15.5 Axial CT views (**a–c**) demonstrating huge paravertebral abscesses without neurological deficit in a 21-year-old patient with L3–L4 spinal TB (Courtesy of P. Fernandes, M.D.)

kyphosis, especially in the presence of involvement of one or two vertebrae, is anticipated. It has been suggested that the success of anti-TB chemotherapy – PZA, INH, EMB and RIF – reduced the role of surgical intervention [2, 33]. Interestingly, however, some authors have reported a paradoxical worsening of present symptoms or the development of new lesions in patients who responded well to anti-TB chemotherapy at first [28]. In such cases, a close monitorization of the patients is very important to prevent the emergence of multiresistant strains [17].

15.9 Modified GATA Classification System

There is no doubt that some guidelines are useful for correct diagnosis and appropriate treatment. To date, there were multiple guidelines for patients with Pott's disease. In 1985, Kumar [34] introduced a new four-point classification system based on the site of the lesion, the stage of the lesion, associated lesions and neurological deficit.

In 2001, Mehta and Bhojraj [35] proposed a new classification system, using information

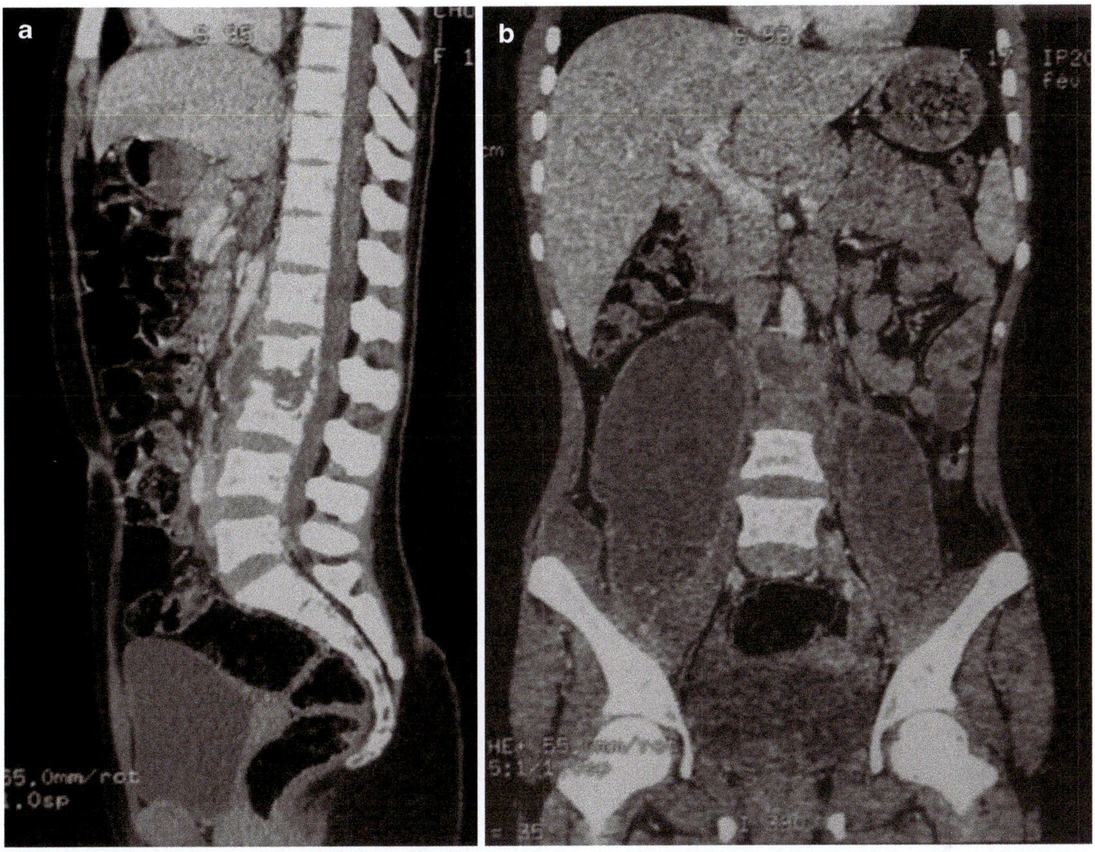

Fig. 15.6 Lumbar spinal CT scan in sagittal (**a**) and coronal (**b**) views showing a L2–L3 Pott's disease associated with bilateral asymmetrical psoas abscess (Courtesy of M. Benzagmout, M.D.)

based on MRI findings, to plan the appropriate surgical treatment for patients with thoracic spinal TB, and they classified in four groups: Group A with involvement of only the anterior column is treated surgically when there is an evidence of spinal cord compression with anterior decompression procedure; Group B with involvement of the anterior and posterior columns was treated with the anterior procedure and then the posterior procedure; Group C with either anterior or global lesions who were at risk if transthoracic surgery was done through the posterior approach; Group D with disease of the posterior column was treated with decompression procedure. In 2008, Oguz et al. [18] suggested a new classification system (Gulhane Askeri Tıp Akademisi [GATA]) for Pott's disease based on some clinical and radiological parameters. They divided Pott's disease in three types (IA/B, II, and III), and they suggested that surgical intervention is indicated for patients of Type IB with no neurological deficit, those of Type II and Type III with or without neurological deficit.

Now, we present a new simple modified classification system from GATA system, as a simple guide for treatment planning in patients with Pott's disease for young spinal surgeons, according to radiological and neurological criteria (Table 15.1) (Fig. 15.14).

15.10 Surgical Techniques

Surgery is necessary to prevent neurological deterioration, to maintain stability and early recovery [3, 4, 18, 31, 34, 35]. And patients

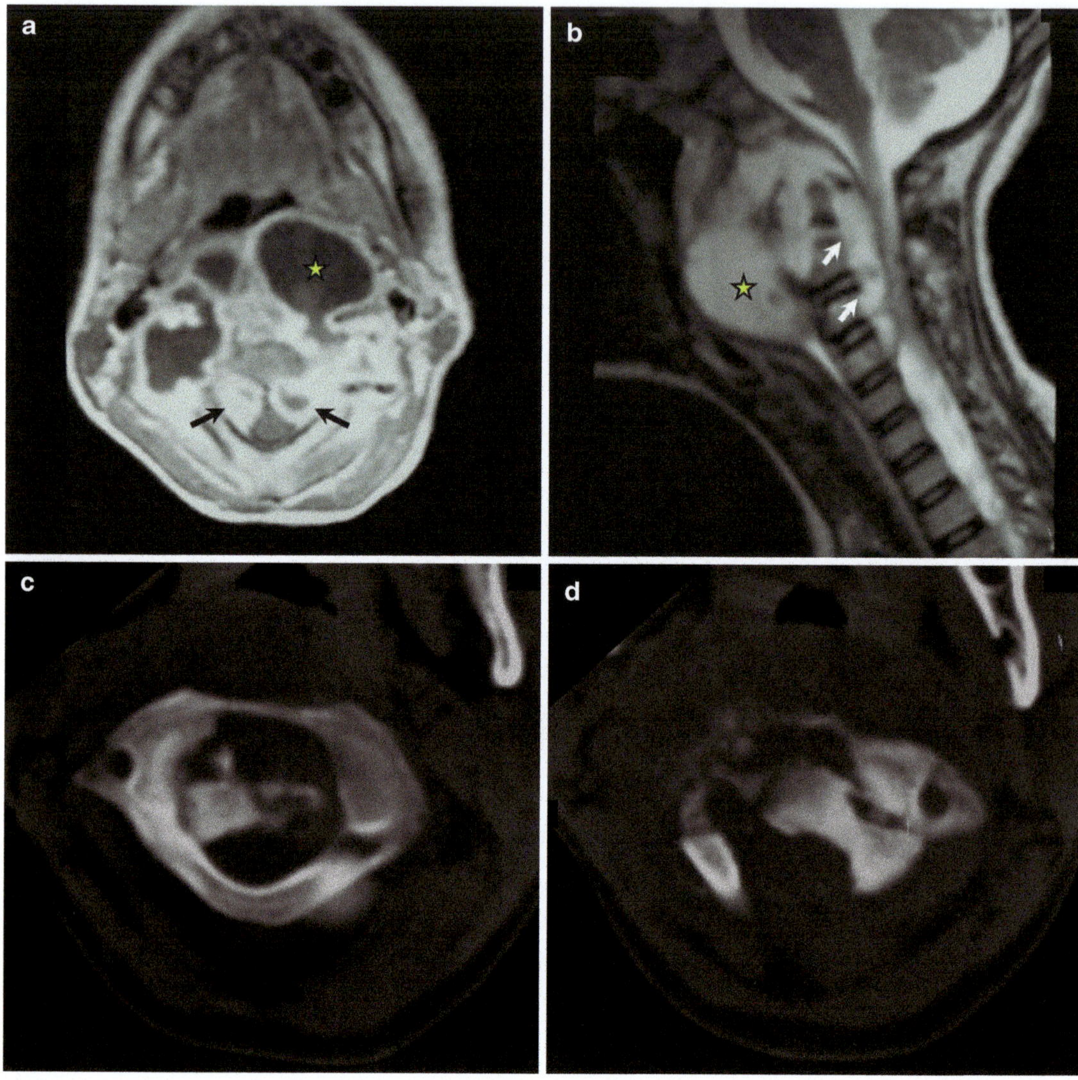

Fig. 15.7 Craniocervical dysjunction, retropharyngeal abscess (*star*) and spinal cord compression (*arrows*) due to suboccipital TB. Axial MRI on T1-weighted image after gadolinium administration (**a**), sagittal view on T2-weighted image (**b**) and axial CT scan on bony windows (**c, d**)

with Pott's disease are treated by neurosurgeons and orthopaedic surgeons specialized in spine surgery in the world. In cases of Pott's disease without evidence of neurological compromise, an attempt to give conservative treatment consisting of anti-TB chemotherapy and bracing for 2–3 months before surgery may be used. In such cases, radiological studies should be obtained during the conservative treatment to exclude any worsening of the kyphosis.

Surgically, an important puzzle in even today's world is the query of which type of surgical intervention is necessary in Pott's paraplegia. In such cases, surgery provides early decompression of the neural structures, correct diagnosis with histological verification and prompt relief of neurological symptoms. But even today, however, there is also still debate on the best surgical approach in patients with Pott's disease. Based on their experience from the surgical treatment of cervical, thoracic and lumbar Pott's disease in 412

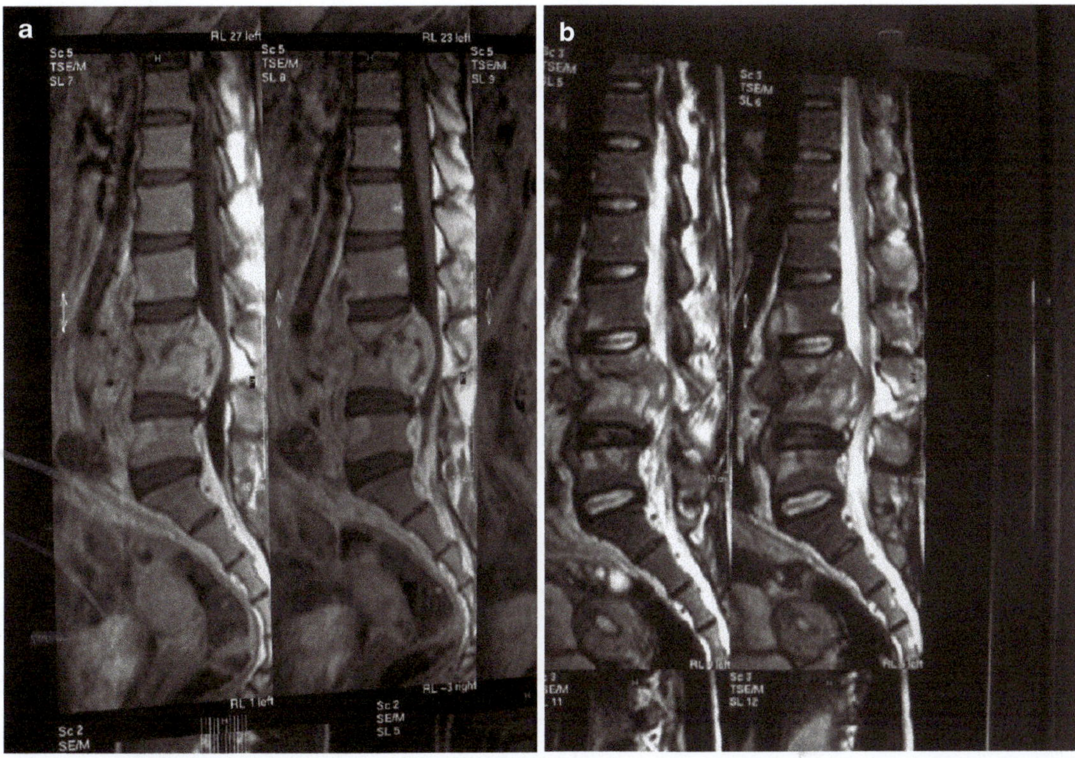

Fig. 15.8 T1-weighted (**a**) and T2-weighted (**b**) sagittal MRIs showing an abscess within the spinal canal in the same patient as in Fig. 15.5 (Courtesy of P. Fernandes, M.D.)

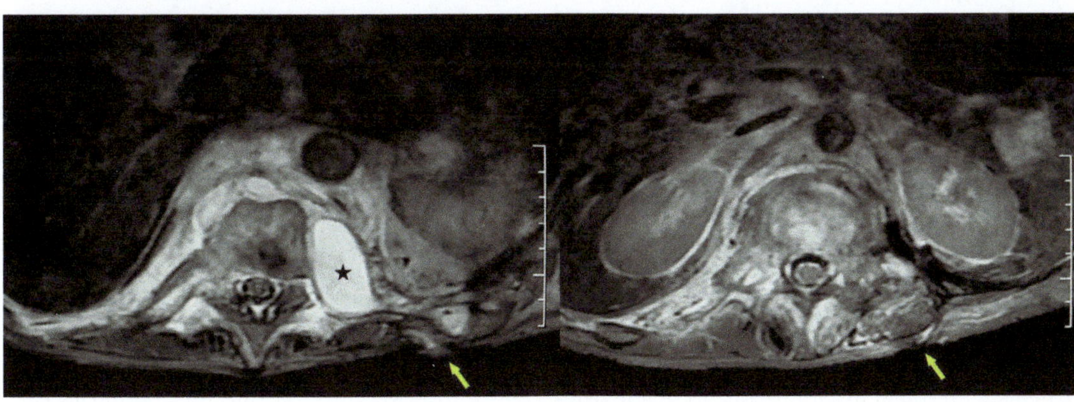

Fig. 15.9 Spinal paraspinal TB abscess (*star*) with superficial cutaneous fistula (*arrows*). Spinal axial MRI on T2-weighted images

patients in 1960, Hodgson et al. [36] described the routine use of debridement consisting of removing purulent necrotic tissues from normal tissue via the anterior approach. In the current literature, most authors suggest surgical decompression combined with medical treatment in patients with Pott's disease having evidence of spinal cord or nerve root compression, extensive abscess formation involving the spinal canal and paraspinal tissues and spinal instability with loss of sagittal alignment of the spine due to extensive osteolysis [3, 4, 17]. Furthermore, debridement of the pre- and intraspinal focus of infection via anterior approach is advised for patients with

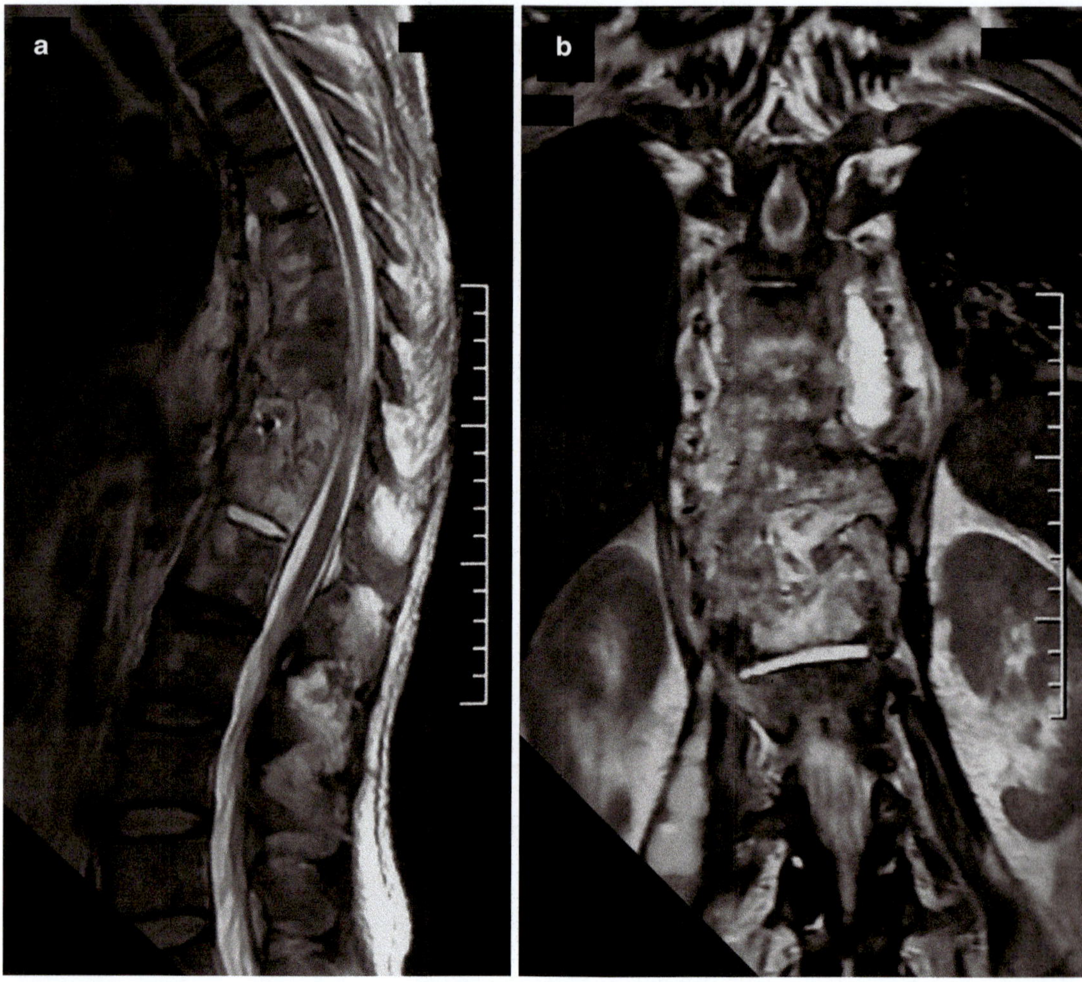

Fig. 15.10 Chronic extensive Pott's disease from T6 to L1 spinal levels in the same patient as in Fig. 15.9. Spinal MRI on T2-weighted images, sagittal (**a**) and coronal (**b**) views

extensive abscess formation but no neurological deficit [37]. Moreover, percutaneous needle aspiration of the caseous necrosis as an alternative has been suggested to ensure decompression in patients with spinal instability due to severe osteolysis requiring posterior fixation [38].

At present, indications of surgical intervention include the existence of cold abscesses, spinal cord compression with neurological deterioration in spite of anti-TB chemotherapy and immobilization and progressive kyphotic deformity [3, 4, 18]. Surgical point of view, technical options include debridement or anterior abscess drainage alone (Fig. 15.15) and laminectomy followed by internal fixation and posterior fusion in the prone position with adjuvant chemotherapy before surgical treatment. In particular, the use of anterior radical debridement and grafting, also called Hong Kong operation, is advised to ensure the stability of anterior column in cases of Pott's disease by many authors [39], while others advocated using the posterior approach alone to perform spinal canal decompression and abscess drainage during the same stage as internal fixation and fusion [40]. Güven et al. [41] described a single-stage instrumentation and fusion in patients with Pott's disease to drain the cold abscess within anterior of the spinal canal with/without lateral extension for decompression of the spinal cord. Accordingly, we also believe

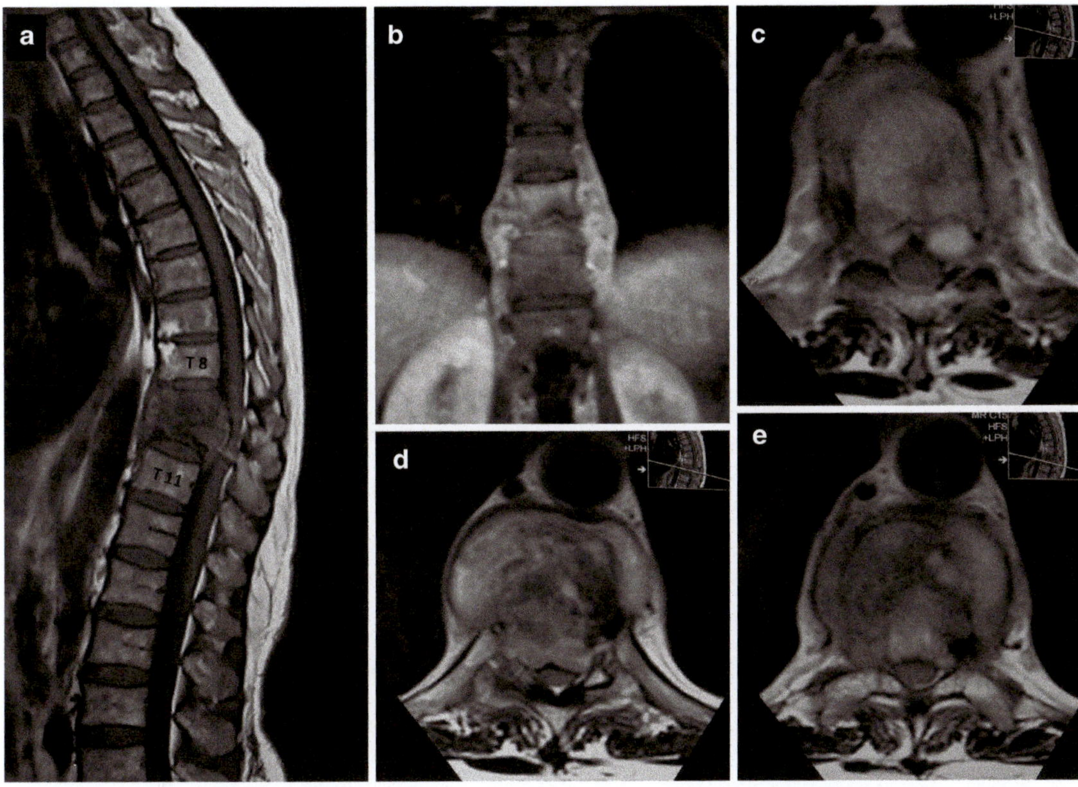

Fig. 15.11 T9–T10 Pott's disease. Spinal MRI on T1-weighted image after gadolinium administration, sagittal (**a**), coronal (**b**) and axial views (**c**–**e**)

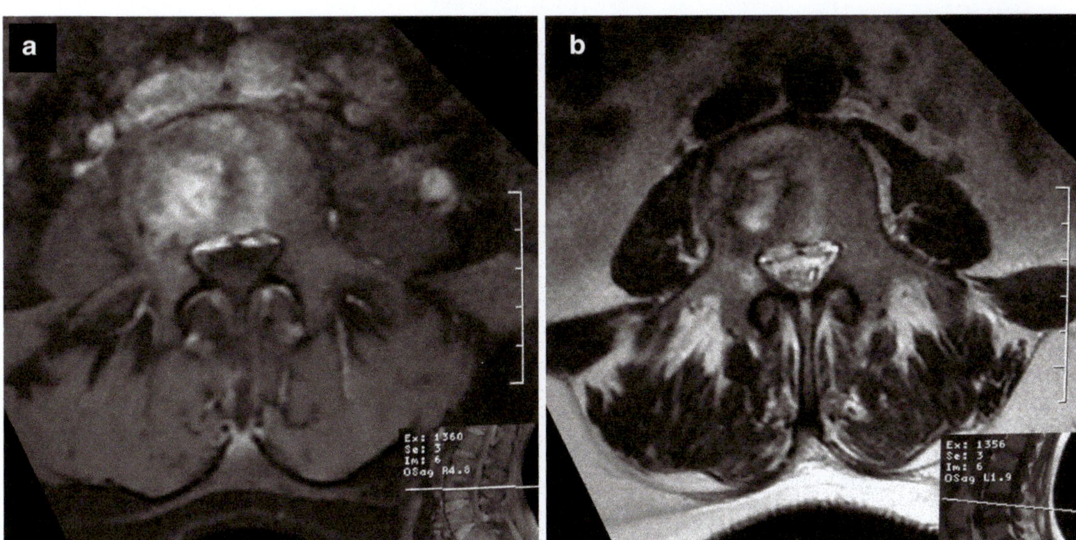

Fig. 15.12 Pott's disease on L4 level with mild intracanalar extension in the same patient as in Fig. 15.2. Axial spinal MRI on T1-weighted image after gadolinium injection (**a**) and on T2-weighted image (**b**)

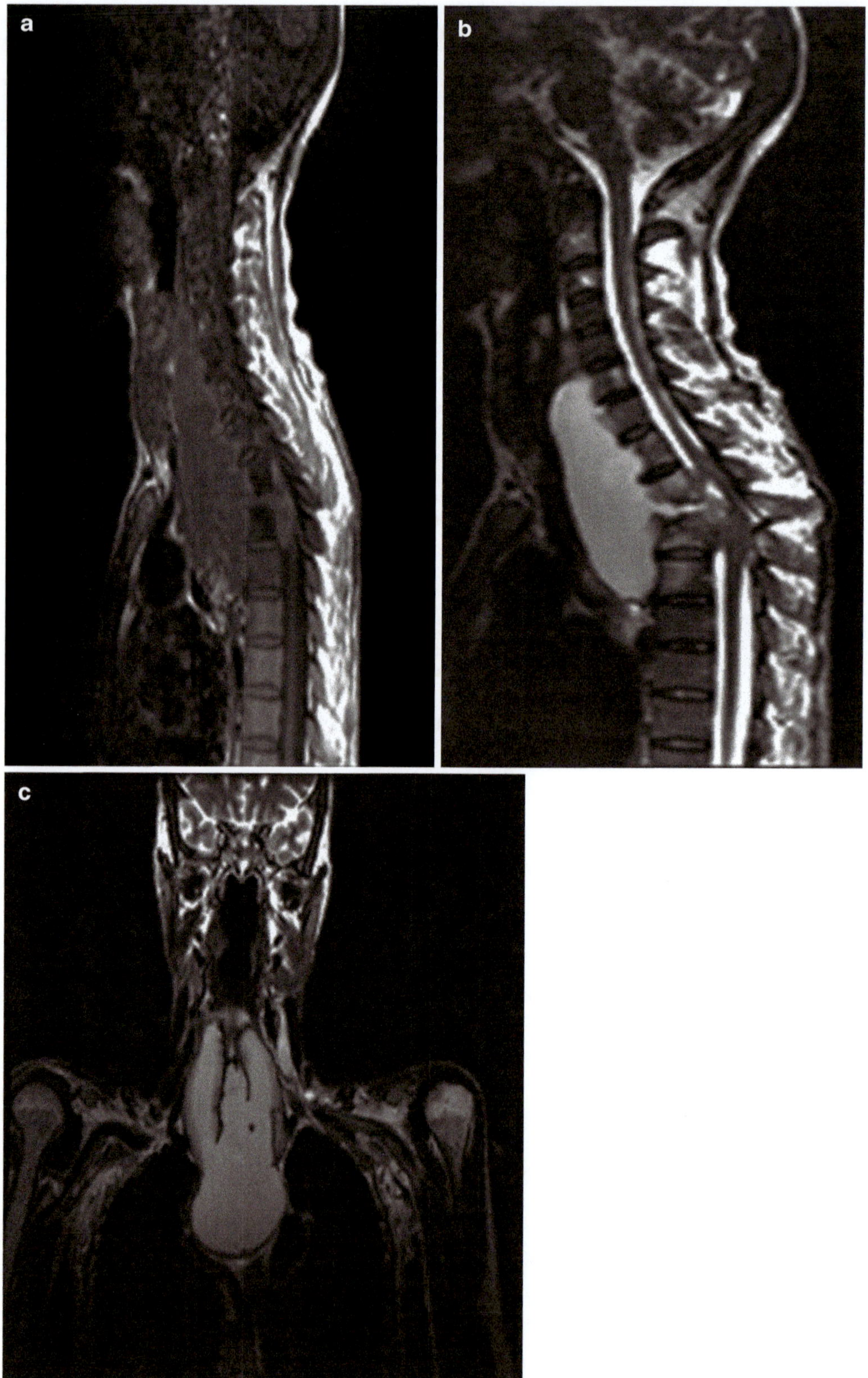

Fig. 15.13 Spinal MRI in T1- (**a**) and T2-weighted (**b**) sagittal and coronal (**c**) views showing a T2–T3 Pott's disease associated with a huge prevertebral cold abscess mimicking goitre (Courtesy of M. Benzagmout, M.D.)

Table 15.1 Modified GATA classification system for Pott's disease

Type of lesion	Degree of vertebral involvement, neurological deficit and abscess formation
Type I	The lesion is limited to the vertebrae with/without abscess formation
Type II	Mild or moderate collapse of vertebrae, stable kyphotic deformity, with/without abscess formation and/or neurologic deficit
Type III	Severe collapse of vertebrae, unstable kyphotic deformity, with/without abscess formation and/or neurologic deficit
Type IV	Severe collapse of vertebrae and paravertebral abscess formation with/without kyphotic deformity and/or neurologic deficit

This classification system is a modification of GATA system described by Oguz et al. [18] in 2008 based on clinical and radiological criteria including abscess formation, vertebral collapse, kyphotic deformity and neurological deficit

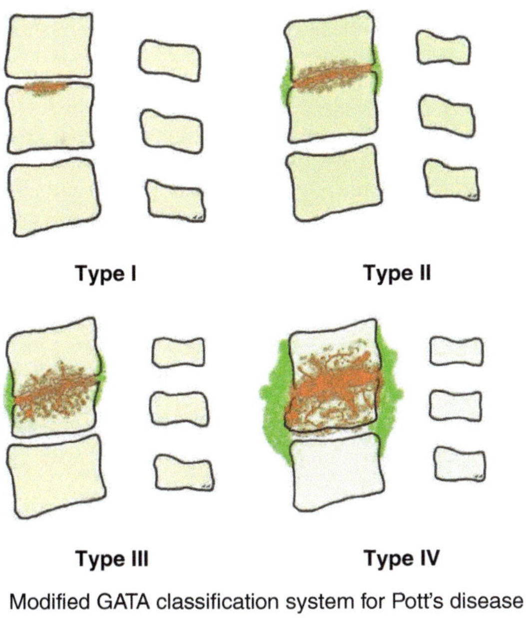

Fig. 15.14 A drawing illustrating modified GATA classification system for Pott's disease

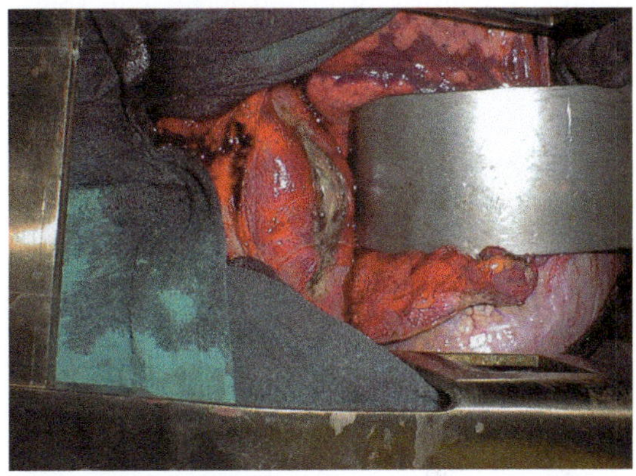

Fig. 15.15 Intraoperative view demonstrating discharge of caseous material following incision of the prevertebral abscess in a case with Pott's disease (Courtesy of M. Benzagmout, M.D.)

that posterior decompressive laminectomy is the surgical approach of choice in patients with involvement of posterior elements. In cases with multisegmental involvement, large abscesses and severe neurological involvement, however, a combined anterior and posterior fusion procedure will be necessary [3]. Based on the findings of a meta-analysis of 694 cases with Pott's disease from the Turkish literature, the senior author of this chapter reported the disease should be treated by anti-TB chemotherapy combined with surgery because of the advanced stage of the disease in most patients [4]. In recent years, the use of open or percutaneous internal fixation techniques and minimally invasive interventional radiology techniques combined with anti-TB chemotherapy have been introduced for high-risk patients with Pott's disease [42]. Unfortunately, it still remains a source of socioeconomic problem in many developing countries, albeit the efforts of WHO [33].

Conclusion

Even today, it is a reality that TB still remains a paramount importance in many developed countries, despite the presence of effective anti-TB drugs. The BCG vaccine should be considered in selected persons who meet specific criteria to help prevent TB infection. Clinical course of Pott's disease is slow; early diagnosis is crucial for proper treatment with anti-TB chemotherapy with/without surgery to avoid its unwanted complications. It should be suspected if the patients present with neurological manifestations of spinal cord and/or nerve root compression or back pain alone. Anatomically, it predominantly affects the thoracic spine, and radiological modalities such as CT and MRI provide a detailed information in the diagnosis of Pott's disease. In patients with Pott's disease, treatment modalities, medical and surgical, with anterior and/or posterior approaches, are necessary to relieve the spinal cord compression due to extensive abscess formation and/or sagittal spinal instability. Surgical management of Pott's disease consists of debridement with spinal cord decompression and stabilization of the spine. Nonetheless, prognosis of patients with Pott's disease is relatively benign when surgical intervention is performed at the onset of the disease. Currently, management in patients with progressive paraplegia requires a multidisciplinary approach including neurosurgeons, orthopaedic spine surgeons, neuroradiologists, infectious disease specialists and rehabilitation specialists.

References

1. Azzam NI, Tammawy M (1988) Tuberculous spondylitis in adults: diagnosis and treatment. Br J Neurosurg 2:85–91
2. Rezai AR, Lee M, Cooper MR, Errico TJ, Koslow M (1995) Modern management of spinal tuberculosis. Neurosurgery 36:87–97
3. Turgut M (2001) Multifocal extensive spinal tuberculosis (Pott's disease) involving cervical, thoracic and lumbar vertebrae. Br J Neurosurg 15:142–146
4. Turgut M (2001) Spinal tuberculosis (Pott's disease): its clinical presentation, surgical management, and outcome. A survey study on 694 patients. Neurosurg Rev 24:8–13
5. World Health Organization (2015) Global tuberculosis report 2015. WHO, Geneva
6. Patankar AP (2016) Tuberculosis of spine: an experience of 30 cases over two years. Asian J Neurosurg 11:226–231
7. Flamm ES (1992) Percivall pott: an 18th century neurosurgeon. J Neurosurg 76:319–326
8. Cambau E, Drancourt M (2014) Steps towards the discovery of Mycobacterium tuberculosis by Robert Koch, 1882. Clin Microbiol Infect 20:196–201
9. Zimmer C (2014) Tuberculosis is newer than thought, study says. New York Times, 21 August
10. Cave AJE (1939) The evidence for the incidence of tuberculosis in ancient Egypt. Br J Tuberc 33:142–152
11. Morse D, Brothwell DR, Ucko PJ (1964) Tuberculosis in ancient Egypt. Am Rev Respir Dis 90:524–541
12. Herzog H (1998) History of tuberculosis. Respiration 65:5–15
13. Kappelman J, Alcicek MC, Kazanci N, Schultz M, Ozkul M, Sen S (2008) First Homo erectus from Turkey and implications for migrations into temperate Eurasia. Am J Phys Anthropol 135:110–116
14. Hershkovitz I, Donoghue HD, Minnikin DE, Besra GS, Lee OY, Gernaey AM, Galili E, Eshed V, Greenblatt CL, Lemma E, Bar-Gal GK, Spigelman M (2008) Detection and molecular characterization of 9,000-year-old Mycobacterium tuberculosis from a Neolithic settlement in the Eastern Mediterranean. PLoS One 3:e3426
15. Dara M, Dadu A, Kremer K, Zaleskis R, Kluge HH (2013) Epidemiology of tuberculosis in WHO European Region and public health response. Eur Spine J 22(Suppl 4):549–555
16. Millet JP, Moreno A, Fina L, del Baño L, Orcau A, de Olalla PG, Caylà JA (2013) Factors that influence current tuberculosis epidemiology. Eur Spine J 22(Suppl 4):539–548
17. Varatharajah S, Charles Y-P, Buy X, Walter A, Steib J-P (2014) Update on the surgical management of Pott's disease. Orthop Traumatol Sur 100:233–239
18. Oguz E, Sehirlioglu A, Altinmakas M, Ozturk C, Komurcu M, Solakoglu C, Vaccaro AR (2008) A new classification and guide for surgical treatment of spinal tuberculosis. Int Orthop 32:127–133
19. Turgut M, Özcan OE, Özgen T, Bertan V (1993) Intradural extramedullary tuberculoma of the spinal cord -a case report. Zentralbl Neurochir 54:197–199
20. Turgut M, Özcan OE, Özgen T, Sağlam S, Bertan V, Erbengi A (1989) Tuberculomas of the craniospinal axis. Turk Neurosurg 1:34–38
21. Batson OV (1940) The function of the vertebral veins and their role in the spread of metastases. Ann Surg 112:138–149
22. Anderson JE (1978) Grant's atlas of anatomy, Seventh edn. Williams and Wilkins, Baltimore
23. Moore SL, Rafii M (2001) Imaging of musculoskeletal and spinal tuberculosis. Radiol Clin North Am 39:329–342
24. Rahman N (1980) Atypical forms of tuberculosis. J Bone Joint Surg Br 62:162–169
25. Kaufman DM, Kaplan JG, Litman N (1980) Infectious agents in spinal epidural abscess. Neurology 30:844–850
26. Tandon PN (1978) Tuberculous meningitis (cranial and spinal). In: Vinken PJ, Bruyn GW (eds) Handbook of clinical neurology, vol 33. Elsevier, Amsterdam, pp 195–262
27. Colmenero JD, Ruiz-Mesa JD, Sanjuan-Jimenez R, Sobrino B, Morata P (2013) Establishing the diagnosis of tuberculous vertebral osteomyelitis. Eur Spine J 22(Suppl 4):579–586

28. Sarmiento OL, Weigle KA, Alexander J, Weber DJ, Miller WC (2003) Assessment by meta-analysis of PCR for diagnosis of smear-negative pulmonary tuberculosis. J Clin Microbiol 41:3233–3240
29. Harisinghani MG, McLoud TC, Shepard J-AO, Ko JP, Shroff MM, Mueller PR (2000) Tuberculosis from head to toe. Radiographics 20:449–470
30. De Roos A, Van Meerten EV, Bloem JL, Bluemm RG (1986) MRI of tuberculous spondylitis. AJR 146:79–82
31. Rivas-Garcia A, Sarria-Estrada S, Torrents-Odin C, Casas-Gomila L, Franquet E (2013) Imaging findings of Pott's disease. Eur Spine J 22(Suppl 4):567–578
32. Rajasekaran S, Khandelwal G (2013) Drug therapy in spinal tuberculosis. Eur Spine J 22(Suppl 4):587–593
33. Medical Research Council Working Party on Tuberculosis of the Spine (1978) A controlled trial of anterior spinal fusion and debridement in the surgical management of tuberculosis of spine in patients on standard chemotherapy: a study in two centers in South Africa. Seventh Rep Tuberc 59:79–105
34. Kumar K (1985) A clinical study and classification of posterior spinal tuberculosis. Int Orthop 9:147–152
35. Mehta JS, Bhojraj SY (2001) Tuberculosis of the thoracic spine A classification based on the selection of surgical strategies. J Bone Joint Surg Br 83:859–863
36. Hodgson AR, Stock FE, Fang HS, Ong GB (1960) Anterior spinal fusion. The operative approach and pathological findings in 412 patients with Pott's disease of the spine. Br J Surg 48:172–178
37. Li M, Du J, Meng H, Wang Z, Luo Z (2011) One-stage surgical management for thoracic tuberculosis by anterior debridement, decompression and autogenous rib grafts, and instrumentation. Spine J 11:726–733
38. Abbas A, Rizvi SR, Mahesri M, Salahuddin HR (2013) Conservative management of spinal tuberculosis: initial series from Pakistan. Asian Spine J 7:73–80
39. Qureshi MA, Khalique AB, Afzal W, Pasha IF, Aebi M (2013) Surgical management of contiguous multilevel thoracolumbar tuberculous spondylitis. Eur Spine J 22(Suppl4):618–623
40. Garg B, Kandwal P, Nagaraja UB, Goswami A, Jayaswal A (2012) Anterior versus posterior procedure for surgical treatment of thoracolumbar tuberculosis: a retrospective analysis. Indian J Orthop 46:165–170
41. Güven O, Yalçın S, Karahan M, Esemenli T (1995) Transpedicular drainage of Pott's abscess. A report of two cases. Am J Orthop 24:421–425
42. Wimmer C (2008) Percutaneous fusion technique on the thoracolumbar spine with the Expedium LIS (in German). Oper Orthop Traumatol 20:511–524

Spinal Dura Mater and Epidural Space

16

Andreas F. Mavrogenis, Vasilios G. Igoumenou, Panayiotis D. Megaloikonomos, Ahmet T. Turgut, Ali Akhaddar, and Mehmet Turgut

Contents

A.F. Mavrogenis, MD (✉) • V.G. Igoumenou, MD
P.D. Megaloikonomos, MD
First Department of Orthopaedics, National and Kapodistrian University of Athens, School of Medicine, ATTIKON University Hospital,
41 Ventouri Street, 15562 Holargos, Athens, Greece
e-mail: afm@otenet.gr; afmavrogenis@med.uoa.gr; vas.igou@gmail.com; panosmeg@hotmail.com

A.T. Turgut, MD
Department of Radiology, Hacettepe University School of Medicine, Ankara, Turkey
e-mail: ahmettuncayturgut@yahoo.com

A. Akhaddar, MD, IFAANS
Department of Neurosurgery, Avicenne Military Hospital of Marrakech, Mohammed V University in Rabat, Rabat, Morocco
e-mail: akhaddar@hotmail.fr

M. Turgut, MD, PhD
Department of Neurosurgery, Adnan Menderes University School of Medicine, Aydın, Turkey
e-mail: drmturgut@yahoo.com

Abbreviations

CNS	Central nervous system
CSF	Cerebrospinal fluid
CT	Computed tomography
EMB	Ethambutol
ESR	Estimated sedimentation rate
INH	Isoniazid
MRI	Magnetic resonance imaging
PZA	Pyrazinamide
RIF	Rifampicin
STR	Streptomycin
TB	Tuberculosis
TBM	Tuberculous meningitis
TBRM	Tuberculous radiculomyelitis
WBC	White blood cell

16.1 Introduction

Infections of the spine have a large spectrum of clinical manifestations; they can affect the vertebrae, the intervertebral disks, the spinal canal, and the paravertebral soft tissues and structures. Spinal canal infections may include the epidural space (epidural abscesses), the meninges (meningitis), the subdural space (subdural abscesses), and the spinal cord (intramedullary abscesses) [1, 2].

Spinal tuberculosis (TB) in human skeletons dates back to the Iron Age [3]. The first spinal fusion was performed in 1911 by Dr. R. Hibbs in a patient with spinal TB to prevent further progression

M. Turgut et al. (eds.), *Tuberculosis of the Central Nervous System*,
DOI 10.1007/978-3-319-50712-5_16

of the spinal curvature [4]; since then, it is an interesting fact that spine surgery was developed as an effort to treat vertebral TB. TB of the central nervous system (CNS) affects about 10% of patients. Non-osseous tuberculomas (extradural, intradural extramedullary, and intramedullary) are rare manifestations of spinal TB; approximately two thirds of them are extradural [5–8].

16.2 Pathophysiology

Spinal TB is classified into four types: Pott's spine (vertebral TB), non-osseous spinal tuberculomas, TB arachnoiditis, and tuberculous meningitis (TBM). Pott's disease is the commonest type accounting for 64% of all cases [9], while TBM is the most common TB manifestation of the CNS. CNS TB is developed in two steps [10]: First, the *Mycobacterium tuberculosis* bacilli infect the host by droplet inhalation, and a localized pulmonary infection is developed within the lungs. When infection is spread to the regional lymph nodes, the primary complex is formed. During this stage, a short but significant bacteremia is present that can seed TB bacilli to other organs. During bacteremia or shortly afterward, lesser TB lesions ("Rich's foci") are developed in the CNS. "Rich's foci" may develop in the meninges, the subpial or subependymal surface of the brain or the spinal cord, and may remain inactive for years. Second, a Rich's focus increases in size until it ruptures into the subarachnoid space causing meningitis; those Rich's foci that have developed and rupture deeper in the brain or spinal cord parenchyma cause tuberculomas or abscesses. Spinal TBM may result from the rupture of Rich's foci into the arachnoid space [11].

TB arachnoiditis accounts for approximately 20% of spinal TB cases [8, 12]. It was previously termed adhesive spinal arachnoiditis or chronic adhesive arachnoiditis and involves the arachnoid lining alongside the spinal cord [8, 12]. Three pathophysiological mechanisms have been suggested: (1) downward extension of intracranial TBM (the most common), (2) a TB lesion primarily arising in the spinal meninges, and (3) transdural extension of TB spondylitis [13]. The thoracic spine and the lumbar and the cervical spines are the most frequently affected spinal sections. Macroscopically, gross granulomatous exudate extends over several segments surrounding without infiltrating the spinal cord and nerve roots. Microscopically, areas of granulomatous inflammation, caseation, tubercles, and fibrous tissue formation are noted. The subdural exudate is accompanied by arterial and venous inflammation (vasculitis) that may result in spinal cord infarction and subsequently damage the neuronal structures [11, 13].

Spinal cord TB may occur in the form of tuberculomas. Dastur et al. [5] studied 74 cases of TB paraplegic patients without evidence of Pott's disease; they reported extradural tuberculomas in 64% of the patients, intradural extramedullary and intramedullary lesions in 8% of the patients, each, and arachnoid lesions with dural involvement in the remaining patients. Most lesions were intracranial, with a cranial to spinal lesions ratio equal to an average of 30:1 [14]. Interestingly, spinal cord tuberculomas may increase in size during anti-TB chemotherapy [11].

Extradural tuberculomas are the most common spinal tuberculomas (approximately 65%), although their pathogenesis is unclear [5]. They are more common in young adults of both sexes, mainly in developing countries [15]. Most patients with extradural tuberculomas do not have evidence of TB infection elsewhere in the body; therefore, it has been suggested that these tuberculomas may represent hematogenous dissemination during primary infection with localization at the epidural space, probably after mild trauma as a predisposing factor [15].

Intramedullary tuberculomas are very rare [16]. They have been more commonly reported at the cervical and thoracic spine, probably due to proximity to the cerebellum. They occur more often in young adults, but there have been also a few cases of children [9, 17, 18]. Multiple sites in the spinal cord may be affected. A ratio of intramedullary to intracerebral tuberculomas of approximately 1:42 has been reported [16]. Intramedullary tuberculomas develop more commonly by hematogenous dissemination or cerebrospinal fluid (CSF) infection, and rarely by the local spread of spinal TB [16]. Exceptionally, paradoxical development or enlargement of intramedullary tuberculomas during anti-TB chemotherapy may occur [19, 20]. Spinal cord compression from intramedullary tuberculomas should also be considered in patients with a history of TB, human immunodeficiency virus infections, and poor socioeconomic status [21, 22].

Intradural extramedullary tuberculomas are usually developed in patients with TBM [23, 24], in contrast to intramedullary tuberculomas that are associated with pulmonary TB [6, 25]. They occur more common in the thoracic spine, in young patients of both genders, and rarely in children [13, 26–28]. An ongoing inflammation in the arachnoid membrane resulting in the development of tuberculomas within 3 weeks to 1 year after initiation of chemotherapy has been reported [6, 29]; probably, this response is due to an interaction between the host immune reaction and mycobacterial products [29]. Intradural extramedullary tuberculomas, probably resulting by a similar inflammatory immunosuppression process, have been reported in approximately 36% of patients with TB and acquired immunodeficiency syndrome (AIDS) during antiretroviral therapy [30]. There have been sparse references of intradural extramedullary tuberculoma cases with concurrent syringomyelia [6, 24, 31]. Some cases of en plaque intradural extramedullary tuberculomas mimicking en plaque meningiomas have also been reported [32–35].

16.3 Presentation

In patients with Pott's disease, neurological defects occur from medullary and radicular inflammation and rarely by compression from an abscess or a tuberculoma [36]. The patients with acute spinal meningitis present with fever, headache, and radicular pain which are signs and symptoms of myelopathy. The patients with chronic localized disease present with progressive spinal cord compression mimicking a spinal cord tumor [11].

TB arachnoiditis commonly presents with thoracic, followed by lumbar and cervical myeloradiculopathy [13]. Often, there is vasculitis, with periarteritis and occlusion of small vessels, and neuronal damage by direct compression or by ischemia. TB arachnoiditis lesions may be focal, multifocal, or diffuse. CSF changes are similar to chronic meningitis; glucose values may be normal and lumbar tap may be dry [11].

The clinical features of spinal tuberculomas are similar to those of extramedullary or intramedullary tumors, although acute deterioration may occur [7, 8, 26, 36–38]. A spinal cord tuberculoma may involve solely to the nervous system; therefore, patients may not report a history of TBM. In the sequel, a minor trauma can produce the symptoms, due to initiation of the inflammation and immune response [26, 36, 37]. The most commonly reported presenting symptoms for extradural tuberculomas are radicular leg pain, numbness, and weakness. Intramedullary and intradural extramedullary tuberculomas may also present with subacute spinal cord compression with motor and sensory deficits related to the level of the lesion, such as back pain, progressive muscle weakness, paresthesia, bladder and bowel dysfunction, and spastic or flaccid paraplegia [7, 8, 38]. Nevertheless, the symptoms of spinal cord compression are mainly attributed to ischemia and edema rather than direct pressure of the granulomas. Due to the relevance of intramedullary tuberculomas and pulmonary TB, these patients should be examined for pulmonary or extrapulmonary TB and TBM in patients with intradural extramedullary tuberculomas.

Wadia and Dastur [39] and others [40, 41] suggested that the term TB radiculomyelitis (TBRM) for cases previously classified as arachnoiditis, intradural spinal tuberculoma or granuloma, and spinal cord complications of TBM. The clinical features are not pathognomonic and include radicular pain, paresthesias, bladder disturbance, muscle wasting, and subacute paraparesis progressing over a time period of 1–2 months. Subsequently, usually within a few days from disease onset, paralysis may occur. In these cases, absent deep tendon reflexes with flaccidity in the lower limbs and extensor plantar response may be observed. Secondary TBRM may occur at the acute stage or in any time period after the initial TBM infection [40, 41].

16.4 Laboratory

Helpful but nondiagnostic laboratory studies include an elevated WBC count and ESR. In most patients, CSF analysis shows an active inflammatory response with pleocytosis (lymphocytosis), hypoglycorrhachia, and increased protein values probably because of CSF flow blockade. These alterations could persist despite CSF sterilization. The diagnosis of dura mater tuberculoma should be documented with imaging studies, CSF protein analysis from purified derivative reactivity, and histopathologic examination.

16.5 Imaging

CT and MRI are critical for the diagnosis of spinal cord TB; MRI is the imaging modality of choice that has replaced myelography in modern era [11, 40, 42]. MRI with pre- and post-gadolinium T1-weighted sagittal and axial views is the most sensitive method for imaging evaluation of patients with an assumptive diagnosis of intraspinal TB, regardless of the stage of the disease [40, 42].

Typical MRI findings of spinal TBM include loculation and obliteration of the subarachnoid space, loss of spinal cord outline in the cervicothoracic region, matting of lumbar nerve roots, and possible syrinx formation [11]. MRI findings of TBRM are similar. Even if enhanced MRI images appear normal, gadolinium contrast administration usually shows nodular, thick, linear intradural enhancement, often completely filling the subarachnoid space. In the chronic disease, gadolinium contrast MRI may not show enhancement, even if images without contrast medium show signs of arachnoiditis. Syrinx formation may be evident in late cases due to chronic arachnoiditis and spinal cord infarction. Tuberculomas are shown as defined lesions with varying degrees of peripheral gadolinium enhancement, with or without compression of the spinal cord. MRI findings of multiple peripherally enhancing lesions after contrast administration should be aware toward the diagnosis of spinal TB lesions [40–42].

Based on the stage and imaging features, three types of tuberculomas have been reported including non-caseating granuloma, caseating granuloma with a solid center, and caseating granuloma with liquid center [7, 16]. In early stages, tuberculomas are characterized by severe inflammation, poor formation of the gel capsule, and severe perilesional edema. During this stage, tuberculomas appear isointense in T1- and T2-weighted MRI images with gadolinium contrast enhancement. As the gel content of the tuberculomas increases, the perilesional edema decreases or may disappear. In this setting, T1-weighted MRI images show isointense signal intensity, and T2-weighted MRI images show low signal intensity or appear isointense. At caseation, T2-weighted MRI images show a typical "target sign" that ranges from the low signal target to the high signal rim. The caseous substance forms the target center, whereas the peripheral infective granulation tissues form the high signal rim (Fig. 16.1) [7, 16].

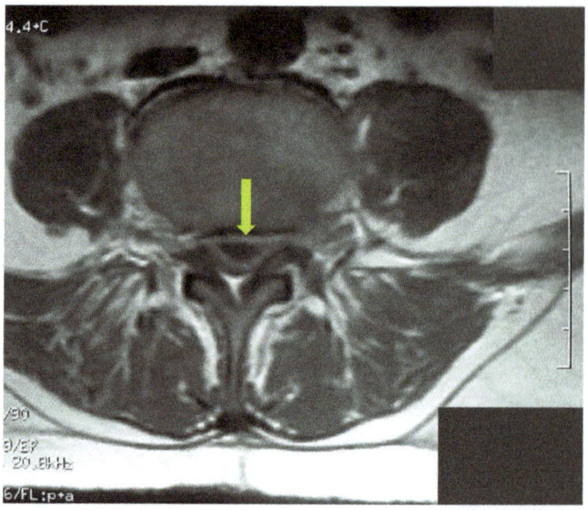

Fig. 16.1 Axial spinal T1-weighted MRI following gadolinium administration shows ring enhancement of an anterior epidural TB abscess at L3-vertebral level (*arrow*) without adjacent bony lesions. This 52-year-old male patient presented with paraparesis and a3-month history of progressive low-back pain radiating to the left leg

The differential diagnosis based on imaging should include tumors, inflammatory or demyelinating diseases, and vascular and granulomatous lesions. If MRI findings are typical for tuberculomas and the patients have systemic TB, spinal tuberculomas are the most probable diagnosis. However, if MRI findings are not typical for tuberculomas and the patients do not have systemic TB, the diagnosis may be extremely difficult to establish, and a high suspicion index is required [8].

According to the World Health Organization [43], "extrapulmonary TB refers to a case of TB involving organs other than the lungs, e.g. pleura, lymph nodes, abdomen, genitourinary tract, skin, joints and bones, meninges. The diagnosis should be based on at least one specimen with confirmed *M. tuberculosis* or histological or strong clinical evidence consistent with active extrapulmonary TB, followed by a decision by a clinician to treat with a full course of TB chemotherapy."

16.6 Treatment

Pulmonary and extrapulmonary TB disease should be treated with the same antibiotic schemes. Because of a high risk of disability and mortality, some infectious disease specialists recommend 9–12 months of anti-TB treatment for TBM; in these cases, unless drug resistance is suspected, adjuvant corticosteroid treatment is recommended, and ethambutol (EMB) should be replaced by streptomycin (STR) [43–46]. The standard 6-month treatment regimens for new patients are 2 months of INH, RIF, PZA, and EMB, followed by 4 months of INH and RIF that can be extended to 7–10 months of treatment for TB of CNS [43].

For patients with spinal arachnoiditis, surgical decompression has been recommended [36]; however, other studies reported that, since arachnoiditis is diffuse, surgery may not be useful [13, 47, 48]. Anti-TB combination therapy should be initiated as soon as the diagnosis is established. Adjuvant medical treatments may also be administered; intrathecal hyaluronidase, an enzyme that hydrolyses the glucosaminidic bonds of hyaluronic acid and other mucopolysaccharides of the ground substance has been reported for the adjuvant treatment of patients who develop spinal arachnoiditis during therapy with systemic steroids and anti-TB drugs [13, 47, 48]. Adjuvant administration of high-dose corticosteroids orally or, rarely, via the intrathecal route for 3–6 weeks has also been reported beneficial for the patients with spinal arachnoiditis [13, 36, 40, 48, 49]. Although the exact mechanism is unclear, steroids most likely suppress the progressive inflammatory process often seen in patients with TBM despite adequate anti-TB therapy [36]. The reduction of CSF protein and globulin levels after the first month of treatment and increase of CSF glucose values in patients treated with steroids compared to the respective of the patients not treated has also been reported [50]. Decompressive laminectomy should be considered in cases where histological diagnosis is necessary, or there is evidence of spinal cord compression with neurological deficit or spinal instability [13, 36, 40, 48–50].

Because of their rare incidence, there are no specific guidelines for the treatment of patients with epidural tuberculomas. Mantzoros et al. [15] reviewed 23 patients who underwent decompressive laminectomy, with ten patients receiving additional anti-TB chemotherapy; the majority of their patients experienced complete recovery [15]. In patients with epidural tuberculomas, surgical resection is indicated when myelopathic symptoms occur, or a histological diagnosis is necessary. Epidural abscesses are mainly of pyogenic origin and associated to spondylitis. They are considered as an indication for urgent surgical treatment, while TB abscesses are nonurgent surgical indication [2].

In patients with intradural extramedullary tuberculomas, medical therapy alone is probably not successful; surgical resection of the tuberculomas followed by anti-TB chemotherapy should be considered for optimal outcome with an improvement of the neurological symptoms and deficits of the patients [6, 25, 36].

Controversy also exists for the treatment of patients with intramedullary spinal tuberculomas; some authors recommended anti-TB therapy alone as appropriate management [51], while others recommended neurosurgical treatment for all symptomatic patients and for those who experience acute or progressive neurological deficits and/or poor response to anti-TB agents [7, 52–54].

Surgical excision of the lesion, combined with anti-TB chemotherapy, has been proved an efficient method of treatment, when properly applied [17, 21, 55–57]. In general, surgical treatment is indicated in patients with (1) uncertain diagnosis, (2) poor response to medical management, (3) neurological deterioration during medical treatment, and (4) progressive enlargement of the lesions on follow-up MRI [7, 54].

In patients with localized arachnoiditis and spinal cord compression, surgical decompression can effectively excise the lesion and provide tissue for histological examination [41]; however, a more extensive adhesive disease usually progresses despite surgical treatment [40]. Surgical excision of a spinal cord tuberculoma has been associated with a higher possibility for a successful outcome if myelopathic symptoms occur [38]. The prognosis for neurological improvement is good with a prompt surgical excision and appropriate anti-TB medication, including EMB, INH, RIF, STR, and/or PZA [35]. Additionally, neurological improvement is more likely to occur if surgical treatment is performed before irreversible spinal cord damage occurs [7].

In the presence of spinal cord TB compression, corticosteroids may arrest the progression of neurological deficits. Most investigators consider that steroids should be administered for cerebral edema, spinal block [36, 40], and enlargement of intramedullary and intradural extramedullary tuberculomas during anti-TB chemotherapy [36]. A possible explanation for this paradoxical enlargement of tuberculomas during chemotherapy is the recovery of patients' delayed hypersensitivity response and increase of response to mycobacterial antigens released after anti-TB treatment initiation [40]. It has also been observed that there is a reduction of patients' mortality in the acute stage of TBM, and a more rapid normalization of WBC counts in CSF and protein content and ESR decreases with the administration of steroids [40].

Table 16.1 Summary of most recent reported cases of intradural extramedullary tuberculomas from the literature

Authors	Age (years)	Gender	Site	TBM	Time from anti-TB medication to surgery	Outcome
Mirzai [32]	40	M	C6-T1	No	NS	Improvement
Luo and Pino [23]	51	M	T3	No	4 months	Improvement
Muthukumar and Sureshkumar [24]	27	F	T11	Yes	8 months	Poor (paraparesis)
Muthukumar et al. [33]	21	M	T6–12	Yes	3 months	Improvement
Kumar et al. [28]	11	F	T11–12	Yes	18 months	Poor (paraparesis)
Takahashi et al. [29]	46	F	T2–3	Yes	2 months	Improvement
Ozek et al. [34]	18	F	T1–9	Yes	6 months	Improvement
Shim et al. [35]	24	M	T2–6	Yes	5 weeks	Improvement
Duan and Mao [27]	14	F	T1–3	Yes	2 months	Improvement
Gul et al. [31]	21	M	T11–12, L1	Yes	3 months	Improvement
Sohn et al. [38]	45	M	T3–7	No	NS	Improvement
Jeong and Kwon [6]	31	F	T1–12	Yes	7 months	Improvement

Abbreviations: *F* female, *M* male, *NS* not stated, *TB* tuberculosis, *TBM* tuberculous meningitis

Table 16.2 Summary of reported cases of intramedullary tuberculomas

Authors	Age (years)	Gender	Site	Time to surgery	Treatment	Outcome
Rhoton et al. [57]	65	M	C3–6	2 months	Excision	Recurrence
Jena et al. [51]	25	F	C2–6	NA	M edication	Improvement
	23	M	C2-T1	NA	Medication	Improvement
Citow and Ammirati [19]	31	M	T11	6 weeks	Excision	Improvement
Lin et al. [20]	36	M	T6–12	5 months	Partial excision	Improvement
Gupta et al. [55]	35	M	T10–11	6 months	Excision	Improvement
	27	M	Conus medullaris	18 months	Not described	Improvement
Ratliff and Connolly [22]	46	F	T10–11	18 months	Biopsy	Improvement
Kayaoglu et al. [21]	65	M	C4	10 weeks	Excision	Improvement
Rao [9]	25	F	T11–12	NA	Medication	Improvement
	16	F	C5–7	NA	Medication	Improvement
	14	M	C5–6, T6	NA	Medication	Improvement
	16	M	C1–6	NA	Medication	Improvement
Nomura et al. [18]	2	F	T6–10	12 months	Partial excision	Improvement
Miyamoto et al. [12]	71	M	C2, T10-L2	6 months	Excision	Improvement
Jaiswal et al. [17]	29	F	T12-L1	NA	Excision	Improvement
	1.5	M	T8–10		Excision	Improvement
	24	M	T3–4		Excision	Improvement
	35	F	T5–6		Excision	Improvement
	45	M	T4–5		Excision	Improvement
	38	M	T6-T9		Excision	Improvement at 3 months
	10	M	L1		Excision	Improvement
	42	M	C3–6		Excision	Partial improvement
	28	F	T5–8		Medication	Improvement
	37	F	L1		Medication	Improvement
	20	M	T12-L1		Medication	Improvement
Liu et al. [56]	28	M	T11	3 weeks	Excision	Improvement

Abbreviations: *F* female, *M* male, *NA* not available

Conclusion

Extradural and intradural extramedullary and intramedullary tuberculomas are rare manifestations of spinal TB. MRI is the imaging modality of choice for the diagnosis. Because of the rarity of the disease, there are no specific guidelines for the treatment of patients. Surgical treatment may be indicated and long-term anti-TB chemotherapy is recommended (Tables 16.1 and 16.2).

References

1. Kim MS, Ju CI, Kim SW, Lee HY (2012) Recurrent bacterial meningitis accompanied by a spinal intramedullary abscess. J Korean Neurosurg Soc 51:380–382
2. Mavrogenis AF, Igoumenou V, Tsiavos K, Megaloikonomos P, Panagopoulos GN, Vottis C, Giannitsioti E, Papadopoulos A, Soultanis KC (2016) When and how to operate on spondylodiscitis: a report of 13 patients. Eur J Orthop Surg Traumatol 26:31–40

3. Tayles N, Buckley HR (2004) Leprosy and tuberculosis in Iron Age Southeast Asia? Am J Phys Anthropol 125:239–256
4. Hibbs RA (2007) An operation for progressive spinal deformities: a preliminary report of three cases from the service of the orthopaedic hospital. 1911. Clin Orthop Relat Res 460:17–20
5. Dastur HM (1983) Diagnosis and neurosurgical treatment of tuberculous disease of the CNS. Neurosurg Rev 6:111–117
6. Jeong DK, Kwon YM (2015) Intradural extramedullary tuberculoma of the spinal cord following tuberculous meningitis. Korean J Spine 12:107–110
7. Lee DY, Kim SP, Kim IS (2015) Coexistence of spinal intramedullary tuberculoma and multiple intracranial tuberculomas. Korean J Spine 12:99–102
8. Mishra SS, Das D, Das S, Mohanta I, Tripathy SR (2015) Spinal cord compression due to primary intramedullary tuberculoma of the spinal cord presenting as paraplegia: a case report and literature review. Surg Neurol Int 6:42
9. Rao GP (2000) Spinal intramedullary tuberculous lesion: medical management. Report of four cases. J Neurosurg 93:137–141
10. Rich AR, McCordock HA (1933) The pathogenesis of tuberculous meningitis. Bull Johns Hopkins Hosp 52:5–37
11. Garg RK (1999) Tuberculosis of the central nervous system. Postgrad Med J 75:133–140
12. Miyamoto J, Sasajima H, Owada K, Odake G, Mineura K (2003) Spinal intramedullary tuberculoma requiring surgical treatment–case report. Neurol Med Chir (Tokyo) 43:567–571
13. Poon TL, Ho WS, Pang KY, Wong CK (2003) Tuberculous meningitis with spinal tuberculous arachnoiditis. Hong Kong Med J 9:59–61
14. Arora B, Sridhar E, Muzumdar D, Jalali R, Munshi A (2010) Spinal tuberculoma in a patient with spinal myxopapillary ependymoma. J Can Res Ther 6:215–217
15. Mantzoros CS, Brown PD, Dembry L (1993) Extraosseous epidural tuberculoma: case report and review. Clin Infect Dis 17:1032–1036
16. Lu M (2010) Imaging diagnosis of spinal intramedullary tuberculoma: case reports and literature review. J Spinal Cord Med 33:159–162
17. Jaiswal M, Gandhi A, Sharma A, Mittal RS (2015) Experiences and conceptualisation of spinal intramedullary tuberculoma management. Korean J Spine 12:5–11
18. Nomura S, Akimura T, Kitahara T, Nogami K, Suzuki M (2001) Surgery for expansion of spinal tuberculoma during antituberculous chemotherapy: a case report. Pediatr Neurosurg 35:153–157
19. Citow JS, Ammirati M (1994) Intramedullary tuberculoma of the spinal cord: case report. Neurosurgery 35:327–330
20. Lin SK, Wu T, Wai YY (1994) Intramedullary spinal tuberculomas during treatment of tuberculous meningitis. Clin Neurol Neurosurg 96:71–78
21. Kayaoglu CR, Tuzun Y, Boga Z, Erdogan F, Gorguner M, Aydin IH (2000) Intramedullary spinal tuberculoma: a case report. Spine (Phila Pa 1976) 25:2265–2268
22. Ratliff JK, Connolly ES (1999) Intramedullary tuberculoma of the spinal cord. Case report and review of the literature. J Neurosurg 90:125–128
23. Luo L, Pino J (2006) An intradural extramedullary tuberculoma of the spinal cord in a non-HIV-infected patient: case report and review of the literature. Lung 184:187–193
24. Muthukumar N, Sureshkumar V (2007) Concurrent syringomyelia and intradural extramedullary tuberculoma as late complications of tuberculous meningitis. J Clin Neurosci 14:1225–1230
25. Turgut M, Özcan OE, Özgen T, Bertan V (1993) Intradural extramedullary tuberculoma of the spinal cord – a case report. Zentralbl Neurochir 54:197–199
26. Compton JS, Dorsch NW (1984) Intradural extramedullary tuberculoma of the cervical spine. Case report. J Neurosurg 60:200–203
27. Duan J, Mao B (2010) Unusual intradural extramedullary tuberculoma of the spinal cord in childhood. Neurol India 58:738–739
28. Kumar R, Kasliwal MK, Srivastava R, Sharma BS (2007) Tuberculoma presenting as an intradural extramedullary lesion. Pediatr Neurosurg 43:541–543
29. Takahashi H, Ito S, Kojima S, Tanno T, Hattori T (2008) Intradural extramedullary tuberculoma of the thoracic spine: paradoxical response to antituberculous therapy. Intern Med 47:797–798
30. Narita M, Ashkin D, Hollender ES, Pitchenik AE (1998) Paradoxical worsening of tuberculosis following antiretroviral therapy in patients with AIDS. Am J Respir Crit Care Med 158:157–161
31. Gul S, Celebi G, Kalayci M, Acikgoz B (2010) Syringomyelia and intradural extramedullary tuberculoma of the spinal cord as a late complication of tuberculous meningitis. Turk Neurosurg 20:561–565
32. Mirzai H (2005) Tuberculoma of the cervical spinal canal mimicking en plaque meningioma. J Spinal Disord Tech 18:197–199
33. Muthukumar N, Sureshkumar V, Ramesh VG (2007) En plaque intradural extramedullary spinal tuberculoma and concurrent intracranial tuberculomas: paradoxical response to antituberculous therapy. Case report. J Neurosurg Spine 6:169–173
34. Ozek E, Iplikcıoglu AC, Erdal M (2009) Intradural extramedullary tuberculoma mimicking en plaque meningioma. Neurol India 57:211–212
35. Shim DW, Oh SK, Kim TK, Chae SU (2010) Intradural extramedullary tuberculoma mimicking en plaque meningioma. Clin Orthop Surg 2:260–263
36. Hristea A, Constantinescu RV, Exergian F, Arama V, Besleaga M, Tanasescu R (2008) Paraplegia due to nonosseous spinal tuberculosis: report of three cases and review of the literature. Int J Infect Dis 12:425–429
37. Kim MS, Kim KJ, Chung CK, Kim HJ (2000) Intradural extramedullary tuberculoma of the spinal cord: a case report. J Korean Med Sci 15:368–370

38. Sohn S, Jin YJ, Kim KJ, Kim HJ (2011) Long-term sequela of intradural extramedullary tuberculoma in the thoracic dorsal spinal cord: case report and review of the literature. Korean J Spine 8:295–299
39. Wadia NH, Dastur DK (1969) Spinal meningitides with radiculo-myelopathy. 1. Clinical and radiological features. J Neurol Sci 8:239–260
40. Hernández-Albújar S, Arribas JR, Royo A, González-García JJ, Peña JM, Vázquez JJ (2000) Tuberculous radiculomyelitis complicating tuberculous meningitis: case report and review. Clin Infect Dis 30:915–921
41. Sree Harsha CK, Shetty AP, Rajasekaran S (2006) Intradural spinal tuberculosis in the absence of vertebral or meningeal tuberculosis: a case report. J Orthop Surg (Hong Kong) 14:71–75
42. Gupta RK, Gupta S, Kumar S, Kohli A, Misra UK, Gujral RB (1994) MRI in intraspinal tuberculosis. Neuroradiology 36:39–43
43. WHO (2010) Treatment of tuberculosis: guidelines, 4th edn. World Health Organization, Geneva
44. American Thoracic Society, CDC, Infectious Diseases Society of America (2003) Treatment of tuberculosis. MMWR Recomm Rep 52(RR-11):1–77
45. National Collaborating Centre for Chronic Conditions (2006) Tuberculosis: clinical diagnosis and management of tuberculosis, and measures for its prevention and control. Royal College of Physicians/NICE (National Institute for Health and Clinical Excellence), London
46. Thwaites GE, Nguyen DB, Nguyen HD, Hoang TQ, Do TT, Nguyen TC, Nguyen QH, Nguyen TT, Nguyen NH, Nguyen TN, Nguyen NL, Nguyen HD, Vu NT, Cao HH, Tran TH, Pham PM, Nguyen TD, Stepniewska K, White NJ, Tran TH, Farrar JJ (2004) Dexamethasone for the treatment of tuberculous meningitis in adolescents and adults. N Engl J Med 351:1741–1751
47. Bhagwati SN, George K (1986) Use of intrathecal hyaluronidase in the management of tuberculous meningitis with hydrocephalus. Childs Nerv Syst 2:20–25
48. Gourie-Devi M, Satishchandra P (1991) Hyaluronidase as an adjuvant in the management of tuberculous spinal arachnoiditis. J Neurol Sci 102:105–111
49. Freilich D, Swash M (1979) Diagnosis and management of tuberculous paraplegia with special reference to tuberculous radiculomyelitis. J Neurol Neurosurg Psychiatry 42:12–18
50. Schoeman JF, Elshof JW, Laubscher JA, Janse van Rensburg A, Donald PR (2001) The effect of adjuvant steroid treatment on serial cerebrospinal fluid changes in tuberculous meningitis. Ann Trop Paediatr 21:299–305
51. Jena A, Banerji AK, Tripathi RP, Gulati PK, Jain RK, Khushu S, Sapra ML (1991) Demonstration of intramedullary tuberculomas by magnetic resonance imaging: a report of two cases. Br J Radiol 64:555–557
52. Li H, You C, Yang Y, He M, Cai B, Wang X, Ju Y (2006) Intramedullary spinal tuberculoma: report of three cases. Surg Neurol 65:185–188
53. Muthukumar N, Venkatesh G, Senthilbabu S, Rajbaskar R (2006) Surgery for intramedullary tuberculoma of the spinal cord: report of 2 cases. Surg Neurol 66:69–74
54. Turgut M (2007) Re: Surgery for intramedullary tuberculoma of the spinal cord: report of 2 cases (Muthukumar et al. SurgNeurol 2006;66: 69–74). Surg Neurol 67:654–656
55. Gupta VK, Sharma BS, Khosla VK (1995) Intramedullary tuberculoma: report of two cases with MRI findings. Surg Neurol 44:241–244
56. Liu J, Zhang H, He B, Wang B, Niu X, Hao D (2016) Intramedullary tuberculoma combined with abscess: case report and literature review. World Neurosurg 89:e1–e4
57. Rhoton EL, Ballinger WE Jr, Quisling R, Sypert GW (1988) Intramedullary spinal tuberculoma. Neurosurgery 22:733–736

Spinal Subdural Space

17

Ahmet T. Turgut, Elif Karadeli, Pelin Demir, Mehmet Turgut, and Ali Akhaddar

Contents

A.T. Turgut, MD (✉)
Department of Radiology, Hacettepe University Faculty of Medicine, 06100 Ankara, Turkey
e-mail: ahmettuncayturgut@yahoo.com

E. Karadeli, MD
Department of Radiology, Baskent University, School of Medicine, Dr. Turgut Noyan Medical and Research Center, Adana, Turkey
e-mail: elifkaradeli@gmail.com

P. Demir, MD
Department of Radiology, Numune Training and Research Hospital, Ankara, Turkey
e-mail: drrpelindemir6@hotmail.com

M. Turgut, MD, PhD
Department of Neurosurgery, Adnan Menderes University School of Medicine, Aydın, Turkey
e-mail: drmturgut@yahoo.com

A. Akhaddar, MD, IFAANS
Department of Neurosurgery, Avicenne Military Hospital of Marrakech, Mohammed V University in Rabat, Rabat, Morocco
e-mail: akhaddar@hotmail.fr

Abbreviations

AIDS	Acquired immuno deficiency syndrome
CNS	Central nervous system
CRP	C-reactive protein
CT	Computed tomography
ESR	Erythrocyte sedimentation rate
MRI	Magnetic resonance imaging
TB	Tuberculosis
WBC	White blood cell count

17.1 Introduction

Approximately 2% of all tuberculosis (TB) cases are spine TB. Anatomically, the sites of involvement are vertebral body, intervertebral disk space, paravertebral soft tissue, and epidural and subdural space. Multiple skip lesions may occur infrequently [1–3]. There are three routes for the development of spinal TB. Hematogenous route, referring to the spread from an origin outside the central nervous system (CNS) via blood stream, is the most common route of infection resulting in radiculo-myelopathy. The second route involves secondary extension caudally from TB meningoencephalitis of the brain. The last route is associated with secondary intraspinal extension from osteoarticular or discal TB [4].

M. Turgut et al. (eds.), *Tuberculosis of the Central Nervous System*,
DOI 10.1007/978-3-319-50712-5_17

17.2 Etiology

The involvement of subdural space by spinal TB is extremely rare. This involvement may present as spinal subdural abscess, spinal subdural empyema, intramedullary and extramedullary tuberculoma, infected spinal subdural cyst, infectious spinal subdural cyst, or arachnoiditis. Sometimes, proper diagnosis with imaging methods may be difficult, and the aforementioned atypical forms of involvement can lead to misdiagnosis and neurological problems, and paraplegia may be seen [5–16]. Anatomically, the subdural space is described as a potential cavity between the dura and arachnoid mater. Radiologically it can been visualized by contrast injection, and epidural catheters have been introduced using radiological techniques [17].

Spinal subdural abscess, which is quite rare, corresponds to a loculated infection between the outermost layer of the meninges, namely, the dura and the arachnoid. Historically, the first case of an adult with a spinal subdural abscess has been reported by Otto Sittig in 1927 [18–20]. There are a few predisposing conditions for the development of spinal subdural infection such as an underlying diseases and impaired immune system. Among the examples of predisposing entities are diabetes mellitus, alcoholism, tumors, chronic renal failure, hemodialysis, infection with human immunodeficiency virus, anatomical abnormalities related to the spinal cord or vertebral column, degenerative joint disease, trauma, surgery, drug injection, and catheters [18–21].

The development of spinal subdural abscess is associated with some possible routes. In this regard, direct seeding of the infection into the subdural space may occur in association with laminectomy, dermal sinus tracts, and decubitus ulcers. Anatomically, the close proximity of ulcers to the sacral dural sac and filum terminale can cause a direct connection to the subdural space. Another route is direct extension from the epidural space where dura perforation during epidural catheter insertion, discography, and lumbar puncture may cause subdural empyema. Also, the contiguous spread of the infection from the epidural space to the subdural region can cause subdural empyema associated with cranial epidural abscess. The other mechanism for the spread of microorganisms involves hematogenous route. Importantly, subdural empyema has been reported after acupuncture and meningitis [22–30].

17.3 Pathogenesis, Clinical, and Radiologic Features

The low incidence of spinal subdural abscesses within the spinal dural layers is due to the absence of dural sinuses, large size of epidural space, and centripetal direction of blood flow in the spinal vasculature. Dural anatomy and perfusion of spinal cord are different from contents of the brain [31]. The most common spinal subdural abscess agents reported in the literature are *Staphylococcus aureus* and anaerobic/microaerophilic streptococci. On the other hand, the involvement of spinal subdural space by TB is extremely rare. It has been pointed out by Velissaris et al. that a total of 65 cases of spinal subdural abscesses has been reported in the literature [12]. *S. aureus*, being detected in 35 patients, has been noted to be the most common bacterial agent for the disease, whereas *Mycobacterium tuberculosis* was reported to be the causative agent in only two cases [12].

Apparently, the diagnosis of abscess should be supported by clinical, laboratory, and imaging findings. However, it is quite difficult to make a distinction between epidural and intradural abscesses both clinically and radiologically. The most common site of spinal involvement is the thoracolumbar region, though the whole spine can be affected. Clinically, back or neck pain, fever, and neurologic manifestations such as para/tetra paresis, bladder dysfunction, impaired rectal tone, and disturbances of consciousness may be presumptive for the diagnosis.

Additionally, radicular chest or abdominal pain and constant pain that worsen at night may be detected. Fever can be detected in 17% of patients with spinal TB, whereas it occurs in 48% of patients with pyogenic spondylodiscitis. On the other hand, dysphagia and torticollis may develop in the patients with cervical involvement of TB [32–35].

The most commonly used laboratory parameters for the assessment of spinal infection are erythrocyte sedimentation rate (ESR), C-reactive protein (CRP), white blood cells (WBC). Increased ESR and CRP values are sensitive markers of infection, though they have low specificity. In addition, they are used in the monitorization of the therapeutic response. In this regard, the return of CRP to normal values after adequate treatment is faster than that of ESR. Of all inflammatory markers, WBC count is the least useful due to its low sensitivity. Furthermore, blood and urine cultures should be obtained prior to antibiotic treatment if there is suspicion for spinal infection. Typically, the microbiologic analysis should include aerobic, anaerobic, fungal, and mycobacterial tests and cultures [36–39].

As a diagnostic interventional tool, percutaneous computed tomography (CT)-guided needle biopsy can be used for revealing the etiology of spinal infection. The specimens should be evaluated with microbiological analysis, such as gram smear, aerobic and anaerobic cultures, and fungal culture particularly for TB infections, acid-fast bacilli smear, polymerase chain reaction, and TB culture [40]. *M. tuberculosis* grows slowly (6–8 weeks), and the use of interferon-gamma release assays measured from whole blood plasma provides faster diagnosis in less than 24 h [41, 42]. Histopathologic analysis is required for distinguishing pyogenic diseases from granulomatous entities, particularly in cases with suspicion of malignancy [43–46].

Cross-sectional imaging such as CT, magnetic resonance imaging (MRI), and myelo-CT can be used for the assessment of the spinal subdural abscess. In this regard, contrast-enhanced MRI is superior to CT in detecting the exact location and extension of the abscess and in diagnosing spinal cord compression [12, 27, 31, 47]. Radiologically, MRI findings of an intradural spinal abscess are usually isointense with the spinal cord in T1-weighted images and hyperintense on T2-weighted images, and it is well demarcated from the other intradural contents. On contrast-enhanced images, ring-enhancing lesion may be detected (Fig. 17.1). However, some of these characteristic features can also be detected in patients with epidural abscess, implying that the diagnosis based solely on imaging findings can be misleading [48, 49].

Tuberculoma is a firm, avascular, granulomatous mass that occurs in the brain, spinal cord, subarachnoid, subdural, or epidural space. Its size ranges from few millimeters to 4 cm. The ratio of the involvement of the spinal cord to that of the brain is 1:42. The incidence for the rare entity of intramedullary tuberculoma is two in 100,000 cases of all TB and constitutes only 0.2–5% of all CNS tuberculomas [50]. On CT, tuberculomas are rounded lesions with an irregular wall of varying thickness and appear hypodense or hyperdense. On contrast-enhanced CT, they have an intense homogenous or ring-enhancement pattern [51]. Sometimes, tuberculomas may be calcified [52].

The MRI findings of spinal tuberculoma are variable depending on different phases of tuberculoma. In early phase, the tuberculoma has equal signal intensity on T1- and T2-weighted images and is enhanced after the administration of gadolinium. This signal is associated with severe infective reactions, poor formation of the gel capsule, and severe edema. In time, the gel content of tuberculoma increases, whereas the peripheral edema is decreased; this results in equal signal intensity on T1-weighted images and isointense or hypointense appearance on T2-weighted images. Also, the rim enhancement and hypointense signal in the central region can be detected

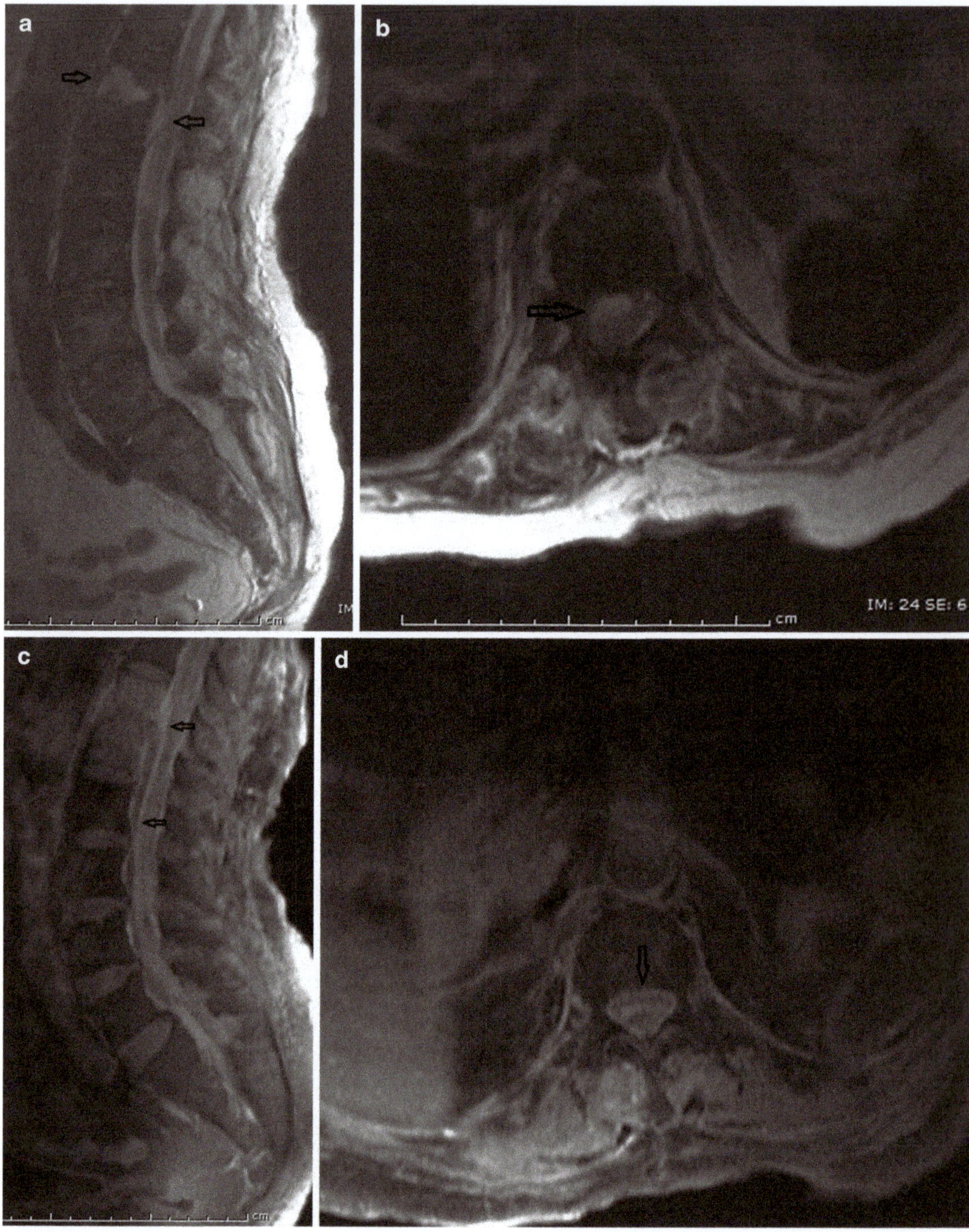

Fig. 17.1 (**a**) Sagittal T2-weighted image shows spondylodiscitis of T12–L1 level (*arrow*) and spinal subdural collection (*arrow*). (**b**) Axial T2-weighted image shows hyperintense subdural collection (*arrow*). (**c**) Sagittal fat-suppressed contrast-enhanced T1-weighted image shows ring-enhancing subdural abscesses at T12–L1 level (*arrow*). (**d**) Axial fat-suppressed contrast-enhanced T1-weighted image shows ring-enhancing subdural abscesses (*arrow*)

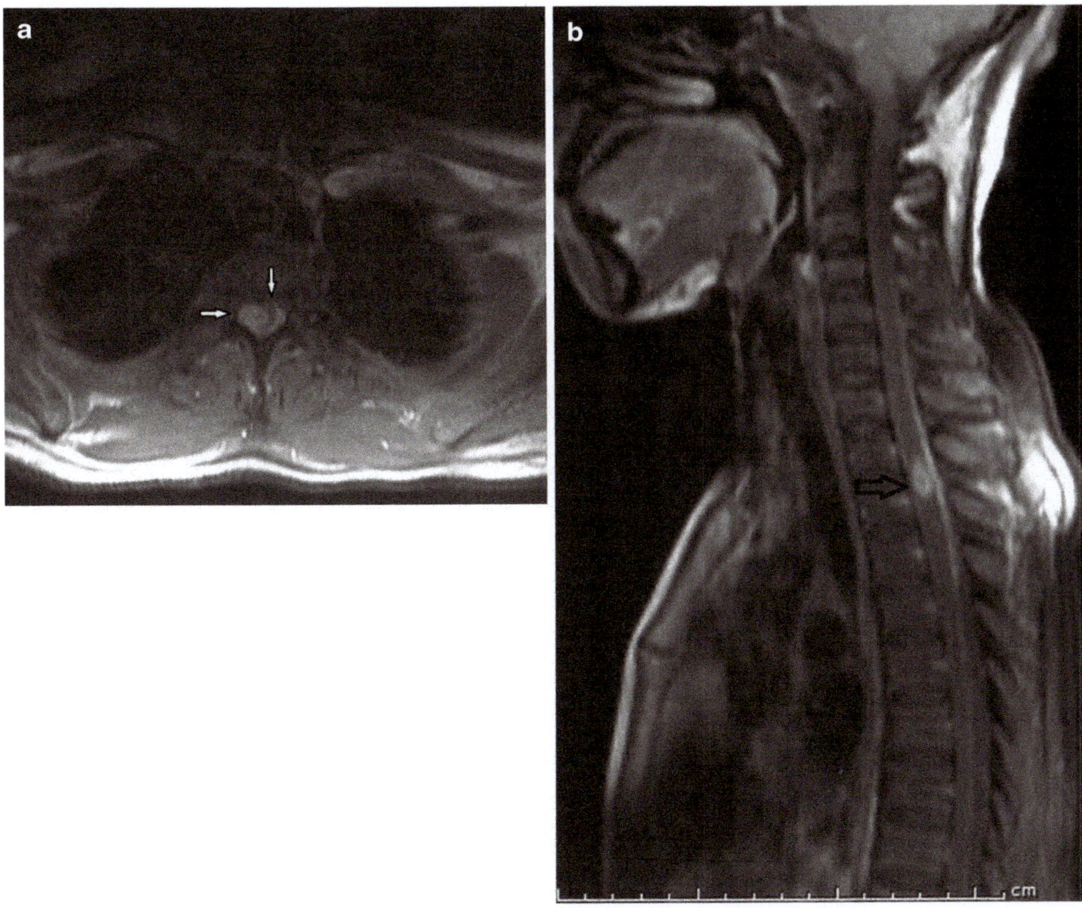

Fig. 17.2 Axial (**a**) and sagittal (**b**) fat-suppressed contrast-enhanced T1-weighted images show a contrast-enhancement lesion (tuberculoma) and displacement of spinal cord at T1–T2 level (*arrows*)

after intravenous contrast material (gadolinium) administration (Figs. 17.2 and 17.3).

On the other hand, "target sign" associated with the development of caseation is a characteristic finding on T2-weighted images. It involves a low-signal target in the central region due to the caseous material and high-signal rim due to the peripheral infective granulation tissues. The external low-signal rim is composed of collagen fibers produced by fibroblasts. The "target sign" is crucial for the differentiation of spinal tuberculoma from other intramedullary lesions. Compared with tumors, spinal tuberculoma has a sharper margin and hypointense signal on T2-weighted images and rim enhancement. Among the entities which should be considered for differential diagnosis of tuberculomas are cysticercal granulomas, pyogenic bacterial abscess, toxoplasmosis, and neoplastic lesions such as astrocytoma, metastasis, or lymphoma.

The TB involvement of spinal cord is due to the inflammatory process and immune reaction, and strangulated spinal cord occurs with progressive constrictive pial fibrosis (so-called spinal arachnoiditis). MRI findings are cerebrospinal fluid loculations, obliteration of the spinal subarachnoid space, and thickened, clumped nerve roots in the lumbar region. The enhancement of chronic fibrotic tissue is poor. Therefore, MRI with

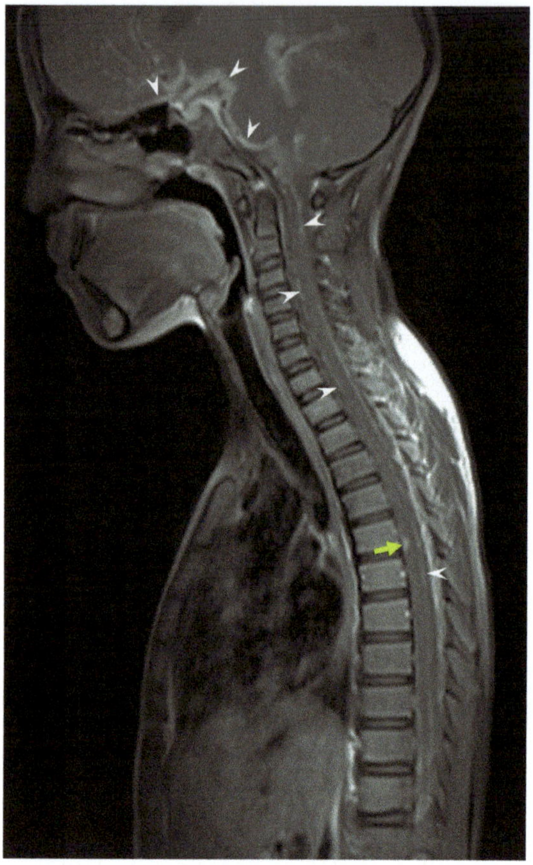

Fig. 17.3 Sagittal craniospinal T1-weighted MRI following gadolinium administration revealing diffuse enhancement of skull base and spinal meninges (*arrowhead*). Note the anterior intradural extramedullary enhancing exudate "tuberculoma" at T4–T5 level (*arrow*)

intravenous gadolinium is valuable in the diagnosis of active TB granulomatous disease and chronic fibrotic adhesion [53, 54] (Figs. 17.4 and 17.5).

17.4 Management

Anti-TB treatment is recommended for tuberculomas [55, 56]. Initially, in patients with spinal TB, anti-TB drugs should be the first choice of treatment. Accordingly, isoniazid and rifampin should be preferred, and additional drugs should be administered during the first 2 months of the treatment. The combination chemotherapy for 6–9 months has been recommended by British Medical Research Council for the treatment of TB of the thoracolumbar spine, though many other experts still recommend chemotherapy for 9–12 months [11, 57–61].

Importantly, early decompression of the spinal cord is important in patients with spinal TB. Therefore, the patients with the diagnosis of subdural TB abscess of the spine must be evaluated by the infectious disease specialist, neurosurgeon, and radiologists. Additionally, neurosurgical or orthopedic treatment is required in approximately 20% of all cases of TB. Clinically, neurological impairment can be extremely rapid, usually full paralysis occurs a few hours after the onset of neurologic deficit. Owing to the fact that the laminectomy with debridement of infected tissues should be performed as soon as possible, it represents a truly neurosurgical emergency. Sometimes, multilevel laminectomy may be necessary because of the extension of the abscess which could cause spinal instability and is associated with poor outcome. The application of surgical procedures may lead to rapid and complete recovery of neurological deficit, though the treatment is performed with drugs in most patients with TB [59, 61–64].

Conclusion

The involvement of subdural space with TB disease is extremely rare. The exact and early diagnosis and adequate treatment before the development of irreversible neurological deficits and spinal deformity are crucial for a satisfactory yield and good prognosis.

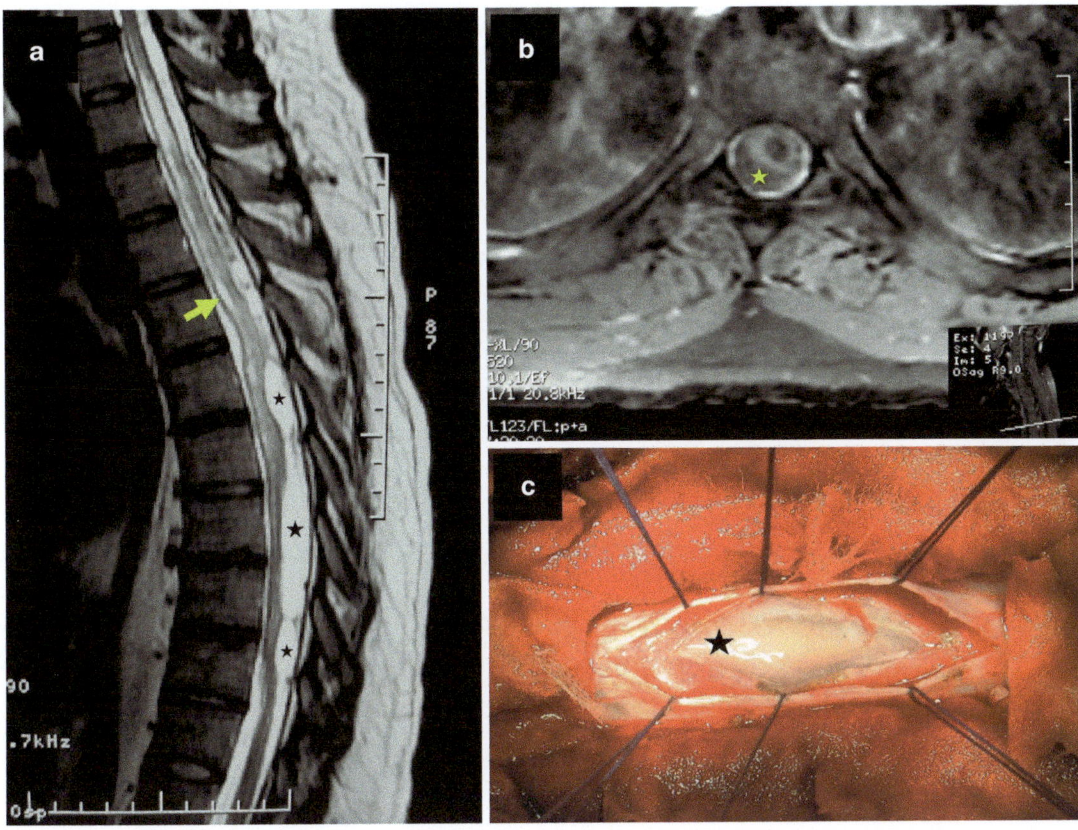

Fig. 17.4 Sagittal spinal T2-weighted MRI (**a**), axial spinal T1-weighted MRI after gadolinium injection (**b**), and operative view (posterior thoracic approach) (**c**). There is a wide posterior reconstructed arachnoid cyst (*stars*) with spinal cord compression. Note the limited intramedullary “syrinx” cavitation (*arrow*)

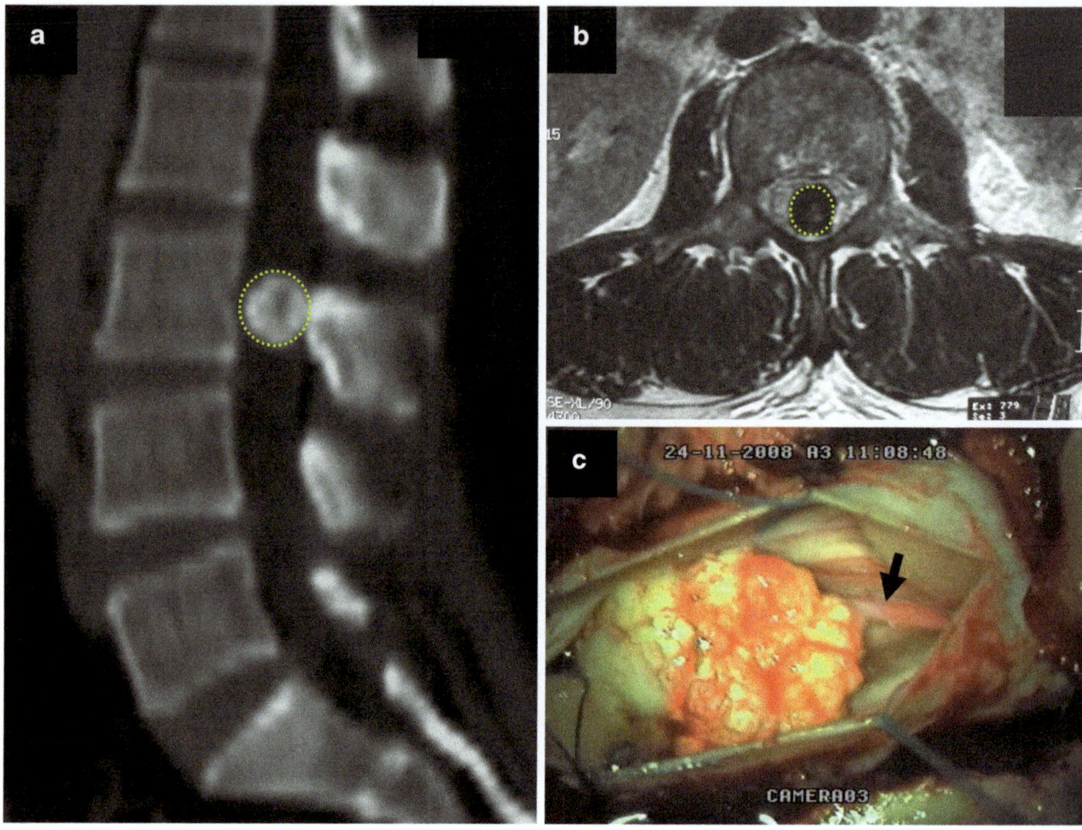

Fig. 17.5 Calcified intradural tuberculoma attached to the filum terminale at L3 spinal level. Spinal CT scan on bone windows after sagittal reconstruction (**a**), axial spinal MRI on T2-weighted image (**b**), and operative view (posterior lumbar approach) (**c**). The mass was fixed to the filum terminale (*arrow*) without dural or nerve root involvement

References

1. Tuli SM, Srivastava TP, Varma BP, Sinha GP (1967) Tuberculosis of spine. Acta Orthop Scand 38:445–458
2. Leibert E, Haralambou G (2004) Tuberculosis. In: Rom WN, Garay SM (eds) Spinal tuberculosis. Lippincott, Williams and Wilkins, Philadelphia, p 56577
3. Azzam NI, Tammawy M (1988) Tuberculous spondylitis in adults: diagnosis and treatment. Br J Neurosurg 2:85–91
4. Wadia NH, Dastur DK (1969) Spinal meningitides with radiculomyelopathy, Part 1: clinical and radiological features. J Neurol Sci 8:239–260
5. Rahman N (1980) Atypical forms of spinal tuberculosis. J Bone Joint Surg Br 162:162–165
6. Miyamoto J, Sasajima H, Owada K, Odake G, Mineura K (2003) Spinal intramedullary tuberculoma requiring surgical treatment-case report. Neurol Med Chir 43:567–571
7. Sree Harsha CK, Shetty AP, Rajasekaran S (2006) Intradural spinal tuberculosis in the absence of vertebral or meningeal tuberculosis: a case report. J Orthop Surg (Hong Kong) 14:71–75
8. Skendros P, Kamaria F, Kontopoulos V, Tsitouridis I, Sidiropoulos L (2003) Intradural, extramedullary tuberculoma of the spinal cord as a complication of tuberculous meningitis. Infection 31:115–117
9. Devi BI, Chandra S, Mongia S, Chandramouli BA, Sastry KV, Shankar SK (2002) Spinal intramedullary tuberculoma and abscess: a rare cause of paraparesis. Neurol India 50:494–496
10. Ozates M, Ozkan U, Kemaloglu S, Hosoglu S, Sari I (2000) Spinal subdural tuberculous abscess. Spinal Cord 38:56–58
11. Semlali S, Akjouj S, Chaouir S, Hanine A, Ben Ameur M (2007) Spinal subdural tuberculous abscess in a patient with tuberculous meningitis (in French). J Radiol 88:280–281
12. Velissaris D, Aretha D, Fligou F, Filos KS (2009) Spinal subdural Staphylococcus Aureus abscess: case

report and review of the literature. World J Emerg Surg 6:31
13. Alessi G, Lemmerling M, Nathoo N (2003) Combined spinal subdural tuberculous empyema and intramedullary tuberculoma in an HIV-positive patient. Eur Radiol 13:1899–1901
14. Tanriverdi T, Kizilkilic O, Hanci M, Kaynar MY, Unalan H, Oz B (2003) Atypical intradural spinal tuberculosis: report of three cases. Spinal Cord 41:403–409
15. Sarangapani A, Fallah A, Provias J, Jha N (2008) Atypical presentation of spinal tuberculosis. Can J Surg 51:E121
16. Wasay M, Arif H, Khealani B, Ahsan H (2006) Neuroimaging of tuberculous myelitis: analysis of ten cases and review of literature. J Neuroimaging 16:197–205
17. Ralph CJ, Williams MP (1996) Subdural or epidural? Confirmation with magnetic resonance imaging. Anaesthesia 51:175–177
18. Bartels RH, de Jong TR, Grotenhuis JA (1992) Spinal subdural abscess. Case report. J Neurosurg 76:307–311
19. Sorar M, Er U, Seckin H, Ozturk MH, Bavbek M (2008) Spinal subdural abscess: a rare cause of low back pain. J Clin Neurosci 15:292–294
20. Sittig O (1927) Metastatischer Rückenmarksabscess bei septi-schem Abortus. Zeitschrift für die gesamte Neurologie und Psychiatrie 107:146–151
21. Hlavin ML, Kaminski HJ, Ross JS, Ganz E (1990) Spinal epidural abscess: a ten year perspective. Neurosurgery 27:177–184
22. Wu AS, Griebel RW, Meguro K, Fourney DR (2004) Spinal subdural empyema after a dural tear. Case report. Neurosurg Focus 17:E10
23. Chen CY, Lin KL, Wang HS, Lui TN (1999) Dermoid cyst with dermal sinus tract complicated with spinal subdural abscess. Pediatr Neurol 20:157–160
24. Park SW, Yoon SH, Cho KH, Shin YS, Ahn YH (2007) Infantile lumbosacral spinal subdural abscess with sacral dermal sinus tract. Spine (Phila Pa) 32:E52–E55
25. Benzil DL, Epstein MH, Knuckey NW (1992) Intramedullary epidermoid associated with an intramedullary spinal abscess secondary to a dermal sinus. Neurosurgery 30:118–121
26. Baker RP, Brown EM, Coakham HB (2003) Overwhelming cranial and spinal subdural empyema secondary infected sacral decubitus ulcers. Br J Neurosurg 17:572–573
27. Pompucci A, De Bonis P, Sabatino G, Federico G, Moschini M, Anile C, Mangiola A (2007) Craniospinal subdural empyema due to S. intermedius: a case report. J Neuroimaging 17:358–360
28. Volk T, Hebecker R, Ruecker G, Perka C, Haas N, Spies C (2005) Subdural empyema combined with paraspinal abscess after epidural catheter insertion. Anesth Analg 100:1222–1223
29. Chern SH, Wei CP, Hsieh RL, Wang JL (2009) Methicillin-resistant Staphylococcus aureus retropharyngeal abscess complicated by a cervical spinal subdural empyema. J Clin Neurosci 16:144–146
30. Chen MH, Chen MH, Huang JS (2004) Cervical subdural empyema following acupuncture. J Clin Neurosci 11:909–911
31. Thomé C, Krauss JK, Zevgaridis D, Schmiedek P (2001) Pyogenic abscess of the filum terminale. Case report. J Neurosurg 95:100–104
32. Carey ME (1996) Infections of the spine and spinal cord. In: Youmans JR (ed) Youmans neurological surgery, vol 4. WB Saunders, Philadelphia, pp 3278–3279
33. Jensen AG, Espersen F, Skinhøj P, Rosdahl VT, Frimodt-Møller N (1997) Increasing frequency of vertebral osteomyelitis following Staphylococcus aureus bacteraemia in Denmark 1980-1990. J Infect 34:113–118
34. Kim CJ, Song KH, Jeon JH, Park WB, Park SW, Kim HB, Oh MD, Choe KW, Kim NJ (2010) A comparative study of pyogenic and tuberculous spondylodiscitis. Spine (Phila Pa 1976) 35:E1096–E1100
35. Schimmer RC, Jeanneret C, Nunley PD, Jeanneret B (2002) Osteomyelitis of the cervical spine: a potentially dramatic disease. J Spinal Disord Tech 15:110–117
36. Carragee EJ, Kim D, van der Vlugt T, Vittum D (1997) The clinical use of erythrocyte sedimentation rate in pyogenic vertebral osteomyelitis. Spine (Phila Pa 1976) 22:2089–2893
37. Beronius M, Bergman B, Andersson R (2001) Vertebral osteomyelitis in Goteborg, Sweden: a retrospective study of patients during 1990-95. Scand J Infect Dis 33:527–532
38. Hsieh PC, Wienecke RJ, O'Shaughnessy BA, Koski TR, Ondra SL (2004) Surgical strategies for vertebral osteomyelitis and epidural abscess. Neurosurg Focus 17:E4
39. Kang BU, Lee SH, Ahn Y, Choi WC, Choi YG (2010) Surgical site infection in spinal surgery: detection and management based on serial C-reactive protein measurements. J Neurosurg Spine 13:158–164
40. Gasbarrini A, Boriani L, Salvadori C, Mobarec S, Kreshak J, Nanni C, Zamparini E, Alberghini M, Viale P, Albisinni U (2012) Biopsy for suspected spondylodiscitis. Eur Rev Med Pharmacol Sci 2:26–34
41. Cheng VC, Yam WC, Hung IF, Woo PC, Lau SK, Tang BS, Yuen KY (2004) Clinical evaluation of the polymerase chain reaction for the rapid diagnosis of tuberculosis. J Clin Pathol 57:281–285
42. Kumar R, Das RK, Mahapatra AK (2010) Role of interferon gamma release assay in the diagnosis of Pott disease. J Neurosurg Spine 12:462–466
43. Michel SC, Pfirrmann CW, Boos N, Hodler J (2006) CT-guided core biopsy of subchondral bone and intervertebral space in suspected spondylodiskitis. AJR Am J Roentgenol 186:977–980

44. Fenollar F, Lévy PY, Raoult D (2008) Usefulness of broad-range PCR for the diagnosis of osteoarticular infections. Curr Opin Rheumatol 20:463–470
45. Fuursted K, Arpi M, Lindblad BE, Pedersen LN (2008) Broad-range PCR as a supplement to culture for detection of bacterial pathogens in patients with a clinically diagnosed spinal infection. Scand J Infect Dis 40:772–777
46. Delogu G, Zumbo A, Fadda G (2012) Microbiological and immunological diagnosis of tuberculous spondylodiscitis. Eur Rev Med Pharmacol Sci 16(Suppl 2):73–78
47. Ko MW, Osborne B, Jung S, Jacobs DA, Marcotte P, Galetta SL (2007) Papilledema as a manifestation of a spinal subdural abscess. J Neurol Sci 260:288–292
48. Murphy KJ, Brunberg JA, Quint DJ, Kazanjian PH (1998) Spinal cord infection: myelitis and abscess formation. AJNR Am J Neuroradiol 19:341–348
49. Kulkarni AG, Chu G, Fehlings MG (2007) Pyogenic intradural abscess: a case report. Spine 32:E354–E357
50. Suzer T, Coskun E, Tahta K, Bayramoglu H, Duzcan E (1998) Intramedullary spinal tuberculoma presenting as a conus tumour: a case report and review of the literature. Eur Spine J 7:168–171
51. Wasay M, Kheleani BA, Moolani MK, Zaheer J, Pui M, Hasan S, Muzaffar S, BakshiR SAR (2003) Brain CT and MRI findings in 100 consecutive patients with intracranial tuberculoma. J Neuroimaging 13:240–247
52. Akhaddar A, Elhamzaoui S, En-nouali H, Albouzidi A, Dami A, Elmostarchid B, Boucetta M (2009) Recurrent pyelonephritis revealing a calcified tuberculoma of the filum terminale. Intern Med 48:1485–1486
53. Moghtaderi A, Alavi Naini R (2003) Tuberculous radiculomyelitis: review and presentation of five patients. Int J Tuberc Lung Dis 7:1186–1190
54. Bernaerts A, Vanhoenacker FM, Parizel PM, Van Goethem JW, Van Altena R, Laridon A, De Roeck J, Coeman V, De Schepper AM (2003) Tuberculosis of the central nervous system: overview of neuroradiological findings. Eur Radiol 13:1876–1890
55. Chang KH, Han MH, Roh JK, Kim IO, Han MC, Choi KS, Kim CW (1990) Gd-DTPA enhanced MR imaging in intracranial tuberculosis. Neuroradiology 32:19–25
56. Gupta VK, Sharma BS, Khosla VK (1995) Intramedullary tuberculoma: report of two cases with MRI findings. Surg Neurol 44:241–243
57. Douglas JG, McLeod MJ (1999) Pharmacokinetic factors in the modern drug treatment of tuberculosis. Clin Pharmacokinet 37:127–146
58. American Thoracic Society; Centers for Disease Control and Prevention; Infectious Diseases Society of America (2005) American Thoracic Society/Centers for Disease Control and Prevention/Infectious Diseases Society of America: controlling tuberculosis in the United States. Am J Respir Crit Care Med 172:1169227
59. Rezai AR, Lee M, Cooper PR, Errico TJ, Koslow M (1995) Modern management of spinal tuberculosis. Neurosurgery 36:87–97
60. Emel E, Güzey FK, Güzey D, Bas NS, Sel B, Alatas I (2006) Noncontiguous multifocal spinal tuberculosis involving cervical, thoracic, lumbar and sacral segments: a case report. Eur Spine J 15:1019–1024
61. Kotil K, Alan MS, Bilge T (2007) Medical management of Pott disease in the thoracic and lumbar spine: a prospective clinical study. J Neurosurg Spine 6:222–228
62. Jain AK (2010) Tuberculosis of the spine: a fresh look at an old disease. J Bone Joint Surg Br 92:905–913
63. Teegala R, Kumar P, Kale SS, Sharma BS (2008) Craniovertebral junction tuberculosis: a new comprehensive therapeutic strategy. Neurosurgery 63:946–955
64. Sucu HK, Ciçek C, Rezanko T, Bezircioğlu H, Erşahin Y, Tunakan M, Minoğlu M (2006) Percutaneous computed-tomography-guided biopsy of the spine: 229 procedures. Joint Bone Spine 73:532–537

18 Spinal Cord

Manish Jaiswal

Contents

M. Jaiswal, MS, MCh
Department of Neurosurgery, King George's Medical University, Lucknow 226003, UP, India
e-mail: manishmlnmc@gmail.com; manishjaiswal@kgmcindia.edu

Abbreviations

Anti-TB	Antitubercular therapy
CNS	Central nervous system
CSF	Cerebrospinal fluid
CT	Computed tomography
CUSA	Cavitron ultrasonic aspirator
ESR	Erythrocyte sedimentation rate
ETB	Ethambutol
HIV	Human immunodeficiency virus
INH	Isoniazid
MF	Moxifloxacin
MRI	Magnetic resonance imaging
RIF	Rifampicin
SEPs	Sensory evoked potentials
STR	Streptomycin
TB	Tuberculosis
TBM	Tubercular meningitis

18.1 Introduction

Tuberculosis (TB) continues as a serious public health problem in developing countries [1–11]. In human immunodeficiency virus (HIV)-infected individual, it is also a common opportunistic infection [12–21]. TB infection that involves the central nervous system (CNS) is rare in the industrialized world. TB involvement of the spinal cord as compared to the brain occurs in the ratio of 1:42 [22–25]. Clinically it may present as compressive myelopathy,

M. Turgut et al. (eds.), *Tuberculosis of the Central Nervous System*,
DOI 10.1007/978-3-319-50712-5_18

radiculopathy or intramedullary mass depending on osseous or non-osseous involvement of the spinal cord [26–29]. Osseous involvement in the form of Pott's spine has been described in detail in this book in Chap. 15. Here we have focussed on non-osseous involvement of the spinal cord which is much rare, and in some patients, diagnosis is almost under question, or anti-TB chemotherapy is not effective, and in some patients, neurological deterioration requires surgical intervention. Clinical and radiological characteristics especially magnetic resonance imaging (MRI) findings of intradural extramedullary tubercular abscess, tubercular arachnoiditis and spinal intramedullary tuberculoma, and post-TB syringomyelia are presented in this chapter. Decision to continue conservative management and surgical indications depending on various factors has been discussed in details to improve the final outcome of these rare entities.

18.2 Spectrum of Spinal Cord Tuberculosis

18.2.1 History

Era Serre (1830) described the tuberculoma of spinal cord for the first time, while first removal seems to have been performed by Krauss and McGuire (1909) [25]. Jennings found only 1 spinal intramedullary tuberculoma among 5344 pulmonary TB patients [30]. Jaff and Schultz disclosed 1 spinal intramedullary tuberculoma in 7000 post-mortems compared with 48 cerebral tuberculomas in the same group [31]. In Kernohan's statistics, the ratio of spinal intramedullary tuberculoma to other spinal cord tumours was 1:48. Among collected 84 cases by Thalhimer and Hassin, only 67 were definitely documented. They added one case of spinal intramedullary tuberculoma [32]. Kupka and Olsen collected 19 more cases since the time of Thalhimer and Hassin's report and added 1 spinal intramedullary tuberculoma [33]. Dastur reviewed 74 patients of paraplegia due to TB without evidence of Pott's spine and revealed that extradural granulomatous lesion occurred in 64%, arachnoiditis in 20%, subdural/extramedullary granuloma in 8% and intramedullary tuberculoma in 8% [34]. Spinal cord involvement compared to that of the brain occurs in the ratio of 1:42 [23]. Spinal intramedullary tuberculomas are rarely reported in developed countries' literature with prevalence of 2 out of 100,000 TB cases. Many cases have been described in literature; however, the contribution of all authors is based on one or very few personal patients. A thorough review of the world literature by Lin in 1960 discovered 105 cases of spinal intramedullary tuberculoma, 88 of which were found during post-mortem examination [35, 36]. Study conducted by Ratliff and Conolly found only 148 cases of spinal intramedullary tuberculomas in the recent literature [37]. Syringomyelia was first described by Charcot and Joffery Vulpian [16, 38, 39]. The first description of syringomyelia attributable to TB is by Marinesco in 1916 [40, 41].

18.2.2 Aetiology and Pathogenesis

The intraspinal tuberculoma are classified (Homi M Dastur 1972) as follows [34]:

1. Extradural with:
   (a) Vertebral body involvement
   (b) Vertebral arch involvement
   (c) Without osseous involvement
   (d) With osseous or dural involvement but within the epidural fatty tissue
2. Subdural:
   (a) Localized
   (b) Diffuse
3. Subdural and extradural
4. Arachnoidal without dural involvement
5. Intramedullary TB granuloma

Non-osseous spinal tuberculoma usually occurs due to spread from a primary pulmonary TB focus via hemopoietic route, but it may also arise by direct extension from TB hilar lymph nodes [23, 34, 42–47]. In most of the reported cases of spinal tuberculoma, the patients have

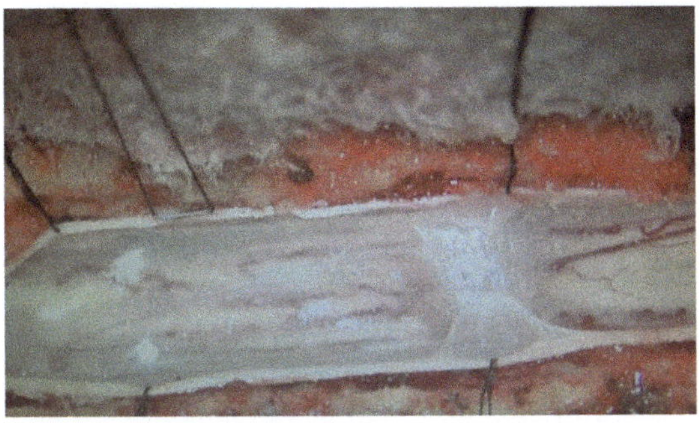

Fig. 18.1 Spinal TB arachnoiditis with web formation causing spinal cord compression

diagnosed following or during treatment for tuberculous meningitis (TBM) [48–52]. In early stage of spinal TB, different degree of inflammatory exudation and congestion may be noted in the meninges (spinal TBM) [53–56]. The spinal cord and its roots may become oedematous (TB myelitis and myeloradiculitis), sometimes surrounded by gelatinous thickened arachnoid and exudates (TB arachnoiditis or web formation) [33, 38, 57, 58]. Three possible pathogeneses for the occurrence of spinal TB arachnoiditis are the following:

1. TB lesion primarily arising in the spinal meninges
2. Extension of TB spondylitis
3. Downward extension of intracranial TBM

Among these, spinal arachnoiditis secondary to intracranial TBM is the most common finding [38, 57]. The most often affected site is the thoracic region, followed by the lumbar and cervical regions of the spine [59]. Macroscopically, TB exudate can be visualized around the spinal cord and nerve roots (Fig. 18.1). The exudate is predominantly noticeable posteriorly, perhaps due to lying in the supine position for a sustained period. Microscopically, inflammatory granulation, caseation, tubercles and fibrous tissue are eminent [36, 60, 61]. In long-lasting cases, the subarachnoid space may be unevenly congested, with the formation of pouches of cerebrospinal fluid (CSF). Variations in arachnoiditis can be documented as either a diffuse-adhesive form or a cystic form [38, 57, 62].

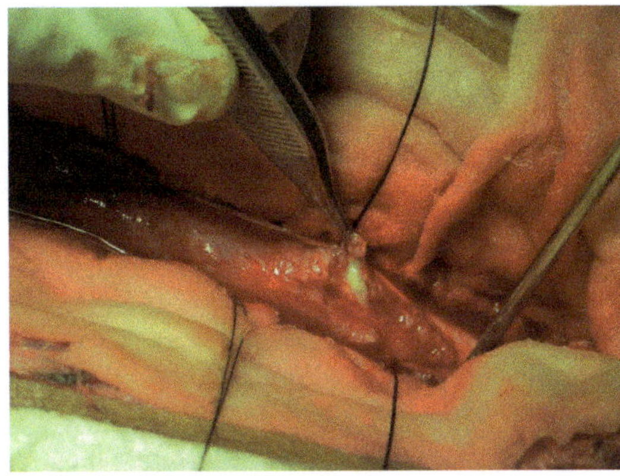

Fig. 18.2 Intradural extramedullary abscess/granuloma causing spinal cord compression

Further increase in exudation leads to the development of abscess or granuloma (intradural extramedullary tuberculoma/abscess) (Fig. 18.2), which is usually densely adhered to the inner side of dura mater and then starts to burrow into the spinal cord called spinal intramedullary tuberculoma. Tuberculoma may be secondary to hematogenous dissemination of systemic diseases or may progress from CSF infection extension into the contiguous spinal cord parenchyma through parenchymal veins and perforating arteries. Sometimes it then becomes difficult to distinguish whether the abscess is intramedullary or extramedullary [36, 61, 63–68]. Necrotic material, debris and caseous material accumulation lead to formation of abscess in the substance of the spinal cord as the disease progresses [47]. Mature tuberculoma has solid caseation necrosis centre surrounded by collagenous tissue capsule, multinucleated giant cells, epithelioid cells and mononuclear inflammatory cells [69]. Outside the capsule is the surrounding oedema. The surrounding oedema is comparatively more noticeable in the early stage of granuloma development, so fusiform swelling of the spinal cord has been eminent in most of the cases of spinal intramedullary tuberculoma [59, 63, 70].

Adhesions between the fibrin-coated nerve roots and meninges lead to CSF loculations and tethering or clumping of nerve roots [33, 58, 62]. The postulated mechanism of development of syrinx cavities has been well described in literature.

The association of syringomyelia with arachnoiditis is well recognized [71–73]. Caplan and Mac Donald have, in fact, suggested that ischemic myelomalacia causes microcystic spinal cord degeneration, which precedes the development of syringomyelia due to arachnoiditis [38, 74]. The microcysts coalesce to produce macrocystic cavities within the cord, which then begin to extend up and down the affected segment of the cord. Further enlargement of the cavity is postulated to be secondary mechanical factors, which increase intracavitary pressure. The development and progression of syringomyelitic cavities are likely to produce delayed neurological deterioration in these patients, even in the absence of the active disease [41].

18.2.3 Clinical Presentation

TB is a chronic bacterial infection produced by *Mycobacterium tuberculosis* [75–78]. TB of the CNS is an unusual entity, affecting 0.5–2% of patients with systemic TB. It is more common in young patients with pulmonary TB (69% of cases) in the developing countries [19, 79, 80]. There may be no proof of extra-neural TB in up to one third cases of neuro-TB. Therefore, even in non-appearance of TB elsewhere in the body, the possibility of TB of CNS cannot be ruled out [63, 81]. In maximum of the described spinal cord TB cases, the patients have presented following or during treatment for TBM [82]. Depending on the various forms of spinal TB, clinical presentation differs in patient to patient [32, 83, 84].

18.2.3.1 Extradural Involvement

Osseous involvement as Pott's spine causes extradural cord compression by vertebral collapse, epidural collection/granulation/debris and kyphotic deformity, leading to compressive myelopathy symptoms and signs along with localized pain, stiffness, local tenderness and muscles spasm, obvious spinal deformity, gibbus and a cold abscess [3, 10]. The advancement of spinal TB is insidious and usually slow [11, 22].

The total period of the disease varies from few months to few years, with usual disease duration extending from 4 to 11 months [29, 85]. Usually, patients pursue opinion only when there is severe pain, obvious spinal deformity or neurological manifestations [26, 28]. Constitutional symptoms are present in around 20–30% of cases of osteoarticular TB [66, 67]. The classical constitutional symptoms of TB indicating the presence of an active disease are loss of weight, malaise, decreased appetite, night sweating, evening rise fever, fatigue and generalized body aches. Back pain is the most common feature of spinal TB. The severity of pain ranges from regular mild dull ache to disabling pain. Pain typically occurs to the site of spinal involvement and is localized and most commonly involves the thoracic region. The pain may be provoked by spinal movement while coughing, and weight-bearing, because of pathological fracture, spinal instability, nerve root compression or advanced disc disruption [22, 68]. Chronic backache as the only presentation was noted in about 61% of cases of Pott's spine.

18.2.3.2 Intradural Involvement

Non-osseous spinal TB as meningitis presents as constitutional fever, headache, backache and sometimes quadriparesis/paraparesis due to vasculitic infarct by involvement of blood vessels or due to thrombus formation (spinal cord syndromes). Intradural extramedullary tuberculoma and abscess cause cord compression leading to upper motor neuron type of weakness below the lesion [43].

TB arachnoiditis causes clumping and adhesion of the roots and presents as radiculitis/radiculopathy [33, 58]. The clinical signs and symptoms are generally restricted to polyradicular or monoradicular pain syndromes that may be complemented by sensory and motor deficits. Symptoms commonly progress over several years, although quickly progressing cases have been mentioned. Sometimes arachnoid thickening forms web and constricting band which compress the cord [Fig. 18.1]. These TB arachnoid web and band ultimately lead to compressive myelopathy and in some cases tethering of cord that leads to tethered cord syndrome features [62, 86].

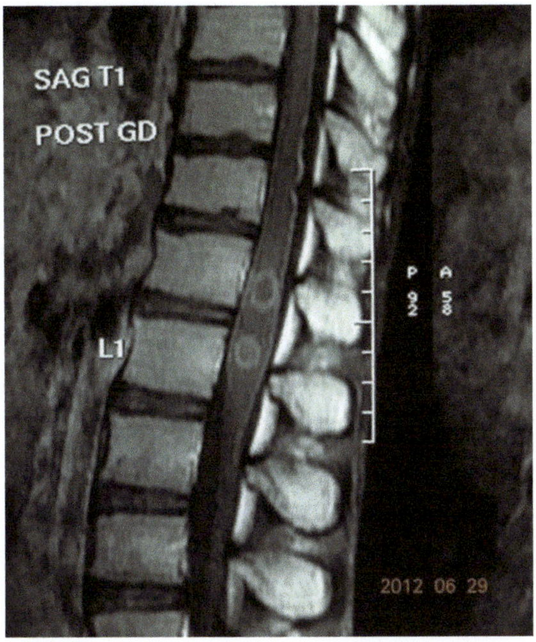

Fig. 18.3 MRI spine showing multiple conglomerate rim-enhancing tuberculomas at conus and epiconus regions

Table 18.1 Mechanisms of paraplegia/tetraplegia in spinal tuberculosis

Causes of neurological involvement	
Early-onset paraplegia	
Mechanical pressure	Mechanical pressure by tuberculous debris, sequestrum of the bone or disc, abscess, subluxation and dislocations, concertina collapse and internal gibbus
Tuberculous granuloma	Tuberculoma in extradural, intradural or intramedullary regions
Tuberculous myelitis	Uncommon. May involve spinal cord parenchyma
Spinal artery thrombosis	Infective thrombosis of anterior spinal artery
Tuberculous arachnoiditis	Meningeal inflammation and fibrosis
Late-onset paraplegia	
Transection of spinal cord by bony bridge	Transverse ridge of bone produced by severe kyphosis
Fibrosis of dura (pachymeningitis)	Formation of tough, fibrous membrane encircling the cord

18.2.3.3 Intramedullary Involvement

Spinal intramedullary tuberculoma and abscess present as spinal tumour syndrome and are very rare [59]. They mimic intramedullary tumour in symptomatology with a rapidly advancing course. If such patient has a TB lesion elsewhere in the body at present or in the past, one can keep this condition in differential diagnosis with non-TB, tumorous and nontumourous lesion [59, 63]. On examination they have no clinical spinal deformity. Spinal intramedullary tuberculoma most commonly involves the thoracic spinal cord. Maximum of the described spinal intramedullary tuberculoma in literature are solitary [1, 2, 13–15, 23, 44, 46]. However, multiple spinal intramedullary tuberculomas have been even more reported after the MRI introduction (Fig. 18.3) [59, 63, 87, 88]. Spinal intramedullary tuberculoma is also reported in HIV patients; patients with auto-immune disease, especially systemic lupus erythematosis; and patients taking immunosuppressive treatment for liver transplantation, so symptomatology of these associated co-morbid conditions may be present [13, 18, 59, 89]. Another manifestation of spinal cord TB is syrinx formation, which pathophysiology is already discussed [38, 74]. Sign and symptoms of central cord syndrome appear in these cases.

Paraplegia is the most upsetting problem of spinal TB [83, 84, 90, 91]. In classical paper of Hodgson on Pott's paraplegia, it is classified into two sets according to the tubercular infection activity:

(a) Paraplegia of active disease (early-onset paraplegia)
(b) Paraplegia of healed disease (late-onset paraplegia) (Table 18.1) [29]

Early-onset paraplegia progresses in the active stage of Pott's spine and requires vigorous management. This category of paraplegia has a better outcome [29]. Late-onset paraplegia, which is a neurological complication in a patient with healed TB, advances after a variable duration. Late-onset paraplegia may occur two to four decades after active stage of infection. Late-onset paraplegia is often accompanying with obvious spinal deformities.

Neurological deterioration is usually more common with thoracic and cervical regions of spine involvement. Early neurological deficit may evolve to complete paraplegia or tetraplegia if left untreated. Paraplegia may develop at whatever time and during any stage of the Pott's spine. The incidence of neurological deficit in Pott's spine varies from 23% to 76% in available literature. The spinal cord level decides the degree of neurological deficits. There are symptoms of cord or root compression in patients having cervical Pott's spine, and it includes neck pain and weakness and numbness of the upper and lower limbs, eventually continuing to quadriplegia. In cases of thoracic or lumbar spine involvement, upper limb function remains full, while lower limb symptoms advances over time ultimately leading to paraplegia [32, 91]. Patients with lumbar and sacral Pott's spine have low backache weakness, numbness and radicular pain due to cauda equina compression and have diminished or absent deep tendon reflexes in involved muscles group. It is just opposite to the hyperreflexia seen with cervical and thoracic spinal cord compression along with bladder symptoms (cauda equina syndrome). Neurological ambulatory status is generally evaluated using the modified McCormick scale [84] [Grade I = normal gait, Grade II = mild gait disturbance not requiring support, Grade III = gait with support, Grade IV = assistance required, Grade V = wheel chair/bedridden (Table 18.2)].

Some patients develop headache with blurring of vision, ataxia and seizure in follow-up, and MRI brain reveals concurrent multiple intracranial tuberculomas (Fig. 18.4) [59, 63, 87, 88]. Concurrent intracranial tuberculoma is extremely rare. We recommend that MRI brain should be advised in the multiple spinal intramedullary tuberculoma cases because the possibility of early asymptomatic intracranial tuberculomas may be there [59]. Early detection of these findings helps in the management of patients with spinal TB.

18.3 Investigation

18.3.1 Evaluation of Primary Focus

All the patients must be completely evaluated in terms of primary focus, site and extent of the lesion and its correlation with manifestations. Usual non-invasive investigative tools are MRI spine with contrast, X-ray chest, X-ray spine, erythrocyte sedimentation rate (ESR) and HIV serological examination [31, 69, 92–95]. Asymptomatic primary focus is common in TB prevalent zone of the world. Skin tests have not much role in making

Table 18.2 Modified McCormick scale for gait assessment in spinal intramedullary lesion

Grade I	Normal gait
Grade II	Mild gait disturbance not requiring support
Grade III	Gait with support
Grade IV	assistance required
Grade V	Wheel chair/ bedridden

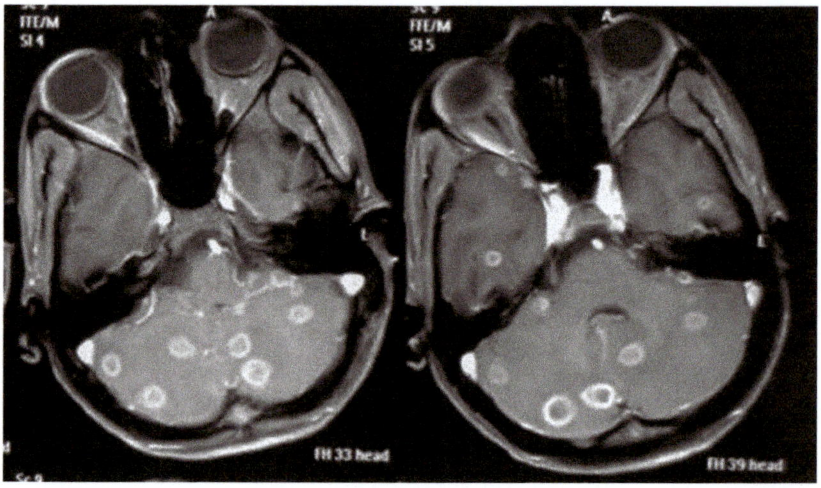

Fig. 18.4 MRI brain with contrast revealed concurrent multiple intracranial tuberculomas in patient with spinal intramedullary tuberculoma

diagnosis especially in juveniles and adults [37, 89, 96–98]. These tests are significant in geographical area where TB is not as frequent [99–101]. The best imaging modality for diagnosis is MRI, because it can precisely show size, location and extent of lesions, in addition to information about degeneration and necrosis surrounding the lesions [59, 102–105]. Etiological approval TB can be done either by demonstration of acid-fast bacilli in pathological sample or histological confirmation of a tubercle or the simple existence of epithelioid cells on the biopsy [106].

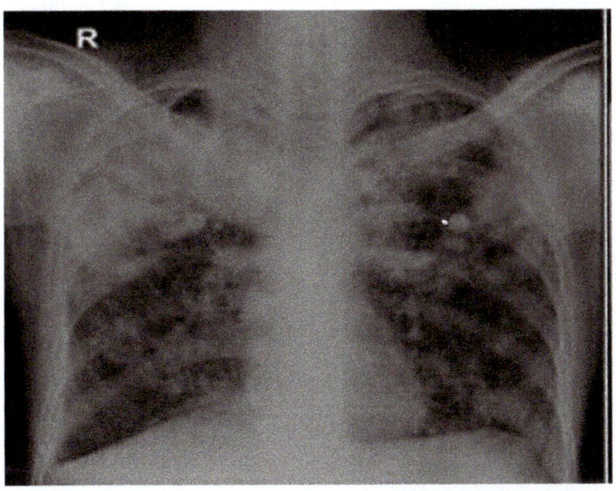

Fig. 18.5 X-ray chest suggestive of associated miliary TB

Plain roentgenograms of chest usually discovered sign of active or healed lung TB in 30–40% of cases which can be supported by CT chest if diagnosis is in doubt (Figs. 18.5 and 18.6) [59, 97]. X-ray of spine or CT of spine reveals osseous involvement, end-plate disruption, bone destruction and paravertebral abscess formation; intrathecal contrast instillation shows the severity of thecal sac obliteration [26, 28, 59]. MRI delineates the extent of cord compression and myelopathic changes, and they are helpful in management of Pott's spine, which is discussed in detail in Chap. 15.

18.3.2 MRI Characteristics of Spinal Tuberculosis

Non-osseous spinal cord involvement is best evaluated by MRI with gadolinium contrast. It is also useful in monitoring the anti-TB chemotherapy response and in follow-up of these patients. It is also helpful in decision making of surgical needs.

18.3.2.1 Tuberculous Spinal Arachnoiditis

MRI is the best investigative tool and may show abolition of the spinal subarachnoid space, with loss of the spinal cord outlining in the cervicothoracic spine and clumping of the cauda

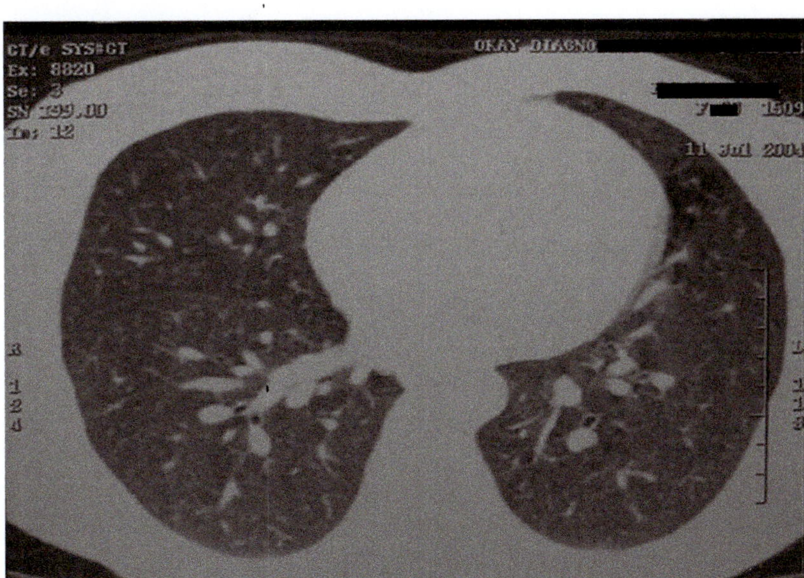

Fig. 18.6 CT thorax suggestive of associated miliary TBs

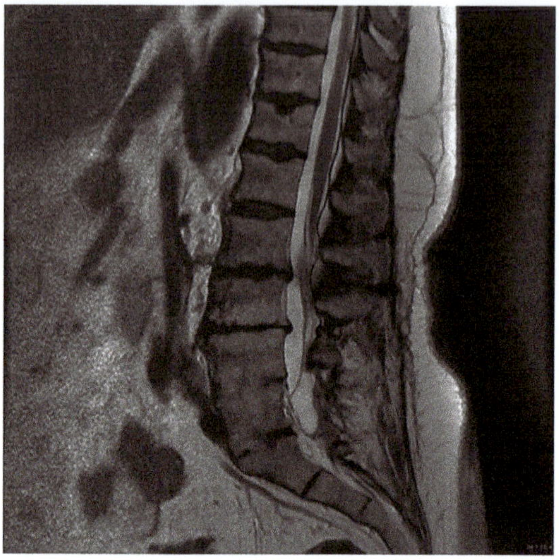

Fig. 18.7 MRI spine suggestive of spinal TB arachnoiditis causing obliteration of subarachnoid space with matting of nerve root and nodular thick intradural enhancement

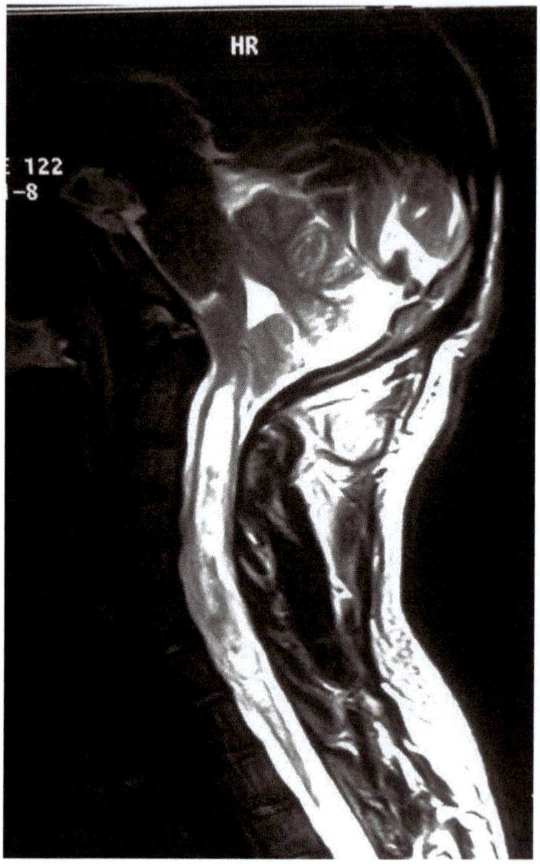

Fig. 18.8 MRI spine showing post-TB meningitis multiloculated syrinx with cord atrophy

equina nerve roots in the lumbar area [30, 61]. Contrast MRI discloses nodular, linear, thick, intradural enhancement, which can entirely block the subarachnoid space, occasionally giving the look of a normal non-enhanced MRI and occasionally shifting the cord ventrally common in dorsal spine (Fig. 18.7) [38, 42, 57]. Chronic spinal TB arachnoiditis may not enhance on contrast MRI. The severity of MRI appearance does not correlate well with symptoms. Classically, three MRI configurations of arachnoiditis have been defined involving the cauda equina region:

Type 1: Central-type roots are matted to the centre of the thecal sac.

Type 2: Peripheral-type roots are adherent to the periphery of the dural sac.

Type 3: Adherent roots to one side of the thecal sac resembling a soft tissue tumour.

Spinal TB arachnoiditis must be differentiated from other probable causes of arachnoiditis.

18.3.2.2 Tuberculous Syringomyelia

Sometimes syringomyelia is associated finding (vasculitic thrombosis of spinal cord vessels leading to ischemic myelomalacia is the mechanism causing postinflammatory syringomyelia) [39]. Usually TB syrinx is multiloculated and significant cord atrophy is seen (Fig. 18.8) [36, 38, 39, 71]. Using different sequences MRI can differentiate myelomalacia and syrinx [41]. Syringomyelia is appreciated as spinal cord cavitation that classically exhibits CSF signal intensity on both T1- and T2-weighted sequences and does not take contrast [72, 73]. T1-weighted, inversion recovery and proton density images are very valuable for making diagnosis of cystic areas due to the arrival of MRI by which tubercular myelopathy and syringomyelia, which are surgically curable, can be noticed in its initial phase.

18.3.2.3 Intradural Extramedullary Tuberculoma

Intradural extramedullary tuberculoma is seen to encase the cord and cause obliteration of the surrounding thecal sac. Epidural fat appears to be compressed by the lesion. The lesions are isointense to

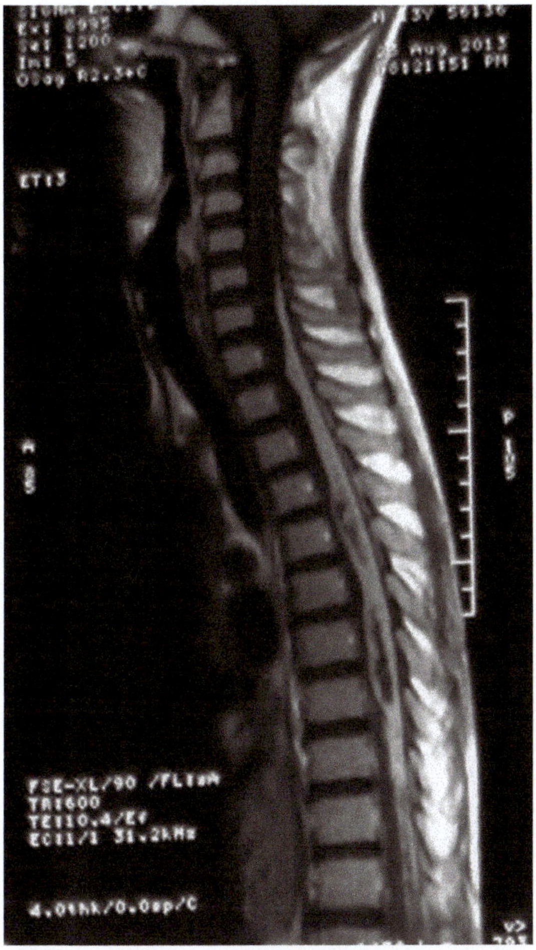

Fig. 18.9 MRI spine showing post-gadolinium-enhancing intradural extramedullary granulomatous collection suggestive of tuberculoma

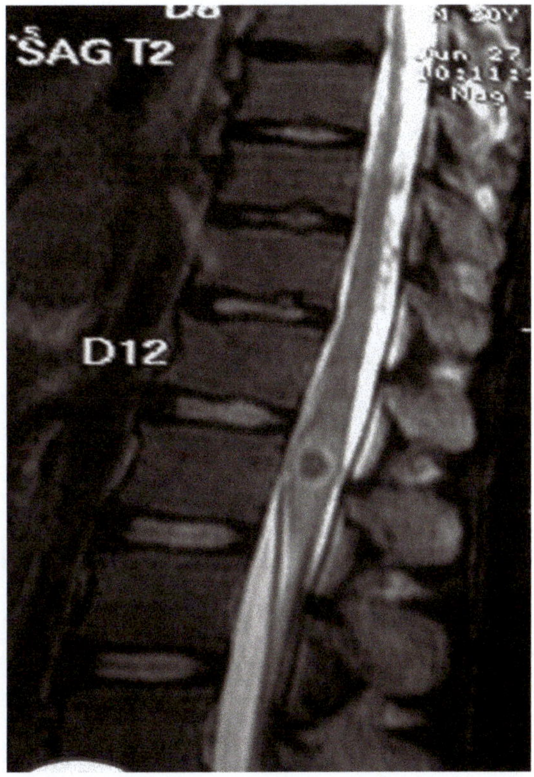

Fig. 18.10 MRI spine showing isointense lesion with hyperintense rim in T2 suggestive of spinal intramedullary tuberculoma

hypointense to the cord parenchyma on T1-weighted sequences and are hypointense on T2-weighted sequences. It usually shows a central hyperintensity on T2-weighted sequence suggestive of necrosis. There is homogenous contrast enhancement after intravenous gadolinium (Fig. 18.9) [42, 43, 55]. It can sometimes present as intradural extramedullary en plaque-shaped mass [56]. There may be also associated syringomyelia both proximal and distal to the lesion.

18.3.2.4 Spinal Intramedullary Tuberculoma

MRI is the gold standard diagnostic tool, as it precisely shows the number and size in such lesion. The first MRI predictable explanation was provided by Rhoton and his colleagues in 1988, and the authors of consequent studies were better capable to depict these lesions as technology advanced [70].

These lesions characterize various phases during the advancement of spinal intramedullary tuberculoma [36, 59, 74, 94]. In early inflammatory stage, there is plenty of giant cells and deprived collagenous capsule with inconstant adjoining oedema. At this stage, spinal intramedullary tuberculoma is isointense on both T1- and T2-weighted sequences with fusiform localized thickening of cord and demonstrates a homogeneous contrast enhancement with gadolinium due to failure of blood-cord barrier. Afterwards surrounding capsule becomes more affluent in collagen, and surrounding inflammatory response starts fading. This results in an isointense or hypointense ring on T1-weighted sequence and as isointense or hypointense signals on T2-weighted sequence of MRI (Fig. 18.10). Post-gadolinium studies demonstrate disc-like or ringlike and

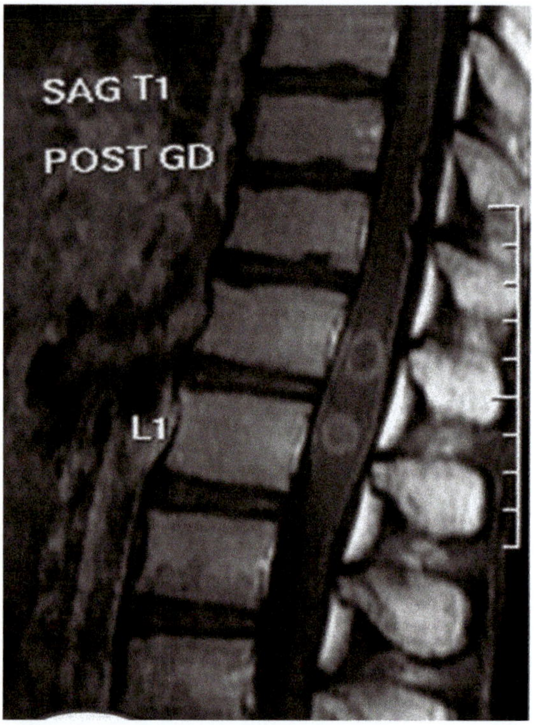

Fig. 18.11 Post-contrast T1 image of MRI spine showing typical "target sign" suggestive of spinal intramedullary tuberculoma

sometimes conglomerate enhancement. With development of caseation, the centre becomes bright on T2-weighted sequences and is typically called the "target sign" (Fig. 18.11) [59, 74, 95, 107]. On treatment with anti-TB chemotherapy, the lesion retrogresses in size and dissolves, to be substituted by gliosis, which perhaps is appreciated as an area of hypodensity on MRI [59, 64]. Follow-up MRI spine becomes essential not only to evaluate the effectiveness of anti-TB chemotherapy but also to identify paradoxical response to medical treatment [18, 59, 85].

The differential diagnosis includes common spinal intramedullary tumours, such as astrocytoma, hemangioblastoma, ependymoma, lymphoma, metastasis, multiple sclerosis, infarction, opportunistic infections and cysticercal granuloma [64, 94, 108–111]. Vascular myelopathy occurs due to HIV virus in HIV patients, and other more common spinal infections in these patients are herpes simplex virus, cytomegalovirus and 92 *Toxoplasma gondii* infections of the spinal cord as compared to tuberculomas. Spinal cord vasculitic infarction and primary non-Hodgkin lymphoma may also be seen in HIV patients [13, 18, 20]. Differentiation between these lesions may be sometimes very difficult, but correlation of history, clinical findings and the peculiar signal changes in MRI can be helpful in making diagnosis of spinal intramedullary tuberculoma very easily [59].

18.4 Management

The ideal management of spinal TB continues debatable and should be customized in each case. The detailed management of Pott's disease, spinal dura mater and epidural space and subdural space TB is discussed in respective chapters of this book (see Chaps. 15, 16 and 17). Assuming the uncommonness of spinal intramedullary tuberculoma, there is no uniform management protocol for this disease. Both surgical and medical management have brought good outcomes in various series.

18.4.1 Medical Management

Several authors have suggested medical management of spinal intramedullary tuberculoma with good outcomes. Pernuate et al. [73] and Jena et al. [105], however, sensed that there was no requirement for surgical interventions, and imaging verdicts were sufficient to start anti-TB treatment. Gupta et al. [103] have described ten cases in which MRI established that spinal intramedullary tuberculoma had responded to medical management. Among other individual case reports of medical management, few cases were described in which paradoxical progression of tuberculoma found even with anti-TB chemotherapy, and these patients needed surgical procedure [59].

Conservative management of spinal intramedullary tuberculoma, if diagnosed early, usually has good response to medical treatment preventing the need for surgical intervention [19, 20, 83, 112, 113]. Anti-TB medications (isoniazid (INH) 5 mg/kg/day, rifampin (RIF) 10 mg/kg/day, etambutol (ETB) 15 mg/kg/day, pyrazinamide (PRZ) 25 mg/kg/day, streptomycin (STR) 15 mg/kg/day and moxifloxacin (MF) 10 mg/kg/day for 3 months in intensive phase of anti-TB chemotherapy followed by two-drug regimen (INH, RIF) in continuance phase range from 12 to 21 months) and a short duration of injectable or oral corticosteroids give an effective, economical, harmless and reasonable choice for treatment of spinal intramedullary tuberculoma, mainly in developing nations [37, 40, 64, 89]. Corticosteroid role is basically not proven [114, 115]. In all three conservatively managed patients, Jaiswal et al. had positive results with oral steroid for a short period, when given along with anti-TB chemotherapy [59]. Indication of conservative management in these three patients was associated pulmonary Koch's for 3–4 months and nonprogressive neurological status in one case and multiple intracranial as well as spinal intramedullary tuberculomas in MRI (Fig. 18.4), clinical feature along with X-ray chest suggestive of pulmonary Koch's in two cases (Fig. 18.5). Especially with perilesional oedema, short-course corticosteroids may be supportive. Generally the conservative management is effective in attaining thorough clinical neurological improvement over a duration of 1–2 years, which is too complemented by resolution of the spinal intramedullary tuberculomas in MRI (Fig. 18.12) [59].

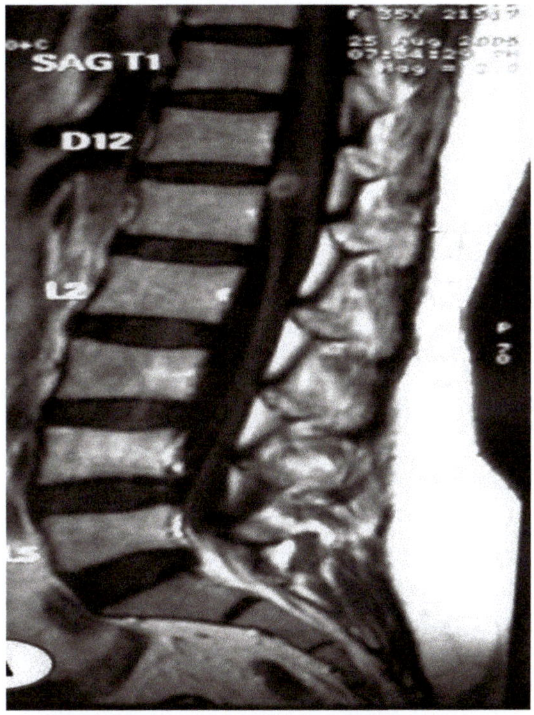

Fig. 18.12 Follow-up MRI spine suggestive of tuberculoma resolution on conservative management

18.4.1.1 Paradoxical Reaction to Anti-tuberculous Chemotherapy

The formation of a new intracranial tuberculoma in patients getting active anti-TB treatment has been well known in the past many decades [35, 116]. This paradoxical reaction, on the other hand, has only in recent times been reported in cases of spinal intraspinal tuberculoma [59, 62]. Similarly, an upsurge in the size of spinal intramedullary tuberculomas in patients taking anti-TB chemotherapy has also been described in recent times. The particular cause for this enlargement in size is not clear but is supposed to be due to the paradoxical reaction of the host to the *M. tuberculosis* yields.

This paradoxical occurrence is supposed to be to the effect of an immunological response: as active TB is under control, immunosuppression settles, and the anti-TB chemotherapy-induced damage of bacilli results in a discharge of disproportionate quantities of tubercular protein. This protein excites the antigen-sensitive lymphocytes in the tuberculoma to multiply, causing in the chain of proceedings that is accountable for enlargement of tuberculoma or conception of formerly barely visible tuberculomas [117, 118]. In an analysis of non-HIV patients with culture-established TB, Cheng et al. [57] evaluated cases in which the reaction to anti-TB chemotherapy was paradoxical compared to cases in which this paradoxical reaction was absent. They obtained that there were lesser absolute lymphocyte counts at the time of diagnosis and more rises in the absolute lymphocyte count after start of anti-TB chemotherapy in patients in whom the paradoxical reaction to anti-TB therapy was lacking. A rise in lymphocyte count, supplemented by an overstated tuberculin skin reaction, was found for the duration of the paradoxical response. These results recommend that enhancements in cell-mediated immune role after start of anti-TB treatment may be relatively accountable for the paradoxical reaction. If such an immune reaction happens at the location of microscopic intracranial and spinal centres, the outcome could be the expansion of tuberculomas at those locations.

18.4.1.2 Paradoxical Reaction to Anti-TB Therapy: Medical or Surgical Management?

Maximum authors have confidence in that continuing anti-TB treatment is suitable when paradoxical response progresses in intracranial tuberculoma. An analysis of the available literature on spinal intramedullary tuberculoma, on the other hand, approves the unresponsiveness of this situation to medical treatment only and points out the requirement for surgical intervention [59]. The cause of unresponsiveness in this situation to anti-TB chemotherapy is not identified. Therefore, when spinal intramedullary tuberculoma takes place as a paradoxical reaction to anti-TB chemotherapy, we consider for surgical intervention.

18.4.2 Surgical Management

Suzer et al. [119] support microsurgical removal of the spinal intramedullary tuberculoma and anti-TB treatment as the management of choice for all patients supposed to have spinal intramedullary tuberculomas. In 15 cases, Ramdurg et al. [64] performed surgical intervention in 12 cases in which 9 showed improvement in neurological function. MacDonnel [74] has stated 65% improvement after surgical treatment. The principle of surgical procedure is the decompression of the cord when continuing neurologic deficits occur and also makes it potential to inspect the tissue histopathologically. Unnecessary postponement due to prolonged medical treatment might produce permanent cord destruction, and the patient might not recover in terms of neurological deficits even though the lesion dissolves in radiological investigation. We trust that surgical management should be well thought out for cases presenting advancing deficits despite satisfactory medical treatment and large lesions causing significant compression. Surgical excision of spinal intramedullary tuberculoma after decompressive laminectomy of the corresponding level was performed in eight cases of author case series [59]. Indication of surgical intervention was the following: (1) unresponsive to anti-TB chemotherapy, (2) diagnosis is in suspicion (MRI finding suggestive of intramedullary tumour in differential diagnosis) in patient with no history of pulmonary TB, (3) there was a rapid deterioration in neurological function, and (4) paradoxical increase in size with mass effect after anti-TB chemotherapy starts.

With capable microsurgical procedures, it is likely to carefully remove the spinal intramedullary tuberculoma as these are well defined [62, 64, 70, 89, 120]. Like any surgical technique, there are associated hazards of anaesthesia and possibility of evolving sinus formation, postsurgical TBM and leftover neurological deficit [59, 119, 121].

18.4.2.1 Basic Steps of Intramedullary Tuberculoma Surgery

Exposure

The exposure of a spinal intramedullary tuberculoma is performed in the prone position. For posterior position, attention should be given to backing the abdomen and thorax adequately to assist venous blood flow to the heart with the aim of limiting extradural venous congestion and to avoid pressure-related harms during surgical intervention that will frequently take many hours. For cervical intramedullary tuberculoma and up to the level of upper two thoracic vertebrae, few persons select the semi-sitting position. Provided an anaesthesiologist team having experience of prone position is near, it does deal significant benefits. Particularly, a fresh surgical exposed area is easy to carry on at all times simply by irrigation. This diminishes the requirement for extra suction adjacent to the spinal cord. Monitoring by sensory evoked potentials (SEPs) can circumvent unwarranted pressure over the spinal cord during this manoeuvre.

After proper positioning, we define the exact spinal level by fluoroscopic exposure. We execute a midline skin incision up to the fascia. The fascia is incised on both sides approximately up to the spinous processes. Next, we separate the paraspinal muscles from spinous processes and laminae with the periosteal elevator. When all laminae are uncovered to about the facet joints, we confirm again the correct spinal level with C-arm (Fig. 18.13). Before bone removal we assure absolute haemostasis. For spinal intramedullary tuberculoma, we do a laminotomy about 10–15 mm wide. For this we cut the lamina with a diamond drill and remove the lamina in one block (Figs. 18.14 and 18.15). We stock en block lamina in tense state to prevent shrinkage till the procedure ends as well as wet with isotonic saline fluid. In this way, we confirm an appropriate fitting of the lamina for reposition after the end of procedure. Traditional laminectomy may be escaped whenever likely to avoid. If a laminectomy is required, we practice a 1 or 2 mm Kerrison punch to prevent the cord injury. Yellow ligament can be left over the dura as cover to prevent epidural venous bleeding during laminectomy.

After the bone removal is over, the ligamentum flavum is cut meticulously. We should avoid pulling of the epidural fat while cutting ligamentum flavum to avoid unnecessary epidural bleed. After exposure of the epidural fat, it can be incised or mobilized to lateral side by bipolar

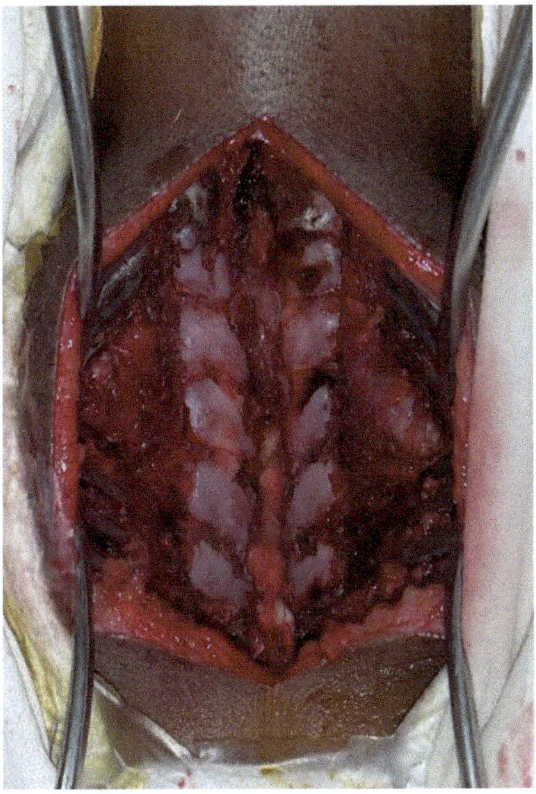

Fig. 18.13 Vertebral arch exposure to about intervertebral joint

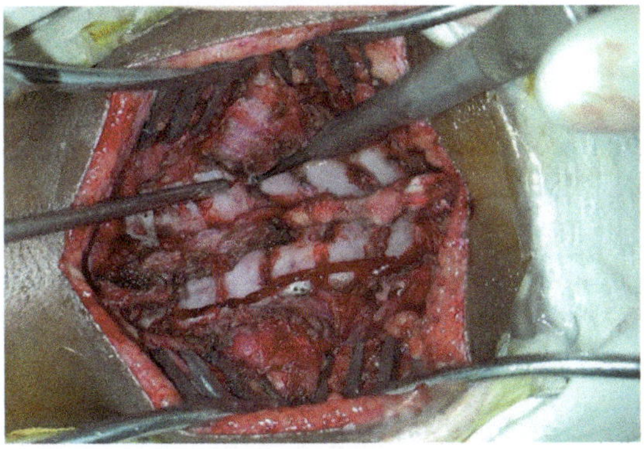

Fig. 18.14 Medial laminotomy by cutting the vertebral arch with small diamond drill

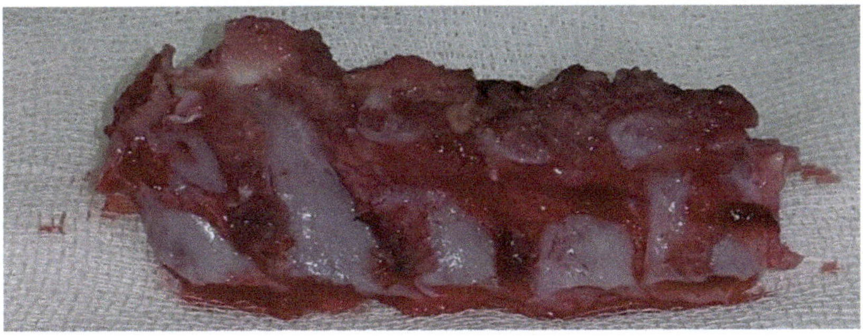

Fig. 18.15 Removal of all laminae including the interspinous and ligamentum flavum as en block

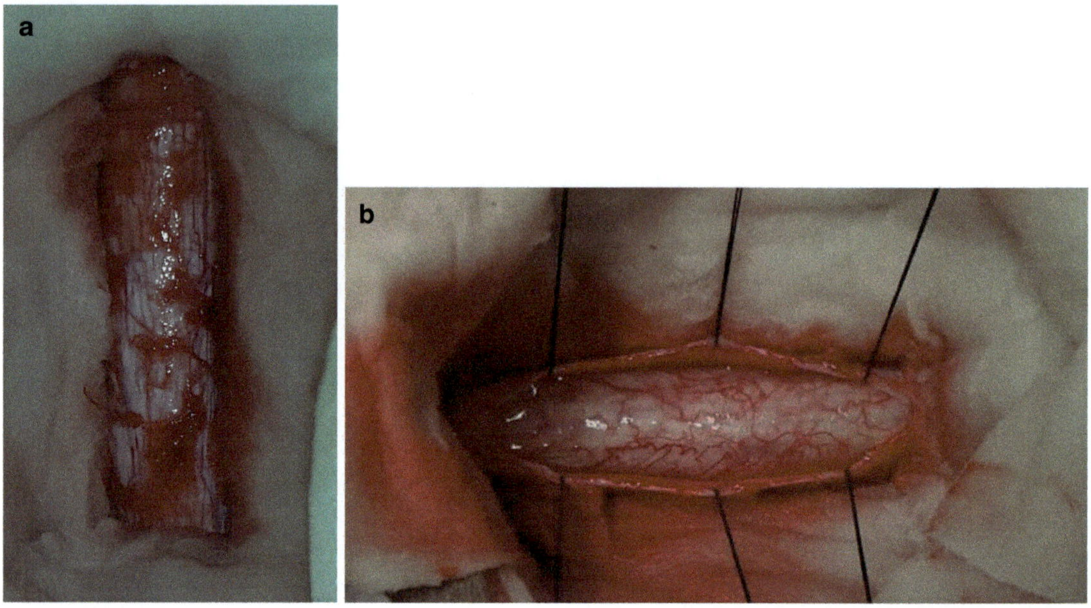

Fig. 18.16 (**a**) Exposed dura mater after haemostasis of epidural venous bleeding. (**b**) Dura mater stay sutures are used to keep dura open

coagulation. All these manoeuvres minimize the blood loss during the exposure of dura.

After dura exposure (Fig. 18.16a), midline dural opening is done under operating microscope. Dural stay sutures are taken to expose the surgical field properly (Fig. 18.16b). The arachnoid membrane should not open along with dura opening to prevent sudden escape of CSF and cord or vascular injury. After the dural opening, the arachnoid membrane is incised with microscissor and arachnoid hook. Arachnoid should be incised in a meticulous manner to prevent injury to the cord and its blood vessels.

Tuberculoma Resection

After the arachnoid layer is opened with microscissors, the spinal cord is looked for an appropriate zone for opening. Most of the time, there is no clue of lesion underlying the dorsum of the spinal cord lest it has extended the pia mater or even grown-up in exophytic manner. Occasionally arachnoidal thickening due to TB arachnoiditis may point to the beneath pathological lesion. In patients with post-TBM syringomyelia, the exact location of spinal intramedullary tuberculoma cannot be predicted only by inspecting of the spinal cord because the spinal cord will be distended over a more widespread region. Therefore, we acclaim ultrasound probe use to confirm that the exposure is satisfactory and to define the precise location of the tuberculoma before myelotomy.

Principally, three alternatives are there for myelotomy. Most of the time, myelotomy is performed in the midline. The dorsal root entry zone may be utilized if the tuberculoma is located laterally. If tuberculoma is encroaching the cord surface or having exophytic component, myelotomy can be done directly over that bulge. Needless coagulation of cord surface vessels should be avoided, because it may lead to substantial sensory deficit. SEPs monitoring is remarkably supportive during myelotomy. Additionally, motor-evoked potential monitoring is helpful during tuberculoma resection.

We advocate myelotomy over the tuberculoma as the first step of resection. We usually perform the dissection with the help of a microneedle hook or microscissors to incise the pia mater. After that, cord opening is done by spreading the cord fibres apart from midline with blunt instruments to avoid sharp dissection.

Best landmark for cord midline is the posterior median septum, which separates the spinal cord in two halves on dorsal aspect. Small conversing blood vessels of both sides into this septum are pointer for median septum.

We use proline 5-0 suture material for anchoring pia mater to keep the myelotomy open. This technique decreases handling of cord parenchyma and prevents injury during tuberculoma resection as well as helps in maintaining the resection plane. For the large tuberculoma, debulking can be done with the help of coagulation and piecemeal removal. Debulking can be achieved by sharp dissection, biopsy forceps or cavitron ultrasonic aspirator (CUSA) as and when required. After adequate debulking, dissection of tuberculoma margins should be performed.

Most of the time, it is likely to almost dissect the tuberculoma capsule from the surrounding cord parenchyma with the help of microforceps and dissectors (Fig. 18.17). In cases where tuberculoma capsule is adherent to cord parenchyma, sharp dissection is to be done to remove the tuberculoma. If there is associated syrinx, it can help in marginalizing the tuberculoma and dissection.

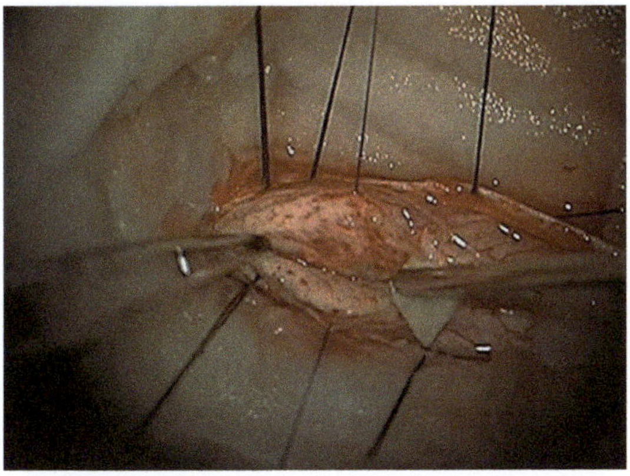

Fig. 18.17 Wipe the covering layer of spinal cord tissue over the tuberculoma capsule

Closure

As tuberculoma is resected and removed, we should look for adequate haemostasis which can be achieved by gentle coagulation, small cottonoids and saline irrigation. Few thin proline sutures can be used to approximate the pia mater to prevent adhesion between arachnoid and cord parenchyma. Some authors recommend to close arachnoid layer to avoid scarring, but it is the surgeon's choice and personal experience. Lastly watertight dura closure is performed.

Laminoplasty can be performed with help of miniplates or sutures. But metallic miniplates cause interface in follow-up MRI so it should be avoided if possible. The paraspinal muscles are approximated with sutures. Deep muscle facia with sheath closure is key to prevent wound gaping and CSF leak. Skin and subcutaneous layer suturing is done in traditional way.

18.4.2.2 Histopathology

The gross pathological specimens are generally encapsulated and/or yellow-grey firm mass. Histopathological evaluation of the resected specimen of tuberculoma in most of the cases has epitheloid cell granulomas with Langerhans giant cells (Fig. 18.18). Areas of caseous necrosis are also a characteristic finding [106]. Along the margin of the lesion, ill-formed granulomas mixed with mononuclear infiltration and are of gliosis are usually seen in histopathological examination [59]. Variable numbers of acid-fast bacilli are often detected in the lesions.

18.4.2.3 Postoperative Outcome and Complications Management

Postoperative MRI shows total resolution of the lesion in most of the operated patients. In some patients, there was postoperative oedema which was resolved in follow-up MRI at 3 months [59, 70, 99]. Few patients develop CSF leak in postoperative period which is successfully managed by acetazolamide, prone position and compression dressing. Sixty percent to 70% of patients improve

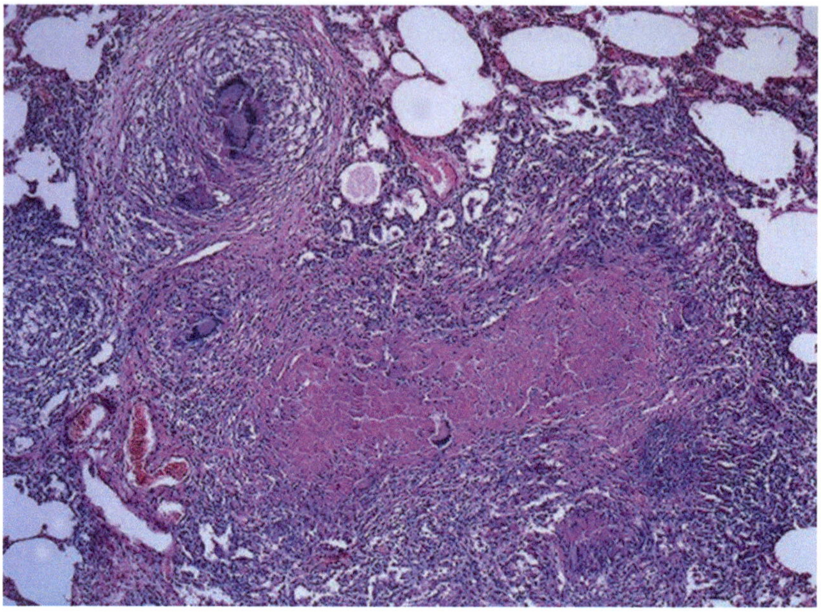

Fig. 18.18 Histopathological examination finding showing multiple epitheloid cell granulomas with Langerhans and foreign body type of giant cells confirming the diagnosis of tuberculoma

significantly and rest gradually in neurological status in terms of ambulation and spasticity in follow-up [119, 121]. Antispastic agent is also advised in postoperative period in dose of baclofen 10 mg thrice a day. Anti-TB chemotherapy is continued postoperatively with follow-up at regular interval of 3 months, 6 months, 1 year and 2 years [59]. Post-TB syringomyelia is managed by syringo-subarachnoid shunt and has good outcome in some patients (Fig. 18.19). Some recent publications related to intramedullary management and outcome are summarized in Table 18.3 [1, 14, 47, 59–61, 64, 83, 89, 91, 107, 116].

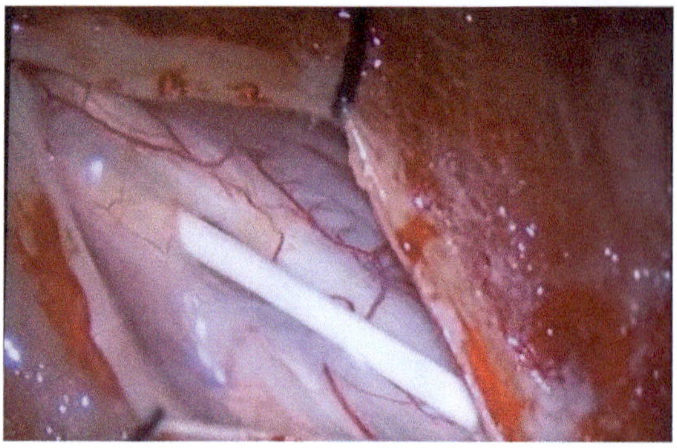

Fig. 18.19 Syringo-subarachnoid shunt for post-TB syringomyelia

Table 18.3 Review literature of patients having spinal intramedullary tuberculoma

Author/year/# of reference	Patient profile	Level	Associated TB	Clinical presentation	Management	Outcome
Jaiswal et al. 2015 [59]	11 cases, mean age 28.5	7 dorsal, 2 lumber, 1 cervical, 1 thoracolumbar, 2 intracranial	5 pulmonary TB	Most common presentation was motor weakness	Laminectomy and excision of lesion in 8 cases, 3 conservative	10 patients have shown improved neurological function. 1 remained same
Li et al. 2012 [83]	23 cases, mean age 30.3	10 dorsal, 6 cervical, 3 cervicothoracic, 1 thoracolumbar, 6 intracranial, 3 patients had multiple lesions	2 Pulmonary TB, 5 TB meningoencephalitis and 1 cervical node	19 patients presented sensory-motor involvement	Laminectomy and excision of lesion in 21 cases	17 patients have shown improved neurological function
Guirado et al. 2011 [60]	29 F	C7 D1	D8 body TB	Paraparesis Grade II and urinary retention	Laminotomy at C7-T1 level was done followed by debulking of the lesion microsurgically	Gradual improvement in power over a period of 6 months
Tyagi et al. 2010 [91]	6 F	D9–10	No	Spastic weakness (Grade III/V) of the lower limbs with exaggerated reflexes	D9–10 laminectomy. Midline durotomy, excision of mass	Recovered completely
Arora et al. 2010 [14]	19 F	Cervicomedullary junction	No	Slight hypoesthesia in the left upper limb	Excision of lesion	At 1 year on follow-up, improved, with complete resolution of the sensory symptoms
Liu et al. 2009 [107]	42 M	D6–7	No	Weakness in lower extremities and urinary retention	Not specified	At 6 months on follow-up, the patient was able to walk with support and regained bladder control
Ramdurg et al. 2008 [64]	15 cases, mean age 31	7 dorsal, 5 cervical, 2 cervicodorsal, 1 dorsolumbar	3 TB meningitis, 1 intracranial granuloma, 1 cervical node, 1 pulmonary TB	14 patients presented	Laminectomy and excision of lesion in 12 cases	9 patients have shown improved neurological function

(continued)

Table 18.3 (continued)

Author/year/# of reference	Patient profile	Level	Associated TB	Clinical presentation	Management	Outcome
Arslantas et al. 2002 [1]	36 M	D10	Pulmonary TB	Paraplegia, spastic reflexes and urinary incontinence	Posterior longitudinal myelotomy	No new neurological deficit
Sharma et al. 2002 [89]	10 cases, mean age 29.7	5 dorsal, 3 cervical, 1 cervicodorsal, 1 dorsolumbar	1 lung, 1 cervical node, 1 brain, 1 TB meningitis	MC presentation was motor weakness (100%)	Laminectomy and excisions of lesion in 8 cases	Six patients have shown improved neurological function
Devi et al. 2002 [47]	5 cases, mean age 23	-	5 pulmonary TB, 1 intracranial tuberculoma	MC presentation was motor weakness	Laminectomy and excision of lesion in four cases	Symptoms improved in all patients
Nomura et al. 2001 [116]	2½ F	Intracranial cisterns and D6–10	TB meningitis	Weakness in both legs, bilateral pes equinus and left pes adductus. The knee and ankle jerks brisk, with ankle clonus. Sensory and bladder function is preserved	Laminectomy was done D7 to D10 the dura was opened. The dorsal mass is incised, but the ventral mass lesions are not addressed	1 year after the operation, she can walk and even run by herself, although the lesions remain
Kayaoglu et al. 2000 [61]	16 M	D4–D5 level	Pulmonary Koch's	Mild paraparesis with hypoactivity in deep tendon reflexes in both low limbs and sensory loss below D6 dermatome	Laminectomy of D4–D5, myelotomy and excision	Improved follow-up neurologic examination was normal

Table 18.4 Management of spinal intramedullary tuberculoma

Intramedullary lesion has high probability of tuberculoma if associated with	
Clinical features	**Investigations**
Constitutional symptoms like Evening rising fever Cough with sputum Weight loss Back or neck pain not responding to analgesics Headache, blurring of vision, neck rigidity suggestive of tubercular meningitis Patient is on anti-TB therapy	Magnetic resonance imaging (MRI) spine with contrast: target sign, disc-like lesion, multiple conglomerate rim enhancements X-ray chest/CT thorax: miliary tuberculosis, cavitation ESR: raised HIV status: positive MRI brain: multiple intracranial tuberculomas Mantoux test: positive
Indications of conservative management with anti-TB therapy	**Indications of surgical intervention along with anti-TB therapy**
1. Small lesion with typical target sign in MRI spine	1. No response to chemotherapy (anti-TB therapy)
2. Neurological status is stable and nonprogressive in nature and responding to anti-TB therapy	2. Diagnosis in doubt (MRI finding suggestive of intramedullary tumour in differential diagnosis) in patient with no history of pulmonary tuberculosis
3. Pulmonary Koch's with MRI spine finding of inflammatory pathology	3. Rapid deterioration in neurological function
4. Multiple intramedullary tuberculomas with or without concurrent intracranial tuberculoma	4. Paradoxical increase in size with mass effect after anti-TB therapy starts
Follow-up:	
6 weeks, 3 months, 6 months, 1 year and 2 years by clinical assessment, liver function test and MRI spine	

Conclusion

- Although rare, spinal intramedullary tuberculoma should be kept in the differential diagnosis of spinal cord lesions.
- Gadolinium-enhanced MRI helps in the accurate diagnosis and monitoring of the treatment response and in the follow-up of spinal intramedullary tuberculoma.
- In cases with early diagnosis of spinal intramedullary tuberculoma, immediate medical treatment with anti-TB treatment is sufficient, and complete resolution of lesions is seen.
- We advocate that patients presenting with progressive neurological deterioration should go through early decompression even with adequate anti-TB chemotherapy, since the spinal intramedullary location and broadening of the cord with demyelination as well as spinal tract damage can aggravate the poor neurological outcome.
- A well-designed prospective study is in need of time to explain the surgical and medical treatment role for the management of tuberculoma.
- Brief conceptualization of the diagnosis and management of spinal intramedullary tuberculoma is tried by us for decision-making (Table 18.4).

References

1. Arslantas A, Faruk A, Kismet B, Esref T (2002) Intramedullary tuberculoma of spinal cord. J Postgrad Med 48:54–55
2. Abercrombie J (1828) Pathological and practical researches on disease of the brain and the spinal cord. Waugh and Innes, Edinburg, pp 371–372
3. Agarwal RP, Mohan N, Garg RK, Bajpai SK, Verma SK, Mohindra Y (1990) Clinicosocial aspect of osteo-articular tuberculosis. J Indian Med Assoc 88:307–309
4. Akhaddar A, Baallal H, Elouennass M, Elgharbaoui H, Mahi M, Boucetta M (2011) Combined Serratia liquefaciens and Mycobacterium tuberculosis in temporal osteitis with brain extension. Surg Infect (Larchmt) 12:329–331
5. Akhaddar A, Boucetta M (2014) Giant brain tuberculoma mimicking a malignant tumor in a child. Pan Afr Med J J17:112
6. Akhaddar A, Boucetta M (2011) Images in clinical medicine. Multiple intracranial tuberculomas. N Engl J Med 365:1527

7. Akhaddar A, Bourazza A, El Mostarchid B, Rouimi A, Boutaleb N, Ouahabi H, Mosseddaq R (2000) Brainstem tuberculomas: two cases. Rev Neurol (Paris) 156:399–402
8. Akhaddar A, Chakir N, El Hassani MY, El Quessar A, Jiddane M, Boukhrissi N (2000) Sub-occipital Pott's disease. Diagnostic imaging in 2 cases. J Neuroradiol 27:144–149
9. Akhaddar A, El Hassani MY, Chakir N, Jiddane M (2001) Optochiasmatic tuberculoma: complication of tuberculous meningitis. Report of a case and review of the literature. J Neuroradiol 28:137–142
10. Akhaddar A, Gazzaz M, Jiddane M, El Hassani MR, Chakir N, El Khamlichi A, Boukhrissi N (2001) Tuberculous osteitis of the posterior vertebral arch: case report. J Radiol 82:257–260
11. Akhaddar A, Gourinda H, Gazzaz M, Elmadhi T, Elalami Z, Miri A (1999) Craniocervical junction tuberculosis in children. Rev Rhum Engl Ed 66:739–742
12. Akhaddar A, Mahi M, Harket A, Elmostarchid B, Belhachemi A, Elasri A, Gazzaz M, Boucetta M (2007) Brainstem tuberculoma in a postpartum patient. J Neuroradiol 34:345–346
13. Alessi G, Lemmerling M, Nathoo N (2003) Combined spinal tuberculous empyema and intramedullary tuberculoma in an HIV-positive patient. Eur Radiol 13:1899–1901
14. Arora B, Sridhar E, Muzumdar D, Jalali R, Munshi A (2010) Spinal tuberculoma in a patient with spinal myxopapillaryependymoma. J Cancer Res Ther 6:215–217
15. Bassoe P (1918) Conglomerate tubercle and combined degeneration of the cord as complications of visceral tuberculosis. Arch Intern Med 21:519–530
16. Charcot JM (1889) Clinical lectures on diseases of the nervous system delivered at the infirmary of la Salpetriere. T. Savill, transl. London: New Sydenham Soc 3: 125–129
17. Garg RK, Malhotra HS, Kumar N (2014) Paradoxical reaction in HIV negative tuberculous meningitis. J Neurol Sci 340:26–36
18. Garg RK, Paliwal V, Malhotra HS (2011) Tuberculous optochiasmatic arachnoiditis: a devastating form of tuberculous meningitis. Expert Rev Anti Infect Ther 9:719–729
19. Garg RK, Sinha MK (2010) Multiple ring-enhancing lesions of the brain. J Postgrad Med 56:307–316
20. Garg RK, Sinha MK (2011) Tuberculous meningitis in patients infected with human immunodeficiency virus. J Neurol 258:3–13
21. Garg RK (2004) Diagnostic criteria for neurocysticercosis: some modifications are needed for Indian patients. Neurol India 52:171–177
22. Bhandari A, Garg RK, Malhotra HS, Verma R, Singh MK, Jain A, Sharma PK (2014) Outcome assessment in conservatively managed patients with cervical spine tuberculosis. Spinal Cord 52:489–493
23. Citow JS, Ammirati M (1994) Intramedullary tuberculoma of the spinal cord: case report. Neurosurgery 35:327–330
24. El Guendouz F, Zajjari Y, Akhaddar A, Belmejdoub G (2012) Cervical Pott's disease revealed by diabetic ketoacidosis. Intern Med 51:681–682
25. Krauss WC, McGuire ER (1909) Intramedullary tuberculoma removed at the level of the fifth thoracic segment of the spinal cord. Note on behaviour of the cerebrospinal fluid. J A M A 53:1911
26. Garg RK, Jain S, Kar AM (1996) Pott's paraplegia like presentation: a neurological complication of lymphatic filariasis. J Assoc Physicians India 44:741–742
27. Garg RK, Karak B, Misra S (1998) Acute paraparesis with tuberculous meningitis. Postgrad Med J74:269–271
28. Garg RK, Raut T, Malhotra HS, Parihar A, Goel M, Jain A, Verma R, Singh MK (2013) Evaluation of prognostic factors in medically treated patients of spinal tuberculosis. Rheumatol Int 33:3009–3015
29. Garg RK, Somvanshi DS (2011) Spinal tuberculosis: a review. J Spinal Cord Med 34:440–454
30. Jennings FL (1984) Tuherculoma of the spinal cord. Ann Intern Med 7:1240–1243
31. Webster R (1938) Pathological reports from the Children's Hospital. Melbourne Med J1:1061–1064
32. Thalhimer W, Hassin GB (1922) Clinico-pathologie notes on solitary tubercle of the spinal cord. J Herr Ment Dis 55:161–193
33. KupkaE ORE (1938) Tuberculoma of the lumbar spinal cord. Am Rev Tuberc 38:517–522
34. Dastur HM (1972) A tuberculoma review with some personal experiences: II. Spinal cord and its coverings. Neurol India 20:127–131
35. Lin SK, Wu T, Wai YY (1994) Intramedullary spinal tuberculoma during treatment of tuberculous meningitis. Clin Neurol Neurosurg 96:71–78
36. Lin TH (1960) İntramedullary tuberculoma of the spinal cord. J Neurosurg 17:497–499
37. Ratliff JK (1999) Intramedullary tuberculoma of spinal cord. J Neurosurg Spine 90:125–128
38. Caplan LR, Norohna AB, Amico LL (1990) Syringomyelia and arachnoiditis. J Neurol Neurosurg Psychiatry 53:106–113
39. Fehling MG, Bernstein M (1992) Syringomyelia as a complication of tuberculous meningitis. Can J Neurol Sci 19:84–87
40. Rao GP (2000) Spinal intramedullary tuberculous lesion medical management. Report of four cases. J Neurosurg Spine 93:137–141
41. Schon F, Bowler JV (1990) Syringomyelia and syringobulbia following tuberculous meningitis. J Neurol 237:122–123
42. Akhaddar A, El Hassani MY, Gazzaz-Rifi M, Chakir N, El Khamlichi A, Jiddane M (2000) MR imaging in the diagnosis of intradural extramedullary tuberculoma. Report of a case and review of the literature. J Neuroradiol l27:107–111
43. Akhaddar A, Elhamzaoui S, En-nouali H, Albouzidi A, Dami A, Elmostarchid B, Boucetta M (2009) Recurrent pyelonephritis revealing a calcified tuberculoma of the filum terminale. Intern Med 48:1485–1486

44. Bertrand I, Guillaume JM, Samson M, Gueguen Y (1958) Tuberculome intramedullaire dorsal. Rev Neurol 98:51–54
45. Bucy PC, Oberhill HR (1950) Intradural spinal granulomas. J Neurosurg 7:1
46. Cascino J, Dibble JB (1956) Tuberculoma of spinal cord. JAMA 162:461–462
47. Devi BI, Chandra S, Mongia S, Chandramouli BA, Sastry KV, Shankar SK (2002) Spinal intramedullary tuberculoma and abscess : a rare cause of paraparesis. Neurol India 50:494–496
48. Anuradha HK, Garg RK, Agarwal A, Sinha MK, Verma R, Singh MK, Shukla R (2010) Predictors of stroke in patients of tuberculous meningitis and its effect on the outcome. QJM 103:671–678
49. Anuradha HK, Garg RK, Sinha MK, Agarwal A, Verma R, Singh MK, Shukla R (2011) Intracranial tuberculomas in patients with tuberculous meningitis: predictors and prognostic significance. Int J Tuberc Lung Dis 15:234–239
50. Garg RK, Malhotra HS, Gupta R (2015) Spinal cord involvement in tuberculous meningitis. Spinal Cord 53:649–657
51. Garg RK, Raut T, Malhotra HS, Jain A (2013) Tuberculous meningitis and hydrocephalus. J Infect 66:541–542
52. Garg RK (2010) Tuberculous meningitis. Acta Neurol Scand 122:75–90
53. Gupta A, Garg RK, Singh MK, Verma R, Malhotra HS, Sankhwar SN, Jain A, Singh R, Parihar A (2013) Bladder dysfunction and urodynamic study in tuberculous meningitis. J Neurol Sci 327:46–54
54. Raut T, Garg RK, Jain A, Verma R, Singh MK, Malhotra HS, Kohli N, Parihar A (2013) Hydrocephalus in tuberculous meningitis: Incidence, its predictive factors and impact on the prognosis. J Infect 66:330–337
55. Sohn S, Jin YJ, Kim K-J, Kim H-J Long-term sequela of intradural extramedullary tuberculoma in the thoracic dorsal spinal cord (2011) case report and review of the literature. Korean J Spine 8:295–299
56. Turgut M (1997) Intradural tuberculous granuloma. Br J Neurosurg 11:264
57. Chang KH, Han MH, Choi YW, Kim IO, Han MC, Kim CW (1989) Tuberculous arachnoiditis of the spine: findings on myelography, CT, and MR imaging. AJNR Am J Neuroradiol 10:1255–1262
58. Gupta R, Garg RK, Jain A, Malhotra HS, Verma R, Sharma PK (2015) Spinal cord and spinal nerve root involvement (myeloradiculopathy) in tuberculous meningitis. Medicine (Baltimore) 94:e404
59. Jaiswal M, Gandhi A, Sharma A, Mittal RS (2015) Experiences and conceptualisation of spinal intramedullary tuberculoma management. Korean J Spine 12:5–11
60. Guirado VM, Welling LC, Meluzzi A, dos Santos ME, Figueiredo EG, Taricco MA, Teixeira MJ (2011) Intramedullary granuloma suggestive of tuberculoma. Arq Neuropsiquiatr 69:848–849
61. Kayaoglu CR, Tuzun Y, Boga Z, Erdogan F, Gorguner M, Aydin IH (2000) Intramedullary spinal tuberculoma: a case report. Spine (Phila Pa 1976) 25:2265–2268
62. Malhotra HS, Garg RK, Lalla R, Gupta A (2012) Paradoxical extensive thoracolumbosacral arachnoiditis in a treated patient of tuberculous meningitis. BMJ Case Rep 2012: pii: bcr2012006262. doi: 10.1136/bcr-2012-006262
63. Jaiswal M, Gandhi A, Purohit D, Mittal RS Concurrent multiple intracranial and intramedullary conus tuberculoma: a rare case report. Asian J Neurosurg. doi:10.4103/1793-5482.143461
64. Ramdurg SR, Gupta DK, Suri A, Sharma BS, Mahapatra AK (2009) Spinal intramedullary tuberculosis: a series of 15 cases. Clin Neurol Neurosurg 111:115–118
65. Turgut M, Ozcan OE, Ozgen T, Bertan V (1993) Intradural extramedullary tuberculoma of the spinal cord – a case report. Zentralbl Neurochir 54:197–199
66. Turgut M (2001) Multifocal extensive spinal tuberculosis (Pott's disease) involving cervical, thoracic and lumbar vertebrae. Br J Neurosurg 15:142–146
67. Turgut M (1997) Pott's disease. J Neurosurg 87:136–138
68. Turgut M (2001) Spinal tuberculosis (Pott's disease): its clinical presentation, surgical management, and outcome. A survey study on 694 patients. Neurosurg Rev 24:8–13
69. Whiteman M, Espinosa L, Post MDJ, Bell MD, Falcon S (1995) Central nervous system tuberculosis in HİV infection patient. Clinical and radiographical finding. AJNR Am J Neuroradiol 16:1319–1327
70. Rhoton EL, Ballinger WE, Quisling R, Sypert GW (1988) Intramedullary spinal tuberculoma. Neurosurgery 22:733
71. GimeÂnez-Roldan S, Esteban A, Benito C (1974) Communicating syringomyelia following cured tuberculous meningitis. J Neurol Sci 23:185–197
72. Kobayashi R, Togashi S, Nagasaka T, Shindo K, Shiozawa Z, Yamada H, Hashizume Y (2000) Intramedullary tuberculoma with syringomyelia. J Spinal Disord Tech 15:88–90
73. Pernuate RS, Berciano J, Rebello M, Pascual J (1996) Intramedullary tuberculoma of the spinal cord with syringomyelia. Neuroradiology 38:105
74. MacDonnell AH, Baird RW, Bronze MS (1990) Intramedullary tuberculomas of the spinal cord: case report and review. Rev Infect Dis 12:432–439
75. Eljebbouri B, Zine M, Akhaddar A, Gazzaz M, Elmoustarchid B (2013) Miliary brain tuberculosis. Rev Prat 63:462
76. Garg RK, Desai P, Kar M, Kar AM (2008) Multiple ring enhancing brain lesions on computed tomography: an Indian perspective. J Neurol Sci 266:92–96
77. Garg RK, Kar AM, Kumar T (2000) Neurocysticercosis like presentation in a case of CNS tuberculosis. Neurol India 48:260–262
78. Garg RK, Karak B, Sharma AM, Ojha R, Misra S (1999) Single CT (ring) lesion in epilepsy patients: a new observation. Indian J Pediatr 66:155–157
79. Garg RK, Singh SK, Malhotra HS, Singh MK (2012) Abnormal head movement in a patient with tuber-

culous meningitis. BMJ Case Rep 2012. doi:pii: bcr2012006663. 10.1136/bcr-2012-006663
80. Garg RK, Singhal P (2007) Primary tuberculosis of the tongue: a case report. J Contemp Dent Pract 8:74–80
81. Naama O, Boulahroud O, Elouennass M, Akhaddar A, Gazzaz M, Elmoustarchid B, Boucetta M (2010) Primary tuberculous cerebellar abscess in an immunocompetent adult. Intern Med 49:875–87610.4103/1793-5482.143461
82. Sharma P, Garg RK, Verma R, Singh MK, Shukla R (2011) Incidence, predictors and prognostic value of cranial nerve involvement in patients with tuberculous meningitis: a retrospective evaluation. Eur J Intern Med 22:289–295
83. Li H, Liu W, You C (2012) Central nervous system tuberculoma. J Clin Neurosci 19:691–695
84. McCormick PC, Stein BM (1990) Intramedullary tumours in adults. Neurosurg Clin N Am 1:609–630
85. Garg RK, Sharma R, Kar AM, Kushwaha RA, Singh MK, Shukla R, Agarwal A, Verma R (2010) Neurological complications of miliary tuberculosis. Clin Neurol Neurosurg 112:188–192
86. Malhotra HS, Garg RK, Gupta A, Saxena S, Majumdar A, Jain A (2012) An unusual cause of visual impairment in tuberculous meningitis. J Neurol Sci 318:174–177
87. Thacker MM, Puri AI (2004) Concurrent intra-medullary and intracranial tuberculomas. J Postgrad Med 50:107–109
88. Yen HL, Lee RJ, Lin JW, Chen HJ (2003) Multiple tuberculomas in the brain and spinal cord: a case report. Spine 28:499–50210.1136/bcr-2012-006262
89. Sharma MC, Arora R, Deol PS, Mahapatra AK, Sinha AK, Sarkar C (2002) Intramedullary tuberculoma of the spinal cord: a series of 10 cases. Clin Neurol Neurosurg 104:279–284
90. Torii H, Takahashi T, Shimizu H, Watanabe M, Tominaga T (2004) Intramedullary spinal tuberculoma: case report. Neurol Med Chir 44:266–268
91. Tyagi DK, Balasubramaniam S, Purandare HR, Savant HV (2010) Intramedullary tuberculoma in a six year old. Neurol India 58:736–738
92. Jha SK, Garg RK, Jain A, Malhotra HS, Verma R, Sharma PK (2015) Definite (microbiologically confirmed) tuberculous meningitis: predictors and prognostic impact. Infection 43(6):639–645
93. Malhotra HS, Garg RK, Raut TP (2012) Pleural involvement in spinal tuberculosis. Am J Trop Med Hyg 86:560
94. Nussbaum ES, Rockswold GL, Bergman TA, Erickson DL, Seljeskog EL (1995) Spinal tuberculosis: a diagnostic and management challenge. J Neurosurg 83:243–247
95. Parmar H, Shah J, Patkar D, Varma R (2000) Intramedullary tuberculomas. MR findings in seven patients. Acta Radiol 41:572–577
96. Patil T, Garg RK, Jain A, Goel MM, Malhotra HS, Verma R, Singh GP, Sharma PK (2015) Serum and CSF cytokines and matrix metalloproteinases in spinal tuberculosis. Inflamm Res 64:97–106
97. Rich AR, McCordock HA (1933) Pathogenesis of tuberculous meningitis. Bull Johns Hopkins Hosp 52:5–13
98. Zohoun A, Ngoh Akwa E, El Ochi M, Oragwu N, Akhaddar A, Albouzidi A, El Ouennass M (2012) Bacteriological features of infectious spondylodiscitis at Mohammed V Military Teaching Hospital of Rabat. Braz J Microbiol 43:1327–1331
99. Shen WC, Cheng TY, Lee SK, Ho YJ, Lee KR (1993) Disseminated tuberculomas in spinal cord and brain demonstrated by MRI with gadolinium-DTPA. Neurosurgery 35:213–215
100. Singh B, Garg RK, Singh MK, Verma R, Malhotra HS, Jain A, Singh R, Kohli N, Phadke RV, Shukla R, Parihar A (2012) Computed tomography angiography in patients with tuberculous meningitis. J Infect 64:565–572
101. Vidhate MR, Singh MK, Garg RK, Verma R, Shukla R, Goel MM, Makker A, Jain A (2011) Diagnostic and prognostic value of Mycobacterium tuberculosis complex specific interferon gamma release assay in patients with tuberculous meningitis. J Infect 62:400–403
102. Gupta RK, Gupta S, Kumar S, Kohli A, Misra UK, Gujral RB (1994) MRI in intraspinal tuberculosis. Neuroradiology 36:39–43
103. Gupta VK, Sharma BS, Khosla VK (1995) Intramedullary tuberculoma: report of two cases with MRI findings. Surg Neurol 44:241–244
104. Huang CR, Lui CC, Chang WN, Wu HS, Chen HJ (1999) Neuroimages of disseminated neurotuberculosis: report of one case. Clin Imaging 23:218–222
105. Jena A, Banerji AK, Tripathi RI, Gulati PK, Jain RK, Khushu S, Supra MI (1991) Demonstration of intramedullary tuberculosis by MRI – a case report of 2 cases. Br J Radiol 64:555–557
106. Elseberg CA (1917) Laminectomy and removal of conglomerate tubercle from the substance of the spinal cord. Ann Surg 65:269
107. Liu YD, Wang FY, Xu JM, Guan Y, Guan H (2010) Intramedullary thoracic tuberculoma. Spinal Cord 48:80–82
108. Garg RK (2002) Proposed diagnostic criteria for neurocysticercosis. Neurology 58:1315. ; author reply 1315–1316
109. Garg RK (2002) Single enhancing computerized tomography-detected lesion in immunocompetent patients. Neurosurg Focus 12:e4
110. Garg RK (1999) Tuberculosis of the central nervous system. Postgrad Med J75:133–140
111. Mohit AA, Santiago P, Rostomily R (2004) Intramedullary tuberculoma mimicking primary CNS lymphoma. J Neurol Neurosurg Psychiatry 75:1636–1638
112. Garg RK, Jain A, Malhotra HS, Agrawal A, Garg R (2013) Drug-resistant tuberculous meningitis. Expert Rev Anti Infect Ther 11(6):605–621
113. Jain A, Dixit P, Jaiswal I, Garg RK, Kumar R (2012) Drug resistance in mycobacterial isolates from meningitis cases. Pediatr Infect Dis J31:1317

114. Karak B, Garg RK (1998) Corticosteroids in tuberculous meningitis. Indian Pediatr 35:193–194
115. Malhotra HS, Garg RK, Singh MK, Agarwal A, Verma R (2009) Corticosteroids (dexamethasone versus intravenous methylprednisolone) in patients with tuberculous meningitis. Ann Trop Med Parasitol 103:625–634
116. Nomura S, Akimura T, Kitahara T, Nogami K, Suzuki M (2001) Surgery for expansion of spinal tuberculoma during antituberculous chemotherapy: a case report. Pediatr Neurosurg 35:153–157
117. Sinha MK, Garg RK, Anuradha HK, Agarwal A, Parihar A, Mandhani PA (2010) Paradoxical vision loss associated with optochiasmatic tuberculoma in tuberculous meningitis: a report of 8 patients. J Infect 60:458–466
118. Sinha MK, Garg RK, Hk A, Agarwal A, Singh MK, Verma R, Shukla R (2010) Vision impairment in tuberculous meningitis: predictors and prognosis. J Neurol Sci 290:27–32
119. Suzer T, Coskun E, Tahta K, Bayramoglu H, Duzcan E (1998) Intramedullary spinal tuberculoma presenting as a conus tumour. A case report and review of literature. Eur Spine J 7:167
120. Muthukumar N, Venkatesh G, Senthilbabu S, Rajbaskar R (2006) Surgery for intramedullary tuberculoma of the spinal cord (report of 2 cases). Surg Neurol 66:69–74
121. Turgut M (2007) Re: Surgery for intramedullary tuberculoma of the spinal cord: report of 2 cases (Muthukumar et al. Surg Neurol 2006;66:69–74). Surg Neurol 67:654

Imaging Findings of Tuberculosis of the Spine and Its Coverings

19

Elif Karadeli and Ahmet T. Turgut

Contents

E. Karadeli, MD
Department of Radiology, Baskent University, School of Medicine, Dr. Turgut Noyan Medical and Research Center, Adana, Turkey
e-mail: elifkaradeli@gmail.com

A.T. Turgut, MD (✉)
Department of Radiology,
Hacettepe University Faculty of Medicine,
06100 Ankara, Turkey
e-mail: ahmettuncayturgut@yahoo.com

Abbreviations

ADC	Apparent diffusion coefficient
AIDS	Acquired immunodeficiency syndrome
CT	Computerized tomography
DW	Diffusion weighted
IVD	Intervertebral disk
MRI	Magnetic resonance imaging
STIR	Short tau inversion recovery
TB	Tuberculosis

19.1 Introduction

Tuberculosis (TB) is an infectious disease caused by *Mycobacterium tuberculosis*, and it usually affects the respiratory system. However, any organ system can be affected by the disease, especially in patients with predisposing conditions such as diabetes, hepatic cirrhosis, corticosteroid treatment, alcoholism, and intravenous drug abuse and in immunocompromised patients [1–5]. Historically, spinal TB was first determined by Percivall Pott in 1779, and thus, the disease was called as "Pott's disease" at present [6].

The hematogenous extension of disease is usually from the lung or other extraosseous regions such as the lymph nodes, gastrointestinal tract, and other viscera. Spinal TB is the most common form of extrapulmonary TB, occurring as osteoarticular TB in 65% of the cases [7]. The most common sites of involvement for the entity are the spinal region, pelvis, hip, and knee. Anatomically, the spine is

M. Turgut et al. (eds.), *Tuberculosis of the Central Nervous System*,
DOI 10.1007/978-3-319-50712-5_19

likely to be involved by *M. tuberculosis* because the agent can easily grow in blood-rich tissues and the spinal region is characterized by slow venous blood and the presence of cancellous bone and terminal arteries being its nutrient artery at this site [8, 9]. TB is seen in any age, though adults of middle age are the most frequently affected group. Men are affected slightly more frequently than women. Unfortunately, severe morbidity and neurologic sequelae may develop due to osteoarticular disease in patients with TB [7, 10–12].

19.2 Imaging Findings

Spinal TB occurs mainly at the upper lumbar and lower thoracic vertebrae, comprising 48–67% of the lesions, by hematogenous dissemination via the venous plexus of Batson. Notably, the cervical and sacral involvement is rare [13, 14]. The disease is usually seen in more than one vertebra, and it usually starts at the anteroinferior region of the vertebral body. The spread of the infection can occur beneath the anterior longitudinal ligament involving the adjacent vertebral bodies or penetration of the subchondral bone plate. Rarely, posterior elements of the spine may be involved too. On the other hand, the narrowing and collapse of intervertebral disk (IVD) space occur secondarily [11].

The lack of proteolytic enzymes in *M. tuberculosis* has been proposed as the cause of relative preservation of the IVD space compared to pyogenic infections [15–17]. The involved vertebral end plates are demineralized and resorbed, which results in the loss of definition of its dense margins on conventional radiographs. After these end plate changes, the spread of the infection to adjacent IVD and other spinal segments becomes easier. Then, the disease involves the paraspinal tissues which may result in the occurrence of paravertebral abscess known as a Pott's abscess. On conventional radiographs, it manifests as lateral bowing of the psoas shadow. Sometimes, the groin and thigh may be affected by psoas abscess. If spinal TB progresses, collapse of partially destructed vertebral bodies and anterior wedging may occur, leading to severe deformities as kyphosis or Gibbus deformity and scoliosis. If spinal TB heals, on the other hand, ankylosis of the vertebral bodies and obliteration of the intervening IVD space may be seen [14, 18–22].

19.2.1 Conventional Radiography

Conventional radiography is usually the first imaging method of choice in patients with spinal TB. The relevant findings are lytic lucencies in anterior portion of the vertebrae, narrowing of the IVD space, end plate erosions, sclerosis secondary to chronic infection, compression fracture, vertebral body collapse, kyphosis, and Gibbus. If bone mineral loss exceeds 30%, a radiolucent lesion is detected on conventional radiography. The earliest radiological feature is narrowing of the IVD space. Then, anterior wedging or collapse occurs, resulting in kyphosis of varying degree and thickening of the prevertebral soft tissue (Fig. 19.1). The tuberculous granulation tissue and necrotic material are fused which results in paravertebral abscess formation. TB abscesses may be accompanied by concave erosions around the anterior margins of

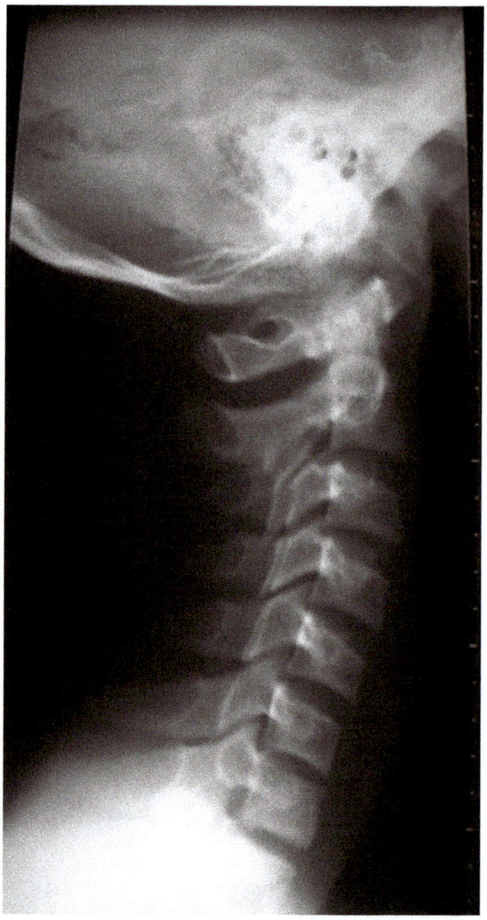

Fig. 19.1 Lateral x-ray of the cervical spine of a patient with spinal tuberculosis (TB) showing thickening of the prevertebral soft tissue (Courtesy of M. Benzagmout)

the vertebral bodies, and this appearance is called as the aneurysmal phenomenon [23].

19.2.2 Computed Tomography

The bone destruction may be determined by using computed tomography (CT) at the beginning. CT depicts irregular lytic bone lesions, sclerosis, collapse of IVD, and disruption of bone circumference much better than conventional radiography (Fig. 19.2). In particular, CT is superior to conventional radiography in depicting lesions with a diameter of less than 1.5 cm. The pattern of bone destruction can be seen well on CT. The patterns of bone destruction are fragmentary (47%), osteolytic (33%), subperiosteal (10%), or localized and sclerotic (10%) [24, 25]. The presence and extent of epidural compression can be determined by CT; the technique is especially helpful for detecting bone fragments within the spinal space in patients with neurological deficit. In addition, CT is quite helpful for defining the shape of paraspinal muscle abscesses (Fig. 19.3). On CT, the granulation tissue is seen as a high-attenuation lesion, whereas an abscess or caseous tissue is depicted with low attenuation. Bone expansion due to destruction and paravertebral abscess with heterotopic bone or calcification is accepted to be a sign of a TB lesion (Fig. 19.4). CT can also be used to guide percutaneous interventions (Fig. 19.5) [11, 24–28].

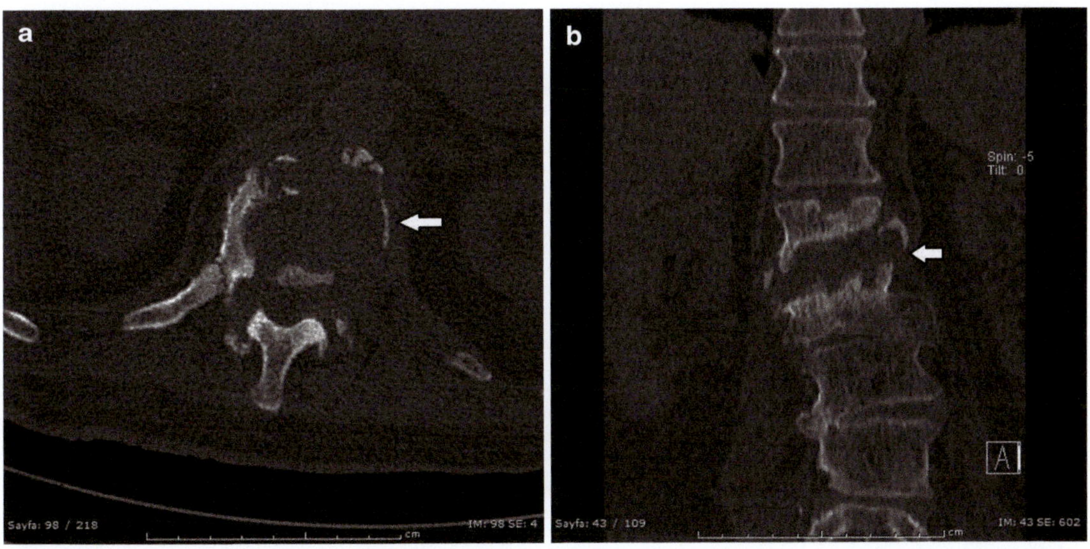

Fig. 19.2 A 67-year-old man. Axial (**a**) and coronal (**b**) CT images demonstrate lytic bone destructions of the vertebral body (*arrow*) with an adjoining soft tissue abscess

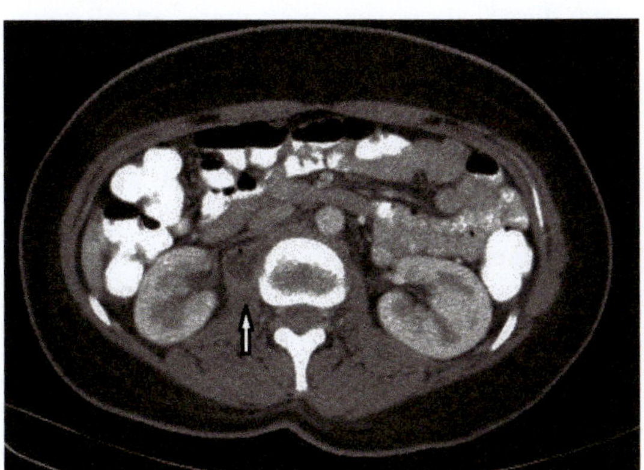

Fig. 19.3 Axial abdominal CT image demonstrates hypodense right TB psoas abscess with peripheral rim enhancement (*arrow*)

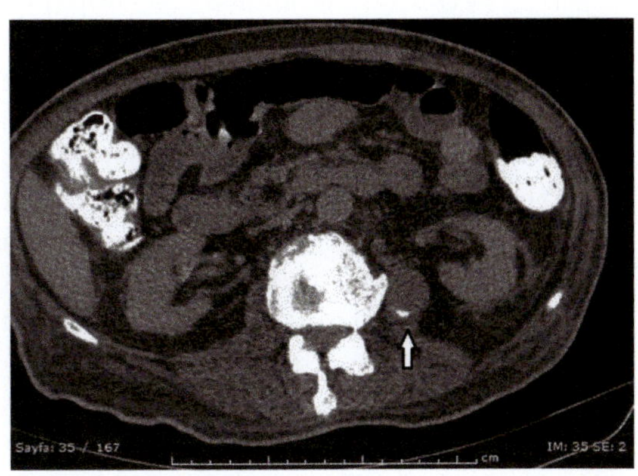

Fig. 19.4 Calcified psoas abscess. Axial noncontrast CT image demonstrates left TB psoas abscess with peripheral calcification (*arrow*)

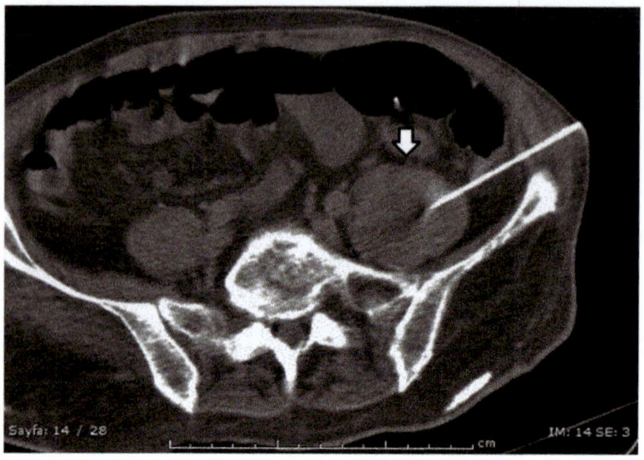

Fig. 19.5 Axial CT image shows left psoas abscess (*arrow*). CT may be used to guide percutaneous interventions

19.2.3 Magnetic Resonance Imaging

Magnetic resonance imaging (MRI) is the gold standard of imaging in spinal TB due to its superior soft tissue resolution and multiplanar capability. MRI is more accurate in determining the epidural and neural extension of the disease in cases with skip lesions [14, 29–32]. MRI sequences used in the evaluation of spinal TB are noncontrast T1-weighted, T2-weighted, short tau inversion recovery (STIR) sequences and contrast-enhanced T1-weighted sequences with gadolinium contrast agent in axial, sagittal, and coronal planes. STIR sequences are helpful for making a distinction between fluid and fatty component in noncontrast sequences [33–38].

The affected vertebral bodies are hypointense on T1-weighted images and hyperintense on T2-weighted images and STIR images, and signal of IVD space is normal [39, 40] (Fig. 19.6). Then, IVD space is affected (Fig. 19.7). Usually, the disease extends to the ligaments and soft tissues from vertebral bodies and IVD space, and this extension frequently occurs anterolaterally. The involvement of posterior peridural region is rare [25, 26]. The cortical destruction and posterior element involvement can be best demonstrated by axial MRI [41]. Khalequzzaman et al. [41] reported that posterior element involvement was found in 55% which is slightly higher than other reported series. The presence of posterior element involvement is important, because this might cause neurological symptoms and necessitate laminectomy for the treatment. In addition, there is a tendency toward pedicular and laminar involvement in patients with spinal TB, whereas pyogenic spondylitis has a predilection for the facet joint. Posterior element involvement is usually seen as an extension of the vertebral body disease, but isolated involvement of posterior element in patients with spinal TB is rare, with an incidence ranging from 0.8% to 10% [42]. Unfortunately, posterior element abnormalities without vertebral body involvement poses as a challenge for the differentiation of an infection from a tumor [20, 42–45].

Paravertebral abscesses are hypointense on T1-weighted images and hyperintense on T2-weighted images (Fig. 19.8). Enhanced coronal images are helpful for delineating these abscesses as well as their communications [46]. The important MRI findings of spinal TB are rim enhancement around intraosseous and paravertebral abscess [17, 47] (Figs. 19.9 and 19.10). The enhancement of the abscess wall related to TB is thin and smooth, and paraspinal abnormal signal is well defined. On the contrary, thick and irregular enhancement of abscess wall and ill-defined paraspinal abnormal signal are seen in spinal pyogenic infections [48, 49]. In addition, the size of the paraspinal abscess related to TB has generally been reported to be bigger than pyogenic abscess. The use of intravenous contrast medium is essential in the differentiation of spinal TB and pyogenic infections [50] (Figs. 19.11 and 19.12). Turgut [51] reported that most of the patients with Pott's disease in Turkey have large abscesses, neurologic involvement, and multisegmental involvement when admitted.

Intracranial tuberculomas are often detected in brain MRI studies. Rarely, intradural extramedullary and intramedullary tuberculomas can be seen on spinal MRI. The MRI findings of spinal tuberculoma are variable depending on different phases of tuberculoma. In early phase, the tuberculoma has equal signal intensity on T1-weighted images and T2-weighted images and enhances after contrast material administration. The reason for this signal is severe infective reactions, poor formation of the gel capsule, and severe edema. In time, the

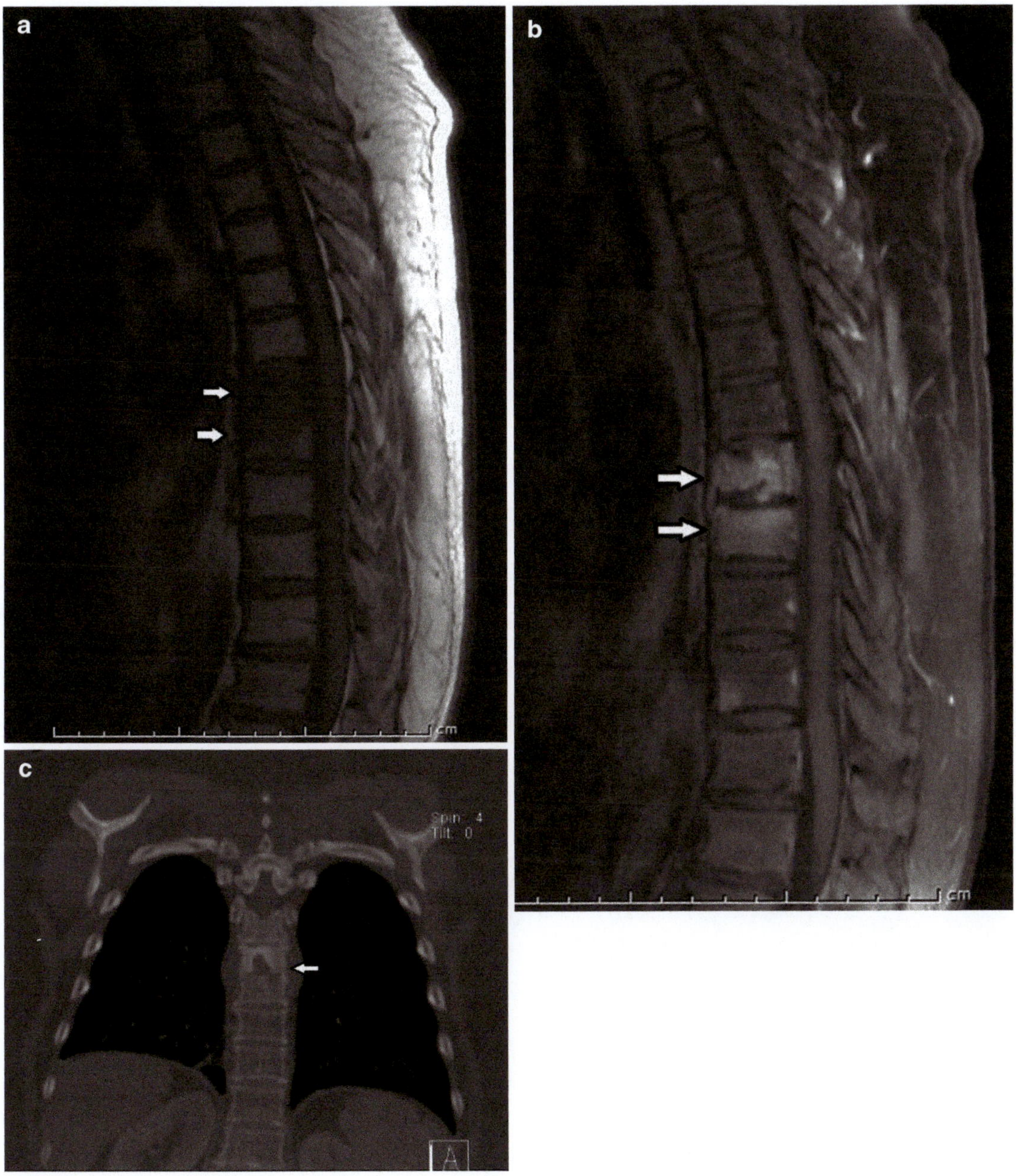

Fig. 19.6 A 55-year-old woman. (**a**) Sagittal T1-weighted MRI shows heterogeneously hypointense signal (*arrow*) in T9–T10 vertebral bodies. (**b**) Sagittal fat-suppressed contrast-enhanced T1-weighted MRI shows heterogeneous enhancement (*arrow*) of T9–T10 vertebral bodies. (**c**) Coronal CT image shows bone destruction

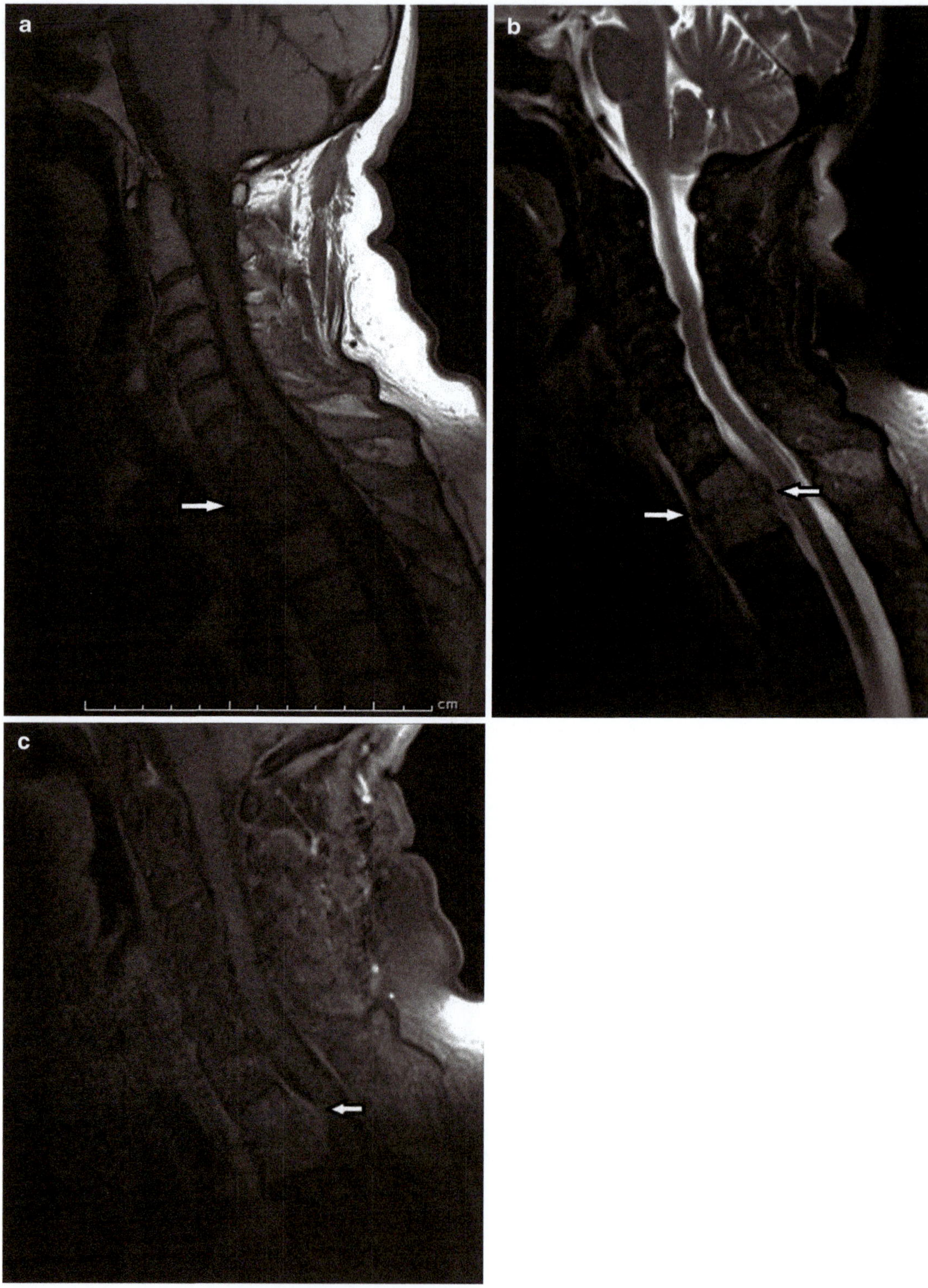

Fig. 19.7 A 75-year-old woman. (**a**) Sagittal T1-weighted MRI shows heterogeneously hypointense signal (*arrow*) in T1–T2 vertebral bodies with epidural mass. (**b**) T1 and T2 vertebral bodies are heterogeneously hyperintense (*arrow*) on sagittal turbo spin-echo T2-weighted MRI. (**c**) Sagittal fat-suppressed contrast-enhanced T1-weighted MRI shows heterogeneous enhancement (*arrow*) of T1–T2 vertebral bodies and the intervertebral disk space

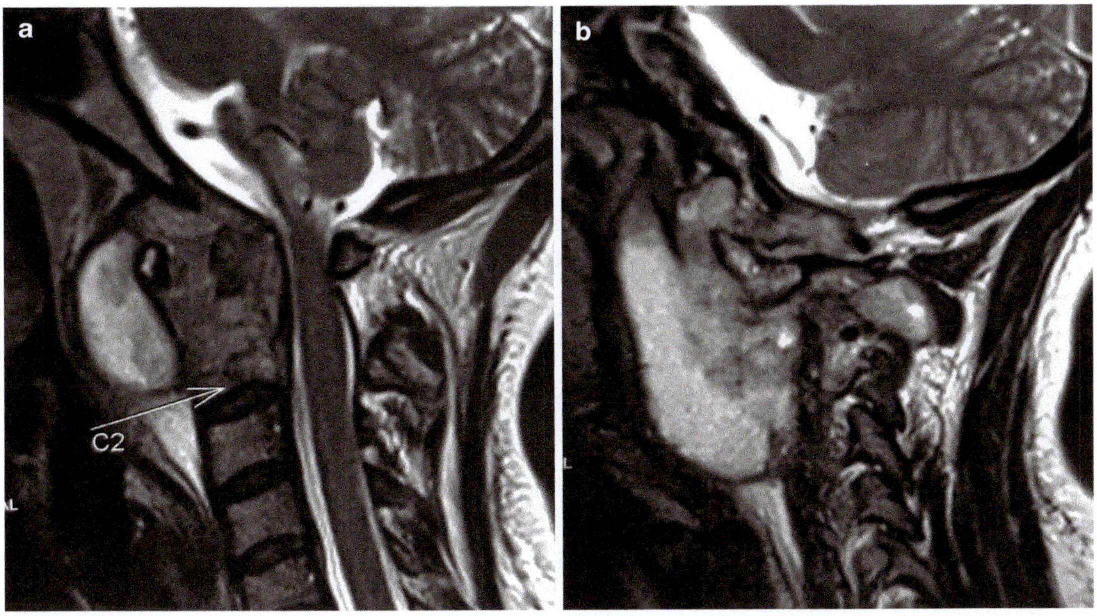

Fig. 19.8 On T2-weighted contrast-enhanced MRI, sagittal (**a**) and parasagittal (**b**) images show craniovertebral junction TB with a large prevertebral abscess (Courtesy of S. Behari)

gel content of tuberculoma increases, and the peripheral edema is decreased. At this phase, it has an isointense appearance on T1-weighted images, whereas it is isointense or hypointense on T2-weighted images. The rim enhancement and hypointense signal in the central region are seen after intravenous contrast material. "Target sign" due to the development of caseation is a characteristic finding on T2-weighted images. It is characterized by a low signal target due to the caseous material and high signal rim due to the peripheral infective granulation tissues. The external low signal rim is composed of collagen fibers produced by fibroblasts. The "target sign" is an important finding which enables the differentiation of spinal tuberculoma from other intramedullary lesions. Compared with tumors, spinal tuberculoma has a sharper margin, and hypointense signal on T2-weighted image signals and rim enhancement can also be seen [52, 53] (Fig. 19.13).

Another radiologic finding in spinal TB is arachnoiditis. Also, the congestive meninges, edematous spinal cord and nerve roots, and peripheral exudate can be seen. Usually, the dorsal spinal region is involved. The spinal cord is hyperintense on T2-weighted images (Fig. 19.14); rarely, cavitation in the spinal cord can occur. The contrast enhancement of the meninges and nerve roots, or spinal cord, clumping of cauda equina roots, and loculation of cerebrospinal fluid are detected (Fig. 19.15). Clinically, paraplegia, quadriplegia, pain, and radicular symptoms may be seen in these patients due to involved segments. The patients usually heal without any sequela in case early diagnosis and proper medical treatment are provided. Sometimes, myelomalacia, moderate to severe cord atrophy, and syringohydromyelia are seen in untreated patients [54, 55]. Recently, diffusion-weighted (DW) MRI and apparent diffusion coefficient (ADC) values are used for the evaluation of the spinal TB and to differentiate TBs from metastatic lesions. The information about tissue composition as well as the physical properties and the microstructure of the tissues can be derived from DW-MRI. ADC values are a measure of the diffusion ability of molecules. High ADC values imply increased diffusion of molecules, and it shows less compact tissue microstructure. Sometimes, ADC values in patients with spinal TB may be similar to metastatic disease. Hence, DW-MRI and ADC values

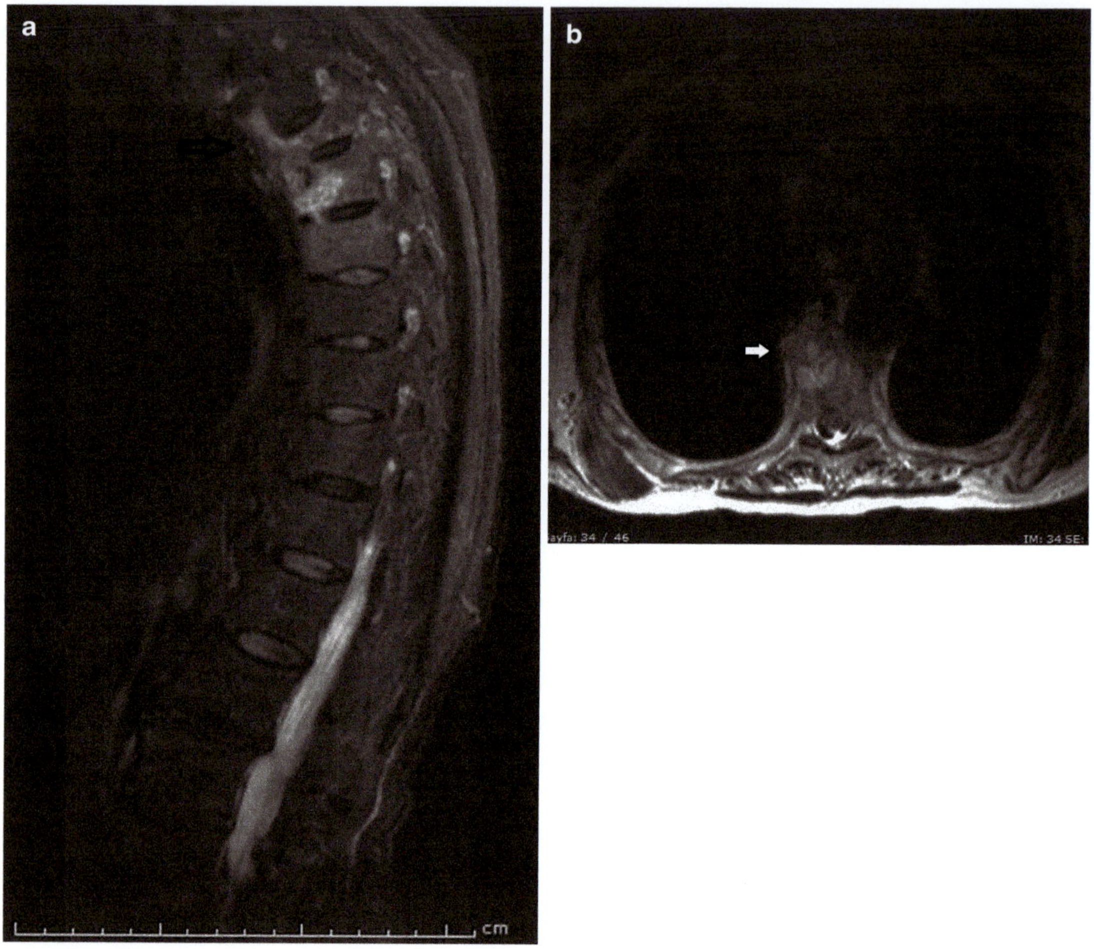

Fig. 19.9 A 80-year-old woman. (**a**) Sagittal STIR MRI shows loss of vertebral body height and increased signal intensity at T4 (*arrow*) and kyphosis at upper thoracal region (**b**) Axial T2-weighted MRI of the upper thoracal spine shows bilateral paraspinal abscesses (*arrow*) with involvement of T4

must be evaluated in association with clinical history and conventional MRI findings [56, 57].

19.2.4 Magnetic Resonance Spectroscopy

Magnetic resonance spectroscopy (MRS) reveals information about the nature and concentration of biochemical metabolites within tissues [58]. MRS is a useful adjunct to routine conventional MRI. However, it is difficult to perform MRS on smaller lesions as partial volume averaging will contaminate the spectra. The MRS findings of many disorders are similar. There is increased choline levels in most neoplastic lesions, tuberculosis, fungal infections, and inflammatory disorders (demyelination). Choline is a cell membrane marker; its elevation indicates high cellularity or cell destruction. Lipid/lactate peak is consistently seen with necrotic tumors, lymphomas, and tuberculomas [58–64].

The MRS findings of tuberculomas are increased peak of lipids, more choline, and less N-acetylaspartate and creatine. In addition, the choline/creatine ratio is also greater than 1 in all tuberculomas [65, 66]. Gupta et al. [63] have demonstrated that high choline level along with the presence of lipid/lactate is a nonspecific finding and may not be useful in the differentiation of tumors from infective/inflammatory intracranial lesions. Therefore, MRS findings should

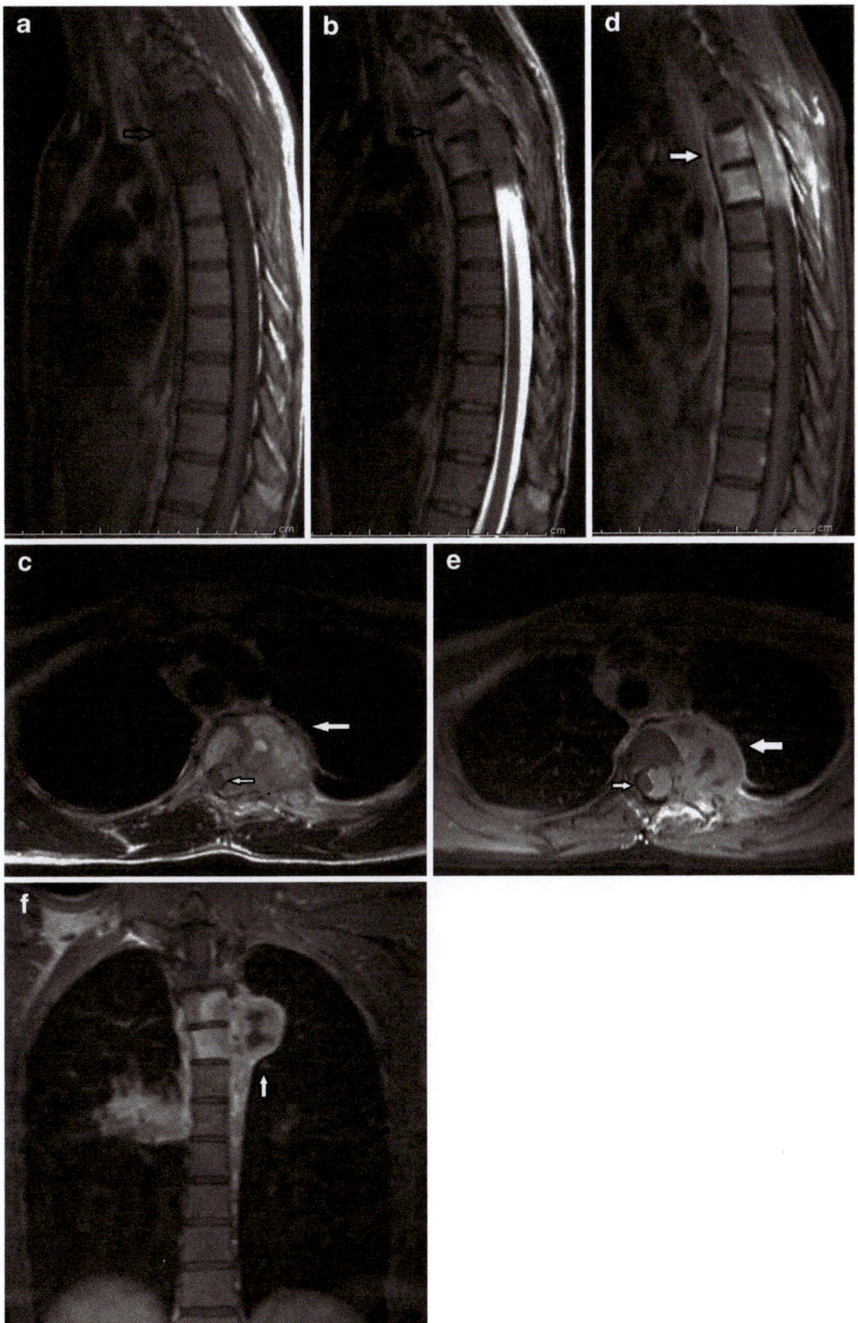

Fig. 19.10 A 24-year-old woman. (**a**) Sagittal T1-weighted MRI shows heterogeneously hypointense signal (*arrow*) in T3–T4 vertebral bodies with epidural mass. (**b**) T3 and T4 vertebral bodies are heterogeneously hyperintense (*arrow*) on sagittal turbo spin-echo T2-weighted image. (**c**) Axial T2 -weighted MRI shows heterogeneous hyperintense signal in T1–T2 vertebral bodies and left pedicle. In addition, there is infiltration of left paraspinal and spinal canal region with abscess formation and displacement of the spinal cord. (**d**) Sagittal fat-suppressed contrast-enhanced T1-weighted MRI shows contrast enhancement (*arrow*) in vertebral bodies and spinal canal. (**e**) Axial fat-suppressed contrast-enhanced T1-weighted MRI shows contrast enhancement (*arrow*) in vertebral bodies and spinal canal. (**f**) Coronal fat-suppressed contrast-enhanced T1-weighted MRI shows enhanced paravertebral abscesses (*arrow*) between T3 and T5 vertebral bodies. A TB lesion is seen at the right lung

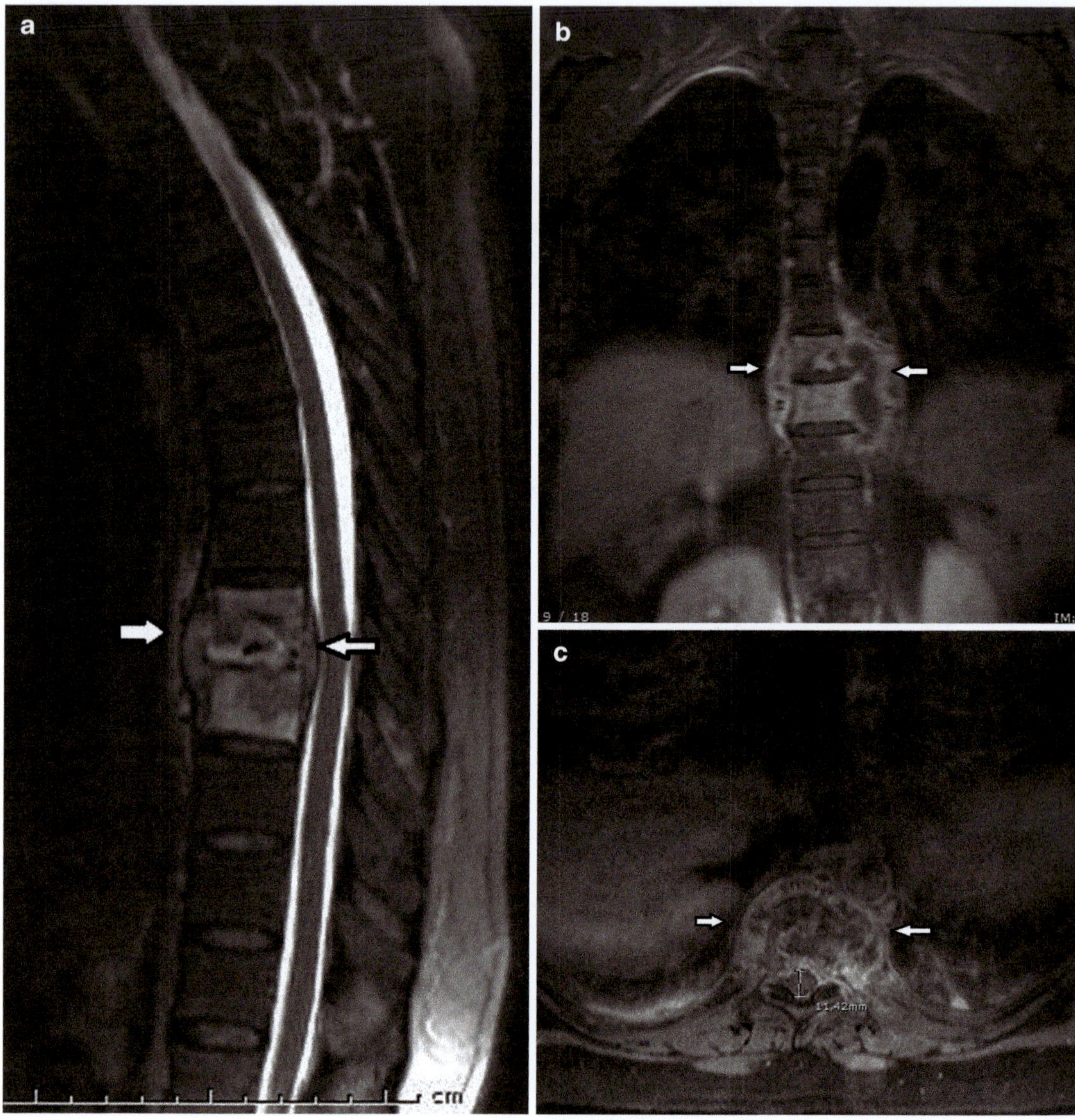

Fig. 19.11 A 47-year-old woman. (**a**) Sagittal T2-weighted MRI shows heterogeneously hypointense signal (*arrow*) in T8–T9 vertebral bodies with epidural mass. (**b**) Coronal fat-suppressed contrast-enhanced T1-weighted MRI shows bilateral paraspinal abscesses (*arrow*) between T8 and T10 vertebral bodies. (**c**) Axial fat-suppressed contrast-enhanced T1-weighted MRI shows contrast enhancement (*arrow*) in vertebral bodies and spinal canal

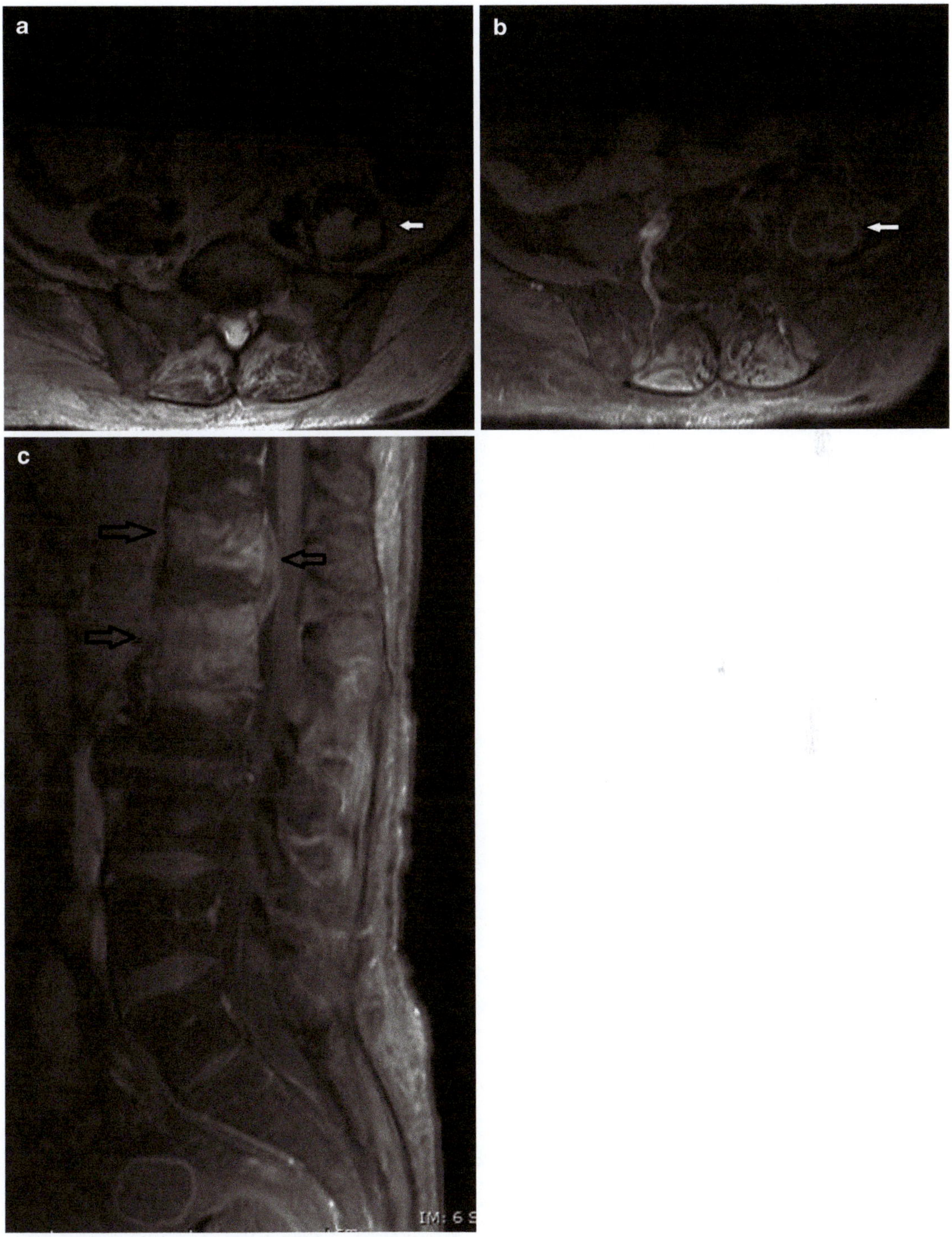

Fig. 19.12 A 67-year-old man. Axial T2-weighted MRI (**a**) shows hyperintense left psoas abscess. Axial (**b**) fat-suppressed contrast-enhanced T1-weighted MRI demonstrates peripheral enhancement of left psoas abscess. Sagittal (**c**) fat-suppressed contrast-enhanced T1-weighted MRI demonstrates involvement of T12, L1, and L2 vertebral bodies (arrow)

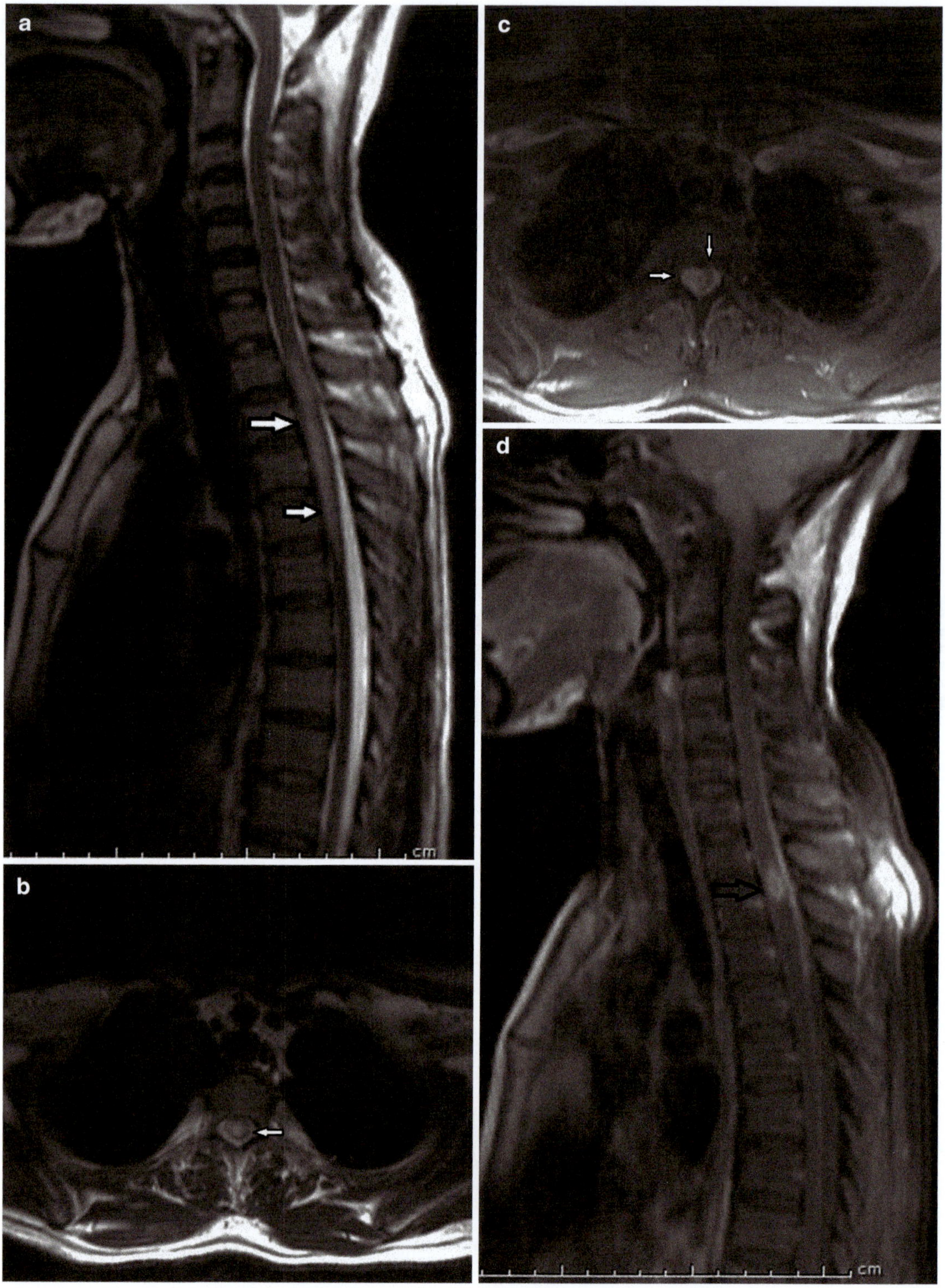

Fig. 19.13 A 36-year-old woman. Sagittal T2-weighted MRI (**a**) and axial T2-weighted MRI (**b**) show hyperintense spinal cord (*arrows*). Axial (**c**) and sagittal (**d**) fat-suppressed contrast-enhanced T1-weighted MRIs demonstrate an enhanced lesion (tuberculoma) and displacement of the spinal cord at T1–T2 level (*arrows*)

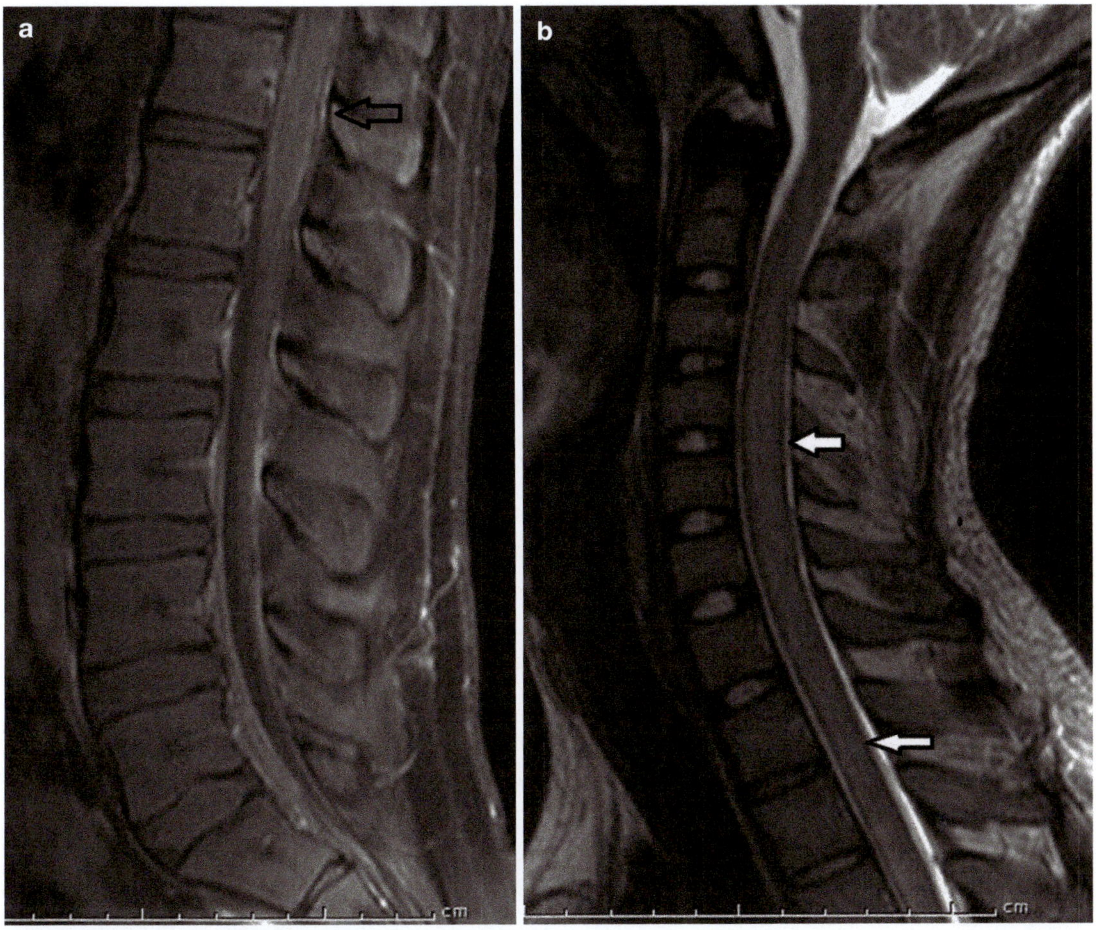

Fig. 19.14 A 23-year-old man. (**a**) Sagittal fat-suppressed contrast-enhanced T1-weighted MRI shows leptomeningeal contrast enhancement (*arrow*) at the lumbar spine. (**b**) Sagittal T2-weighted MRI shows hyperintense signal and expansion of the cervical spinal cord due to edema (*arrow*)

be evaluated with the data derived conventional MRI as well as the patient history; if there is a suspicion, biopsy must be performed.

19.3 Differential Diagnosis

The differential diagnosis for spinal TB involves metastatic disease and low-grade pyogenic infection like brucellosis, fungal infection, and sarcoidosis. In the early stage of infection, radiologic findings are nonspecific. However, some clinical and radiologic features may aid in the diagnosis of spinal TB [67].

Posterior vertebral elements are often abnormal in metastatic disease, whereas they are rarely involved in spinal TB. The anterior scalloping due to subligamentous spread of infection may be seen with paravertebral lymphadenopathy, secondary to metastases and lymphoma. Anterior scalloping of the vertebral bodies due to psoas abscess is similar to that seen with lymphoma or abdominal aortic aneurysm. The calcification within the abscess is important in the diagnosis of spinal TB [11, 14].

Unfortunately, the differentiation between spinal TB and pyogenic infection based on clinical and imaging findings is often difficult. The slow course of the disease, normal erythrocyte sedimentation rate, and pulmonary findings and symptoms are related to spinal TB infection. Especially, involvement of one or more segments,

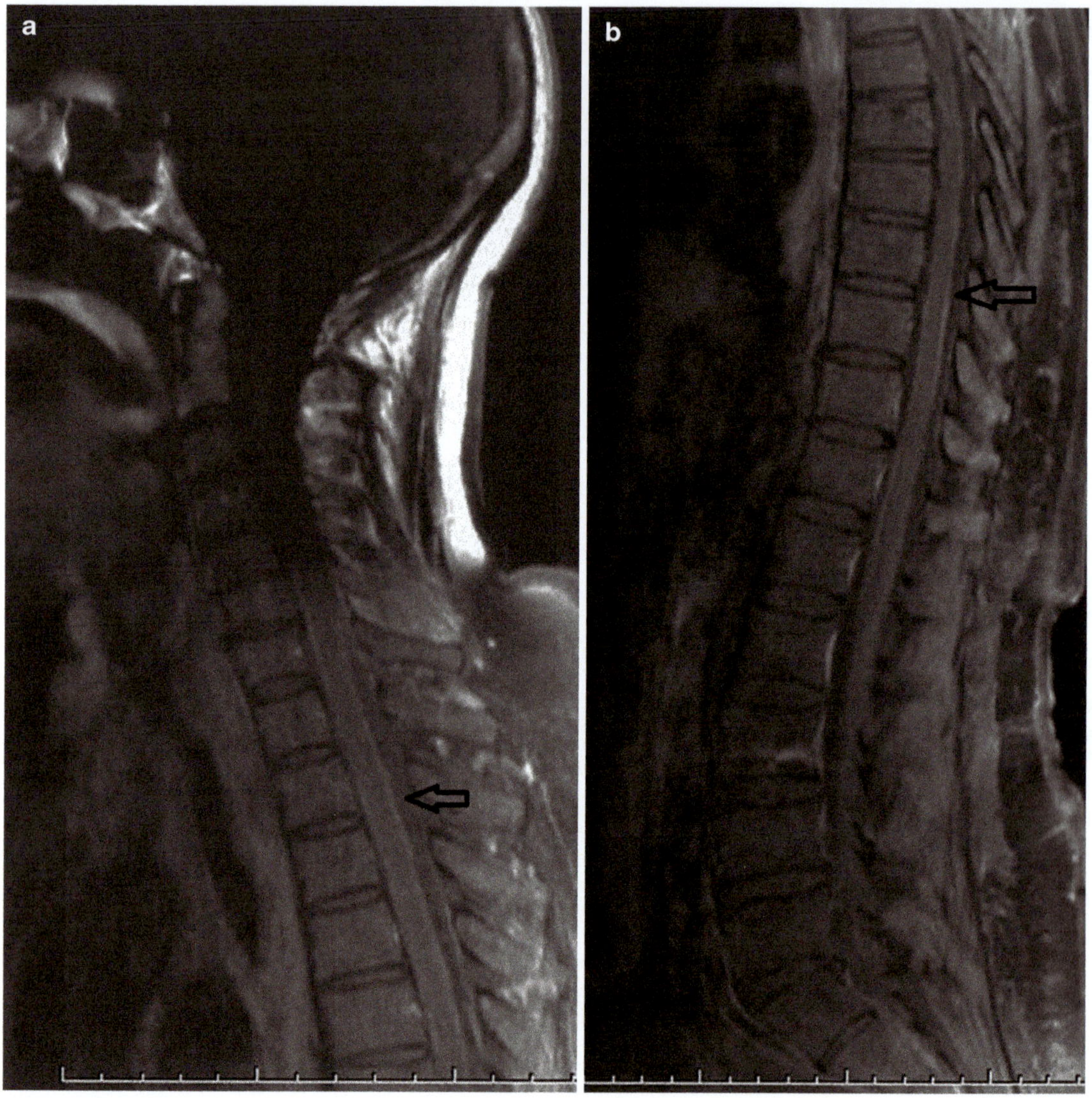

Fig. 19.15 A 63-year-old woman. Sagittal fat-suppressed contrast-enhanced T1-weighted MRI shows leptomeningeal contrast enhancement (*arrows*) around cord at the whole cervical (**a**) and thoracal (**b**) spine

delay in destruction of the IVD space, large calcified paravertebral mass, and absence of sclerosis are more specific for spinal TB. At the beginning, the IVD space is not destroyed in spinal TB; therefore, the signal of the IVD space is normal on T2-weighted images. On the contrary, the increased signal at the IVD space on T2W images is detected in spinal pyogenic infections. Radiologically, the enhancement of the abscess wall related to TB is thin and smooth, and paraspinal abnormal signal is well defined, whereas thick and irregular enhancement of abscess wall and ill-defined paraspinal abnormal signal are seen in spinal pyogenic infections. Additionally, the size of the paraspinal abscess related to TB has generally been reported to be larger than pyogenic abscess. Importantly, the use of intravenous contrast medium for MRIs is essential in the differentiation of spinal TB and pyogenic infections [48–50, 68].

Spinal brucellosis often affects the lower lumbar region without causing kyphosis. Usually, the radiologic findings of spinal brucellosis are gas in the IVD space and small paraspinal abscess

[25]. Sarcoidosis is similar to spinal TB, with multiple focal lesions of the vertebrae and IVD spaces and the formation of paravertebral abscesses. Medullary involvement of sarcoidosis is rarely seen. The lesions tend to regress with the utilization of corticosteroid. Correlation with laboratory tests and imaging findings is crucial for making a distinction from TB [69–72].

Conclusion

TB usually affects the respiratory system. However, it can affect any organ system, especially in patients with predisposing conditions as diabetes, hepatic cirrhosis, corticosteroid treatment, alcoholism, intravenous drug abuse, and immunocompromised patients. Severe morbidity and neurologic sequelae may develop in untreated patients. Spinal TB has a variety of radiologic findings which may be similar to other diseases such as brucellosis, metastasis, lymphoma, sarcoidosis, and pyogenic infections. The positive culture or histologic analysis of biopsy specimens is still required in diagnosis of spinal TB. Conventional radiography, CT, and MRI clearly demonstrate the extensions of spinal TB. CT is useful for the evaluation of the type and extent of bone destruction. MRI is the gold standard imaging tool in spinal TB due to its superior soft tissue resolution and multiplanar capability and the lack of ionizing radiation. MRI is especially superior to CT in the evaluation of the epidural and foraminal extension of the disease and involvement of the spinal cord and the nerve root in the asymptomatic patients. MRI shows findings of spinal TB earlier than conventional methods, and this provides earlier detection and treatment. In addition, the response to treatment and regression of the disease may be followed with serial MRI.

References

1. Davies PD, Humphries MJ, Byfield SP, Nunn AJ, Darbyshire JH, Citron KM, Fox W (1984) Bone and joint tuberculosis. A survey of notifications in England and Wales. J Bone Joint Surg Br 66:326–330
2. Halsey JP, Reeback JS, Barnes CG (1982) A decade of skeletal tuberculosis. Ann Rheum Dis 41:7–10
3. Jaffle RB, Koshman EB (1970) Intravenous drug abuse: pulmonary, cardiac, and vascular complications. AJR Am J Roentgenol 109:107–120
4. Newton P, Sharp J, Barnes KL (1982) Bone and joint tuberculosis in Greater Manchester 1969–79. Ann Rheum Dis 41:1–6
5. Lauzardo M, Peloquin CA (2012) Antituberculosis therapy for 2012 and beyond. Expert Opin Pharmacother 13:511–526
6. Thrush A, Enzmann D (1990) MR Imaging of infectious spondylitis. AJNR Am J Neuroradiol 11:1171–1180
7. Liu ZX, Zhu H, Qi QL, Liu J (2010) Analysis of the curative effect of 162 cases of thoracic and lumbar tuberculosis. Zhongguo Gu Shang 23:497–499
8. Jin D, Qu D, Chen J, Zhang H (2004) One-stage anterior interbody autografting and internal fixation in primary surgical management of thoracolumbar spinal tuberculosis. Eur Spine J 13:114–121
9. Gu XF, Cheng L, Zhou YY (2009) The analysis of therapeutic effect with posterior debridement and bone grafting fusion internal fixation of thoracic lumbar tuberculosis. Chin Med J (Engl) 89:2898–2901
10. Davidson PT, Horowitz I (1970) Skeletal tuberculosis: a review with patient presentations and discussion. Am J Med 48:77–84
11. Resnick D (2002) Tuberculous infection. In: Resnick D (ed) Diagnosis of bone and joint disorders, 3rd edn. Saunders, London, pp 2524–2545
12. Liu GC, Chou MS, Tsai TC, Lin SY, Shen YS (1993) MR evaluation of tuberculous spondylitis. Acta Radiol 34:554–558
13. Jain R, Sawhney S, Berry M (1993) Computed tomography of vertebral tuberculosis : patterns of bone destruction. Clin Radiol 47:659–664
14. Weaver P, Lifeso RM (1984) The radiological diagnosis of tuberculosis of the adult spine. Skeletal Radiol 12:178–186
15. Smith AS, Weinstein MA, Mizushima A, Coughlin B, Hayden SP, Lakin MM, Lanzieri CF (1989) MR imaging characteristics of tuberculous spondylitis vs vertebral osteomyelitis. AJR Am J Roentgenol 153:399–405
16. Gouliamos AD, Kehagias DT, Lahanis S, Athanassopoulou AA, Moulopoulou ES, Kalovidouris AA, Trakadas SJ, Vlahos LJ (2001) MR imaging of tuberculous vertebral osteomyelitis: pictorial review. Eur Radiol 11:575–579
17. Arizono T, Oga M, Shiota E, Honda K, Sugioka Y (1995) Differentiation of vertebral osteomyelitis and tuberculous spondylitis by magnetic resonance imaging. Int Orthop 19:319–322
18. Boxer DI, Pratt C, Hine AL, McNicol M (1992) Radiological features during and following treatment of spinal tuberculosis. Br J Radiol 65:476–479
19. al-Mulhim FA, Ibrahim EM, el-Hassan AY, Moharram HM (1995) Magnetic resonance imaging of tuberculous spondylitis. Spine 20:2287–2292
20. Chapman M, Murray R, Stocker D (1979) Tuberculosis of the bones and joints. Semin Roentgenol 14:266–282

21. Resnik D, Niwayama G (1988) Diagnoses of bone and joint disorders, vol 4. Saunders, Philadelphia
22. Desai SS (1994) Early diagnosis of spinal tuberculosis by MRI. J Bone Joint Surg Br 76:863–869
23. Watts HG, Lifeso RM (1996) Tuberculosis of bones and joints. J Bone Joint Surg Am 78:288–298
24. Jain R, Sawhney S, Berry M (1993) Computed tomography of vertebral tuberculosis: patterns of bone destruction. Clin Radiol 47:196–199
25. Sinan T, Al-Khawari H, Ismail M, Ben-Nakhi A, Sheikh M (2004) Spinal tuberculosis: CT and MRI feature. Ann Saudi Med 24:437–441
26. Chauhan A, Gupta BB (2007) Spinal tuberculosis. Indian Acad Clin Med 8:110–114
27. Yao DC, Sartoris DJ (1995) Musculoskeletal tuberculosis. Radiol Clin North Am 33:679–689
28. Resnick D (1996) Bone and joint imaging, 2nd edn. Saunders, Philadelphia, pp 684–716
29. Hoffman EB, Crosier JH, Cremin BJ (1993) Imaging in children with spinal tuberculosis: a comparison of radiography, computed tomography and magnetic resonance imaging. J Bone Joint Surg Br 75:233–239
30. Modic MT, Feiglin DH, Piraino DW, Boumphrey F, Weinstein MA, Duchesneau PM, Rehm S (1985) Vertebral osteomyelitis: assessment using MR. Radiology 157:157–166
31. Varma R, Lander P, Assaf A (2001) Imaging of pyogenic infectious spondylodiskitis. Radiol Clin North Am 39:203–213
32. Prasad A, Manchanda S, Sachdev N, Baruah BP, Manchanda V (2012) Imaging features of pediatric musculoskeletal tuberculosis. Pediatr Radiol 42:1235–1249
33. Zamiati W, Jiddane M, El Hassani MR, Chakir N, Boukhrissi N (1999) Contribution of spiral CT scan and MRI in spinal tuberculosis. J Neuroradiol 26:27–34
34. Omari B, Robertson JM, Nelson RJ, Chiu LC (1989) Pott's disease: a resurgent challenge to the thoracic surgeon. Chest 95:145–150
35. Narlawar RS, Shah JR, Pimple MK, Patkar DP, Patankar T, Castillo M (2002) Isolated tuberculosis of posterior elements of spine: Magnetic resonance imaging findings in 33 patients. Spine (Phila Pa 1976) 27:275–281
36. Yusof MI, Hassan E, Rahmat N, Yunus R (2009) Spinal tuberculosis: the association between pedicle involvement and anterior column damage and kyphotic deformity. Spine (Phila Pa 1976) 234:713–717
37. Zaidi H, Akram MH, Wala MS (2010) Frequency and magnetic resonance imaging patterns of tuberculous spondylitis lesions in adults. J Coll Physicians Surg Pak 20:303–306
38. Mohammadreza E, Fariborz S, Gholamreza B (2010) Pott's disease: a review of 58 cases. Med J Islam Repub Iran 23:200–206
39. Sharif HS, Clark DC, Aabed MY, Haddad MC, al Deeb SM, Yaqub B, al Moutaery KR (1990) Granulomatous spinal infections: MR imaging. Radiology 177:101–107
40. Sharif HS (1992) Role of MR imaging in the management of spinal infections. AJR Am J Roentgenol 158:1333–1345
41. Khalequzzaman S, Hoque HW (2012) Tuberculosis of spine. Magnetic resonance imaging (MRI) evaluation of 42 cases. Med Today 24:59–62
42. Babhulkar SS, Tayade WB, Babhulkar SK (1984) Atypical spinal tuberculosis. J Bone Joint Surg 66:239–242
43. Ur-Rahman N (1980) Atypical forms of spinal tuberculosis. J Bone Joint Surg 62:162–165
44. Travlos J, du Toit G (1990) Spinal tuberculosis: beware the posterior elements. J Bone Joint Surg 72:722–723
45. Loke TK, Ma HTG, Chan CS (1997) Magnetic resonance imaging of the tuberculous spinal infection. Australas Radiol 4:7–12
46. de Roos A, van Persijn van Meerten EL, Bloem JL, Bluemm RG (1986) MRI of tuberculous spondylitis. AJR Am J Roentgenol 147:79–82
47. Sharif HS, Morgan JL, al Shahed MS, al Thagafi MY (1995) Role of CT and MR imaging in the management of tuberculous spondylitis. Radiol Clin North Am 33:787–804
48. Jung NY, Jee WH, Ha KY, Park CK, Byun JY (2004) Discrimination of tuberculous spondylitis from pyogenic spondylitis on MRI. AJR Am J Roentgenol 182:1405–1410
49. Hong SH, Kim SM, Ahn JM, Chung HW, Shin MJ, Kang HS (2001) Tuberculous versus pyogenic arthritis: MR imaging evaluation. Radiology 218:848–853
50. Moorthy S, Prabhu NK (2002) Spectrum of MR imaging findings in spinal tuberculosis. AJR Am J Roentgenol 179:979–983
51. Turgut M (2001) Spinal tuberculosis (Pott's disease): its clinical presentation, surgical management, and outcome. A survey study on 694 patients. Neurosurg Rev 24:8–13
52. Chang KH, Han MH, Roh JK, Kim IO, Han MC, Choi KS, Kim CW (1990) Gd-DTPA enhanced MR imaging in intracranial tuberculosis. Neuroradiology 32:19–25
53. Gupta VK, Sharma BS, Khosla VK (1995) Intramedullary tuberculoma: report of two cases with MRI findings. Surg Neurol 44:241–243
54. Jain AK, Jena A, Dhammi IK (2000) Correlation of clinical course with magnetic resonance imaging in tuberculous myelopathy. Neural India 48:132–139
55. Sharma A, Goyal M, Mishra NK, Gupta V, Gaikwad SB (1997) MR imaging of tubercular spinal arachnoiditis. AJR Am J Roentgenol 168:807–812
56. Palle L, Reddy B, Reddy KJ (2010) Role of magnetic resonance diffusion imaging and apparent diffusion coefficient values in the evaluation of spinal tuberculosis in Indian patients. Indian J Radiol Imaging 20:279–283
57. Basser PJ (2002) Diffusion and diffusion tensor imaging. In: Atlas SW (ed) Magnetic resonance imaging of

brain and spine, 3rd edn. Lippincot Williams and Wilkins, Philadelphia, pp 197–212
58. Bertholdo D, Watcharakorn A, Castillo M (2013) Brain proton magnetic resonance spectroscopy: introduction and overview. Neuroimaging Clin N Am 23:359–380
59. Venkatesh SK, Gupta RK, Pal L, Husain N, Husain M (2001) Spectroscopic increase in choline signal is a nonspecific marker for differentiation of infective/inflammatory from neoplastic lesions of the brain. J Magn Reson Imaging 14:8–15
60. Wirt MD, Petermann GW (2003) Magnetic resonance spectroscopy: a basic guide to data acquisition and interpretation. Appl Radiol 32:25–32
61. Pandya HG, Wilkinson ID, Agarwal SK, Griffiths PD (2005) The nonspecific nature of proton spectroscopy in brain masses in children: a series of demyelinating lesions. Neuroradiology 47:955–959
62. Rovira A, Alonso J (2013) 1H magnetic resonance spectroscopy in multiple sclerosis and related disorders. Neuroimaging Clin N Am 23:459–474
63. Gupta RK, Vatsal DK, Husain N, Chawla S, Prasad KN, Roy R, Kumar R, Jha D, Husain M (2001) Differentiation of tuberculous from pyogenic brain abscesses with in vivo proton MR spectroscopy and magnetization transfer MR imaging. AJNR Am J Neuroradiol 22:1503–1509
64. Luthra G, Parihar A, Nath K, Jaiswal S, Prasad KN, Husain N, Husain M, Singh S, Behari S, Gupta RK (2007) Comparative evaluation of fungal, tubercular, and pyogenic brain abscesses with conventional and diffusion MR imaging and proton MR spectroscopy. AJNR Am J Neuroradiol 28:1332–1338
65. Mishra AM, Gupta RK, Jaggi RS, Reddy JS, Jha DK, Husain N, Prasad KN, Behari S, Husain M (2004) Role of diffusion-weighted imaging and in vivo proton magnetic resonance spectroscopy in the differential diagnosis of ring-enhancing intracranial cystic mass lesions. J Comput Assist Tomogr 28:540–547
66. Pretell EJ, Martinot C Jr, Garcia HH, Alvarado M, Bustos JA, Martinot C, Cysticercosis Working Group in Peru (2005) Differential diagnosis between cerebral tuberculosis and neurocysticercosis by magnetic resonance spectroscopy. J Comput Assist Tomogr 29:112–114
67. Harisinghani MG, McLoud TC, Shepard JA, Ko JP, Shroff MM, Mueller PR (2000) Tuberculosis from head to toe. Radiographics 20:449–470
68. Jain AK (2010) Tuberculosis of the spine: a fresh look at an old disease. J Bone Joint Surg Br 92:905–913
69. Burrill J, Williams CJ, Bain G, Conder G, Hine AL, Misra RR (2007) Tuberculosis: a radiologic review. Radiographics 27:1255–1273
70. Bradley DA, Lower EE, Baughman RP (2006) Diagnosis and management of spinal cord sarcoidosis. Sarcoidosis Vasc Diffuse Lung Dis 23:58–65
71. Sakushima K, Yabe I, Nakano F, Yoshida K, Tajima Y, Houzen H, Maruo Y, Sasaki H (2011) Clinical features of spinal cord sarcoidosis: analysis of 17 neurosarcoidosis patients. J Neurol 258:2163–2167
72. Cohen-Aubart F, Galanaud D, Grabli D, Haroche J, Amoura Z, Chapelon-Abric C, Lyon-Caen O, Valeyre D, Piette JC (2010) Spinal cord sarcoidosis: clinical and laboratory profile and outcome of 31 patients in a case-control study. Medicine 89:133–140

Surgical Therapy

20

Rajab Ali and Amir Jalil

Contents

Abbreviations

GATA	Gulhane Askeri Tıp Akademisi
MIS	Minimal invasive surgery
MRC	Medical research council
PCR	Polymerase chain reaction
TB	Tuberculosis
TMC	Titanium mesh cage
VATS	Video-assisted thoracoscopic surgery

R. Ali, FCPS (✉) • A. Jalil, FCPS
Department of Orthopedic Surgery,
Abbasi Shaheed Hospital, Karachi Medical
and Dental College, Karachi, Pakistan
e-mail: drrajabali@gmail.com; dramirjalil@yahoo.com

M. Turgut et al. (eds.), *Tuberculosis of the Central Nervous System*,
DOI 10.1007/978-3-319-50712-5_20

20.1 Introduction

Spinal tuberculosis (TB) is one of the most challenging diseases for surgeons to treat. Spinal TB is a serious type of skeletal TB, as it can be associated with very harmful complications such as neurologic deficit and spinal deformity due to spinal collapse. Hence, early detection and proper management of this disease are important in preventing its grave complications.

Although chemotherapy is the mainstay treatment, surgery has its significant role with definite indications. A variety of surgical procedures/techniques is in use today for treatment of spinal TB and its associated complications with a successful outcome. A brief account of commonly applied procedures with radiograph figures is presented in this chapter. Just like other surgical areas today, minimal invasive surgery (MIS) techniques using endoscopy and modern instrumentation are also frequently applied in spinal TB surgery. Some currently reported MIS techniques and their indications are also mentioned in this chapter.

20.2 History of Spinal Tuberculosis Treatment

TB has been prevalent in the human population since antiquity. Its treatment has been varied over the time. The management protocol for musculoskeletal TB has evolved through different phases [1]. In the pre-anti-TB period, patients were treated by orthodox nonoperative methods and few early surgical procedures. The orthodox treatment was entirely constitutional and based mainly on recumbence and immobilization in the form of body casts, plaster beds, and several types of braces. The main objective of these treatment modalities before the availability of chemotherapy was to limit the spread of the disease and to prevent the development of spinal deformity, but the results were highly unsatisfactory [2, 3]. Few early surgical procedures developed for this disease included a simple aspiration or drainage of the abscesses and removing the lesion through the limited posterior route [4, 5]. In 1895, Menard used an anterolateral extrapleural approach to decompress TB abscess around the spinal cord with gratifying results [6]. In 1911, Hibbs and Albee introduced posterior spinal fusion with bone grafting [7, 8]. In 1937, McKee and Seddon proved that posterior bone grafting alone was not beneficial and was even damaging in the presence of active TB [9, 10]. Though anterior radical debridement and non-instrumented fusion were initially reported by Ito and Asami in 1934 [2], however, Hodgson and Stock are being accredited for their extensive work and publishing the detailed technique of this procedure [11].

The standard treatment practiced during 1950–1960 was universal excisional surgery combined with anti-TB drugs [12–15]. Simultaneously, all the same, many reports showed excellent results by anti-TB drugs alone and limiting surgery to those patients who failed to respond to drugs or those with complications. With the development of the so-called middle path regime, the indications of surgery became more selective and mainly aimed for prevention and correction of spinal deformity and neural complications [16, 17].

To resolve the debate over various treatment options, the Medical Research Council (MRC) working party on TB of the spine conducted the prospective multicenter clinical trials in Hong Kong, Korea, Rhodesia, and South Africa [19]. Various combinations of conservative treatment were compared to debridement, and debridement was compared to radical debridement with strut grafting. In the earlier reviews, comparable results were reported with the different treatment protocols used. The ambulatory treatment was in general as effective as inpatient bed confinement treatment. The results of ambulatory chemotherapy were comparable to the debridement surgery group. Similarly, no significant difference was found between debridement alone and radical surgery group in early reports. However, when these data were examined in greater details, it was evident that the radical surgery group treated in Hong Kong did have a distinct advantage over the other two groups. The symptoms of the disease were resolved earlier, and there was no neurological involvement during treatment in this group. A comparatively higher rate of bone fusion and improvement of the deformity were seen at 5 years and were maintained till the final 15 years follow-up [19, 20]. Nevertheless, in succeeding years it became evident that even anterior radical surgery with bone grafting alone without instrumentation was not often successful in achieving reasonable correction and in preventing progression of deformity. Therefore, instrumented correction was recommended to bring the best possible outcomes for surgery [21].

Major advances in spinal surgery have been accomplished in recent years. With the application of the modern segmental instrumentation system, newer interventional radiological techniques, and percutaneous methods of debridement and internal fixation, a variety of surgical procedures are done today for spinal TB management with excellent outcomes. These procedures include several combinations of MIS techniques, open limited and radical debridement, different bone grafting methods, and stabilization with specialized spinal instruments [22–25].

20.3 Classification System

Presently, there are only few classification systems based on objective data that can steer the choice of the proper treatment approach for patients with spinal TB.

Kumar [26] proposed a 4-point classification system for posterior spinal TB based on location and stages of the disease. The main limitation to this classification scheme was its description of posterior disease alone and not including the relatively common anterior spinal lesions.

The classification system of Mehta and Bhojraj [27] uses MRI findings and classifies the spinal TB patients into four groups according to the employed surgical technique:

1. Group A consisted of patients with stable anterior lesions and no kyphotic deformity, which were managed with anterior debridement and strut grafting.
2. Group B consisted of patients with global lesions, kyphosis, and instability and these patients were managed with posterior instrumentation using a closed-loop rectangle with sublaminar wires plus anterior strut grafting.
3. Group C patients had anterior or global lesions along with a high operative risk for transthoracic surgery due to medical comorbidities and possible anesthetic complications. Therefore, these patients underwent posterior decompression with the anterior aspect of the cord being approached through a transpedicular route and posterior instrumentation performed using a closed-loop rectangle held by sublaminar wires.
4. Group D patients had isolated posterior lesions that needed only a posterior decompression.

This classification addresses only the thoracic lesions and that is its most important limitation. To overcome these limitations, Oguz et al. presented [28] GATA (Gulhane Askeri Tıp Akademisi) classification based on seven clinical and radiological criteria including abscess formation, disc degeneration, vertebral collapse, kyphosis, sagittal index, instability, and neurological problems (Table 20.1). They also recommended specific techniques for each type [29]. Even though it is a more practical classification system, it is not widely accepted because it holds no special consideration for posterior lesions and its type-specific treatment recommendations are not universally agreed upon [5, 30].

Table 20.1 GATA classification system

Type	Lesion
Type IA	The lesion is limited to the vertebra, one level disc degeneration, no collapse, no abscess, no neurologic deficit
Type IB	Abscess formation; one- or two-level disc degeneration, no collapse, no neurologic deficit
Type II	Collapse of vertebrae; abscess formation; kyphosis (correctable with anterior surgery); stable deformity with or without neurologic deficit; sagittal index is less than 20°
Type III	A more severe vertebral collapse; abscess formation; severe kyphosis; instable deformity with or without neurologic deficit; sagittal index is more than 20°

20.4 Indications for Surgery

Chemotherapy is the mainstay treatment for all types of TB [31]. Surgery plays a significant role in the management of spinal TB. Properly indicated and timely done surgical procedures are the cornerstone in the prevention of neurological complications, maintenance of stability, and early recuperation [18, 28].

Main indications for surgery are [19, 32–35]:

1. Progression of neurologic deficit
2. Progression of spinal deformity (either coronal or sagittal)
3. Failure of conservative treatment (indicated by progressive increase in neurologic deficit and/or spinal deformity or severe pain due to spinal abscess or instability)
4. For diagnostic purpose

20.4.1 Neurologic Deficit

These include a newly onset or worsening neural complications in patients receiving anti-TB chemotherapy, paraplegia of rapid onset, painful paraplegia in elderly, neural arch disease, and spinal tumor syndrome (epidural spinal tuberculoma without osseous involvement).

20.4.2 Spinal Instability or Deformity

When the anterior column of the spine is destroyed by the infectious focus, severe kyphosis may develop due to progressive anterior collapse. Besides obvious deformity, severe kyphosis may cause late-onset paraplegia and cardiopulmonary compromise. Timely done operative procedures would prevent a serious deformity. Patients at risk of developing severe kyphotic deformity should be identified early. The following guidelines help clinicians to identify the patients at risk [22, 34, 36, 37]:

1. Younger patients (less than 11 years of age)
2. Location of lesion between seventh cervical to first lumbar vertebrae
3. Multiple vertebral bodies' destruction (three or more)
4. If vertical height of the spinal column is lost equal to or more than 1.5 vertebral bodies
5. If progression of the kyphotic deformity is seen in serial X-rays

There is rapid progression in kyphosis with acute and severe curves. The intact posterior arch of the spinal column acts like a tension band and prevents "buckling collapse of the spine. Surgical treatment is generally indicated in 50° or more severe kyphosis as it is associated with the most morbidity. As compared to the lumbar spine, more kyphosis can be accepted in the thoracic spine. Even a simple loss of lumbar lordosis is not easily tolerated. Involvement of junctional (cervicothoracic, dorsolumbar, and lumbosacral) areas of the spine leads to severe discomfort and instability; hence, surgery is frequently indicated in these lesions [38–41].

For children especially younger than 11 years, growth may be a cause of further deterioration, and it can lead to progress in kyphotic angles despite healing of infection. Children at risk of developing severe deformity can readily be identified by few plain radiographic signs proposed by Rajasekaran [42]. As shown in Fig. 20.1, these signs include:

(a) Facet joints separation
(b) Retropulsion
(c) Lateral translation
(d) Toppling

The main pathology is the dislocation of the facet joint that leads to spinal instability and produces this characteristic radiographic appearance. One score is attributed to each sign. A score of three or more predicts an increase in the kyphosis by more than 30° and a final deformity of more than 60°. These signs can be detected very early in the course of the disease, and early surgical intervention can halt the progression of the deformity [39, 42].

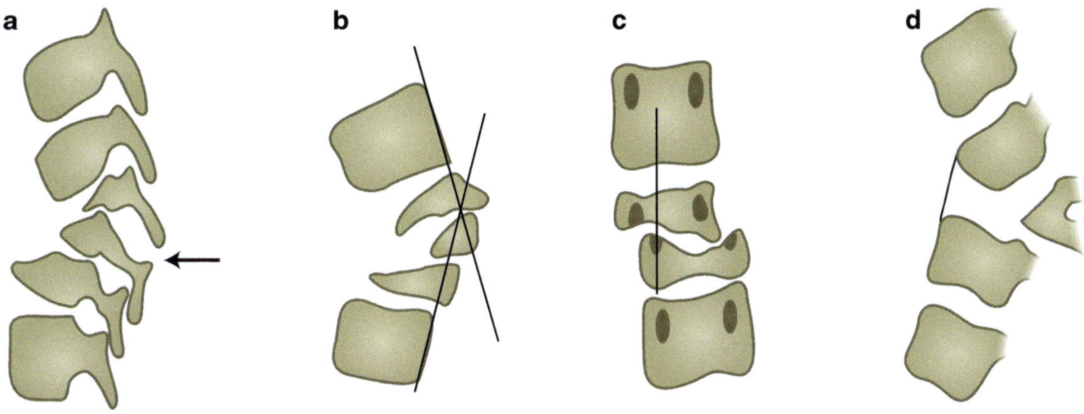

Fig. 20.1 "Spine at risk" radiological signs. (**a**) Separation of the facet joint, (**b**) retropulsion, (**c**) lateral translation, and (**d**) toppling

20.4.3 Failure of Conservative Management

Surgery is indicated by the failure of conservative treatment, which may manifest as an increase in the intensity of pain or progressive neurologic deficit after at least 3–4 weeks course of chemotherapy. The possible causes of pain in spinal TB are a persistent infection, a large abscess, spinal instability and deformity due to progressive destruction of vertebral structures, and nerve root compression. Though most of the spinal TB abscesses can be managed adequately by CT-guided drainage, anterior cervical and some thoracic abscesses may prove to be excessively difficult to aspirate and may need surgical drainage [43].

20.4.4 Uncertain Diagnosis

In some difficult cases of spinal TB, open biopsy may be needed to establish the diagnosis. The specimen is subjected to acid-fast bacilli staining, culture studies, polymerase chain reaction (PCR), and histopathology. Histopathology may be the sole evidence of disease in certain cases [44].

20.5 Surgical Approaches

The spine can be approached from anterior, posterior, or anterolateral or posterolateral sides. Choice of an approach is dictated and decided by various factors including the availability of appropriate facilities, site, development and extent of infection, the plan of action, and the experience and individual choice of the surgeon.

The main goals of surgery in spinal TB are proper decompression and debridement of the lesion, maintenance and reinforcement of stability to prevent deformity, and correction of existing deformity. Since the anterior spinal column including the vertebral bodies and disk spaces is the predominant site of spinal TB, the anterior approach has been favored throughout the spine to achieve these goals. It allows direct access to the infected focus and is convenient for debridement and reconstruction of the defect [45–48]. There is universal agreement on an anterior approach to the cervical spine, and all modalities of surgery such as abscess drainage, corpectomy, and internal fixation can be performed via the anterior approach alone. Additional posterior stabilization is required only in patients with extensive bone destruction [49]. The selection of anterior versus posterior or combined anterior and posterior approach for thoracolumbar TB is still a matter of debate. Conventional surgical approaches to the ventral aspect of the dorsal spine include thoracotomy with extrapleural or transpleural access, lateral extracavitary and costotransversectomy approaches, and retroperitoneal approaches for the lumbar spine [50–53]. Recent data, however, associates the best outcomes with the posterior or combined surgical approaches [54, 55]. A combined anterior and posterior approach helps to overcome stability-related drawbacks of anterior approach alone [56–60]. However, it entails two surgeries (single event or staged) with additional morbidity [33, 61, 62].

20.5.1 Anterior Transthoracic Approach to the Dorsal Spine

The anterior approach remains the reference standard. It is the most suitable approach for most cases of spinal TB and serves to achieve everything that is desired in the radical treatment of the disease. It allows direct debridement of the prevertebral and intraspinal focus of infection. With this approach, skip lesions, double lesions, and extensive lesions involving a number of vertebrae can be managed at the same sitting. This is a good approach for anterior decompression of the cord, for the correction of mild to moderate kyphotic deformity and as an initial step in the serial correction of severe kyphotic deformity [63–65]. However, it is through major body cavities and is associated with increase morbidity. It needs a team of well-trained surgeons and operation room staff, a well-equipped operation theater, and intensive care facilities.

20.5.2 Anterolateral Approach/Extrapleural Approach

Anterolateral approach for a dorsal or dorsolumbar lesion is an extension of costotransversectomy. It is a simpler and safe technique. It is a time-tested approach that is suitable for most of the lesions of anterior complex [4, 66]. The access to spinal lesion is adequate, excision of the disease is near complete, full decompression of the cord is possible, and subsequent fusion is satisfactory. There are no risks of anterior spinal surgery and problem of opening and closure of the chest. Not only it allows anterior debridement and fusion, posterior aspect of the spine can also be approached by turning the patient prone, and even posterior instrumentation can be done simultaneously through this single approach alone [47].

20.5.3 Posterior Approach/Transpedicular Approach

Conventionally, the posterior approach was applied for the cases with destruction of posterior structures of the spine accompanied by an epidural abscess or the involvement of neural arch, causing posterior spinal cord compression. Recently, posterior approach has gained popularity with the application of MIS techniques to the spine. It provides opportunity for transforaminal debridement, interbody bone graft fusion, and posterior instrumentation all from one approach in one stage [67–69]. It delivers the advantages of minimal surgical invasion and little hazard of focal neurological injury due to easy access to the spinal canal. It, therefore, obviates the need for anterior exposure and its associated complications [70, 71].

20.6 Surgical Techniques/Procedures

Diverse surgical techniques for treatment of spinal TB and their associated complications are described. These range from simple aspiration of an abscess to radical debridement and fusion with variable combinations of instrumentation and minimal invasive techniques using endoscopy and modern instrumentation [70]. The main aim of surgery in spinal TB is adequate decompression/debridement of lesion, to correct the deformity and to stabilize the spine to halt the progress of deformity. These aims are achieved by different combinations of undermentioned procedures along with proper chemotherapy [49]:

- Debridement/decompression of lesion
- Bone grafting
- Anterior fusion
- Posterior fusion
- Combined anterior and posterior fusion
- Spinal osteotomies
- Spinal shortening
- Anterior instrumentation
- Posterior instrumentation
- Combined anterior and posterior instrumentation

Commonly described methods to achieve these aims are briefly described here.

20.6.1 Abscess Drainage

Most of the small- and medium-size cold abscesses resolve spontaneously with anti-TB chemotherapy. Drainage is not recommended as a routine practice [22]. Evacuation of abscesses did not alter patients' general condition and may result in persistent discharge from abscess cavity. However, some large abscesses in cervical area (e.g., retropharyngeal abscess) and some thoracic abscesses may be painful and need urgent surgical drainage. Iliopsoas abscesses can be drained by CT-guided percutaneous drainage [43, 72, 73].

20.6.2 Debridement/Surgical Decompression

Debridement of spinal focus involves surgical removal of whole pus, sloughs, caseous material, and sequestra without removal of the unaffected and healthy bone. It provides adequate access to the infectious focus to decompress the cord [74]. Isolated anterior decompression without bone grafting and instrumentation traditionally had a poor outcome in comparison to radical debridement and bone grafting. Posterior laminectomy for debridement of anterior body lesion was also condemned [75, 76], but due to recent advances in spinal surgery and application of MIS techniques and modern spinal instrumentation, the role of focal debridement of TB lesion has reemerged. It can be done by anterior less invasive mini-open approach or by posterior transpedicular approach combined with posterior segmental instrumentation [77–79].

20.6.3 Anterior Radical Debridement and Bone Grafting (Hong Kong Operation)

Anterior radical debridement with strut bone graft fusion is the standard in the surgical treatment of spinal TB [63, 70]. This technique was originally described by Hodgson and Stock in 1956, the so-called Hong Kong operation [11]. In the radical debridement, the excision of the bone extends upward and downward until healthy, bleeding cancellous bone is reached with a surface suitable for reception of bone graft and posteriorly until the dura matter is reached. In widespread involvement where a healthy bleeding bone cannot be shaped, the intervertebral disks and end plates proximal and distal to the lesions are sacrificed. Slots are made in the healthy bleeding bones of vertebral bodies above and/or below the affected ones as a bed for bone graft. At the end of debridement, the length of the defect is measured. A strut graft few mm longer than the defect is inserted into the defect by gentle pushing on the kyphosis posteriorly and opening up the defect. Bone grafting after anterior radical debridement is a safe procedure in spinal TB [74, 80].

A wide variety of grafting materials is available for the reconstruction of the anterior column. The traditional approach is to use rib grafts in the dorsal spine and tricortical iliac crest for the reconstruction of the spine at all levels. However, the donor site morbidity is great if the length of the graft needed is greater than 5 cm or if the patient is elderly. Rib grafts are readily available after thoracotomy, but they are structurally weak and do not contain cancellous bone. Vascularized rib grafts have been used successfully but they also suffer from structural weakness [81]. The fibula takes a longer time to incorporate. Allograft from the humerus, tibia, and femur has been used successfully [82, 83]; they need supplementation with cancellous bone grafting. Titanium mesh cage (TMC) filled with cancellous bone is also in general use these days. The potential advantage is the healing that can occur between the host bone and the cancellous bone in the TMC. Though it is a foreign body in an infected environment, it has been shown to be safe [84]. After surgery patient is kept on strict bed rest for 6–8 weeks and subsequently mobilized in brace.

Though the anterior radical surgery without instrumentation was once advised as the treatment of choice for spinal TB, it later became evident that it has limitation in achieving reasonable deformity correction and a tendency to halt progression in kyphotic deformity due to high possibility of graft failure [12, 85, 86]. Non-instrumented anterior fusion is associated with higher rate of deformity progression when compared even to nonoperative treatment [21].

20.6.4 Debridement and Fusion with Instrumentation

Panvertebral (circumferential involvement of vertebral bodies) TB lesions are potentially unstable and may not be able to resist transitory stresses, thereby leading to pathological subluxation or dislocation of the spinal column with resultant neural deficit and progressive kyphosis. Surgical decompression may cause further instability [40, 87]. Though anterior debridement and bone graft fusion lessen the kyphotic deformity to some extent, there is a high incidence of recurrence and progression of deformity due to graft-related complications, and also the rehabilitation is slower [64, 67, 88]. Addition of spinal instrumentation to the reconstruction helps to regain the height of the collapsed vertebra and to withstand the shearing forces across the spine. It also stabilizes the graft and accelerates the graft incorporation and fusion. It promotes early mobilization of patient [88, 89].

Though the insertion of implants in the infected bony areas is generally contraindicated, due to risk of harboring pyogenic bacteria which forms a biofilm on the implant surfaces and then, are very difficult to eradicate, however, in the case of bone TB, there is less risk of such bond formation between TB organism and implant, because *M. tuberculosis* divides very slowly with minimal glycocalyx slime production and exists in a planktonic form, which responds well to chemotherapy. Hence, the use of metal or other reconstruction biomaterial is not contraindicated even in the presence of active TB infection. Instrumented stabilization is found to be safe in spinal TB [90, 91].

Junctional areas of the spine show more biomechanical stresses. These are the junction of a fixed and a mobile segment, and spinal curvature is changed from kyphosis to lordosis and vice versa. Therefore, instrumented stabilization is advised in such cases [37]. Some general indications for spinal instrumentation in spinal TB are:

- Panvertebral disease
- Long segment of disease (vertebral loss of two or more)
- Surgical correction of kyphosis
- TB of junctional areas (cervicodorsal, dorsolumbar, or lumbosacral spine) [40, 47, 87]

The choice of particular implant depends on individual cases. It depends on surgical approach, level and extent of lesion, availability of implant, facility, and experience of surgeon. A large range of implants are available for fixation of the anterior column of the spine including plates, rod system, and different types of meshes. The anterior plates, screws, and rods are used in short-segment disease. As healthy vertebral bodies are necessary above and below the diseased segment to acquire purchase, this system can be used in mild to moderate kyphosis only. Anterior instrumentation can only be used when disease is confined to the anterior and middle columns and the posterior column is healthy. In panvertebral disease, anterior instrumentation alone does not provide mechanical stability. Hence, stabilization by posterior instrumentation is indicated [87].

In recent days, cages are frequently being used in anterior reconstruction. The material strength and toughness of cages provide adequate immediate stability for a reconstructed segment. The cages are filled with crushed autograft, allograft, artificial bone graft, or even hybrid graft as per need. The availability of these cages offers more choices for anterior reconstruction and ensures satisfactory osseous healing [92]. These cages can be divided into metallic and nonmetallic types. TMC is a typical example of metallic cage. It was first introduced in 1986, since then it is broadly used in spinal reconstruction [93]. TMC has proved its superiority in providing good mechanical support with a satisfactory outcome [94, 95]. Few complications associated with the use of TMCs are the stress shielding, postoperative radiographic interference, and implant subsidence [93, 96]. To overcome these material defects of metallic cages, nonmetallic cages are developed with equal efficacy. More recently, a bionic nonmetallic hollow cylindrical cage n-HA/PA66 cage (nano-hydroxyapatite/polyamide-66) has been used in anterior cervical reconstruction. It is made by covalent miscibility of the nano-hydroxyapatite and polyamide-66 which simulates the constituent form of the natural bone (Fig. 20.2) [92]. With isolated insertion of a cage, there is risk of dislodgement; therefore, whenever possible, it should be supported by anterior and/or posterior instrumentation [87].

The use of sublaminar wiring and Hartshill loop rectangle in spinal surgery had fallen out of favor in comparison to the third-generation implants. The main reasons are high incidence of neurological complications due to the wires; inadequate corrective forces, especially rotatory control in the instrumented segment; and sagittal profile correction and maintenance [97, 98]. At present, the posterior pedicle screw system (Fig. 20.3) is the most widely used implant system in the spinal surgery. It has been proven effective for the treatment of many thoracic spinal disorders associated with segmental instability and neurologic impairment. It provides extremely stable and rigid fixation [77, 99].

20.6.5 Anterior Radical Surgery and Anterior Instrumentation

Conventionally, the infected spine has been approached anteriorly as the TB pathology mainly affects the anterior column of the spine. It permits direct access to the infected focus for

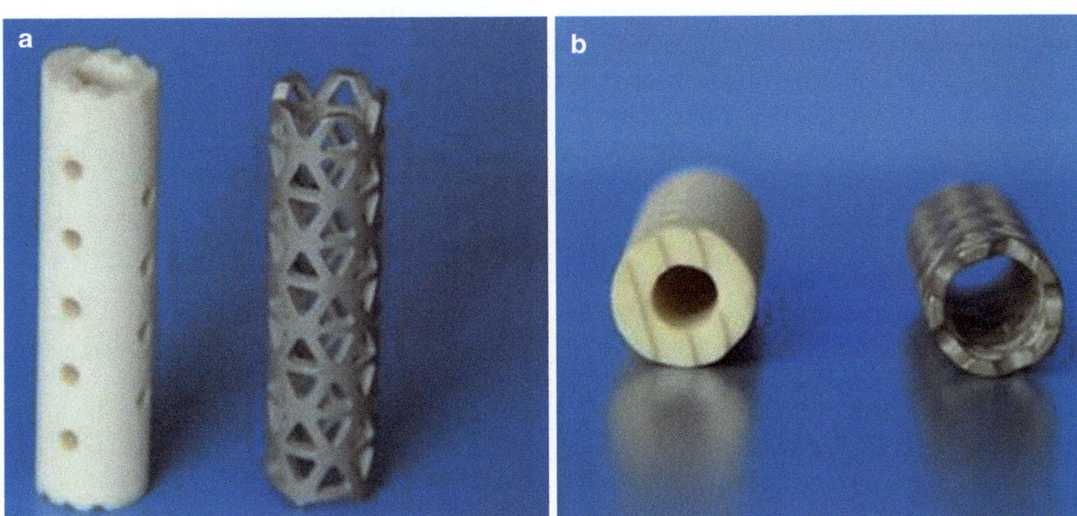

Fig. 20.2 Frontal (**a**) and transverse (**b**) view of cervical nano-hydroxyapatite/polyamide-66 cage (n-HA/PA66) (*left side*) and titanium mesh cage (TMC) (*right side*). There are several shallow recesses designed on the rims of the n-HA/PA66 cage to prevent cage translocation (**a**). The rims of the n-HA/PA66 cage are wider than TMC which reduce cutting of the cage into the end plates and preventing subsidence (**b**)

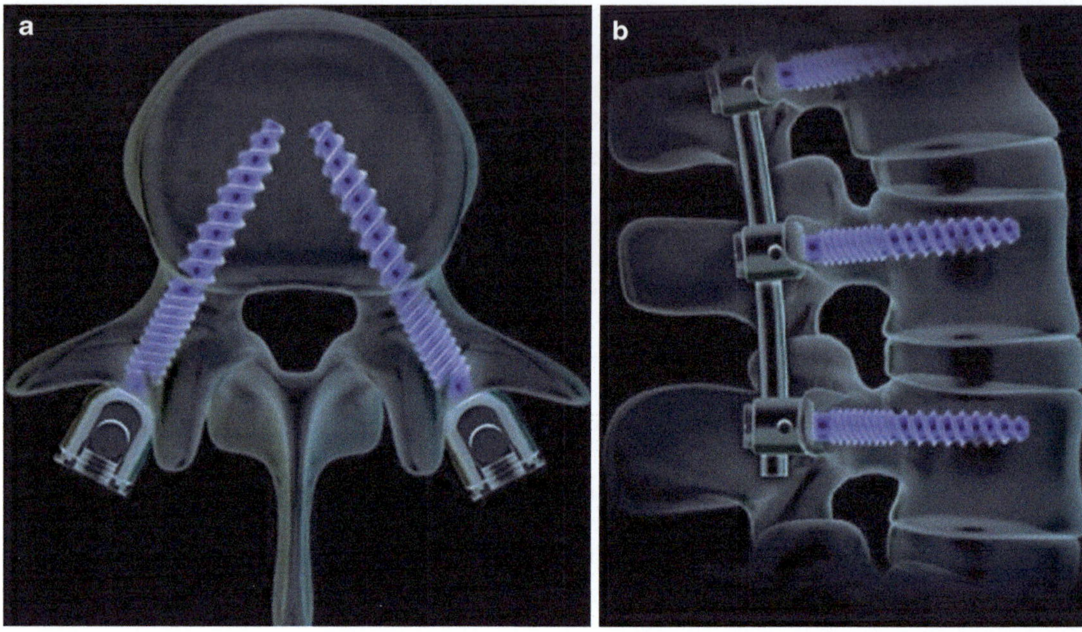

Fig. 20.3 Segmental spinal pedicle screw system

debridement and reconstruction of the defect [46, 47, 100]. The safety and efficacy of anterior fixation in surgical treatment of spinal TB via both open and endoscopic approaches in different regions of the spine especially in the dorsal and cervical spine have well been established [55, 64, 65, 101]. The use of anterior instrumentation alone is indicated only if the posterior elements are intact. Anterior instrumentation and grafting are done as single-stage surgery through the same incision, minimizing total blood loss and surgery time with no risk of the graft slipping out. It also prevents fusing an unnecessarily large number of levels, and postoperatively, immobilization in orthosis is not needed [46, 102]. However, there is some difficulty in inserting the implants anteriorly and chances of prominent hardware impaling the great vessels, particularly in the thoracic spine. The retrieval of dislodged anterior implant also carries the risk of fatal bleeding due to extensive scarring near major vessels [103, 104]. Both anterior plating and mesh cages are used in combination or alone for anterior reconstruction (Figs. 20.4 and 20.5). However, due to risk of dislodgement, isolated insertion of cages should be avoided, and it should be supported by anterior plating whenever possible [105].

20.6.6 Anterior Radical Surgery with Posterior Instrumentation

This combined procedure includes anterior radical surgery with posterior instrumented stabilization of the spine. This can be done as a one-stage simultaneous anterior debridement with bone grafting and then posterior instrumentation by turning the patient prone [47, 80, 106] or as a two-stage procedure with anterior surgery done first, followed in second stage by posterior instrumentation (Fig. 20.6) [107]. Alternatively with severe kyphosis deformity, posterior instrumental stabilization can be done first followed later by anterior debridement and fusion [24]. Each method has its distinct advantages. Pedicle screw system is the most commonly used implant for posterior stabilization. When the infection and destruction of the

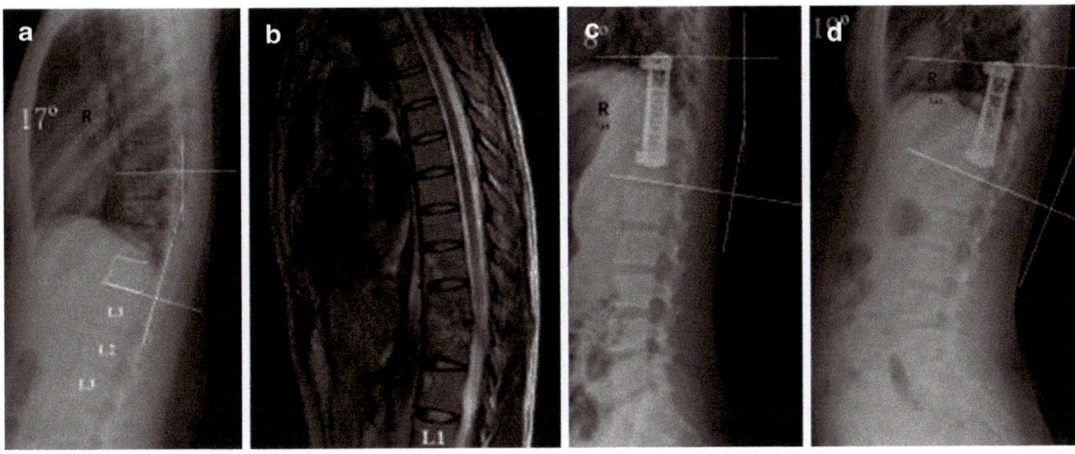

Fig. 20.4 (**a–d**) A 33-year-old woman with spinal tuberculosis (TB) in the T9–T12 vertebrae, especially T10–T11. Three mobile segments were instrumented anteriorly, and 9° correction of kyphosis deformity was obtained after anterior radical debridement and titanium cage filled with morsellised rib-bone grafting and instrumentation in the sagittal plane. There was an 11° loss of correction in local kyphosis angle at the last visit. Preoperative (**a**) lateral radiograph and (**b**) sagittal magnetic resonance image (MRI) and (**c**) postoperative lateral and (**d**) 12-month follow-up lateral radiographs

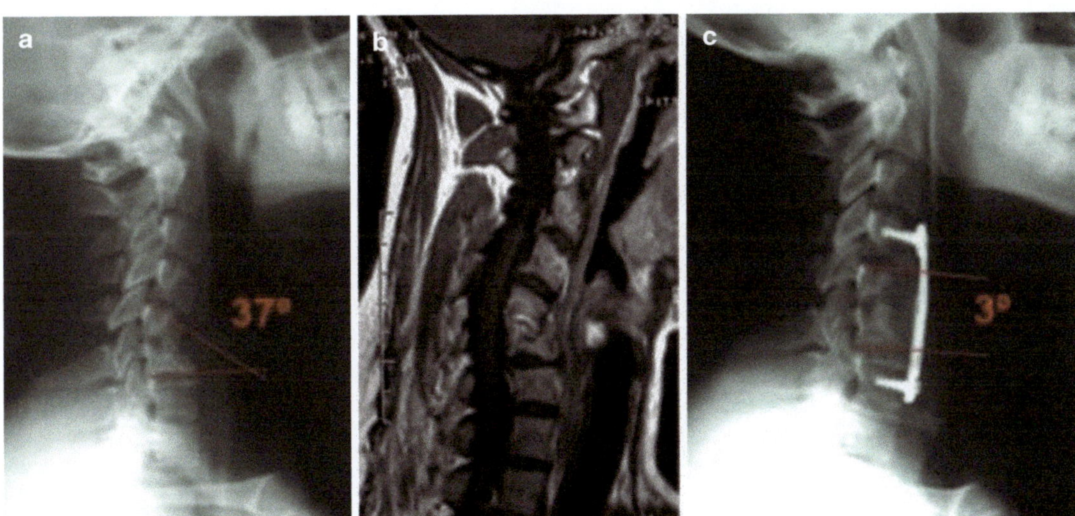

Fig. 20.5 A 51-year-old female with C5/6 TB lesion with marked kyphosis reconstructed by an iliac crest autograft and anterior cervical plating. (**a**) Preop X-rays with a 37° kyphosis, (**b**) preop MRI, and (**c**) final correction to 3°

vertebral body is severe, pedicle screw is fixed one level above or below the infected segment. Patients presenting late with extensive, multi-segment TB involving more than two vertebral bodies and progressive kyphosis are suitable candidates for the two-stage procedure. Anterior radical debridement and strut grafting combined with posterior instrumentation and fusion shorten the postoperative immobilization period and hospital stay, obtain good and long-lasting correction of kyphosis, and prevent further collapse and graft failure [60, 107, 108].

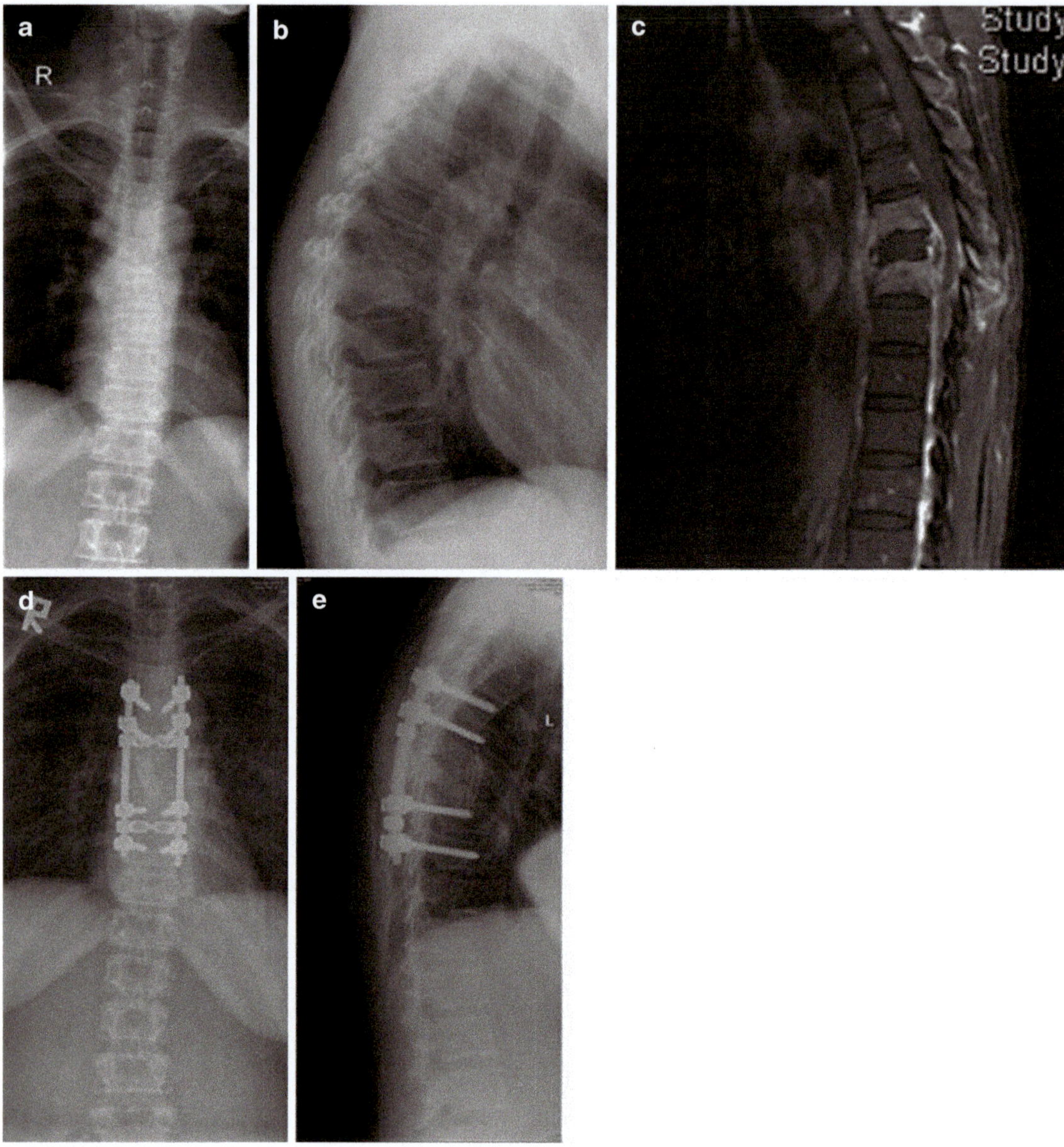

Fig. 20.6 A case requiring anterior debridement and rib strut grafting (the "Hong Kong operation") combined with posterior instrumentation to preserve the sagittal alignment in a case with multilevel infection. Preoperative X-rays (**a**, **b**) and the MRI (**c**) showing the extent of involvement and postoperative X-rays (**d**, **e**) showing restoration of normal kyphosis

20.6.7 Anterior Radical Surgery with Combined Anterior and Posterior Instrumentation

The combined anterior and posterior instrumentation used in cervical and thoracic tuberculous lesions results in satisfactory clinical outcomes [55, 109–111]. When the anterior approach is combined with posterior approaches, it significantly reduces the stress on plate and graft and increases the stability of the spine, thereby reducing the graft and/or the fixation-related complications (Fig. 20.7). Anterior instrumented fusion can be combined with posterior fusion as well as with instrumentation [55]. Due to long operation time, long hospitalization time, more bleeding,

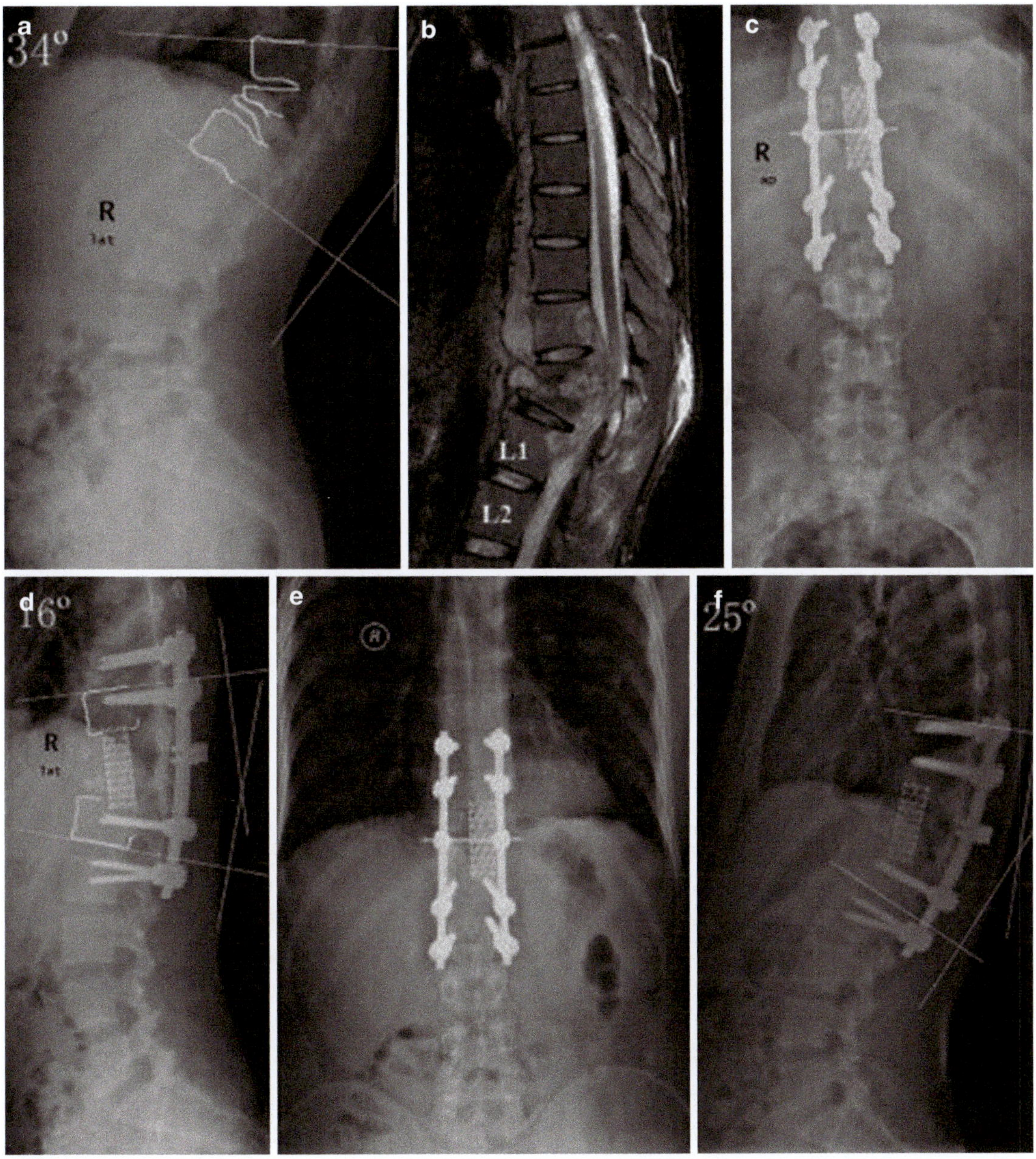

Fig. 20.7 (**a–f**) A 23-year-old man with spinal TB in the T10–L1 vertebrae, especially in T11–12. Three mobile segments were instrumented posteriorly, and 18° correction of kyphosis deformity was obtained after anterior radical debridement and titanium cage filled with morsellised rib-bone grafting and posterior instrumentation in the sagittal plane. There was a 9° loss of correction in local kyphosis angle at the last visit. Preoperative (**a**) lateral radiograph and (**b**) sagittal MRI, postoperative (**c**) anteroposterior and (**d**) lateral radiographs, and12-month control (**e**) anteroposterior and (**f**) lateral radiographs

and routine anterior-posterior approach-related complications, this combined procedure is reserved for certain case of spinal TB such as multilevel segmental lesion, severe spinal destruction, and complex kyphosis deformity [112]. Progressive increase in kyphosis can continue in children with spinal TB even after solid anterior fusion due to posterior longitudinal overgrowth [42, 113]. Therefore, supplemental posterior fusion is recommended sooner or later after anterior radical surgery in children to keep a mechanical balance between anterior and posterior spinal elements [65].

20.6.8 Debridement, Reconstruction, and Instrumentation by Posterior-Only Approach

One-stage posterior transpedicular debridement, interbody fusion with or without posterior fusion, and posterior instrumentation with pedicular screw system are the present-day treatments of choice for many spinal TB lesions [68, 77, 114]. The technique has been successfully used at all levels of the spine from the upper cervical (Fig. 20.8) to the lower lumbar spine [78, 115]. It is a MIS intervention that assures an early neurological recovery and a good correction of kyphosis [27, 114]. This posterior-only approach provides sufficient operating space through resection of both sides of the facet joint, diapophysis, and laminae. It allows operation on the vertebral body at a 360° angle under direct visualization of the outside of the dura mater for thorough removal of the sequestrum, collapsed vertebra, and intervertebral disk. A complete spinal decompression is possible without injuring the spinal cord. Associated paraspinal abscess can be evacuated by adequate pressure washing and postural drainage. Supplemented posterior instrumentation, combined with posterior interbody and posterolateral intertransverse fusion, serves to correct the angular deformity and to minimize the loss of correction [68, 109].

20.6.8.1 Minimally Invasive Surgical (MIS) Approaches in the Management of Tuberculosis of the Thoracic and Lumbar Spine

MIS approaches are frequently used for various spinal disorders, such as degenerative spine, trauma, and tumors [71, 116, 117]. Video-assisted thoracoscopic anterior surgery (VATS) is a MIS technique used in the management of the dorsal

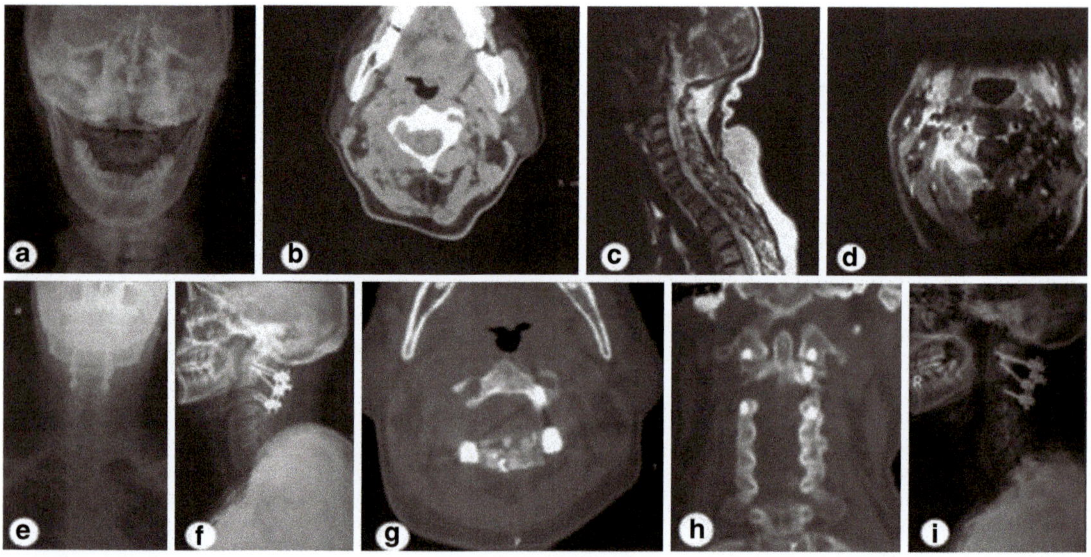

Fig. 20.8 A 14-year-old female, axis destruction and formation of epidural cold abscess, posterior debridement, short-segment fusion, and posterior instrumentation in C1–C3. Preoperative radiography showed destructive segments located at C2, and preoperative CT and MRI showed C2 vertebral body was almost vanished and abscess was localized (**a–d**). Postoperative roentgenographs and CT showed atlas with bilateral pedicle screws, axis with left pedicle screw and C3 with bilateral lateral mass screw (**e–h**). Twenty-five month's postoperative roentgenographs showed internal fixation with good bone fusion (**i**)

spinal TB [79, 118, 119]. Some other MIS techniques used for evacuation of spinal abscesses include nucleotome-based percutaneous aspiration [120, 121], endoscopic suction and drainage [122], and open transpedicular decompression [123]. VATS is considered as a surgical alternative to conventional thoracotomy. Alone it can be used for decompression and biopsy of the lesion [79, 118, 124], or it can be combined with percutaneous posterior transpedicular fixation [119]. It is associated with minimal morbidity [118, 124–126]. However, there is a steep learning curve for this technique, and it is associated with some pulmonary complications such as lung collapse and pleural adhesions. To facilitate further, less invasive mini-thoracotomy (mini-open or using tubular retractor ports) techniques have been developed. They use small 3–4 cm mini incisions to provide direct visualization of the thoracic spine including vessels, nerves, and visceral structures. Due to a direct three-dimensional view, it is easy to perform procedures like corpectomy with direct spinal canal decompression, bone grafting, and placement of anterior instrumentation. The operative time is significantly reduced (Fig. 20.9) [79, 127, 128].

Posterior-only MIS procedures to approach posterior part of the spine include MIS transpedicular debridement and percutaneous transpedicular screw fixation for thoracic spine levels and MIS hemilaminectomy and debridement, followed by internal fixation using percutaneous transpedicular screws for the lumbar spine (Fig. 20.10) [71, 129, 130].

In hybrid MIS techniques, combined ventral and dorsal procedures are done using limited exposures. The ventral decompression and fusion is performed in lateral position using mini-thoracotomy transpleural approach. Drainage of abscess and debridement of necrotic tissues is done to achieve adequate cord decompression and ventral column reconstruction is done using iliac crest or rib autograft or TMC filled with autograft. This is supplemented with posterior fixation using posterior transpedicular screws inserted percutaneously in the prone position in the same sitting as a single stage (Figs. 20.11 and 20.12). This hybrid MIS method helps to achieve all the aims of conventional approaches using MIS principles [71, 119].

20.7 Procedures for Kyphosis Correction

Kyphosis is the most common spinal deformity produced by the TB dorsal spine. TB of the cervical and lumbar spine starts with reversal of lordosis and followed by kyphosis. Kyphosis continues to increase in adult patients if they are treated nonoperatively and even in operated cases if surgery is not supplemented with spinal instrumentation. In children, kyphotic deformity can continue to increase even after healing of the primary disease, due to the remaining growth potential. The sequel to residual healed kyphosis is painful costo-pelvic impingement, reduced vital capacity and eventual respiratory failure, spinal canal stenosis proximal to the kyphosis, and paraplegia. Patient's life span is reduced. These complications can be avoided by early diagnosis and proper intervention according to the stage of the disease. A kyphotic deformity of more than 50° is a severe one, and is likely to progress further, if urgent intervention is not done. Some risk factors for exponential increase in kyphosis in children are age less than 7 years at the time of diagnosis, dorsolumbar disease, loss of two or more vertebral body height, and the presence of two or more spine at risk signs described above. These children are potential candidate for surgical correction of their deformity and should be kept under strict observation [36, 38, 42, 66].

20.7.1 Kyphosis Correction in Active Disease

Spinal TB patients with a kyphotic deformity of 50° or more should be evaluated for kyphosis correction surgery [66]. Kyphotic deformity extending from D2 to L2 can be corrected by single-stage correction by the extrapleural or extraperitoneal anterolateral approach with patient in a lateral position. Anterior decompression and corpec-

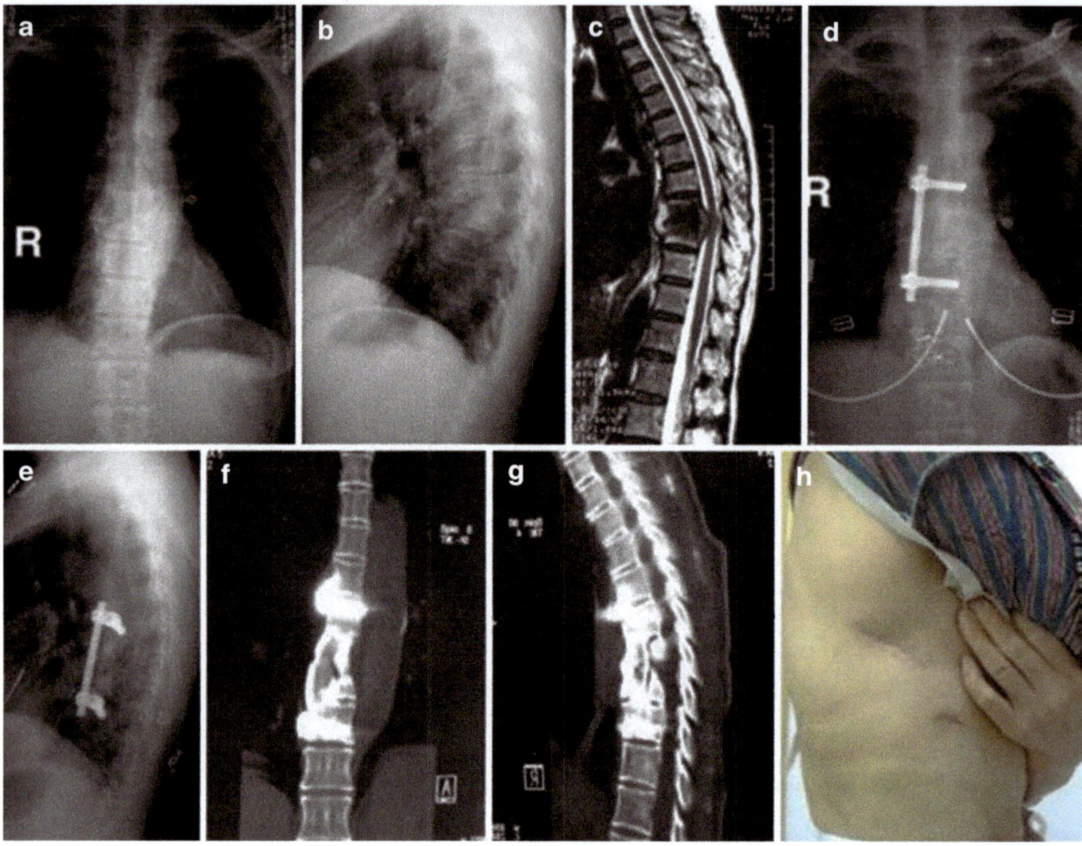

Fig. 20.9 **A** 53-year-old female with T8–T9 TB underwent thoracoscopic-assisted anterior debridement, iliac bone autograft, and fixation with single-rod Ventrofix system (Synthes Spine, Switzerland). (**a, b**) AP X-ray shows paraspinal shadow, and lateral plain radiograph demonstrates a narrowed disk space at T8–T9 and a kyphotic angle of 39°. (**c**) MRI demonstrates vertebral destruction and paravertebral and epidural abscess with compression of the spinal cord. (**d, e**) AP X-ray and lateral plain radiograph of final follow-up show that there was no fixation failure, and the postoperative kyphotic angle is measured 22° at final follow-up. (**f, g**) Three-dimensional CT scan in *coronal* and *sagittal planes* demonstrates a solid fusion. (**h**) Postoperative clinical photograph demonstrates the size of the skin incision

tomy are done first followed by posterior column shortening, instrumented stabilization, and reconstruction of anterior gap by bone graft sequentially in one stage (Fig. 20.13) [37].

The combined anterior and posterior approaches enable access to all three columns of the spine and encourage correction of both neurologic deficit and kyphosis. Anterior decompression with bone grafting is done first, followed by correction of kyphosis and posterior instrumentation or in vice versa fashion where posterior instrumentation is done first followed by anterior surgery (Fig. 20.14) [55, 60, 88, 131–133].

Single posterior debridement, bone grafting and instrumentation is an alternative option where both the anterior and posterior aspects of the spine can be approached through a single incision from behind. It avoids the possible hazards of violating the thoracic and abdominal cavities [39, 134]. A midline incision is made centering at kyphosis. A costotransversectomy and excision of pedicle are carried out at the apex of the kyphosis. The abscess is drained, granulation tissue and bony sequestrum are debrided off, and spinal cord is decompressed. All bony tissues and soft tissues preventing the correction of kyphosis are removed. Segmental

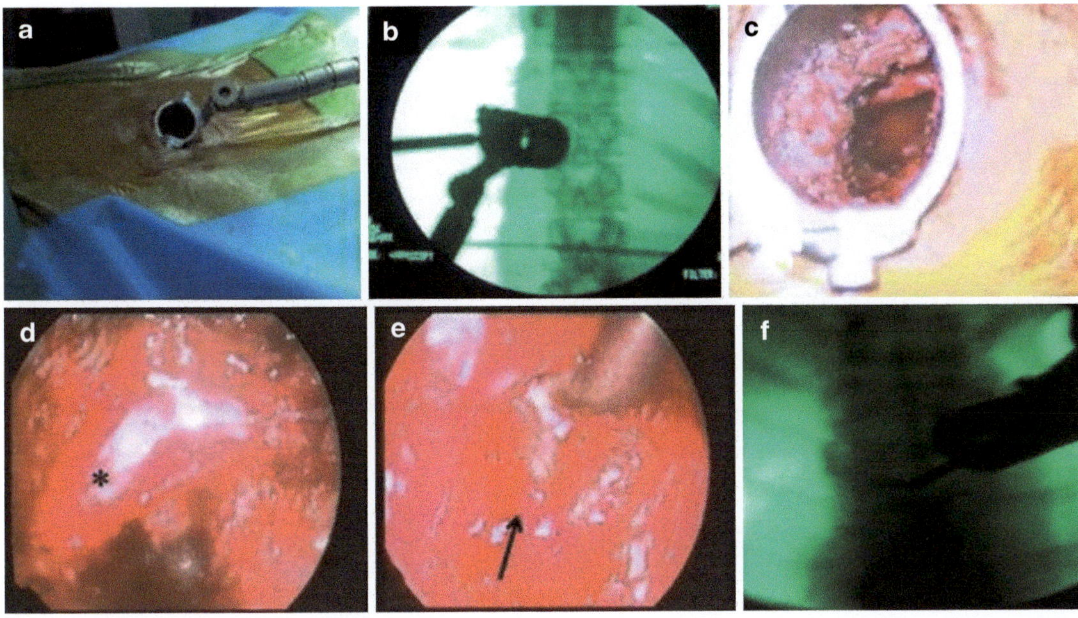

Fig. 20.10 MIS transpedicular decompression and percutaneous fixation (posterior-only MIS method) are illustrated. (**a**) The X-Tube is positioned. (**b**) The position of the X-Tube is confirmed with the C-arm. (**c**) An intraoperative microscopic view after decompression of the thecal sac is shown. (**d**) An endoscopic view allows better visualization of the ventrolateral aspect of the dura using the 30° forward-angled 4-mm telescope. *Asterisk* = thecal sac. (**e**) Endoscope-assisted decompression of the ventral aspect of the thecal sac is performed using an angled curette. *Arrow* = necrotic bone. (**f**) A C-arm image shows the extent of decompression with angled curettes

spinal instrumentation using Hartshill rectangle with sublaminar wiring or pedicle instrumentation is done, and kyphosis is gradually corrected. The anterior defect is subsequently grafted [58]. This is supposed to be the best technique to treat single-segment thoracic and lumbar spinal TB, especially for patients in early phase of bone destruction or ones with mild kyphosis (Fig. 20.15) [67, 135]. In children with advanced thoracolumbar spinal TB with kyphosis, one-stage posterior focus debridement and interbody or combined interbody and posterior fusion with posterior instrumentation have achieved good correction of kyphosis [78, 114].

20.7.2 Kyphosis Correction in Healed Disease

In healed disease with residual kyphosis, the bony anatomy is distorted, and the cord in this area is ischemic, deformed, and less mobile. It is often trapped in the deformed, narrow, hypoplastic canal and is adherent to the dura [46, 136]. Several surgical procedures are described for correction of rigid TB kyphosis. These include different types of osteotomies, decancellation procedures, and vertebral column resection [22, 137–140]. The choice of operation depends on the magnitude of correction required. Long-segment stabilization and fusion are required in this surgery (Fig. 20.16).

20.8 Surgery-Related Complications

Like all surgeries, surgical procedures for spinal TB are also associated with several complications (Table. 20.2) [141–143]. A large number of intraoperative and postoperative complications including vascular, neurological, chest, local, graft, and implant-related complications are reported in the literature [60, 113, 131, 144–146]. When the main surgical goals of deformity correction and neural recovery are not achieved, the

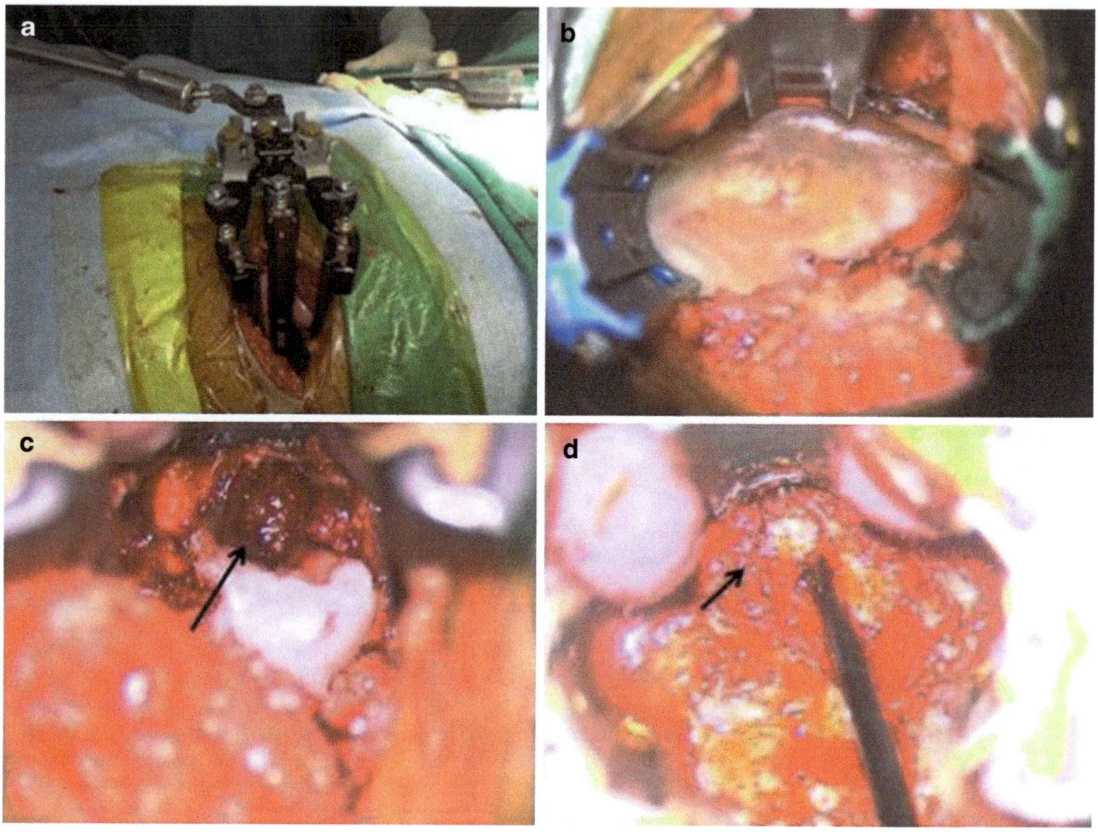

Fig. 20.11 Intraoperative images illustrate mini-thoracotomy with expandable tubular retractors. (**a**) A three-blade retractor is positioned, with one blade retracting the lung. (**b**) Paravertebral pus is drained. (**c**) A defect (*arrow*) remains after debridement. (**d**) Fusion is performed with iliac crest autograft (*arrow*)

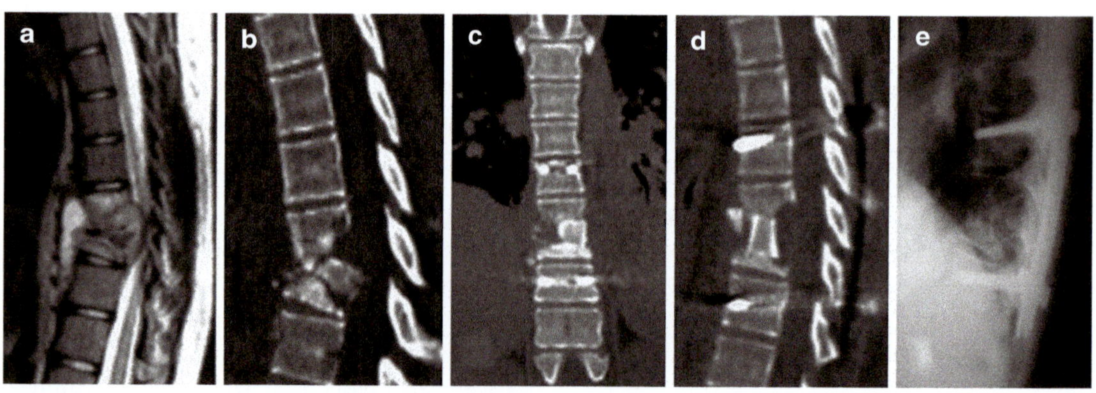

Fig. 20.12 Images illustrate the case of a spinal TB patient treated by hybrid MIS techniques. (**a**) A preoperative T2-weighted sagittal MR image shows destruction of the vertebral body, kyphosis, and epidural and paravertebral abscess with cord compression. (**b**) A preoperative sagittal CT scan shows sequestered bone compromising the canal. Postoperative (**c**) AP and (**d**) sagittal CT scans show the spine after intracorporeal decompression and iliac crest graft in situ and correction of deformity. (**e**) A lateral follow-up radiograph shows bony fusion without deformity progression

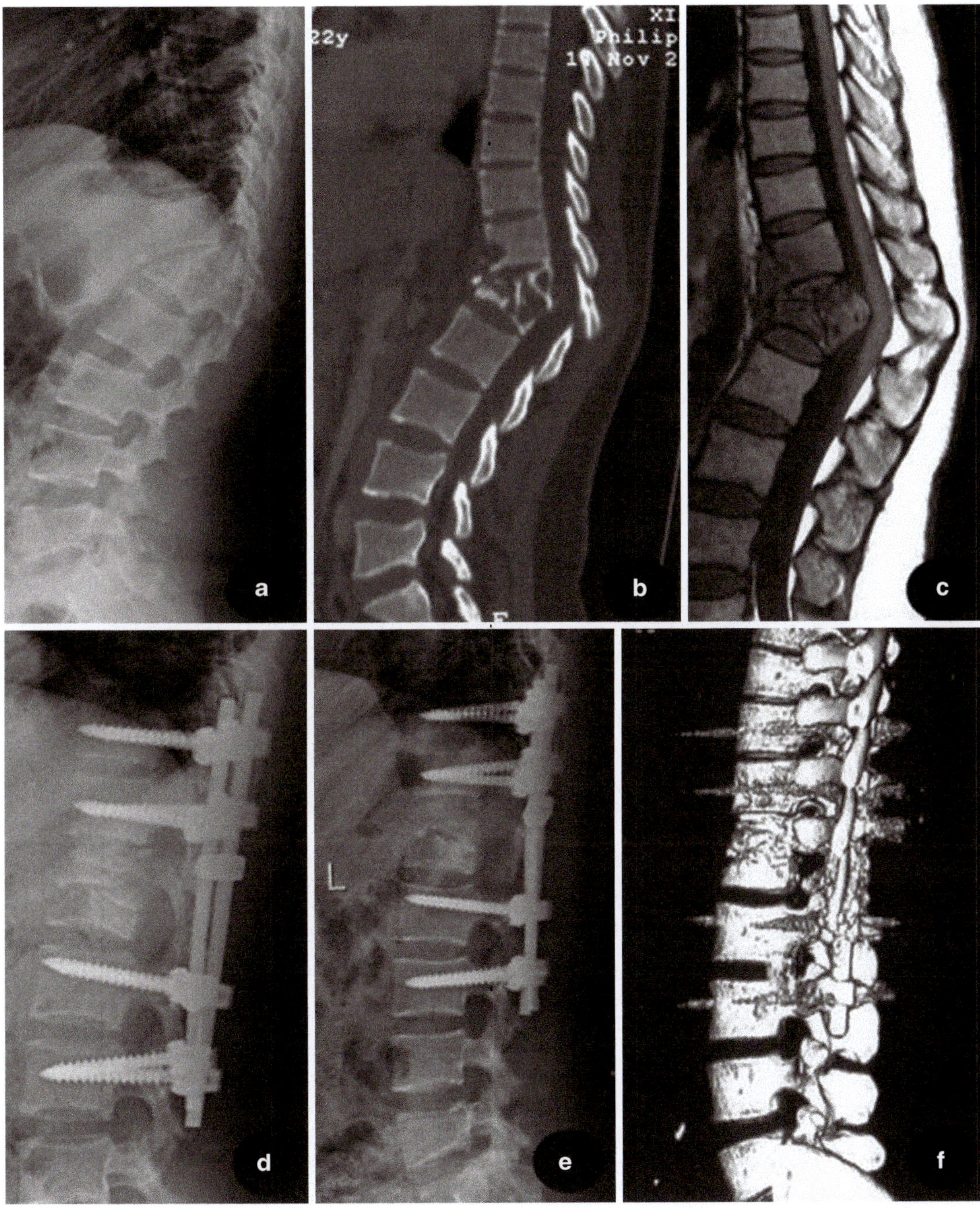

Fig. 20.13 (**a**) A preoperative X-ray of a 45-year-old male demonstrated the destruction of T12 and L1, with a kyphosis angle of 43°. CT and MRI (**b**, **c**) show vertebral bone destruction and paravertebral abscess formation, with, severe spinal cord compression. The patient underwent one-stage anterior debridement, autologous bone grafting, and posterior instrumentation. (**d**) A lateral X-ray indicates that kyphosis was corrected to 6° 3 months after surgery. (**e**, **f**) At 18-month follow-up, fixation was in good shape, without signs of TB recurrence

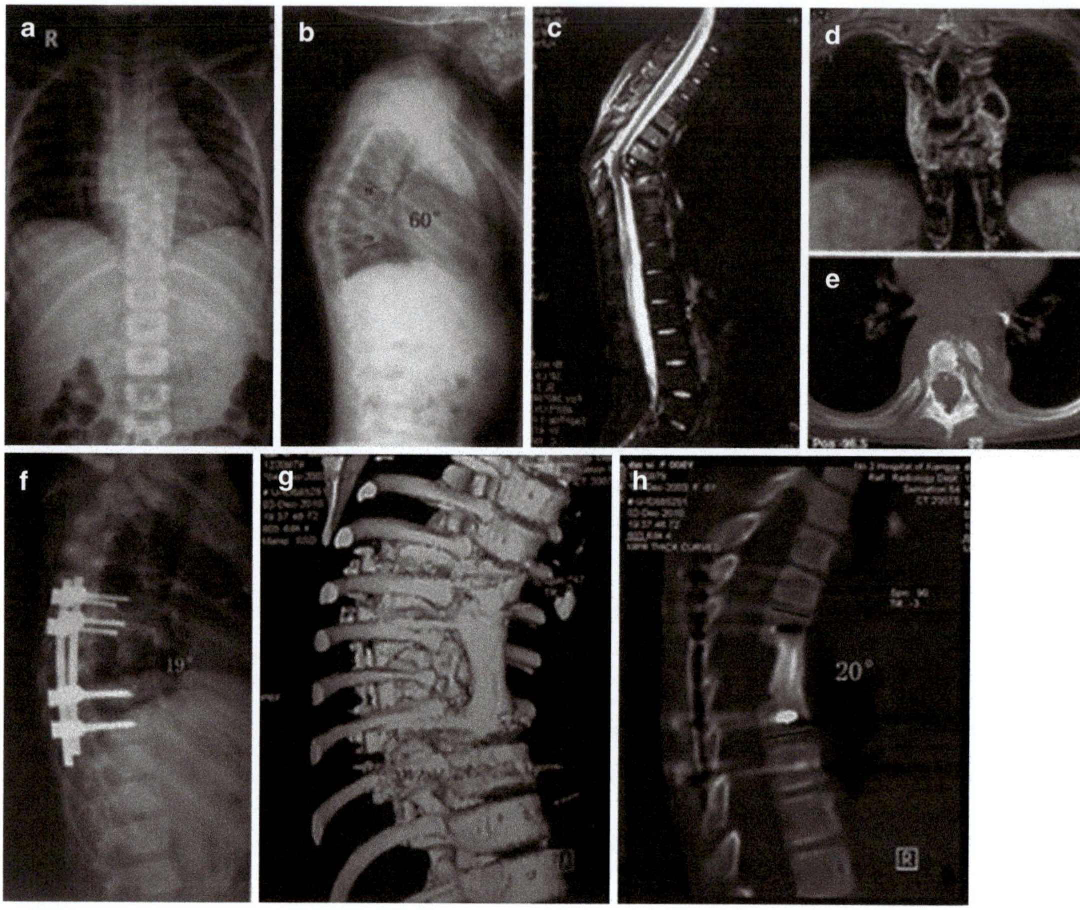

Fig. 20.14 A six-year-old girl. (**a**, **b**) Preoperative X-ray demonstrated destruction of T7 and T8, with a 60° kyphosis measured between T6 and T9. MRI reveals (**c**) protrusion of dead bone fragments and granulation tissue into the canal, leading to compression of the dural sac. (**d**) Pronounced paravertebral abscesses. (**e**) A cross-sectional CT scan shows moth-eaten bone destruction. patient underwent single stage posterior instrumentation, anterior debridement and bone grafting with tricortical iliac crest graft.. (**f**) At the 3-month follow-up, a lateral X-ray indicates that kyphosis was corrected to 19°. (**g**, **h**) At the 9-month follow-up, a CT scan shows successful fusion at the grafted site, and the kyphosis was 20°

results are labeled as a failure in spite of the healed disease.

The development of surgical complications is related to the patient and surgeon factors including the patient's age and general condition, cord condition, severity of deformity, emergency surgery, unjustified surgical indication, and surgeon's skills. Generally, the surgical complication rates are higher in the deformity correction surgery [38, 147].

Careful preoperative surgical planning and patient care, using appropriate surgical technique, and proper postoperative patient management are some important factors to avoid these complications. Any decision to operate should be based on clear goal of treatment for each individual and must weigh the high complication and reoperation rates against the anticipated improvement. Surgical risks and complications must be fully explained to the patient, and ultimately the patient should choose between the risks and his/her quality of life. Highly evolved surgical techniques, improved surgical tools, and newly developed anti-TB drugs have contributed greatly in reducing the complications of surgery in spinal TB [141, 147, 148].

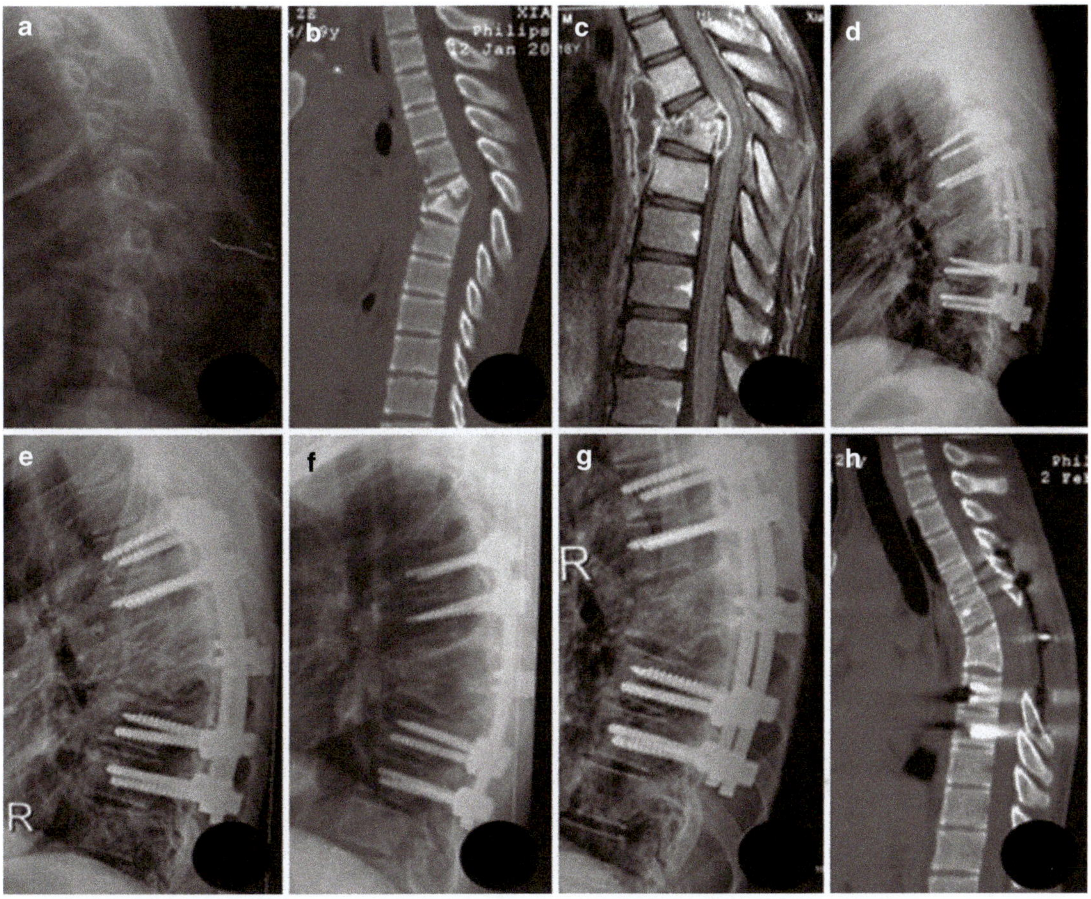

Fig. 20.15 (**a**) A preoperative X-ray of a 22-year-old male demonstrated the destruction of T6 and T7, with a kyphosis angle of 32°. CT and MRI (**b**, **c**) show vertebral bone destruction, paravertebral abscess formation, and spinal cord compression. (**d**, **e**) 3 months after single posterior debridement, bone grafting and instrumentation, a lateral X-ray indicated that kyphosis was corrected to 26°. (**f–h**) At final follow up Xrays and CT revealed successful fusion and a kyphosis angle of 27°

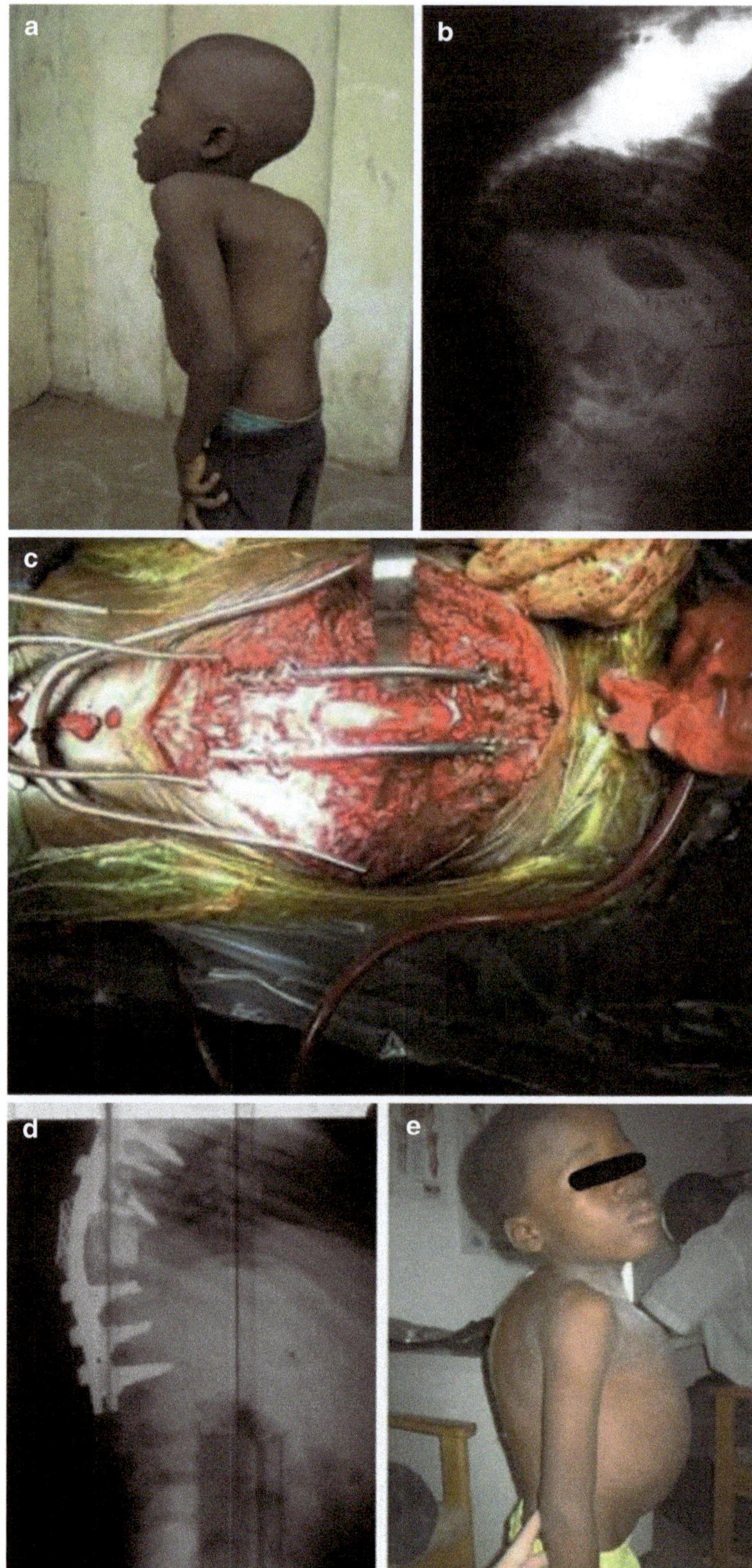

Fig. 20.16 An 8-year-old boy with spinal TB treated medically. He developed a progressive severe kyphosis and bilateral leg weakness. (**a**) Clinical appearance preoperatively demonstrating skin breakdown over the gibbus deformity. (**b**) Lateral radiograph shows sharp (140°) angular deformity of the thoracolumbar spine with spinal cord compression. (**c**) Appearance after decompression and vertebral column resection. (**d**) Lateral radiograph shows anterior cage support with bone graft and posterior instrumented fusion. (**e**) Clinical appearance postoperatively

Table 20.2 Surgery-related complications

Intraoperative	
Vascular injury	Aorta, vena cava, iliac vein
Neural injury	Cord injury, dural tear, root injury, intercostal nerve cut, symphatheticolysis
Esophagus perforation	
Lung damage	
Ureteric injury	
Peritoneal perforation	
Postoperative	
Death	Cerebral embolism due to thromboembolism in a paraparetic
Respiratory complication	ARDS, pneumothorax, hemothorax, pleural effusion, lung atelectasis, pulmonary edema, pneumonia, hiccup (diaphragmatic crus irritation)
Neurological complications	Transient re-paralysis (below T8), recurrent laryngeal nerve palsy (transient), peroneal palsy, intercostal neuroma, intercostal neuralgia, symphatheticolysis in the lower extremity, Sudeck's atrophy in the upper extremity, no neurological recovery
Local complications	Surgical site infection, wound disruption, thrombophlebitis in the lower extremity, incisional hernia
Ileus	
Urinary retention	
Retrograde ejaculation	
Graft problems	Absorption, fracture, bed failure, graft slip-out
Implant loosening	
Increase in deformity (kyphosis)	
Fusion failure/pseudoarthrosis	

Conclusion

The primary treatment of spinal TB is chemotherapy. Surgery is mainly indicated for the failure of conservative treatment, progressive neurologic deficit, and prevention and correction of spinal deformity. There are different surgical procedures for treatment of spinal TB. Each has its own indication and advantage. The main aim of surgery is debridement/decompression of lesion and stabilization of the spine. Anterior radical debridement (Hong Kong procedure) with bone graft fusion is the standard in spinal TB surgery. Instrumented stabilization of the spine produces a better outcome. Posterior segmental stabilization with pedicle screw system has changed the trend in spinal surgery. Posterior-only approach as MIS technique is effectively employed for debridement, fusion, and instrumented stabilization in dorsal and lumbar spinal TB. Video-assisted mini-open approaches are developed to avoid the complications of conventional thoracotomy. Kyphosis correction in healed lesion is difficult surgery and is associated with serious complications. Any decision to operate on should be based on clear goals for each individual and must weigh the high complication and reoperation rates against the anticipated improvement.

References

1. Agrawal V, Patgaonkar PR, Nagariya SP (2010) Tuberculosis of spine. J Craniovertebr Junction Spine 1:74–85
2. Ito H, Asami T (1934) A new radical operation for Pott's disease: report of ten cases. J Bone Joint Surg Br 16:499–515

3. Duraiswami PK, Tuli SM (1971) 5000 years of orthopaedics in India. Clin Orthop Relat Res 75:269–280
4. Tuli SM (2007) Tuberculosis of the spine: a historical review. Clin Orthop Relat Res 460:29–38
5. Rasouli MR, Mirkoohi M, Vaccaro AR, Yarandi KK, Rahimi-Movaghar V (2012) Spinal tuberculosis: diagnosis and management. Asian spine J 6:294–308
6. Moon MS (2006) Development in the management of tuberculosis of the spine. Curr Orthop 20:132–140
7. Albee FH (1911) Transplantation of a portion of the tibia into the spine for Pott's disease: a preliminary report. JAMA 57:885–886
8. Hibbs RA (1911) An operation for Pott's disease of the spine. JAMA 59:433–436
9. McKee GK (1937) A comparison of the results of spinal fixation operation and non-operative treatment in Pott's disease in adults. Br J Surg 24:456–468
10. Seddon HJ (1938) Pott's paraplegia: prognosis and treatment. Br J Surg 22:769–799
11. Hodgson AR, Stock FE (1956) Anterior spinal fusion. A preliminary communication on the radical treatment of Pott's disease and Pott's paraplegia. Br J Surg 44:266–275
12. Hodgson AR, Stock FE (1960) Anterior spine fusion for the treatment of tuberculosis of the spine: the operative findings and results of treatment in the first 100 cases. J Bone Joint Surg Am 42:295–310
13. Kondo E, Yamada K (1957) End results of focal debridement in bone and joint tuberculosis and its indications. J Bone Joint Surg Am 39:27–31
14. Wilkinson MC (1995) The treatment of tuberculosis. J Bone Joint Surg Br 37:382–391
15. Deroy MS, Fisher H (1952) The treatment of tuberculous bone disease by surgical drainage combined with streptomycin. J Bone Joint Surg Am 34:299–330
16. Tuli SM (1975) Results of treatment of spinal tuberculosis by middle path regime. J Bone Joint Surg Br 57:13–23
17. Martin NS (1970) Tuberculosis of the spine-A study of the results of treatment during the last twenty-five years. J Bone Joint Surg Br 52:613–628
18. Moon MS, Moon YW, Moon JL, Kim SS, Sun DH (2002) Conservative treatment of tuberculosis of the lumbar and lumbosacral spine. Clin Orthop Relat Res 398:40–49
19. Mak KC, Cheung KM (2013) Surgical treatment of acute TB spondylitis: indications and outcomes. Eur Spine J 22:603–611
20. Tuli SM (2011) Tuberculosis of spine: a historical perspective and evolution of treatment. In: Rajasekaran S (ed) Spinal infections and trauma. Jaypee brothers medical publishers (P) Ltd, New Dehli, pp 55–63
21. Rajasekaran S, Soundarapandian S (1989) Progression of kyphosis in tuberculosis of the spine treated by anterior arthrodesis. J Bone Joint Surg Am 71:1314–1323
22. Moon MS (2014) Tuberculosis of spine: current views in diagnosis and management. Asian Spine J 8:97–111
23. El-Sharkawi MM, Said GZ (2012) Instrumented circumferential fusion for tuberculosis of the dorso-lumbar spine. A single or double stage procedure? Int Orthop 36:315–324
24. Varatharajah S, Charles YP, Buy X, Walter A, Steib JP (2014) Update on the surgical management of Pott's disease. Orthop Traumatol Surg Res 100:229–235
25. Wang Z, Yuan H, Geng G, Shi J, Jin W (2012) Posterior monosegmental fixation, combined with anterior debridement and strut graft, for treatment of the mono-segmental lumbar spine tuberculosis. Int Orthop 36:325–329
26. Kumar K (1985) A clinical study and classification of posterior spinal tuberculosis. Int Orthop 9:147–152
27. Mehta JS, Bhojraj SY (2001) Tuberculosis of the thoracic spine A classification based on the selection of the surgical strategies. J Bone Joint Surg Br 83:859–863
28. Oguz E, Sehirlioglu A, Altinmakas M, Ozturk C, Komurcu M, Solakoglu C, Vaccaro AR (2008) A new classification and guide for surgical treatment of spinal tuberculosis. Int Orthop 32:127–133
29. Ekinci S, Tataa O, Akpancar S, Bilgic S, Ersen O (2015) Spinal tuberculosis. J Exp Neurosci 9:89–90
30. Samuel S (2010) Comment on Oguz et al.: a new classification and guide for surgical treatment of spinal tuberculosis. Int Orthop 34:613
31. Ekinci S, Akyildiz F, Ersen O (2015) Response to: Surgery related complications and sequel in management of tuberculosis of spine. Asian Spine J 9:153–154
32. Gill JB, Levin A, Burd T, Longley M (2008) Corrective osteotomies in spine surgery. J Bone Joint Surg Am 90:2509–2520
33. Okada Y, Miyamoto H, Uno K, Sumi M (2009) Clinical and radiological outcome of surgery for pyogenic and tuberculous spondylitis: comparisons of surgical techniques and disease types. J Neurosurg Spine 11:620–627
34. Tuli SM (2013) Historical aspects of Pott's disease (spinal tuberculosis) management. Eur Spine J 22:S529–S538
35. Muhammad T, Baloch NA, Khan A (2015) Management of spinal tuberculosis – a metropolitan city based survey among orthopaedic and neurosurgeons. J Pak Med Assoc 65:1256–1260
36. Rajasekaran S (2002) The problem of deformity in spinal tuberculosis. Clin Orthop Relat Res 398:85–92
37. Jain AK, Maheshwari AV, Jena S (2007) Kyphus correction in spinal tuberculosis. Clin Orthop Relat Res 460:117–123
38. Rajasekaran S (2007) Buckling collapse of the spine in childhood spinal tuberculosis. Clin Orthop Relat Res 460:86–92
39. Rajasekaran S (2012) Kyphotic deformity in spinal tuberculosis and its management. Int Orthop 36:359–365
40. Jain AK (2010) Tuberculosis of the spine: a fresh look at an old disease. J Bone Joint Surg Br 92:905–913
41. Tuli SM (1995) Severe kyphotic deformity in tuberculosis of the spine. Int Orthop 19:327–331
42. Rajasekaran S (2001) The natural history of post-tubercular kyphosis in children Radiological signs

which predict late increase in deformity. J Bone Joint Surg Br 83:954–962
43. Dinc H, Ahmetoglu A, Baykal S, Sari A, Sayil O, Gumele HR (2002) Image-guided percutaneous drainage of tuberculous iliopsoas and spondylodiskitic abscesses: midterm results. Radiology 225:353–358
44. Cheng VC, Yam WC, Hung IF, Woo PC, Lau SK, Tang BS, Yuen KY (2004) Clinical evaluation of the polymerase chain reaction for the rapid diagnosis of tuberculosis. J Clin Pathol 57:281–285
45. Garg B, Kandwal P, Nagaraja UB, Goswami A, Jayaswal A (2012) Anterior versus posterior procedure for surgical treatment of thoracolumbar tuberculosis: a retrospective analysis. Indian J Orthop 46:165–170
46. Benli IT, Kaya A, Acaroglu E (2007) Anterior instrumentation in tuberculous spondylitis: is it effective and safe? Clin Orthop Relat Res 460:108–116
47. Jain AK, Dhammi IK, Prashad B, Sinha S, Mishra P (2008) Simultaneous anterior decompression and posterior instrumentation of the tuberculous spine using an anterolateral extrapleural approach. J Bone Joint Surg Br 90:1477–1481
48. Hodgson AR, Stock FE, Fang HS, Ong GB (1960) Anterior spinal fusion: the operative approach and pathological findings in 412 patients with Pott's disease of the spine. Br J Surg 48:172–178
49. Soares Do Brito J, Tirado A, Fernandes P (2014) Surgical treatment of spinal tuberculosis complicated with extensive abscesss. Iowa Orthop J 34:129–136
50. Jain AK (2002) Treatment of tuberculosis of the spine with neurological complications. Clin Orthop Relat Res 398:75–84
51. Pu X, Zhou Q, He Q, Dai F, Xu J, Zhang Z, Branko K (2012) A posterior versus anterior surgical approach in combination with debridement, interbody autografting and instrumentation for thoracic and lumbar tuberculosis. Int Orthop 36:307–313
52. Sharkawi MM, Said GK (2012) Instrumented circumferential fusion for tuberculosis of the dorso-lumbar spine: a single or double stage procedure? Int Orthop 36:315–324
53. Soundararaj GD (2009) Simultaneous anterior decompression and posterior instrumentation of the tuberculous spine using anterolateral extrapleural approach. J Bone Joint Surg Br 91:702–703
54. Guerado E, Cerván AM (2012) Surgical treatment of spondylodiscitis. An update. Int Orthop 36:413–420
55. Ma YZ, Cui X, Li HW, Chen X, Cai XJ, Bai YB (2012) Outcomes of anterior and posterior instrumentation under different surgical procedures for treating thoracic and lumbar spinal tuberculosis in adults. Int Orthop 36:299–305
56. Hee HT, Majd ME, Holt RT, Pienkowski D (2002) Better treatment of vertebral osteomyelitis using posterior stabilization and titanium mesh cages. J Spinal Disord Tech 15:149–156
57. Fukuta S, Miyamoto K, Masuda T, Hosoe H, Kodama H, Nishimoto H, Sakaeda H, Shimizu K (2003) Two stage (Posterior and anterior) surgical treatment using posterior spinal instrumentation for pyogenic and tuberculotic spondylitis. Spine (Phila Pa 1976) 28:E302–E308
58. Laheri VJ, Badhe NP, Dewnany GT (2001) Single stage decompression, anterior interbody fusion and posterior instrumentation for tuberculous kyphosis of the dorso-lumbar spine. Spinal Cord 39:429–436
59. Moon MS (1991) Combined posterior instrumentation and anterior interbody fusion for active tuberculous kyphosis of the thoraco-lumbar spine. Curr Orthop 5:177–179
60. Moon MS, Woo YK, Lee KS, Ha KY, Kim SS, Sun DH (1995) Posterior instrumentation and anterior interbody fusion for tuberculous kyphosis of dorsal and lumbar spines. Spine (Phila Pa 1976) 20:1910–1916
61. Jain AK, Dhammi IK (2007) Tuberculosis of the spine: a review. Clin Orthop Relat Res 460:39–49
62. Güven O, Kumano K, Yalçin S, Karaham M, Tsuji S (1994) A single stage posterior approach and rigid fixation for preventing kyphosis in the treatment of spinal tuberculosis. Spine (Phila Pa 1976) 19:1039–1043
63. Upadhyay SS, Sell P, Saji MJ, Sell B, Hsu LC (1994) Surgical management of spinal tuberculosis in adults Hong Kong operation compared with debridement surgery for short and long term outcome of deformity. Clin Orthop Relat Res 302:173–182
64. Dai LY, Jiang LS, Wang W, Cui YM (2005) Single-stage anterior autogenous bone grafting and instrumentation in the surgical management of spinal tuberculosis. Spine (Phila Pa 1976) 30:2342–2349
65. Jin D, Qu D, Chen J, Zhang H (2004) One-stage anterior interbody autografting and instrumentation in primary surgical management of thoracolumbar spinal tuberculosis. Eur Spine J 13:114–121
66. Jain AK, Dhammi IK, Jain S, Mishra P (2010) Kyphosis in spinal tuberculosis–prevention and correction. Indian J Orthop 44:127–136
67. Wang X, Pang X, Wu P, Luo C, Shen X (2014) One stage anterior debridement, bone grafting and posterior instrumentation vs. single posterior debridement, bone grafting and instrumentation for the treatment of thoracic and lumbar spinal tuberculosis. Eur Spine J 23:830–837
68. Rathinavelu B, Arockiaraj J, Krishnan V, Amritanand R, Sundararaj GD (2014) The extended posterior circumferential decompression technique in the management of tubercular spondylitis with and without paraplegia. Asian Spine J 8:711–719
69. Zhang H, Sheng B, Tang M, Guo C, Liu S, Huang S, Gao Q, Liu J, Wu J (2013) One-stage surgical treatment for upper thoracic spinal tuberculosis by internal fixation, debridement, and combined interbody and posterior fusion via posterior-only approach. Eur Spine J 22:616–623
70. Huag J, Zhang H, Zeng K, Gao Q (2014) The clinical outcomes of surgical treatment of non contiguous spinal tuberculosis: a retrospective study in 23 cases. PLoS One 9(4):e93648. doi:10.1371/journal.pone.0093648

71. Garg N, Vohra R (2014) Minimally invasive surgical approaches in the management of tuberculosis of the thoracic and lumbar spine. Clin Orthop Relat Res 472:1855–1867
72. Gupta S, Suri S, Gulati M, Singh P (1997) Ilio-psoas abscesses: percutaneous drainage under image guidance. Clin Radiol 52:704–707
73. Behari S, Nayak SR, Bhargava V, Banerji D, Chhabra DK, Jain VK (2003) Craniocervical tuberculosis: protocol of surgical management. Neurosurgery 52:72–80
74. Upadhyay SS, Sell P, Saji MJ, Leong JC (1993) Radical and débridement surgery for tuberculosis of the spine in children: a preliminary analysis of results from a 17-year prospective study. Eur Spine J 1:231–235
75. Jain AK (2008) Tuberculosis of spine: Neurological deficit. In: Kulkarni GS (ed) Textbook of orthopedic and Trauma. Jaypee brother's medical publishers (P) Ltd, New Dehli, pp 423–445
76. Jarrett CD, Heller JG, Tsai L (2009) Anterior exposure of the lumbar spine with and without an "access surgeon": morbidity analysis of 265 consecutive cases. J Spinal Disord Tech 22:559–564
77. Shen X, Liu H, Wang G, Liu X (2015) Single-stage posterior-only approach treating single-segment thoracic tubercular spondylitis. Int J Clin Exp Pathol 1:11051–11059
78. Hu X, Zhang H, Yin X, Chen Y, Yu H, Zhou Z (2015) One-stage posterior focus debridement, fusion, and instrumentation in the surgical treatment of lumbar spinal tuberculosis with kyphosis in children. Childs Nerv Syst 32:535–539
79. Lu G, Wang B, Li J, Liu W, Cheng I (2012) Anterior debridement and reconstruction via thoracoscopy assisted mini-open approach for the treatment of thoracic spinal tuberculosis: minimum 5 year follow up. Eur Spine J 21:463–469
80. Wang XB, Li J, Lu GH, Wang B, Kang YJ (2012) Single stage posterior instrumentation and anterior debridement for active tuberculosis of the thoracic and lumbar spine with kyphotic deformity. Int Orthop 36:373–380
81. Govender S, Kumar KP, Med PC (2001) Long-term follow-up assessment of vascularized rib pedicle graft for tuberculosis kyphosis. J Pediatr Orthop 21:281–284
82. Govender S, Kumar KP (2003) Cortical allograft in spinal tuberculosis. Int Orthop 27:244–248
83. Govender S, Parbhoo AH (1999) Support of the anterior column with allografts in tuberculosis of the spine. J Bone Joint Surg Br 81:106–109
84. Zhang H, Zeng K, Yin X, Huang J, Tang M, Guo C (2015) Debridement, internal fixation, and reconstruction using titanium mesh for the surgical treatment of thoracic and lumbar spinal tuberculosis via a posterior-only approach: a 4-year follow-up of 28 patients. J Orthop Surg Res 10:150. doi:10.1186/s13018-015-0292-7
85. Upadhyay SS, Saji MJ, Yau AC (1996) Duration of antituberculosis chemotherapy in conjunction with radical surgery in the management of spinal tuberculosis. Spine (Phila Pa 1976) 21:1898–1903
86. Jiang T, Zhao J, He M, Wang K, Fowdur M, Wu Y (2015) Outcomes and treatment of lumbosacral spinal tuberculosis: a retrospective study of 53 patients. PLoS One 10:e0130185. doi:10.1371/journal.pone.0130185
87. Jain AK, Jain S (2012) Instrumented stabilization in spinal tuberculosis. Int Orthop 36:285–292
88. Uvaraj NR, Bosco A, Gopinath NR (2015) Global reconstruction for extensive destruction in tuberculosis of the lumbar spine and Lumbosacral junction. A case report. Global Spine J 5:e17–e21
89. Pun WK, Chow SP, Luk KDK, Cheng CL, Hsu LCS, Leong JCY (1990) Tuberculosis of the lumbosacral junction. Long-term follow-up of 26 cases. J Bone Joint Surg Br 72:675–678
90. Ha KY, Chung YG, Ryoo SJ (2005) Adherence and biofilm formation of *Staphylococcus epidermidis* and Mycobacterium tuberculosis on various spinal implants. Spine (Phila Pa 1976) 30:38–43
91. Oga M, Arizono T, Takasita M, Sugioka Y (1993) Evaluation of the risk of instrumentation as a foreign body in the spinal tuberculosis: clinical and biologic study. Spine (Phila Pa 1976) 18:1890–1894
92. Yang X, Chen Q, Liu L, Song Y, Kong Q, Zeng J, Xue Y, Ren C (2013) Comparison of anterior cervical fusion by titanium mesh cage versus nano-hydroxyapatite/polyamide cage following single-level corpectomy. Int Orthop 37:2421–2427
93. Riew KD, Rhee JM (2002) The use of titanium mesh cages in the cervical spine. Clin Orthop Relat Res 394:47–54
94. Majd ME, Vadhva M, Holt RT (1999) Anterior cervical reconstruction using titanium cage with anterior plating. Spine (Phila Pa 1976) 24:1604–1610
95. Eck KR, Bridwell KH, Ungacta FF, Lapp MA, Lenke LG, Riew KD (2000) Analysis of titanium mesh cages in adults with minimum two-year follow-up. Spine (Phila Pa 1976) 25:2407–2415
96. Chen Y, Chen D, Guo Y, Wang X, Lu X, He Z, Yuan W (2008) Subsidence of titanium mesh cage: a study based on 300 cases. J Spinal Disord Tech 21:489–492
97. Wilber RG, Thompson GH, Shaffer JW, Brown RH, Nash CL Jr (1984) Postoperative neurological deficits in segmental spinal instrumentation. J Bone Joint Surg Am 66:1178–1187
98. Bhjraj SY, Verma RG, Nene AM, Mohite S (2010) Spinal loop rectangle and sublaminar wiring as a technique for scoliosis correction. Indian J Orthop 44:50–56
99. Zhang HQ, Lin MZ, Shen KY, Ge L, Li JS, Tang MX, Wu JH, Liu JY (2012) Surgical management for multilevel noncontiguous thoracic spinal tuberculosis by single-stage posterior transforaminal thoracic debridement, limited decompression, interbody fusion, and posterior instrumentation (modified TTIF). Arch Orthop Trauma Surg 132:751–757

100. Benli IT, Acaroglu E, Akalin S, Kiş M, Duman E, Un A (2003) Anterior radical debridement and anterior instrumentation in tuberculosis spondylitis. Eur Spine J 12:224–234
101. Regan JJ, Guyer RD (1997) Endoscopic techniques in spinal surgery. Clin Orthop Relat Res 335:122–139
102. Benli IT, Alanay A, Akalin S, Kis M, Acaroglu E, Ates B, Aydin E (2004) Comparison of anterior instrumentation systems and the results of minimum 5 years follow-up in the treatment of tuberculosis spondylitis. Kobe J Med Sci 50:167–180
103. Chen CL, Chou CW, Su WW, Cheng CY, Yu CT (2008) Dislodged upper thoracic cage in the gastrointestinal tract: a case report and literature reviews. Spine 33:E802–E806
104. Korovessis P, Petsinis G, Koureas G, Iliopoulos P, Zacharatos S (2006) Anterior surgery with insertion of titanium mesh cage and posterior instrumented fusion performed sequentially on the same day under one anesthesia for septic spondylitis of thoracolumbar spine: is the use of titanium mesh cages safe? Spine 31:1014–1019
105. Koptan W, Elmiligui Y, Elsharkawi M (2011) Single stage anterior reconstruction using titanium mesh cages in neglected kyphotic tuberculous spondylodiscitis of the cervical spine. Eur Spine J 20:308–313
106. Suh KT, Seong YJ, Lee JS (2008) Simultaneous anterior and posterior surgery in the management of tuberculous spondylitis with psoas abscess patients with neurological deficits. Asian Spine J 2:94–101
107. Talu U, Gogus A, Ozturk C (2006) The role of posterior instrumentation and fusion after anterior radical debridement and fusion in the surgical treatment of spinal tuberculosis: experience of 127 cases. J Spinal Disord Tech 19:554–559
108. Sundararaj GD, Behera S, Ravi V, Venkatesh K, Cherian VM, Lee V (2003) Role of posterior stabilisation in the management of tuberculosis of the dorsal and lumbar spine. J Bone Joint Surg Br 85:100–106
109. Zeng H, Shen X, Luo C, Xu ZY, Liu Z, Wang X (2015) Comparison of three surgical approaches for cervicothoracic spinal tuberculosis: a retrospective case –control study. J Orthop Surg Res 10:100. doi:10.1186/s13018-015-0238-0
110. Wang XT, Zhou CL, Xi CY, Sun CL, Yan JL (2012) Surgical treatment of cervicothoracic junction spinal tuberculosis via combined anterior and posterior approaches in children. Chin Med J (Engl) 125:1443–1447
111. Nottmeier EW, Deen HG, Patel N, Birch B (2009) Cervical kyphotic deformity correction using 360-degree reconstruction. J Spinal Disord Tech 22:385–391
112. Jain AK, Aggarwal PK, Arora A, Singh S (2004) Behaviour of the kyphotic angle in spinal tuberculosis. Int Orthop 28:110–114
113. Fountain SS, Hsu LCS, Yau AC, Hodgson AR (1975) Progressive kyphosis following solid anterior spine fusion in children with tuberculosis of the spine. J Bone Joint Surg Am 57:1104–1107
114. Zhang HQ, Wang YX, Guo CF, Liu JY, Wu JH, Chen J, Guo D, Tang MX (2010) One-stage posterior approach and combined interbody and posterior fusion for thoracolumbar spinal tuberculosis with kyphosis in children. Orthopedics 33:808. doi:10.3928/01477447-20100924-10
115. Zhang HQ, Lin MZ, Guo HB, Ge L, Wu JH, Liu JY (2013) One-stage surgical management for tuberculosis of the upper cervical spine by posterior debridement, short-segment fusion, and posterior instrumentation in children. Eur Spine J 22:72–77
116. De Iure F, Cappuccio M, Paderni S, Bosco G, Amendola L (2012) Minimally invasive percutaneous fixation of thoracic and lumbar spine fractures. Min Invasive Surg 2012:141032. doi:10.1007/s00586-009-0989-6
117. McLain RF (2001) Spinal cord decompression: an endoscopically assisted approach for metastatic tumors. Spinal Cord 39:482–487
118. Jayaswal A, Upendra B, Ahmed A, Chowdhury B, Kumar A (2007) Video assisted thoracoscopic anterior surgery for tuberculous spondylitis. Clin Orthop Relat Res 460:100–107
119. Kandwal P, Garg B, Upendra BN, Chowdhury B, Jayaswal A (2012) Outcome of minimally invasive surgery in the management of tuberculous spondylitis. Indian J Orthop 46:159–164
120. Hanaoka N, Kawasaki Y, Sakai T, Nakamura T, Nanamori K, Nakamura E, Uchida K, Yamada H (2006) Percutaneous drainage and continuous irrigation in patients with severe pyogenic spondylitis, abscess formation and marked bone destruction. J Neurosurg Spine 4:374–379
121. Yu MY, Siu C, Wing PC, Schweigel IF, Jetha N (1991) Percutaneous suction aspiration for osteomyelitis: report of two cases. Spine (Phila Pa 1976) 16:198–202
122. Ito M, Sudo H, Abumi K, Kotani Y, Takahata M, Fujita M, Minami A (2009) Minimally invasive surgical treatment for tuberculous spondylodiscitis. Minim Invasive Neurosurg 52:250–253
123. Chacko AG, Moorthy RK, Chandy MJ (2004) The trans-pedicular approach in the management of thoracic spine tuberculosis: a short term follow up study. Spine (Phila Pa 1976) 29:E363–E567
124. Kapoor S, Kapoor S, Agrawal M, Aggarwal M, Jain BK Jr (2012) Thoracoscopic decompression in Pott's spine and its long-term follow-up. Int Orthop 36:331–337
125. Zong W, Xiong G, Wang B, Lu C, Dai Z, Lv G (2015) Surgical management for thoracic spinal tuberculosis posterior only versus anterior video- assisted thoracoscopic surgery. PLoS One 10:e0119759. doi:10.1371/journal.pone.0119759
126. Singh R, Gogna P, Parshad S, Karwasra RK, Karwasra PK, Kaur K (2014) Video-assisted thoracic surgery for tubercular spondylitis. Minim Invasive Surg 2014:963497–963498. doi:10.1155/2014/963497

127. Kossmann T, Jacobi D, Trentz O (2001) The use of a retractor system (SynFrame) for open, minimal invasive reconstruction of the anterior column of the thoracic and lumbar spine. Eur Spine J 10:396–402
128. Levin R, Matusz D, Hasharoni A, Scharf C, Lonner B, Errico T (2005) Mini-open thoracoscopically assisted thoracotomy versus video-assisted thoracoscopic surgery for anterior release in thoracic scoliosis and kyphosis: a comparison of operative and radiographic results. Spine J 5:632–638
129. Lee BH, Lee HM, Kim TH, Kim HS, Moon ES, Park JO, Chong HS, Moon SH (2012) Transpedicular curettage and drainage of infective lumbar spondylodiscitis: technique and clinical results. Clin Orthop Surg 4:200–208
130. Ringel F, Stoffel M, Stuer C, Meyer B (2006) Minimally invasive transmuscular pedicle screw fixation of the thoracic and lumbar spine. Neurosurgery 59:361–367
131. Lee JS, Moon KP, Kim SJ, Suh KT (2007) Posterior lumbar interbody fusion and posterior instrumentation in the surgical management of lumbar tuberculous spondylitis. J Bone Joint Surg Br 89:210–214
132. Panchmatia JR, Lenke LG, Molloy S, Cheung KM, Kebaish KM (2015) Review article: surgical approaches for correction of posttubercular kyphosis. J Orthop Surg (Hong Kong) 23:391–394
133. Klöckner C, Valencia R (2003) Sagittal alignment after anterior debridement and fusion with or without additional posterior instrumentation in the treatment of pyogenic and tuberculous spondylodiscitis. Spine (Phila Pa 1976) 28:1036–1042
134. Issack PS, Boachie-Adjej O (2012) Surgical correction of kyphotic deformity in spinal tuberculosis. Int Orthop 36:353–357
135. Lee SH, Sung JK, Park YM (2006) Single-stage transpedicular decompression and posterior instrumentation in treatment of thoracic and thoracolumbar spinal tuberculosis: a retrospective case series. J Spinal Disord Tech 19:595–602
136. Moon MS (2007) Tuberculosis of spine: contemporary thoughts on current issues and perspective views. Curr Orthop 21:364–379
137. Moon MS, Moon JL, Moon YW, Kim SS, Kim SS, Sun DH, Choi WT (2003) Pott's paraplegia in patients with severely deformed dorsal or dorsolumbar spines: treatment and prognosis. Spinal Cord 41:164–171
138. Yau AC, Hsu LC, O'Brien JP, Hodgson AR (1974) Tuberculous kyphosis: correction with spinal osteotomy, halo-pelvic distraction, and anterior and posterior fusion. J Bone Joint Surg Am 56:1419–1434
139. Wang Y, Zhang Y, Zhang X, Wang Z, Mao K, Chen C, Zheng G, Li G, Wood KB (2009) Posterior-only multilevel modified vertebral column resection for extremely severe Pott's kyphotic deformity. Eur Spine J 18:1436–1441
140. Wang Y, Zhang Y, Zhang X, Huang P, Xiao S, Wang Z, Liu Z, Liu B, Lu N, Mao K (2008) A single posterior approach for multilevel modified vertebral column resection in adults with severe rigid congenital kyphoscoliosis: a retrospective study of 13 cases. Eur Spine J 17:361–372
141. Moon MS, Kim SS, Moon YW, Moon H, Kim SS (2014) Surgery-related complications and sequelae in management of tuberculosis of spine. Asian Spine J 8:435–445
142. Sengupta DK, Grevitt MP, Mehdian SM (1999) Hypoglossal nerve injury as a complication of anterior surgery to the upper cervical spine. Eur Spine J 8:78–80
143. Yilmaz C, Selek HY, Gurkan I, Erdemli B, Korkusuz Z (1999) Anterior instrumentation for the treatment of spinal tuberculosis. J Bone Joint Surg Am 81:1261–1267
144. Cheung KM, Al Ghazi S (2008) Approach-related complications of open versus thoracoscopic anterior exposures of the thoracic spine. J Orthop Surg (Hong Kong) 16:343–347
145. Moon MS, Ha KY, Sun DH, Moon JL, Moon YW, Chung JH (1996) Pott's Paraplegia: 67 cases. Clin Orthop Relat Res 323:122–128
146. Moon MS (1997) Tuberculosis of the spine Controversies and a new challenge. Spine (Phila Pa 1976) 22:1791–1797
147. Moon MS, Kim SS, Lee BJ, Moon JL, Moon YW (2011) Surgical management of severe rigid tuberculous kyphosis of dorsolumbar spine. Int Orthop 35:75–81
148. Rajasekaran S, Vijay K, Shetty AP (2010) Single-stage closing-opening wedge osteotomy of spine to correct severe post-tubercular kyphotic deformities of the spine: a 3-year follow-up of 17 patients. Eur Spine J 19:583–592

Video-Assisted Thoracic Surgery for Tubercular Spondylitis

21

Roop Singh

Contents

R. Singh, MD
Department of Orthopaedics, Organization/University, Pt. B.D. Sharma Postgraduate Institute of Medical Sciences, Rohtak 124001, Haryana, India
e-mail: drroopsingh@rediffmail.com; drroopsingh08@gmail.com

Abbreviations

(D4-D9)	Dorsal 4th–9th vertebrae
ICS	Intercostal space
MRI	Magnetic resonance imaging
TB	Tuberculosis
TS	Tubercular spondylitis
VATS	Video-assisted thoracic surgery

21.1 Introduction

Tuberculosis (TB) is the most common infectious disease worldwide [1], with the spine being one of the most common sites of extrapulmonary involvement. Although anti-TB chemotherapy is the mainstay of treatment for spinal TB [2], it may not be applicable to all patients such as those with worsening neurological deficit, where surgery would be required in addition [3]. The standard surgical method of decompression of TB dorsal spine is either the anterolateral extrapleural or open transthoracic transpleural approach. The application of thoracoscopy to treat spinal lesions is a relatively recent development [4–11]. This chapter elaborates its use in tubercular spondylitis (TS), viz., indications, contraindications, surgical technique, and complications. At the end of the chapter, there is a thorough presentation of the current relevant literature of video-assisted thoracic surgery (VATS) in TS.

M. Turgut et al. (eds.), *Tuberculosis of the Central Nervous System*,
DOI 10.1007/978-3-319-50712-5_21

21.2 VATS for Tubercular Spondylitis

The thoracic spine is most often involved spinal area in TS, followed by lumbar and cervical spine [12, 13]. Neurological involvement is highest in the patients who have the mid-thoracic spinal TB involvement. It is thought due to highest cord/canal ratio, and precarious blood supply in dorsal spine (D_4–D_9) spinal cord is at risk in this region. Good outcome in spinal TB is observed with anti-TB drug treatment, alone or in combination with surgical decompression. Absolute indications for surgery in patients with spinal TB under active treatment are approximately 6% in those without neurological deficit and approximately 60% in those with neurological deficit [14]. VATS has been used in various spinal procedures with the most frequently reported applications being in the management of rigid scoliosis releases or thoracic disc herniations [15–17]. Now, VATS is being used in active TB of dorsal spine in many centers [5, 6, 8, 9, 11].

21.2.1 History

Thoracic cavity was inspected endoscopically for the first time by Bozzini in 1806 [18]. Jacobaeus from Stockholm, Sweden, was credited to perform thoracoscopic procedures in human beings for the first time. He introduced in 1910 the use of thoracoscopy in the diagnosis and management of pulmonary TB [19–21]. Open surgical procedures replaced thoracoscopy from the 1950s until the 1980s [19]. In 1991, Lewis popularized VATS for pulmonary diseases. The first description of VATS for thoracic spinal diseases was published by Mack and others in 1993 [15, 17, 22–24].

Reagan et al. successfully used endoscopic techniques to perform interbody grafting and, more recently, instrumentation in diverse thoracic spinal pathology, including deformity and degenerative disease [22, 23, 25]. Rosenthal et al. reported the use of VATS for ventral decompression and stabilization in patients with metastatic tumors of the thoracic spine [26]. Huang et al. in 2000 published first report of the use of VATS in TS. They also introduced the concept of extended manipulating channel method [5]. Later on more authors reported their experience with VATS in TS [5, 6, 8, 9, 11]. Thoracoscopy has emerged as a safe surgical technique with a wide field of application.

21.2.2 Indications and Contraindications

Indications Clinically, TB of the spine can mimic other infections or tumorous (either primary or metastatic) conditions. It continues to be a scourge in the developing world, contributing to spinal deformity and neurological deficit. TB pathology, such as inflammatory focus, debris, and caseation, compresses the spinal cord from the anterior aspect. Therefore, it is better to approach the spinal cord anteriorly to decompress it from this anterior pathology. Anterolateral decompression and transthoracic anterior decompression have been the two favored approaches. VATS can be a valuable alternative to those conventional approaches. VATS can be employed for biopsy, debridement, decompression, and reconstruction in TS.

Contraindications VATS is contraindicated in TS in the following situations:

- Significant morbid cardiopulmonary condition with limited cardiopulmonary reserve and other contraindications for single-lung anesthesia.
- Expected difficulty in visualization and manipulation of instruments through a scarred chest cavity especially in patients with pleural symphysis, failed prior open ventral surgery, or bullous lung pathology.
- Significant hemostatic disturbances.
- Relative contraindications include empyema, previous thoracotomy, or previous tube thoracostomy.

21.2.3 Preoperative Evaluation

Important information on the anatomical as well as the patho-anatomical structure; three dimensional position of the spine, including malpositioning; and

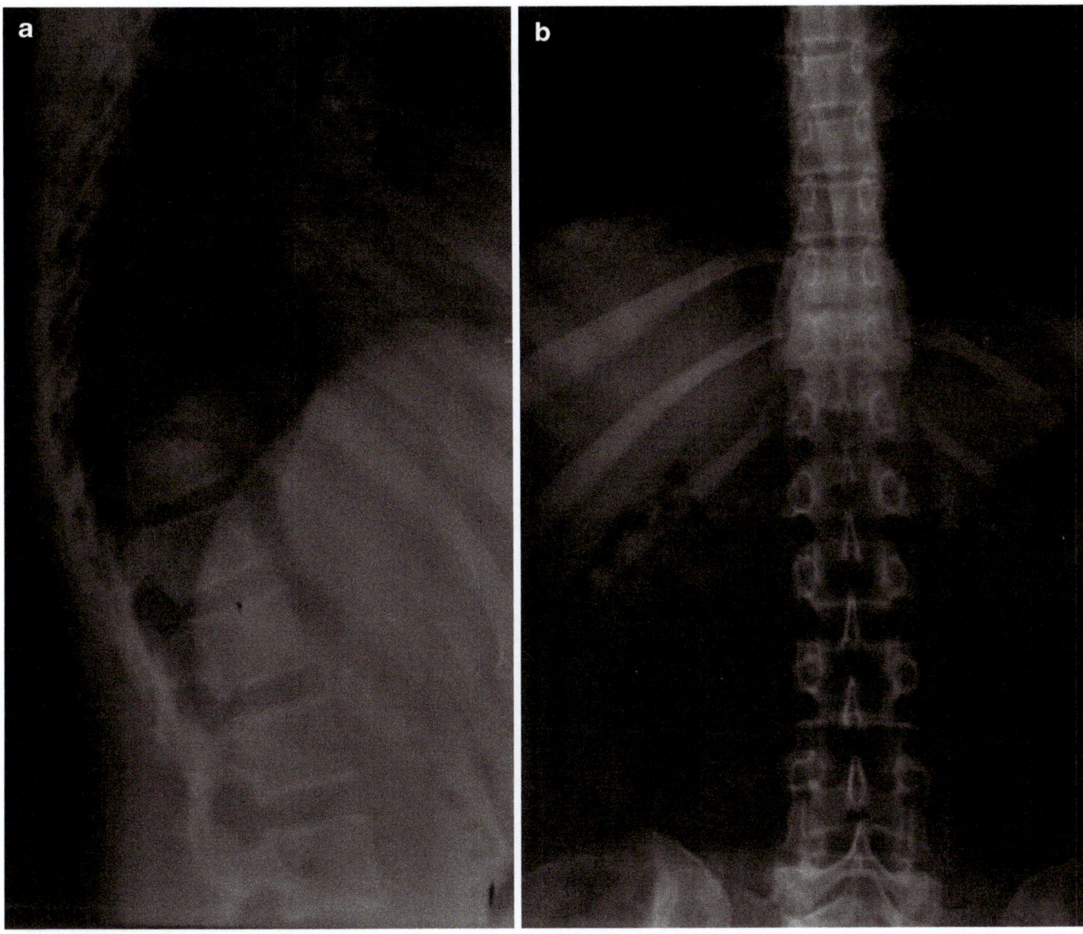

Fig. 21.1 Preoperative radiographs lateral (**a**) and anteroposterior (**b**) are essential in preoperative planning as these can depict any deviation in the curvature of the spine and configuration of the vertebral bodies

the topographical anatomy of the diseased area require well-planned preoperative imaging (Fig. 21.1). Assessment of the curvature of the spine and configuration of the vertebral bodies requires standard spinal x-rays (AP and lateral) [27]. It is also desirous to include magnetic resonance imaging (MRI) in preoperative planning, as it better delineates paraspinal soft tissues, the neural structures including the situation within the spinal cord, as well as the localization and course of the greater vessels in relation to spine (Fig. 21.2) [27].

Posteroanterior and lateral chest radiographs are required to evaluate any associated pathology, viz., pleural fluid, fibrinous membranes, or adhesions in the pleural space. Electrocardiogram is used to exclude any recent myocardial infarction or significant arrhythmia. In addition, laboratory investigations including the coagulation parameters, serum electrolytes, blood group typing, and platelet count should be carried out preoperatively [4].

21.2.4 Anesthetic Considerations

General anesthesia using a double-lumen endotracheal tube is given to the patient to achieve single-lung ventilation for maximal surgical exposure during thoracoscopy (Fig. 21.3). Single-lumen tube with an endotracheal block is an alternative to difficult double-lumen endotracheal intubation. The correct position of the endotracheal tube is confirmed with a bronchoscope before and after final positioning [5, 28].

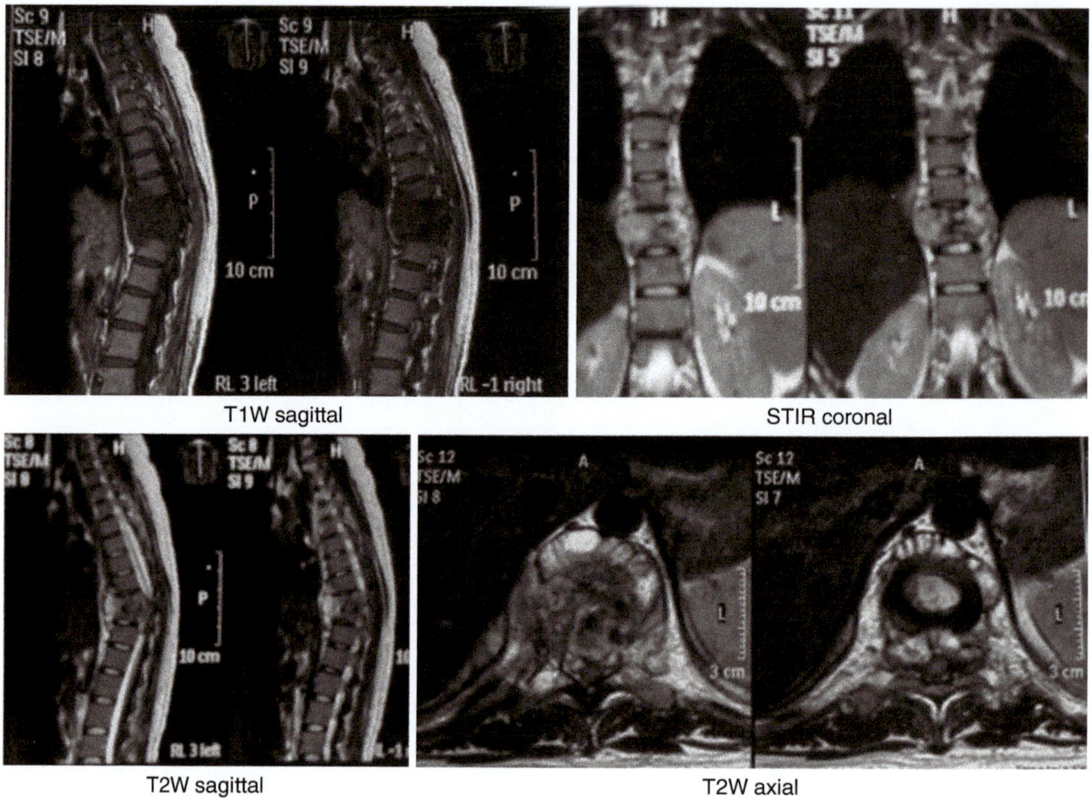

Fig. 21.2 MRI showing body destruction, paravertebral abscesses, spinal cord condition, and location of great vessels

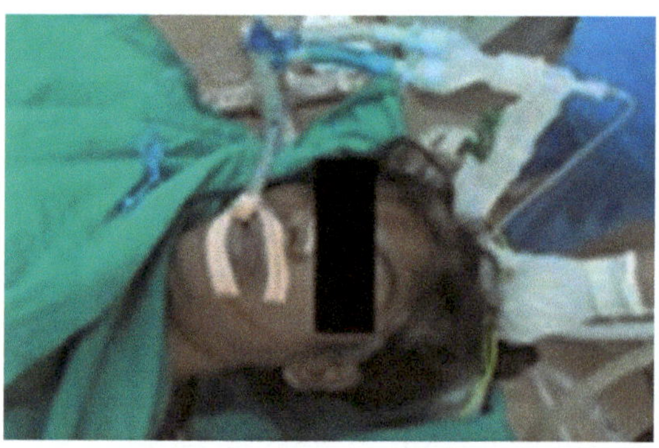

Fig. 21.3 Shows use of double-lumen endotracheal tube for general anesthesia purpose. It helps in achieving single-lung ventilation and maximal surgical exposure

Hypotensive anesthesia should be avoided in myelopathic patients or in those undergoing segmental artery sacrifices [2, 12]. In addition, a Foley catheter and arterial and central venous lines are placed.

21.2.5 Positioning

Lateral decubitus position of the patient is obtained by securing the patient on a radiolucent operation table with legs flexed slightly and an axillary roll placed under the axilla. Right/left lateral decubitus position during surgery is decided depending on the radiologic findings (i.e., bulk of abscess and caseating tissue and destruction of the body). Cleaning and draping is done as for a standard posterolateral thoracotomy (for conversion to standard thoracotomy in circumstance of intraoperative complications or the presence of severe pleural adhesion).

Prone positioning may be used during a simultaneous anterior-posterior approach [25, 29]. Simultaneous surgical exposures eliminate the need to stage the procedure, along with the added time and costs for repositioning, redraping, and a new operating room setup [28].

21.2.6 Thoracoscopic Access and Exposure

The correct placement of the portals is of particular importance. With selective collapse of right/left lung, the initial trocar incision (2 cm) is usually made at the fifth or sixth intercostal space (ICS) or higher along the anterior axillary line depending upon the site of lesion [9, 27]. The first portal site is opened using a blunt dissection technique to minimize possible injury to the lung. The subcutaneous tissues and intercostal muscles are dissected bluntly without removing any rib, which minimizes local trauma. The pleural space is the exposed and palpation is used to detect any pleural adhesions. There may be a higher rate of pleurodesis secondary to inflammation, requiring either meticulous thoracoscopic release of adhesions (Fig. 21.4) or conversion to an open procedure (Fig. 21.5). The parietal pleura is opened under direct visualization to ensure proper lung deflation. Once this structure is deflated securely, the first trocar (11 mm) is used to introduce the operating thoracoscope, and the exploratory thoracoscopy is performed (Fig. 21.6). The lesion site is identified and displayed on the video monitor. Two other stab incisions, the extended manipulating channel, usually 3–4 cm in length, are done 2–3 ICS above and below the first port, slightly posterior to the posterior axillary line (Fig. 21.7). The correct placement of these portals is of utmost importance to ensure the correct working direction and avoid loss of orientation.

Visualization of the spine can be enhanced by tilting the patient forward so that the lungs fall

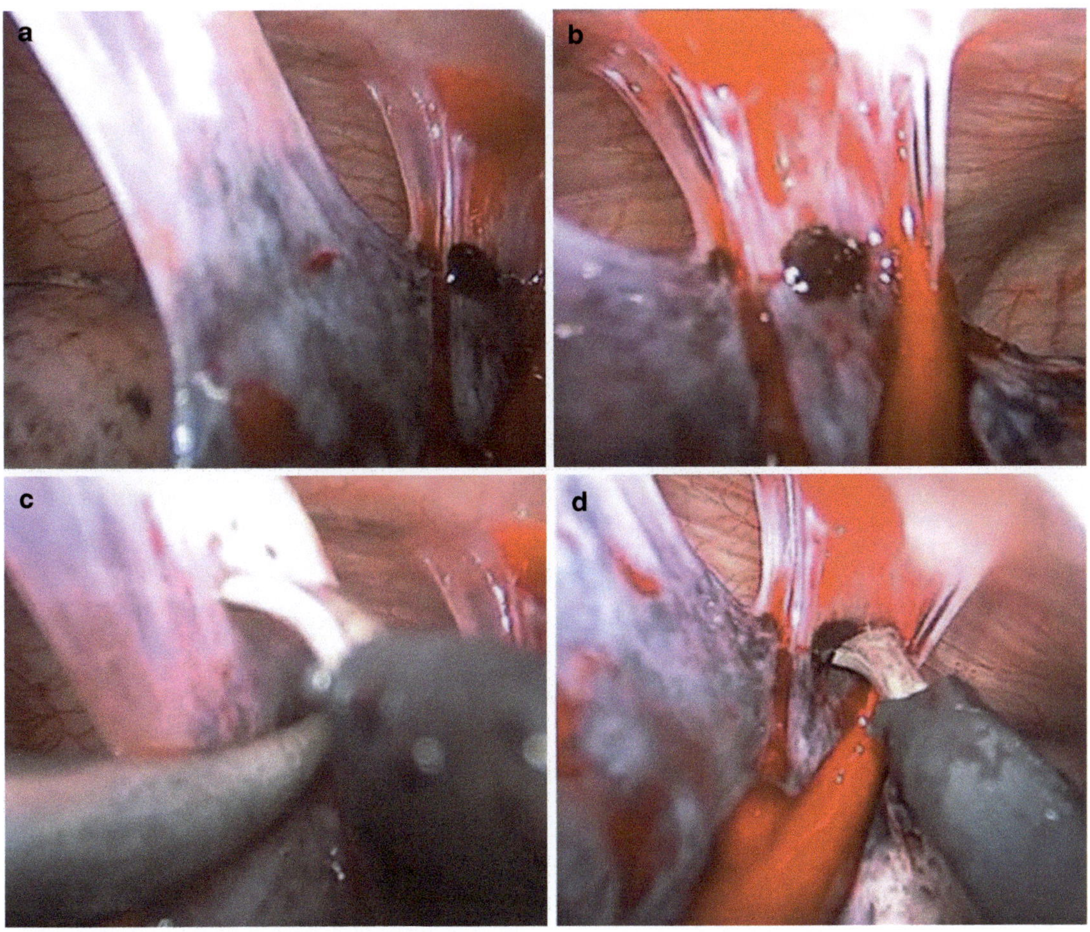

Fig. 21.4 Shows lung adhesions (**a**, **b**) being separated with thoracoscopic release of adhesions (**c**, **d**)

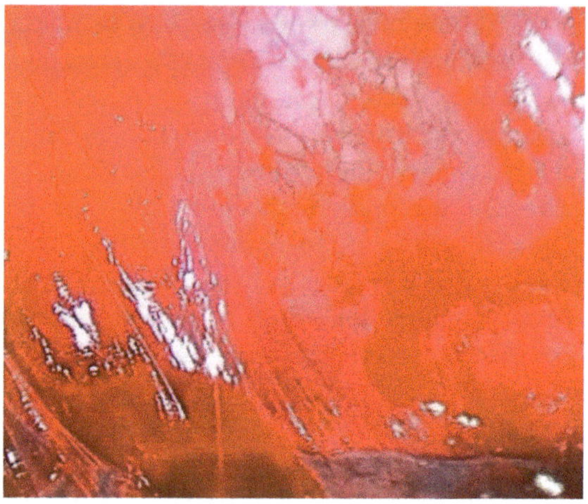

Fig. 21.5 Shows extensive lung adhesions and the patient-required mini-thoracotomy for adhesiolysis

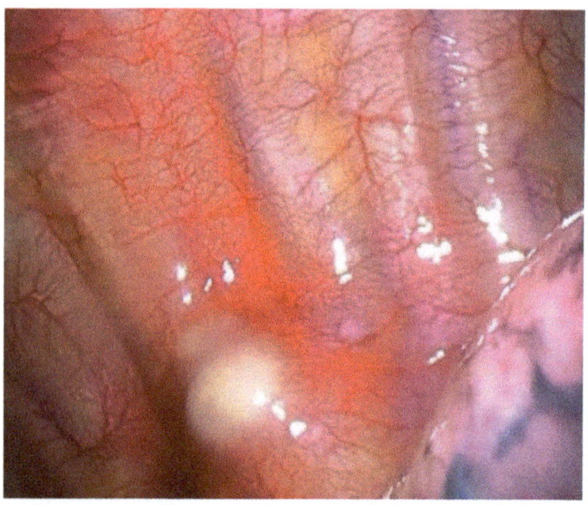

Fig. 21.6 Shows view of exploratory thoracoscopy localizing site of lesion (pus pointing underneath the pleura)

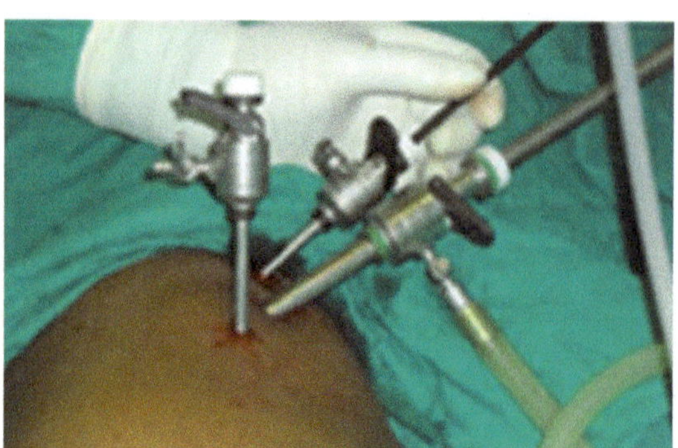

Fig. 21.7 Shows classical three portals for the VATS

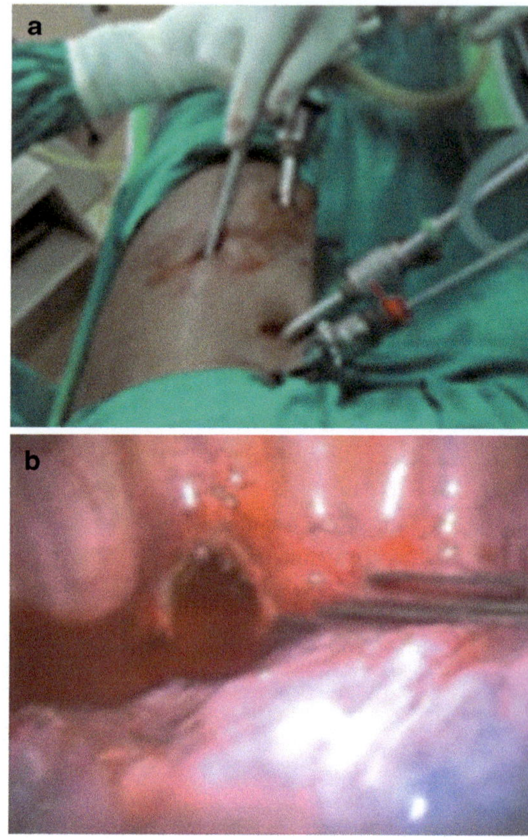

Fig. 21.8 Shows additional portal (**a**) being used for the fan retractor to retract the lung (**b**)

anteriorly and, if required, a fan retractor for further retraction of ipsilateral lung is inserted (Fig. 21.8) [8]. Brief insufflations of carbon dioxide at a pressure of 8 cm H_2O can be used if descriptive atelectasis of the ipsilateral lung is found incomplete.

21.2.7 Debridement, Decompression, Reconstruction, and Fusion

The correct level of diseased vertebrae is determined by counting the ribs as seen through the endoscope. Putting a spinal needle from the preoperative marker site and visualizing the tip of needle through the thoracoscope further confirm the correct level. With monopolar electrocautery accompanied by a suction tube the parietal pleura overlying the rib head is incised. Alternatively, the

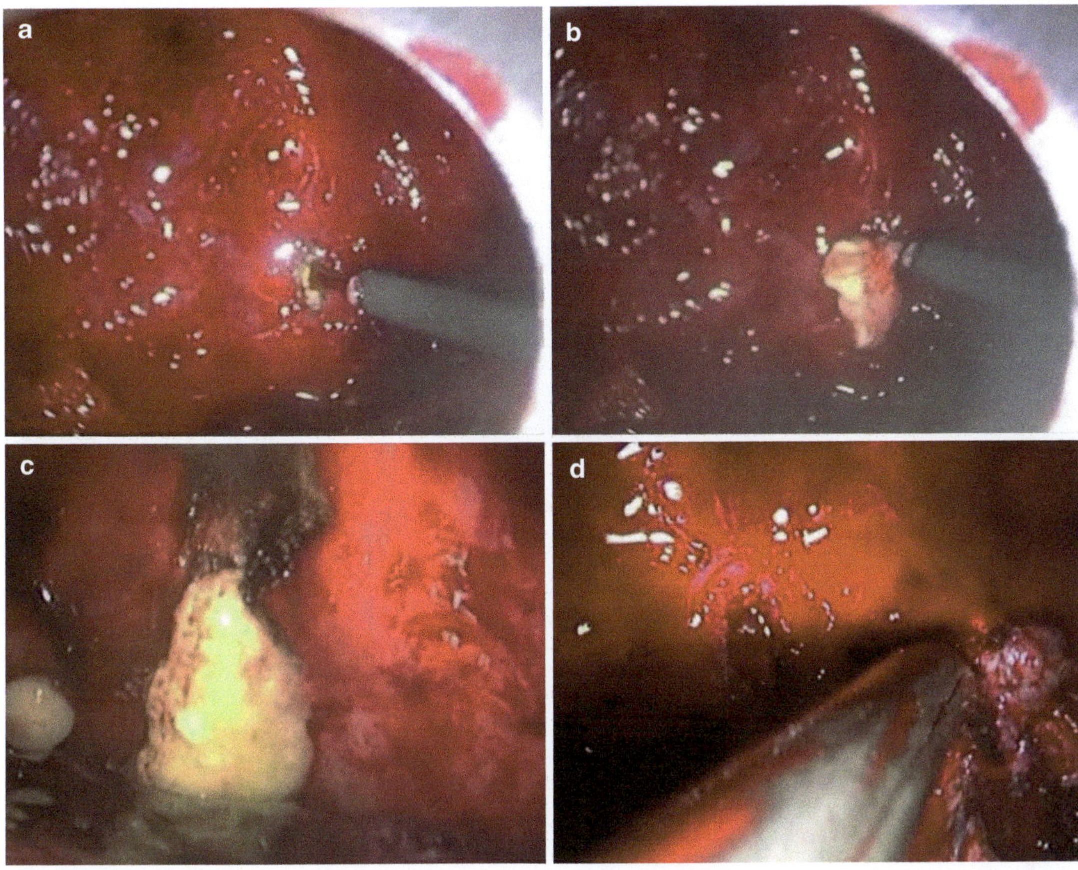

Fig. 21.9 Shows pleura over the lesion being divided (**a**, **b**) using electrocautery. Pus is drained (**c**) and granulation tissue is removed (**d**)

harmonic scalpel can dissect with less smoke and char. Avoid monopolar cautery at inferior margin of the rib where intercostal nerve may be injured. The degree of pleural dissection depends on the extent of the intended surgery but may include longitudinal approaches parallel to the spine or transverse approaches parallel to each disc space [28]. Pleura over the lesion is divided longitudinally/transversely; pus is drained and granulation tissue is removed (Fig. 21.9). Suction should be available before incising the pleura to suck the pus immediately to avoid contamination. A thorough debridement is performed to remove necrotic disc, sequestra, infected granulation tissue, and caseous material under direct vision through the thoracoscope (Fig. 21.10). The working portals are enlarged to be used as extended manipulating channels, facilitating the used conventional instruments (Fig. 21.11). Of late, various manufacturers now also offer sets of instruments for soft tissue and bone preparation. These instruments are ergonomically designed for good control and handling with depth scale on the sides of each instruments. The decompression is considered complete only when dura is exposed in the involved segment and appears to be devoid of compression. Epidural granulation tissue can be adherent to the dura mater and surrounding tissues, requiring careful dissection.

Essentially the steps of biopsy, decompression, discectomy, and reconstruction are same as with open procedures.

The specimen is obtained for Ziehl-Neelsen staining, gram staining, and culture for TB and pyogenic organisms. The paravertebral incision is extended by a smaller horizontal incision, parallel to the ribs and starting from the center of the longitudinal incision in a T-shaped manner [8]. The larger intercostal arteries and veins

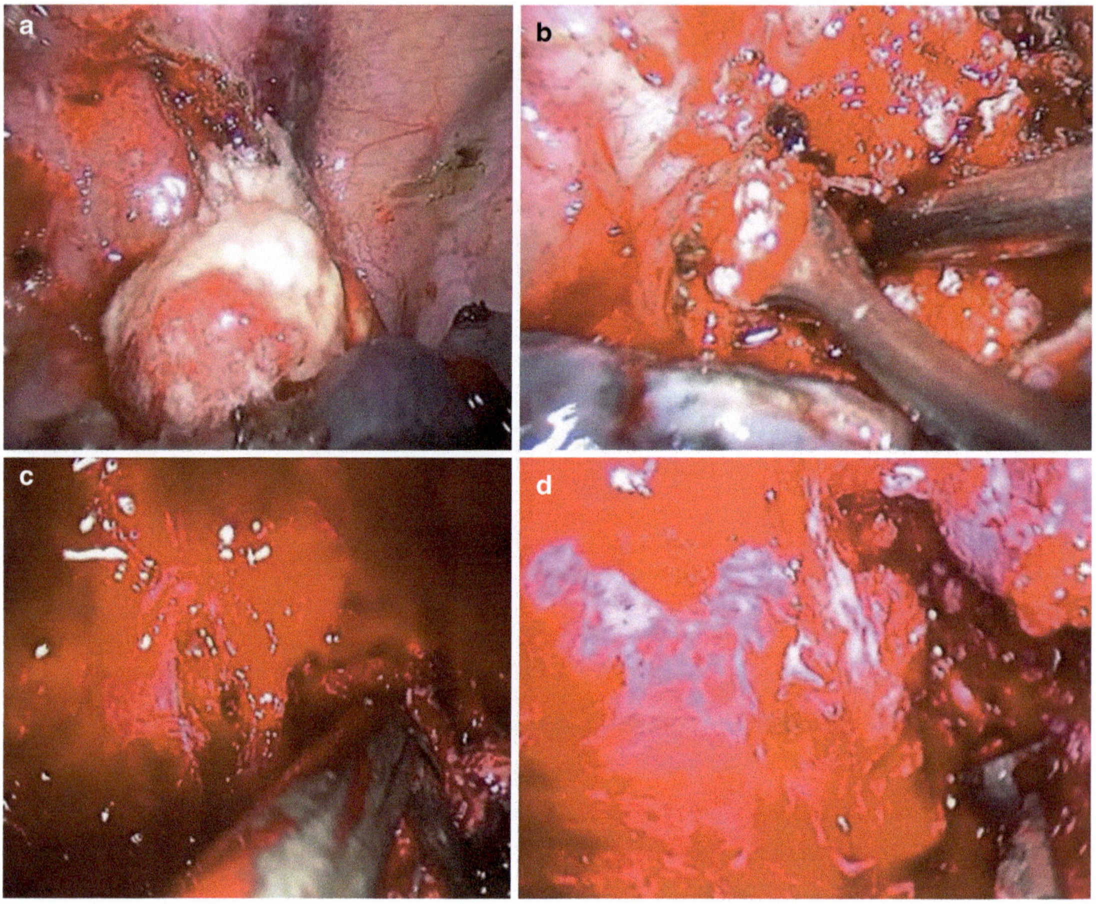

Fig. 21.10 Shows thorough debridement is being performed to remove caseous material (**a**), infected granulation tissue (**b**), necrotic disc (**c**), and sequestra (**d**) under direct vision through the thoracoscope

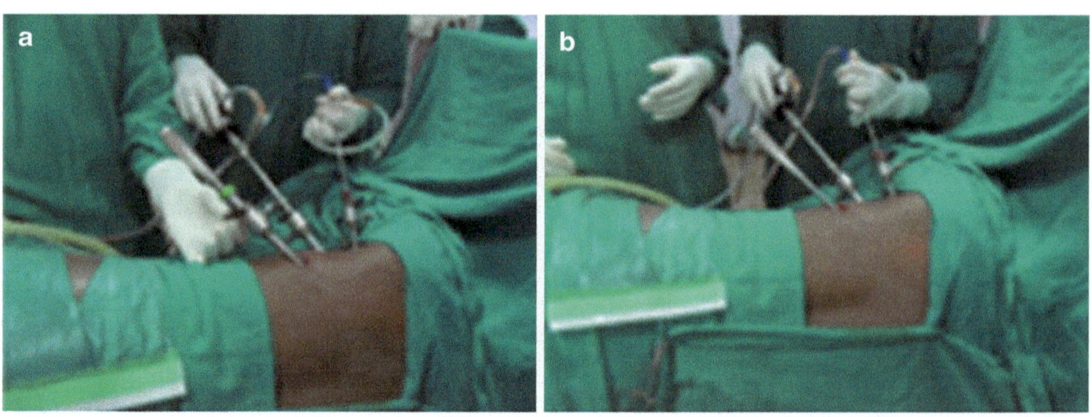

Fig. 21.11 Shows conventional long curette being used through thoracoscopic port (**a**) and through extended manipulation channel (**b**)

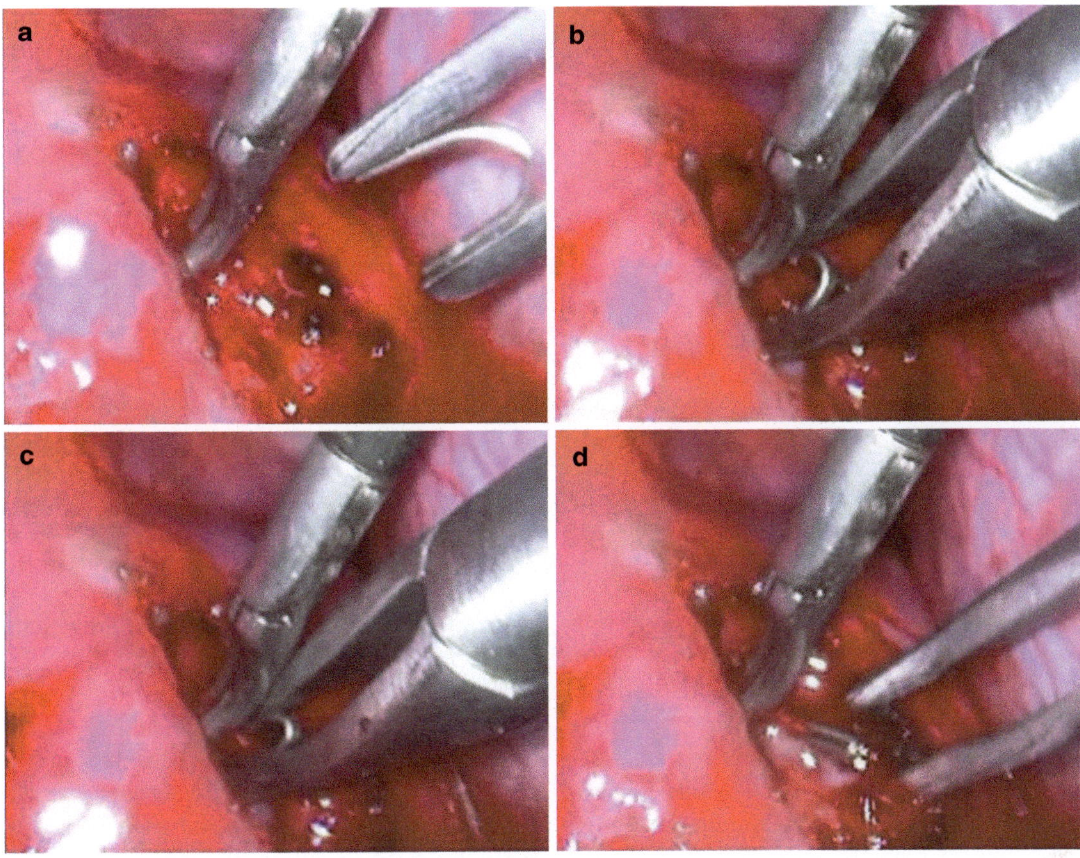

Fig. 21.12 Shows segmental vessel being isolated (**a**) and ligated using ligaclips (**b–d**)

are isolated, ligated, and divided if needed (Fig. 21.12). The remainder of the surgery is conducted from beneath the incised pleural that, along with the anterior longitudinal ligament, had been distal from the vertebral body by abscess and granulation tissue. This precaution ensures that the important structures, i.e., artery, inferior vena cava, azygos vein, sympathetic trunk, and thoracic duct, are not damaged.

Reconstruction of anterior column depends on the extent of bone defect. Small defects can be reconstructed using rib grafts or tricortical iliac crest grafts (Fig. 21.13). Anterior rib grafts are harvested by subcutaneous dissection of the rib through portal incision. Larger anterior defects can be filled with titanium mesh cages. These can be stabilized with anterior instrumentation with screw-rod construct. The portal for screw insertion is made carefully, with C-arm guidance using strict lateral views, and an attempt should be made to make the working portals exactly coaxial with the tributary of the planned screws. Sometimes open posterior instrumentation using a pedicle screw-rod construct can be completed first, and in the same setting, thoracoscopic-assisted anterior debridement and anterior column reconstruction can be done.

After irrigating the thoracic cavity and removal of blood clots, hemostasis is achieved. Chest tube drain of appropriate size is inserted through one of the port sites in the 7th or 8th ICS in midaxillary line and is connected to underwater seal. The small wounds are closed.

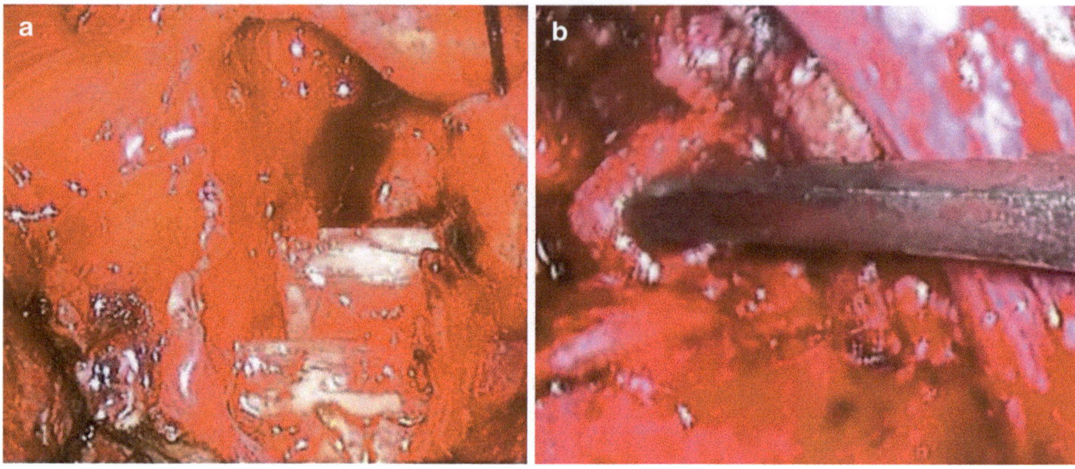

Fig. 21.13 Shows anterior column reconstruction after thorough debridement with rib (**a**) and tricortical iliac bone crest graft (**b**)

21.2.8 Postoperative Care

Patient is monitored closely for heart rate, arterial pressure, respiratory rate, oxygen saturation, blood loss (in water seal bag), and any respiratory complication. Postoperative plain chest radiograph is taken to check adequate lung inflation. Chest tube is removed once collection in the chest tube bag is <50–100 mL in the last 24 h. With radiological evidence of complete lung inflation, postoperative chest physiotherapy with incentive spirometer is started in the first day to allow early lung expansion and minimize atelectasis [8, 19].

Antitubercular drugs are continued and patient mobilized with brace depending on the individual patient's situation.

21.3 Advantages and Disadvantages of VATS

VATS confers many proven potential advantages to both the surgeon and patient, including improved visualization through magnification and lighting, decreased perioperative morbidity, and shorter hospital stay. In addition, thoracoscopic surgery provides small thin incisions without the need for rib resection or retraction. This procedure offers reduction in pain, better cosmetic effect, lower perioperative morbidity, and earlier return to normal activities [5, 6, 9, 10, 28, 29].

The most significant disadvantage of VATS procedure is an extremely steep learning curve for proper thoracoscopic surgery technique, such as establishing proper operative orientation and performing the operation through small portals with long surgical instruments at longer distances from the target area [6, 10, 28].

21.4 Results and Complications Relevant to VATS in Tubercular Spondylitis

Very few studies have been reported about the role of VATS in TS in the literature. Authors of other studies have shared their experience, results, and complications about VATS [6, 11, 12, 26, 27].

In 2000, Huang et al. reported first study of VATS in TS in ten cases. At the mean follow-up of 24 months, four patients had an excellent result, five had a good result, one had a poor result, and one had a fair result [5]. The average neurological recovery was 1.1 grades on Frankel's grade. Postoperative complications included one-lung atelectasis. Pleural adhesions, owing to local inflammation or paravertebral abscess, were seen in four patients, in one patient with severe pleural diagnosis who needed an open technique for treatment. Postoperative air leaks were seen in 40% of the cases but all were transient. They concluded that VATS has diagnostic and therapeutic role in the management of TB [5].

In 2005, Kapoor et al. reported a prospective, observational study in 16 patients with middorsal TS with paraplegia/paraparesis [8]. Eighty-eight percent of patients had good neurological recovery. In one patient, thoracoscopy was abandoned, and open thoracotomy was performed because of persistent bleeding; in one patient anterolateral decompression was performed 10 weeks after thoracoscopy due to non-recovery; and in patient there was a rib fracture. They concluded that video-assisted thoracoscopic decompression of TB dorsal spondylitis was a viable option to achieve significant neurological recovery with less morbidity, blood requirement, and hospital stay compared to the open thoracotomy procedures [8].

In 2007, Jayaswal et al. reported a retrospective review of 23 patients with single-level thoracic spinal TB (T4-T11) treated with VATS [6]. Twenty two of 23 patients achieved flexion with no recurrence. Complications occurred in seven patients and one patient had superficial wound infection. Two had prolonged intercostal drainage tube in situ for 5 days due to persistent air leak. Conversion to open thoracotomy was undertaken in three patients; the cause was extensive pleural adhesion in two patients and uncontrolled bleeding in one patient. Pneumonitis occurred in one patient [6].

In 2012, Kapoor et al. reported long-term follow-up results of VATS-consisted treatment of dorsal spinal TB in 30 patients [9]. All patients had neurological improvement and one return of ambulatory power. Ninety-six percent of patients achieved an excellent or good subjective outcome. There were ten complications including two cases of superficial wound infection, six with pulmonary complications, and one with postoperative air leak [9].

The author of the present chapter reported VATS for TS in a patient in 2014. At the time of final follow-up, fusion was achieved in all patients, the VAS score for back pain improved from a pretreatment 8.3–2, and the functional assessment yielded excellent ($n = 4$) to good ($n = 5$) results. In two patients mini-thoracotomy had to be reported due to extensive pleural adhesions ($n = 1$) or difficulty in placement of graft ($n = 1$) [11].

In addition to these complications in TS, general intraoperative complications of VATS, viz., risk of injury to the aorta or vena cava, spinal cord or nerve root, dural tear, etc., are always there. Postoperative complications like intrathoracic bleeding, lung atelectasis, pneumothorax, and splenic injury should always be kept in mind.

Conclusion

- Among the infectious diseases, TB is the most prevalent disease worldwide. The spine is one of the most common sites of extrapulmonary TB.
- Anti-TB drugs are the mainstay of treatment in spinal TB. In patients with worsening neurological deficit alone, it may not be sufficient.
- Anterolateral extrapleural and open transthoracic transpleural are the standard surgical procedures used to decompress dorsal spine in TB. Significant morbidity and mortality is associated with these open approaches.
- VATS is a relatively recent development in the treatment of TS and can be a valuable alternative to conventional approaches.
- VATS can be employed for biopsy, debridement, cord decompression, and reconstruction in TS.
- VATS is contraindicated in significant cardiopulmonary disease of associated contraindication for single lung disease, scarred chest cavity, and failed prior open ventral surgery.
- VATS requires a proper preoperative evaluation and planning to prevent complications and for a better surgical outcome.
- VATS is a safe and effective procedure in the management of spinal TB. Inherent advantages of VATS are decreased blood loss and minimum postoperative morbidity and complications.

References

1. World Health Organization (2008) Global tuberculosis control: surveillance, planning, financing. Publication no. WHO/HTM/TB/ 2008.393. World Health Organization, Geneva
2. Tuli SM (1975) Results of treatment of spinal tuberculosis by "middle-path" regime. J Bone Joint Surg Br 57B:13–23
3. Rajasekaran S, Soundarapandian S (1989) Progression of kyphosis in tuberculosis of spine treated by anterior arthrodesis. J Bone Joint Surg Am 71:1314–1323
4. Amini A, Beisse R, Schmidt MH (2005) Thoracoscopic spine surgery for decompression and stabilization of the anterolateral thoracolumbar spine. Neurosurg Focus 19:E4
5. Huang TJ, Hsu RW, Chen SH, Liu HP (2000) Video-assisted thoracoscopic surgery in managing tuberculous spondylitis. Clin Orthop Relat Res 379: 143–153
6. Jayaswal A, Upendra B, Ahmed A, Chowdhury B, Kumar A (2007) Video-assisted thoracoscopic anterior surgery for tuberculous spondylitis. Clin Orthop Relat Res 460:100–107
7. Kandwal P, Garg B, Upendra BN, Chowdhury B, Jayaswal A (2012) Outcome of minimally invasive surgery in the management of tuberculous spondylitis. Indian J Orthop 46:159–164
8. Kapoor SK, Agarwal PN, Jain BK Jr, Kumar R (2005) Videoassisted thoracoscopic decompression of tubercular spondylitis: clinical evaluation. Spine (Phila Pa 1976) 30:E605–E610
9. Kapoor SK, Kapoor S, Agarwal M, Agarwal P, Jain BK Jr (2012) Thoracoscopic decompression in Pott's spine and its long-term follow-up. Int Orthop 36:3331–3337
10. Kim SJ, Sohn MJ, Ryoo JY, Kim YS, Whang CJ (2007) Clinical analysis of video-assisted thoracoscopic surgery in the thoracic or thoracolumbar spinal pathologies. J Korean Neurosurg Soc 42:293–297
11. Singh R, Gogna P, Parsad S, Karwasra RK, Karwasra PK, Kaur K (2014) Video-assisted thoracic surgery for tubercular spondylitis. Minim Invasive Surg. Article ID 963497, 8 pages. http://dx.doi.org/10.1155/2014/963497
12. Hodgson AR, Stock FE (1960) Anterior spinal fusion for the treatment of tuberculosis of the spine. The operative findings and results of treatment in the first one hundred cases. J Bone Joint Surg Am 42A:295–310
13. Lifeso RM, Weaver P, Harder EH (1985) Tuberculous spondylitis in adults. J Bone Joint Surg Am 67A:1405–1413
14. Bakalim G (1960) Tuberculosis spondylitis a clinical study with special reference to the significance of spinal fusion and chemotherapy. Acta Orthop Scand (Suppl)47: 1-111
15. Mack MJ, Regan JJ, Bobechko WP, Acuff TE (1993) Application of thoracoscopy for diseases of the spine. Ann Thorac Surg 56:736–738
16. McAfee PC, Regan JJ, Zdeblick T (1995) The incidence of complications in endoscopic anterior thoracolumbar spinal reconstructive surgery: a prospective multicentre study comprising the first 100 consecutive cases. Spine 14:1624–1632
17. Regan JJ, Mack MJ, Picetti GD (1995) A technical report on video-assisted thoracoscopy in thoracic spinal surgery—preliminary description. Spine 20:831–837
18. Bloomberg AE (1978) Collective reviews: thoracoscopy in perspective. Surg Gynecol Obstet 147:433–443
19. Dickman CA, Rosenthal DJ, Perin NI (1999) Thoracoscopic spine surgery, 1st edn. Thieme-Verlag, New York
20. Jacobaeus HC (1910) Possibility of the use of cystoscope for investigations of serous cavities. Munch Med Wochenschr 57:2090–2092
21. Jacobaeus HC (1921) The practical importance of thoracoscopy on surgery of the chest. Surg Gynecol Obstet 32:493–500
22. Regan JJ, Guyer RD (1997) Endoscopic technique in spinal surgery. Clin Orthop 225:122–139
23. Regan JJ, Ben-Yishay A, Mack MJ (1998) Video-assisted thoracoscopic excision of herniated thoracic disc. Description of technique and preliminary experience in first 29 cases. J Spinal Disord 11(13):183–191
24. Rosenthal D, Rosenthal R, de Simone A (1994) Removal of a protruded thoracic disc using microsurgical endoscopy. A new technique. Spine 19:1087–1091
25. Regan JJ, Mack MJ (1995) Endoscopic approach strategies. In: Regan JJ, McAffee PJ, Mack MJ (eds) Atlas of endoscopic spine surgery, 1st edn. Quality Medical Publishing, St. Louis, pp 117–136
26. Rosenthal D, Marquardt G, Lorenz et al (1996) Anterior decompression and stabilization using a microsurgical endoscopic technique for metastatic tumours of the thoracic spine. J Neurosurg 84:565B–572B
27. Heider F, Beisse R (2012) Anterior thoracoscopic approaches, including fracture treatment. In: Hartl R, Korge A (eds) Minimally invasive spine surgery- technique, evidence, and controversies. Thieme Verlag, New York, pp 191–207
28. Lieberman IH, McLain RF, Truumees E, Brebach GT (2004) Positioning and approaches to the thoracolumbar spine. Endoscopic and minimally invasive approaches. In: Frymore JW, Weisel SW (eds) The adult and pediatric spine, 3rd edn. Lippincott Williams & Wilkins, Philadelphia, pp 1061–1080
29. Lieberman IH, Salo PT, Orr RD, Brenda K (2000) Prone position endoscopic transthoracic release with simultaneous posterior instrumentation for spinal deformity: a description of technique. Spine 25:2251–2257

Part IV

Tuberculosis of the Cranial and Peripheral Nerves

Optochiasmatic Tuberculosis

22

Neeraj Kumar, Ravindra K. Garg, and Hardeep Singh Malhotra

Contents

N. Kumar, MD, DM (✉) • R.K. Garg, MD, DM
H.S. Malhotra, MD, DM
Department of Neurology, King George's Medical University, Lucknow, UP, India
e-mail: drneeraj2903@gmail.com; garg50@yahoo.com; drhsmalhotra@yahoo.com

Abbreviations

CNS	Central nervous system
CSF	Cerebrospinal fluid
CT	Computed tomography
EMB	Ethambutol
IL	Interleukin
INH	Isoniazid
MMP	Matrix metalloproteinases
OCA	Optochiasmatic arachnoiditis
OCT	Optochiasmatic tuberculoma
PAS	Para-aminosalicylic sodium
PCEG	Pneumocisterno-encephalography
PL	Perception of light
RIF	Rifampicin
RIHSA	Radioactive human serum albumin
STR	Streptomycin
TB	Tuberculosis
TBM	Tuberculous meningitis
TNF	Tumor necrosis factor
WHO	World Health Organization

22.1 Introduction

Tuberculous meningitis (TBM) is a serious form of extrapulmonary TB. Recently in 2015, the World Health Organization (WHO) released the 20th edition of its global TB report. In 2014, 9.6 million people were estimated to have TB, but only six million new cases were reported to WHO. The death due to TB was 1.5 million

M. Turgut et al. (eds.), *Tuberculosis of the Central Nervous System*,
DOI 10.1007/978-3-319-50712-5_22

people during the same year. In a major shift, the earlier Stop TB Strategy is being changed to the End TB Strategy from 2016 onwards [1].

TBM presents with various manifestations and complications. Cranial nerve involvement is common, including frequent affection of vision. Optochiasmatic TB can present either as optochiasmatic arachnoiditis (OCA) or optochiasmatic tuberculoma (OCT). Optochiasmatic TB is a dreaded complication of TBM and requires meticulous work-up and treatment. In 1929, Balado et al. gave the first detailed description of OCA in a case with visual deterioration [2]. The surgical intervention and release of adhesions around optochiasmatic region lead to excellent visual recovery, and later on the disease was named as "syndrome of Balado" [3]. Soon many such cases with good surgical results were published [4, 5]. In 1951, Yuhl et al. reported the first case of proven TB OCA. Though the visual loss improved markedly after surgery the patient succumbed due to disseminated disease status [6]. Both surgical and medical treatment has been reported with good prognosis. A review of all the reported cases of optochiasmatic TB in the literature till date has been summarized in Table 22.1.

22.2 Anatomy of Optochiasmatic Region

Anatomy of optochiasmatic region is very complex. Involvement in TB OCA due to basal exudates is not confined to chiasmatic region only. Cisterns are the subarachnoid cerebrospinal fluid (CSF) space at places where adherent pia mater is separated from overlying arachnoid mater. The basal exudates in subarachnoid space may extend from one to another cisternal space depending upon the inflammatory response.

The chiasm is surrounded by chiasmatic cistern, which extends around the optic nerves too. Chiasmatic cistern is bounded laterally by the medial carotid membrane and adjoining carotid cisterns, anteroinferiorly by the arachnoid membrane over diaphragma and tuberculum sellae, and posteriorly by a membrane of Liliequist over diencephalon [38, 39]. The suprasellar cistern comprises chiasmatic cistern, cistern of lamina terminalis, and interpeduncular cistern. The exudates in this region may extend to involve as far as Sylvian fissure, ambient cistern, and occasionally prepontine cistern too (Figs. 22.1, 22.2, and 22.3). The blood supply to optic chiasm is via small branches arising from vessels of the circle of Willis (anterior cerebral, anterior communicating artery, posterior cerebral, posterior communicating and basilar arteries). Sometimes, TB vasculitic involvement of these branches or vasa nervorum may lead to optic nerve and chiasm infarcts.

22.3 Etiopathogenesis and Pathology

Central nervous system (CNS) TB occurs secondary to some primary focus (most commonly lungs) [40]. The postulated mechanism suggests initial lung involvement via the inhalational route and then dissemination to the brain. Other primary sites like the intestine, lymph node, and bones may also spread the *Mycobacterium tuberculosis* to the brain.

Brain involvement occurs either via the hematogenous route or via direct extension of a focus like mastoids [41] and Pott's spine. The hematogenous spread commonly leads to the formation of a Rich focus at the cortex or less commonly choroid plexus involvement [42–45]. The Rich focus may either rupture into subarachnoid CSF space, resulting in TBM, or extend deeper into brain parenchyma and thus leading to the formation of tuberculoma or TB abscess [46]. Even choroid involvement leads to TB ventriculitis and TBM. Characteristically, TBM is associated with basal exudates. The ventral cranial nerves exiting from the brainstem are commonly involved. Optochiasmatic region involvement is also common, resulting in visual loss. Sellar and suprasellar region involvement leads to pituitary and hypothalamic dysfunction [47, 48]. Visual involvement may occur due to entrapment of optic chiasm in thick exudates. Additionally, occlusion and vasculitis of blood vessels supplying the optic nerve may also lead to visual loss.

Table 22.1 Reported cases of tubercular optochiasmatic arachnoiditis and optochiasmatic tuberculomas with clinical features, investigations, radiology, treatment, and outcome

Author (year)	Patients	Age (in years)/sex	Clinical presentation	Paradoxical gap	CSF	Imaging	Treatment	Outcome (last follow-up)	Ref
Idriraj et al. (2015)	1	5/M	Meningitis FUP 2 months Visual loss	2 mts	NA	Baseline MRI OCT	HRZE Steroid	Improvement	[7]
Ahmetgjekaj et al. (2014)	1	5/M	Meningitis FUP 3 months Visual loss	3 mts	CSF: NA	Baseline MRI: NA FUP MRI (3 months) OCT	HRZE Steroids FUP 3 months Steroids addition	NA	[8]
Nema et al. (2014)	2	6/M	Meningitis, FUP 1 month Visual loss BE: NLP	1 mts	Cells: 910 Diff: NA Protein: 230 Glucose: 30 AFB: NA PCR: NA	Baseline MRI: NA FUP MRI: basal exudates and OCA	HRZE MPS	Improvement RE: 6/18 LE: 6/12 (18 months)	[9]
		4/M	Meningitis FUP 3 weeks Visual loss BE: NLP	3 wks	Cells: 120 Diff: P(10)L(90) Protein: 20 Glucose: NA AFB: NA PCR: NA	Baseline CT Hydrocephalous FUP MRI: OCA	HRZE MPS VP shunt	Improvement BE: 6/18 (1 year)	[9]
Verma et al. (2014)	8	NA	Meningitis, FUP 1 month Visual loss	1 mts	NA	Baseline MRI OCA (6), OCT (2)	HRZS	NA	[10]
Verma et al. (2014)	1	25/M	Meningitis Visual loss BE: NLP	No	PCR + ve	Baseline MRI OCA and OCT	ATT	NA	[11]

(continued)

Table 22.1 (continued)

Author (year)	Patients	Age (in years)/sex	Clinical presentation	Paradoxical gap	CSF	Imaging	Treatment	Outcome (last follow-up)	Ref
Joseph et al. (2013)	3	20/F	Meningitis, seizures, hemiparesis, facial palsy FUP 1 year RE: 6/6 LE: 6/18	1 year	Cells: 470 Diff: P(59)L(41) Protein: 182 Glucose: 20 AFB: −ve PCR: NA	Baseline MRI Tuberculoma in left parietal region FUP MRI OCT, suprasellar tuberculoma and arachnoiditis	HRZE Steroid AED MPS X 5 d	Improvement in vision RE: 6/6 LE: 6/9 (2 months)	[12]
		26/F	Meningitis, FUP 2 months Visual loss RE: 6/12 LE: 6/60	2 mts	Cells: NA Diff: NA Protein: 190 Glucose: NA AFB: NA PCR: NA	Baseline MRI Normal FUP MRI OCT, OCA with basal exudates	HRZE Steroid AED MPS X 5 d	Improvement RE: 6/9 LE: 6/24 (1 week)	[12]
		16/F	Pulmonary tuberculosis FUP 2 months Visual loss RE: 6/24 LE: 6/60	2 mts	NA	Baseline MRI OCT	ATT Steroid	Improvement BE: 6/6 (1 week)	[12]
Verma et al. (2013)	1	27/F	Meningitis, visual loss BE: NLP	No	Cells: 85 Diff: L(100) Protein: 92 Glucose: 40 AFB: –ve PCR: NA	Baseline MRI Leptomeningeal and basal exudates, OCA	ATT Steroid	No improvement in vision BE: NLP	[13]
Lima et al. (2012)	1	32/F	Headache, vomiting Visual loss RE: 20/60 LE: NLP Past history of culture-positive pulmonary tuberculosis	8 years	Cells: 8 Diff: NA Protein: 55 Glucose: 40 AFB: –ve PCR: NA	Baseline MRI OCT FUP MRI (14 months) Complete resolution	HRZE Steroids	Visual disability (14 months) BE: blindness	[14]

Author (year)	Patients	Age (in years)/sex	Clinical presentation	Paradoxical gap	CSF	Imaging	Treatment	Outcome (last follow-up)	Ref
Wani et al. (2012)	1	56/M	Meningitis FUP 2 months Visual loss BE: 20/200	2 mts	NA	Baseline MRI: NA FUP MRI: OCT and perimesencephalic tuberculomas	HRZE Dexamethasone	Improvement RE: 20/60 LE: 20/70 (5 months)	[15]
Sharma et al. (2011)	27	31.95 ± 13.96 years	NA	NA	NA	Baseline MRI: OCA	HRZS Steroid	NA	[16]
Sinha et al. (2010)	40	30 ± 13	Meningitis Visual loss	No	NA	Baseline MRI OCA (22) OCT (18)	HRZS Steroid	Improvement or stabilization in majority (6 months)	[17]
Behari et al. (2009)	1	F	Headache Visual loss RE: 5/60 LE: FC	No	NA	Baseline MRI Sellar and suprasellar tuberculoma, arachnoiditis	HRZE Steroid Operative debulking	Improvement with stabilized vision	[18]
Ghosh et al. (2009)	1	25/F	Meningitis FUP 2 months III, IV, VI cranial nerve palsy Visual loss BE: NLP	1 mts	NA	Baseline MRI Hydrocephalous, OCA, thick exudates	ATT Steroid	No visual improvement	[19]
Stefan et al. (2009)	1	7/M	Pulmonary TB, acute lymphoblastic leukemia, meningitis Papilledema	No	Cells: 201 Diff: P(1)L(99) Protein: 225 Glucose: 19 AFB: –ve PCR: NA	Baseline MRI: OCA, basal exudates, hydrocephalous	HRZE Steroid Aspirin VP shunt Thalidomide	Improvement in vision RE: FC LE: 6/30 (3 months)	[20]
Yeh et al. (2009)	1	18/F	Pregnant, headache, altered sensorium, B/l abducens Visual loss RE: NLP LE: PL+	No	Traumatic RBCs: 5800 Cells: 506 Diff: P(46)L(54) Protein: 367 Glucose: 53 AFB: NA PCR: +ve	Baseline MRI OCA and OCT, basal exudates, cerebral convexities enhancement, hydrocephalous	Vancomycin Ceftriaxone Clindamycin Acyclovir HRZE MPS (250 mg iv 6hrly X 3 days) VP shunt	Visual disability (4 months) BE: NLP	[21]

(continued)

Table 22.1 (continued)

Author (year)	Patients	Age (in years)/sex	Clinical presentation	Paradoxical gap	CSF	Imaging	Treatment	Outcome (last follow-up)	Ref
Aliyu et al. (2007)	1	34/M	Altered sensorium Oculomotor nerve palsy	No	Cells; 160 Diff: P(30)L(70) Protein: 60 Glucose: 36 AFB: –ve PCR: NA	Baseline MRI OCA, Exudates at Sylvian fissure and prepontine space	HRZE Dexamethasone Thalidomide VP shunt	Improvement in vision (1 year)	[22]
Sunbul et al. (2007)	1	18/F	Meningitis Vision loss	No	NA	Baseline MRI Hydrocephalous, OCA	ATT Steroid	No visual improvement	[23]
Kalkan et al. (2006)	1	15/F	Meningitis Bilateral abducens palsy, papilledema	1 mts	Cells: 140 Diff: P(35)L(65) Protein: 85 Glucose: 35 AFB: NA PCR: NA	Baseline MRI Multiple brain tuberculoma FUP MRI- OCT	HRZS Steroid	Improvement BE: 6/6 (28 months)	[126]
Meyer et al. (2006)	1	4/F	Meningitis Seizure Visual loss	No	Lymphocytic pleocytosis PCR + ve	Baseline MRI Multiple OCT and cerebral tuberculoma	ATT Steroid	Visual loss (3 months)	[24]
Tsai et al. (2004)	1	6/M	Fever, lethargy FUP 7 weeks Visual loss RE: 24/60 LE: 6/60 Bitemporal hemianopsia	2 mts	Cells: 475 Diff: P(6)L(76) Protein: 124 Glucose: 39 AFB: +ve PCR: NA	Baseline CT Mild hydrocephalous FUP MRI (7 weeks) OCA and multiple tuberculomas, hydrocephalous	Penicillin G Acyclovir HRZS Dexamethasone VP shunt Steroid and streptomycin added again	Normal vision BE: 6/6 (18 months)	[25]
Aversa do Souto et al. (2003)	1	20/M	Seizures, drowsiness, visual loss BE: NLP	No	NA AFB + ve on HPx tissue	Baseline MRI: OCA	HRE	No improvement in vision BE: NLP (15 months)	[26]
Roberts et al. (2003)	1	23/F	Pulmonary TB, meningitis FUP 1 year Visual loss Bitemporal hemianopia	1 year	PCR + ve	Baseline CT Basal exudates FUP MRI Multiple OCT	HRZE Steroid Thalidomide	Improvement in visual field (2 years)	[27]

Author (year)	Patients	Age (in years)/sex	Clinical presentation	Paradoxical gap	CSF	Imaging	Treatment	Outcome (last follow-up)	Ref
Sharma et al. (2003)	1	14/F	Meningitis Visual loss BL: NLP	No	Cells: 175 Diff: P(5)L(95) Protein: 61 Glucose: 7 AFB: –ve PCR: NA	Baseline MRI Multiple OCA	HRZS Steroid Surgical debulking	No visual improvement (6 months)	[28]
Sodhi et al. (2001)	1	29/F	Headache, vomiting, visual loss RE: 6/6 LE: NLP	No	Cells: NA Diff: NA, L(9) Protein: 65 Glucose: 52 AFB: –ve PCR: +ve	Baseline MRI OCA, tuberculoma	HRZE Steroid	Improvement Vision BE: 6/6	[29]
Silverman et al. (1995)	1	11/M	Meningitis, altered sensorium, facial palsy Visual loss, BE: NLP	No	Cells: 407 Diff: P(50)L(40) Protein: 215 Glucose: 26 AFB: –ve PCR: +ve	Baseline MRI Basal and Sylvian exudates, infarct (basal ganglia) FUP MRI (3 months) OCA and basal exudates, left parietal infarct	HRZS Dexamethasone Dexamethasone again restarted at 3 months	Death (7 months)	[30]
Poon et al. (1993)	1	5/F	Meningitis, Visual loss BE: 20/200	2 wks	Cells: 250 Diff: P(60)L(40) Protein: 180 Glucose: 14 AFB: +ve PCR: NA	Baseline CT: OCT FUP CT: normal	HRZS Steroid	Improvement RE: 20/25 LE: 20/40	[31]
Teoh et al. (1988)	1	22/M	Meningitis FUP 1 month Visual loss RE: 20/200 LE: PL + ve	1 mts	Cells: 75 Diff: P(84)L(16) Protein: 112 Glucose: 16 AFB: +ve PCR: NA	Baseline CT: normal FUP CT: suprasellar tuberculoma with OCA	HRZS Dexamethasone Surgical debulking	Improvement BE: 20/25 (3 months)	[32]
Kingsley et al. (1987)	8	1–70 years	Meningitis, seizures, visual loss	NA	NA	Baseline CT Hydrocephalous, OCA, exudates	ATT Surgery	Poor visual outcome (6)	[33]

(continued)

Table 22.1 (continued)

Author (year)	Patients	Age (in years)/sex	Clinical presentation	Paradoxical gap	CSF	Imaging	Treatment	Outcome (last follow-up)	Ref
Navarro et al. (1981)	8	3/F	Meningitis Left III nerve palsy, left hemiparesis, Visual loss BE: NLP	No	CSF: NA HPx: evidence of OCA	Baseline CT Hydrocephalous PCEG: blockage of chiasmatic cistern	HRZE Steroids VP shunt	Death	[34]
		11 mts/M	Meningitis, hemiparesis, seizures FUP 5 months Visual loss BE: NLP	5 mts	CSF: NA HPx: evidence of OCA	Baseline CT: normal FUP CT (5 months) CT: hydrocephalous PCEG: blockage of chiasmatic cistern	HRZE Steroids VP shunt	Improvement in vision BE: 20/30 (27 months)	[34]
		12/F	Meningitis, altered sensorium Visual loss RE: 20/45 LE: 20/40	No	CSF: NA HPx: evidence of OCA	Baseline CT Hydrocephalous PCEG: blockage of chiasmatic cistern	HRZE Steroids VP shunt	Improvement in vision BE: 20/35 (3 years)	[34]
		11mts/M	Meningitis, Seizures, visual loss BE: PL + nt	No	CSF: NA HPx: evidence of OCA	Baseline CT hydrocephalous PCEG: blockage of chiasmatic cistern	HRZE Steroids VP shunt	Improvement in vision BE: 20/30 (2 years)	[34]
		18mts/M	Meningitis Seizures FUP 4 months Visual loss	4 mts	CSF: NA HPx: evidence of OCA	CT: hydrocephalous	HRZE Steroids VP shunt	Improvement in vision RE: 20/35 LE: 20/30 (8 months)	[34]
		2/F	Meningitis Seizures, visual loss	No	CSF: NA HPx: evidence of OCA	PCEG: blockage of chiasmatic cistern and hydrocephalous	HRZE Steroids VP shunt	Improvement in vision BE: 20/20 (18 months)	[34]
		2/M	Meningitis, Akinetic mutism, hemiparesis, visual loss	No	CSF: NA HPx: evidence of OCA	Baseline CT hydrocephalous PCEG: blockage of chiasmatic cistern and hydrocephalous	HRZE Steroids VP shunt	Improvement in vision (2 months)	[34]
		3/M	Meningitis Seizures, visual loss BE: NLP	No	CSF: NA HPx: evidence of OCA	PCEG: blockage of chiasmatic cistern and hydrocephalous	HRZE Steroids VP shunt	Improvement in vision RE: 20/25 LE: 20/20 (1 year)	[34]

Author (year)	Patients	Age (in years)/sex	Clinical presentation	Paradoxical gap	CSF	Imaging	Treatment	Outcome (last follow-up)	Ref
Iraci et al. (1980)	1	25/M	Meningitis FUP 7 months Visual loss RE: NLP LE: PL + ve	7 mts	Histopathological	PCEG: block at chiasmatic cistern	ATT Steroid Surgical debulking	Improvement in vision BE: 6/6	[35]
Scott et al. (1977)	1	5/M	Meningitis, seizures, III nerve palsy FUP 2 months Visual loss RE: 2/400 LE: PL + ve	2 mts	Cells: 100 Diff: P(35)L(65) Protein: 144 Glucose: 38 AFB: +ve PCR: NA	PCEG: obliteration of chiasmatic cistern, hydrocephalous	HES Surgical debulking	Improvement BE: 20/30 (4 months)	[36]
Coyle et al. (1969)	1	14/M	Meningitis, hemiparesis, FUP 3 months Visual loss RE: 20/20 LE: PL + ve	14 mts	Cells: 30 Diff: NA Protein: 65 Glucose: NA HPx: evidence of OCA	PCEG: blockage of chiasmatic and interpeduncular cistern	PAS, HS, Steroid Surgical intervention at optic chiasm	Improvement in vision BE: 20/20 (3 years)	[37]
Yuhl et al. (1951)	1	25/M	Meningitis Facial palsy FUP 9 months Visual loss Bitemporal hemianopsia	9 mts	Cells: 913 Diff: P(25)L(75) Protein: 368 Glucose: 25 AFB: +ve PCR: NA HPx: evidence of OCA	NA	PAS, Streptomycin Steroid Surgical intervention at optic chiasm	Death after 18 months	[6]

Abbreviations: *+ve* present, *−ve* absent, *AED* antiepileptic drug, *AFB* acid-fast bacilli, *BE* both eyes, *CT* computed tomography, *Diff* differential counts in CSF, *E* ethambutol, *F* female, *FC* finger counting, *FUP* follow-up, *L* lymphocytes in CSF, *H* isoniazid, *HPx* histopathology, *LE* left eye, *mts* months, *M* male, *MPS* methyl prednisolone, *MRI* magnetic resonance imaging, *NA* not available, *NLP* no light perception, *OCA* optochiasmatic arachnoiditis, *OCT* optochiasmatic tuberculoma, *P* polymorphs in CSF, *PAS* Para-aminosalicylic acid, *PCR* polymerase chain reaction, *PL* perception of light, *PCEG* pneumo-cisterno-encephalography, *R* rifampicin, *RBC* red blood cells, *RE* right eye, *S* streptomycin, *VP* ventriculoperitoneal, *wks* weeks, *Z* pyrazinamide

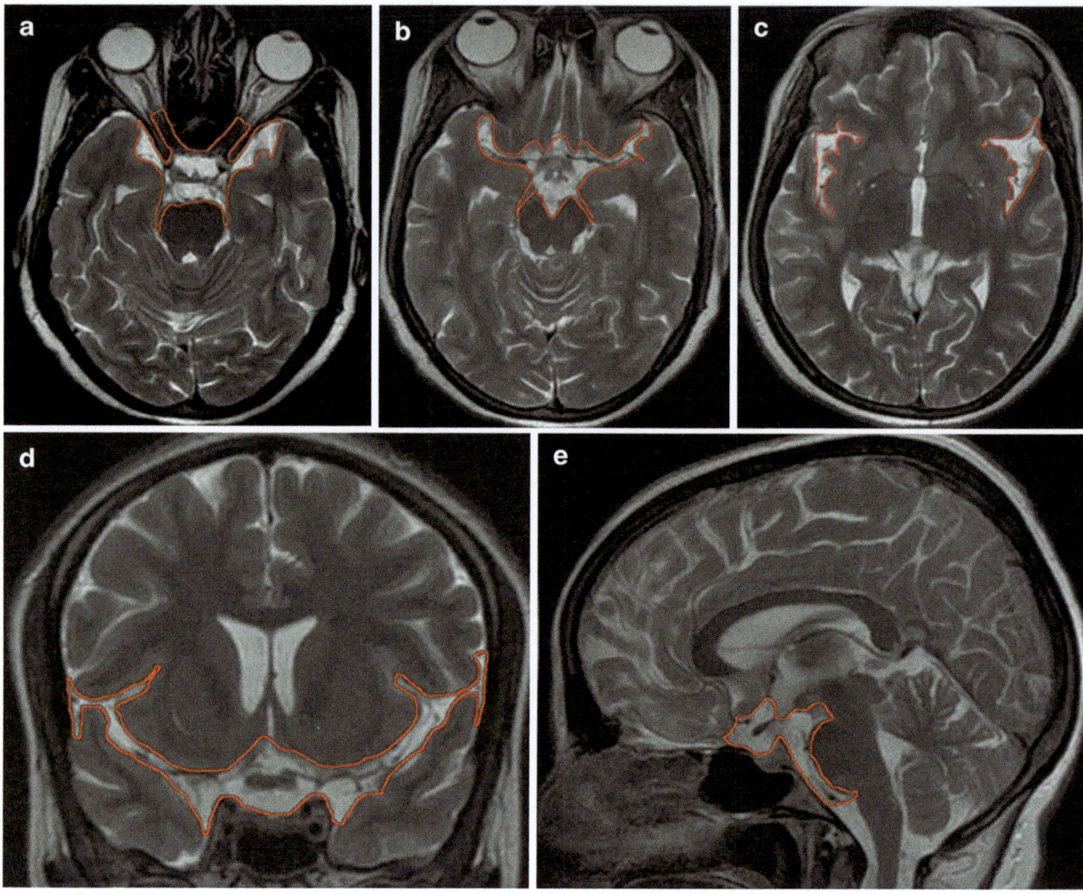

Fig. 22.1 Normal anatomy and extension of optochiasmatic region cisterns (*outlined in red*). (**a**) Axial T2 sequence shows optochiasmatic region with extension of cerebrospinal fluid (CSF) spaces around optic nerves and medial portion of anterior temporal lobes (Sylvian fissure). (**b, c**) Axial T2 sequence shows optochiasmatic region with CSF space around middle cerebral artery (Sylvian fissure) and extension to perimesencephalic cistern. (**d**) Coronal T2 sequence shows optochiasmatic region with Sylvian fissure. (**e**) Sagittal T2 sequence shows optochiasmatic, suprasellar, perimesencephalic, and prepontine CSF spaces

Gross pathological examination reveals thick, gelatinous, grayish exudates involving most commonly basal region, including optochiasmatic region, interpeduncular cistern, Sylvian fissure, prepontine space, and less commonly superficial sulcus [18, 49].

Sometimes, rather than arachnoiditis, OCT is the prominent radiological presentation. Histopathologically, these tuberculomas show caseation, epitheloid granuloma, lymphocytes, and Langerhans giant cells. Acid-fast bacilli positivity is uncommon [18].

Paradoxical reaction in TBM is a common phenomenon despite adequate treatment [8, 32, 50–52]. This paradoxical reaction may manifest as a clinical deterioration with the radiological appearance of new tuberculomas, increased exudates, optochiasmatic involvement [8, 28], raised CSF proteins, lumbosacral arachnoiditis, and even extracranial involvement. The exact cause of development of optochiasmatic granulomas or paradoxical reaction is not known, but role of pro-inflammatory cytokines and chemokines has been postulated. *M. tuberculosis* interacts with the CNS microglial cells and leads to production of pro-inflammatory cytokines and chemokines. T-helper cell 1 produces tumor necrosis factor (TNF)-α, interferon (IFN)-γ, and interleukin (IL) 2. T-helper cell 2 produces IL2, 4, 5, 10,

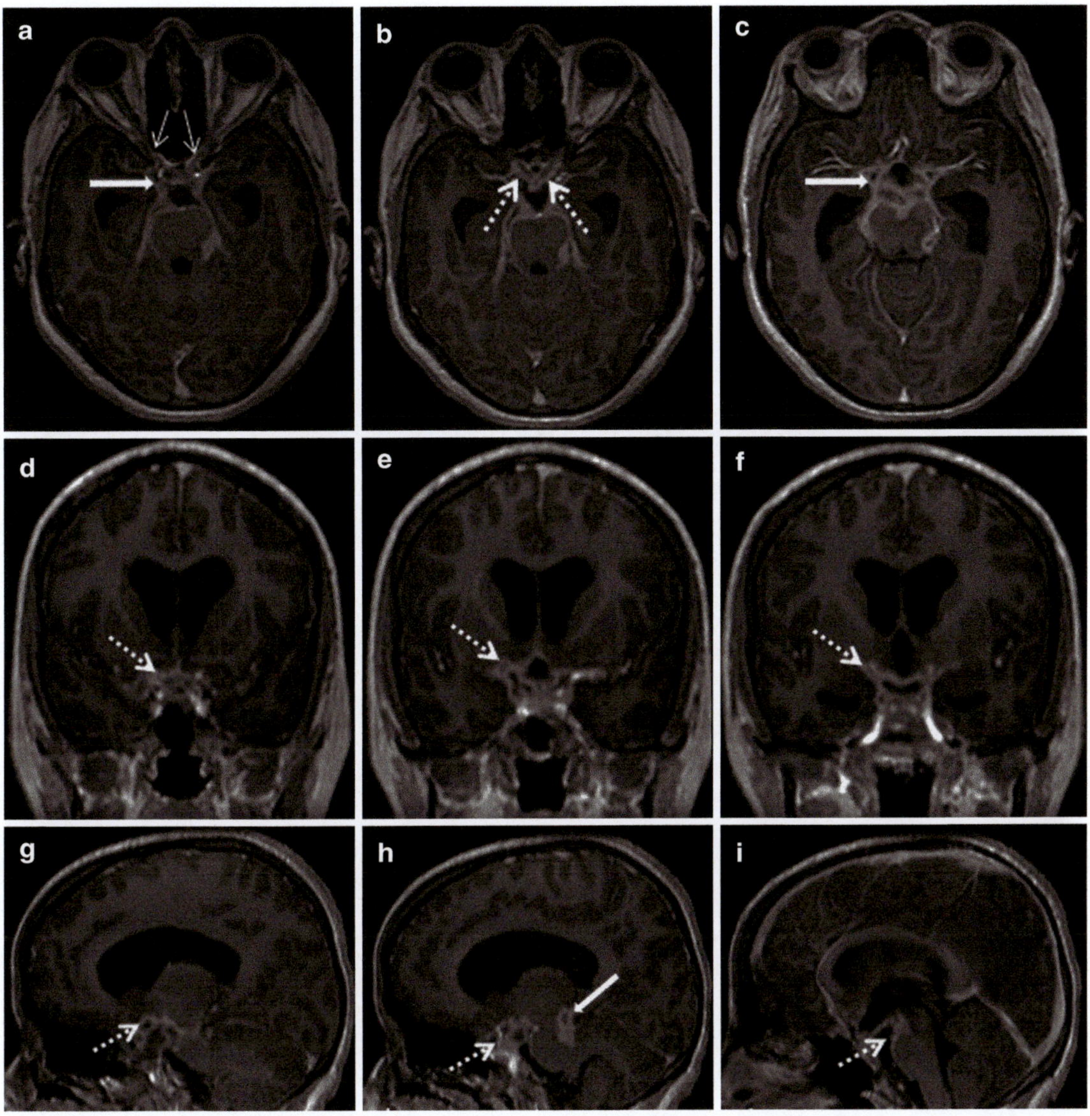

Fig. 22.2 Contrast-enhanced spoiled gradient-recalled-echo (*SPGR*) imaging shows TB optochiasmatic arachnoiditis (OCA) and optochiasmatic tuberculoma (OCT). Axial SPGR contrast shows (**a**) exudates in optochiasmatic (*bold arrow*) and perimesencephalic region and around optic nerves (*thin arrows*), (**b**) exudates around optic chiasm (*dotted arrows*), and (**c**) exudates in optochiasmatic region and around middle cerebral artery (*bold arrow*). Coronal SPGR contrast shows (**d–f**) exudates in optochiasmatic and Sylvian fissures along with basal exudates (*dotted lines*). Sagittal SPGR contrast shows (**g**) OCT (*dotted line*), (**h**) perimesencephalic exudates and tuberculoma (*dotted and bold lines*), (**i**) perimesencephalic exudates (*dotted line*)

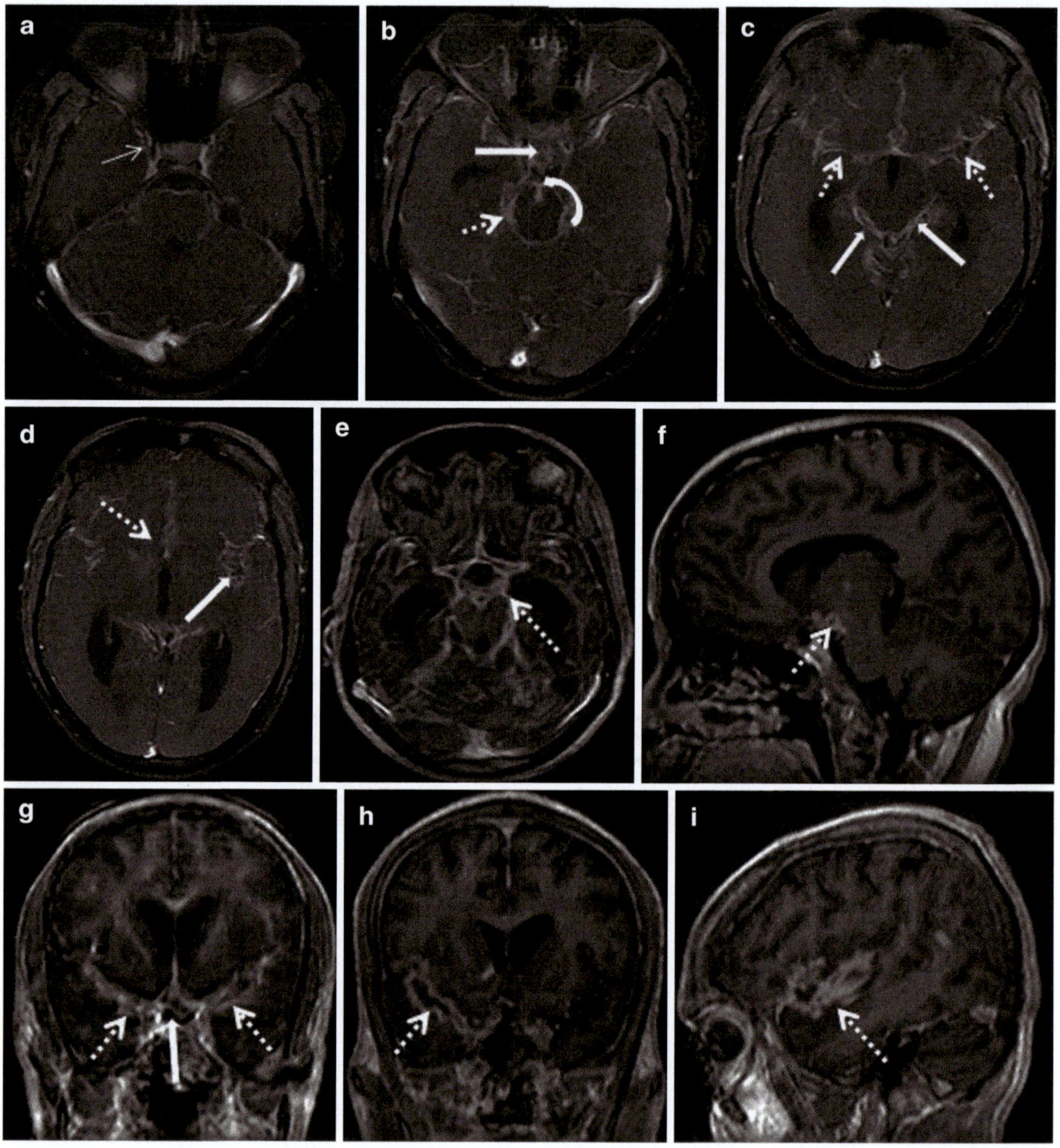

Fig. 22.3 Contrast-enhanced T1 and spoiled gradient-recalled-echo (*SPGR*) imaging shows exudates in optochiasmatic and other cisterns. Axial T1 contrast shows (**a**) exudates in Sylvian fissure (*thin line*); (**b**) OCA (*bold arrow*), perimesencephalic exudates (*dotted arrow, curved arrow*); (**c**) exudates in Sylvian fissure (*dotted lines*) and quadrigeminal plate cistern (*bold arrows*); (**d**) exudates in interhemispheric CSF space (*dotted arrow*) and Sylvian fissure (*bold arrow*); (**e**) exudates in optochiasmatic region, Sylvian fissure, and perimesencephalic and ambient cisterns (*dotted line*); (**f**) tuberculoma in perimesencephalic region (sagittal view); (**g–i**) exudates in Sylvian fissure (*dotted lines*)

and 13. Matrix metalloproteinases (MMPs) have role in blood–brain barrier breakdown as well as in brain tissue damage. MMP2 and MMP9 are especially associated with hydrocephalus, tuberculoma formation, and prognosis. Other ILs have also been analyzed in various studies and were found to be raised in TBM [53–57].

22.4 Clinical Features and Presentation

Cranial nerve involvement is a common presentation of TBM. It can appear during the initial presentation or as a complication later on. Even during treatment, paradoxical manifestation with the appearance of new cranial nerve deficits is commonly reported. Various studies have shown cranial nerve involvement ranging from 23% to 51% [16, 58–62]. The most common nerve to be involved is abducens [60] owing to its long intracranial course in the subarachnoid space and acute bend over petrous portion of temporal bone. Second common nerve affected is oculomotor owing to its course in basal region of the brain with easy susceptibility to exudates. Apart from the facial nerve, lower cranial nerve involvement has also been reported in literature. Some rare case reports have demonstrated the involvement of vestibulocochlear nerve too [60], but no report is present, documenting the involvement of olfactory nerve.

Visual involvement is the most devastating and dreaded complication of TBM. Though the involvement of other cranial nerves improve or recover completely with time, the visual loss may persist. This disability has a profound bearing on patient's personal and social life. Ocular and visual involvement can occur due to the involvement of several structures. Ocular involvement may present with or without visual impairment. Numerous case reports and a review [63] have mentioned ocular involvement [64–66] as adnexal, lid or conjunctival disease [67, 68], orbital tuberculoma or abscess [69], iris nodules [70], ciliary mass [71], keratitis [36], uveitis [72], scleritis [73], choroidal tubercle [74], choroiditis [75], optic disk tuberculoma [76], panophthalmitis [77], neuroretinitis [78, 79], and Eales disease [80].

In CNS TB, the visual involvement [81] may manifest as monocular or binocular blindness, optic neuritis, scotomas, concentric filed defects, bitemporal hemianopia, palinopsia [82], and cortical blindness. The onset is usually gradual but may be an acute onset in few cases.

The clinical examination may reveal pupillary reaction abnormalities [83]; diminution of vision; fundus changes like choroid tubercle, papilledema, or optic atrophy [13]; and field defects such as scotoma or hemianopias. Visual axis involvement can be divided into anterior and posterior visual pathways. Apart from orbital causes, other sites and etiologies of anterior visual involvement may be due to tubercular optic neuritis, optic nerve tuberculoma [35, 84, 85], vasculitic infarct of optic nerve, drug induced, OCA [6], and tuberculomas [18, 30]. Posterior visual pathway involvement has been reported as optic tract, optic radiation tuberculoma [82, 86], and cortical lesions. TB OCA and OCT develop gradually either during the initial course of disease or later on as a paradoxical manifestation. The visual complains are similar as discussed earlier.

The literature review shows lack of prospective studies focusing on optochiasmatic involvement in TBM. Most reports are as case reports and case series. Even studies on visual involvement in TBM are few. In a study by Aaron et al. [87], out of 163 TBM patients, OCA was present in 23 patients (14%) and cranial nerve involvement in 61% of these 23 OCA patients. Associated spinal arachnoiditis was present in 48% of OCA patients. This complication of optochiasmatic involvement was late, and the study showed mean interval between the TBM diagnosis and onset of visual symptoms to be 6.4 (± 1.27) months. This delay may be due to paradoxical phenomenon. Visual assessment at presentation showed blindness (<3/60 according to WHO) in 82%, papilledema in 39%, and optic atrophy in 52% of OCA patients. Almost 43% of these patients were in stage III, thus associating OCA with advanced state of TBM. In another such study by Sinha et al. [17], 101 adult TBM patients were evaluated for visual involvement. Around 27% patients presented with low vision (between 6/18 and 3/60) or blindness (<3/60 according to WHO). The cause for visual involvement was found to be OCA in 40% and OCT in 22%. But, radiologically, OCA was present in 21.8% and OCT in 17.8% of all TBM patients. They concluded that visual impairment was related with poor outcome either as disability or death. Moreover, baseline cranial nerve palsies, papilledema, markedly raised CSF proteins, and OCA on magnetic resonance imaging (MRI) were associated with visual deterioration during follow-up.

Paradoxical reactions and development or enlargement of tuberculoma is commonly reported [12, 15]. In a case series, Sinha et al. [88] reported eight cases of paradoxical vision loss due to OCT developing in TBM patients with normal baseline visual acuity. Out of these eight cases, three patients were having baseline OCA on MRI along with normal vision. Paradoxical development of OCT occurred after a mean of 41 days. This was associated with severe vision loss ($\leq$ 6/60) in six patients and death of two patients.

22.5 Diagnostic Investigations and Differential Diagnosis

Diagnosis of TB OCA firstly requires establishment of TBM and then diagnosis of OCA.

22.5.1 Diagnosis of Tuberculous Meningitis

Clinical diagnosis of TBM requires investigative support too. Brain neuroimaging is an essential part of this diagnostic endeavor. Though MRI is better than computed tomography (CT), both these modalities are sufficient to detect hydrocephalous, exudates, and tuberculomas. Vasculitic infarcts, conglomerate granuloma, and abscess may be additional imaging findings.

CSF plays a vital role in diagnosis. Classically, CSF in TB is yellowish in color with raised cells (up to 1000), lymphocytic predominance, increased proteins, and decreased glucose. Routine microscopy may demonstrate AFB positivity on ZN staining. Culture and sensitivity are helpful in demonstrating mycobacterium and drug sensitivity. Polymerase chain reaction is now widely used owing to its high detection rate. Recently, for rapid detection of rifampicin (RIF) resistance, GeneXpert MTB/RIF assay is a new tool for the diagnosis of TB [89].

Other supportive investigations for evidence of TB like tuberculin test, X-ray chest, ultrasound abdomen, and IGRA assay may be helpful to some extent. Interleukins and cytokines are raised in TBM but due to its non-specific character, utility for diagnosis is lacking.

22.5.2 Diagnosis of Optochiasmatic Tuberculosis

First clue to OCA or OCT is vision impairment, and complete visual assessment is an integral part of diagnosis of OCA. Radiological and histopathological features also support OCA diagnosis.

22.5.2.1 Visual Assessment

Visual complains of a patient is the first clue to OCA. Clinical examination includes visual acuity and fundus examination. Field charting can be done to ascertain the type of scotoma and field defects. Classical patterns of optic chiasm involvement is lacking as the arachnoiditis is a diffuse process involving chiasm, optic nerve, and to some extent optic tracts too. Fundus photography and OCT help in evaluation of retinal layers. Visual evoked potential is another modality to assess the visual pathway and is usually abnormal in OCA. Prospective study evaluating these parameters in OCA is lacking, and available literature such as case reports and case series

[17, 87, 88, 90] mentions only visual acuity or field defects.

22.5.2.2 Radiological Evaluation

Since 1929 when Balado gave the first description of OCA, the radiological diagnosis of OCA has changed a lot. During the initial days, indirect evidence of OCA pathology was suspected on direct roentgenogram either as a calcification within adhesions or an associated sinusitis (initially linked to OCA). Cerebral angiography provided no better evidence and only clue to an OCA pathology used to be traction and constriction of carotid siphon or A1 segment of anterior cerebral artery. Cisternography with radioactive human serum albumin (RIHSA) was used to demonstrate slowing and delayed circulation of CSF in anterior circulation. The best aid available at that time was pneumo-cisterno-encephalography (PCEG). The features suggestive of OCA were (a) a slowing or failure of air passage from the basal cistern into the subarachnoid space, (b) changes in shape and increase in size of the chiasmatic or interpeduncular cisterns and of the lamina terminalis, and (c) scanty or irregular filling of frontal subarachnoid spaces. Even these diagnostic findings were challenged later on owing to such features in normal individuals too. It was also postulated that arrest of air was due to Liliequist membrane [91].

The invention and medical use of CT provided a big boost in diagnosis of diseases. Brain CT was helpful in showing brain parenchyma, ventricles, and CSF spaces. Administration of contrast was vital in providing additional information. For decades, the contrast enhanced CT was the imaging of choice for OCA. CT was able to demonstrate basal exudates and exudates in various cisterns including optochiasmatic region. Though subjective findings of basal exudates on CT in TBM are described in numerous studies and reports, objective defining criteria were given by Andronikou et al. [92] in 2004. Such a criterion exclusively for defining exudates in perichiasmatic region is still lacking. Out of the nine criteria for exudates, four are relevant for defining exudates in perichiasmal region, namely, (a) filling of cistern with contrast and obliteration of normal CSF space around the vessels, (b) double and triple line signs, (c) linear enhancement in the middle cerebral artery cistern, and (d) Y sign. MRI is better than CT in detecting parenchymal tuberculomas, hydrocephalus, and exudates at an earlier stage. Vascular anatomy and exudates in perichiasmal region is also better delineated. An objective criterion for OCA has not been defined yet, but literature shows numerous pictures of OCA. In a study by Aaron et al. [87] on TBM, 23 patients of OCA were found. The basal exudates, perichiasmal tuberculomas, and parenchymal tuberculomas were detected in 87%, 13%, and 35%, respectively. In another study by Raut et al. [61], basal exudates were found in 52% cases. Commonly, optochiasmatic region shows exudates which extend anteriorly along the anterior cerebral vessels and CSF space between the two frontal lobes, along middle cerebral artery reaching as far as Sylvian fissure, in sellar and suprasellar region, and along the clivus to ambient as well as prepontine cistern (Figs. 22.2 and 22.3). Secondary complications like infarct and hydrocephalus can also be detected well on MRI. In a study by Anuradha et al. [93], significant association was found between stroke and exudates in and around optic chiasm, Sylvian fissure, and posterior fossa.

22.5.2.3 Histopathological Evaluation

Initially, the concept of OCA was substantiated and established by histopathological diagnosis rather than imaging. In 1945, Hartmann [81] published a beautiful review and description of histopathological findings in OCA. Though chronic serous meningitis and pockets of fluid collection in the brain were reported in the later part of nineteenth century, the turning point in the recognition of OCA was a case reported by Balado in 1929 [2, 6]. Histopathological description of his case of bilateral primary optic atrophy showed a milky appearance of arachnoid and exudates in basal region and around

Table 22.2 Etiology and differential diagnosis of optochiasmatic involvement

Etiology		Author	References
Infection	Syphilis	Bruetsch et al.	[3]
		Vail et al.	[94]
		Bollack et al.	[95]
		Bruetsch et al.	[4]
	Tubercular	Behari et al.	[18]
	Cryptococcal	Maruki et al.	[96]
	Epstein–Barr virus	Purvin et al.	[127]
	Sinus infection Middle ear infection Mastoid infection	Bruetsch et al.	[3]
	Meningeal infections	Bruetsch et al.	[3]
Trauma		Bruetsch et al.	[3]
		Iraci et al.	[97]
Sarcoidosis		Tang et al.	[98]
		Hosseini et al.	[46]
Multiple sclerosis		Bruetsch et al.	[3]
		Bell et al.	[99]
Pick's disease		Bruetsch et al.	[3]
Rheumatic fever		Bruetsch et al.	[3]
Cerebral tumors		Bruetsch et al. Gruber et al.	[3] [100]
Postsurgical		Carreras et al.	[101]
Differential diagnosis of optochiasmatic arachnoiditis			
Suprasellar meningioma		Bruetsch et al.	[3]
Pituitary adenoma		Bruetsch et al.	[3]
Craniopharyngioma		Bruetsch et al.	[3]
Glioma of the chiasm		Bruetsch et al.	[3]
Suprasellar aneurysm		Bruetsch et al.et al	[3]

optic nerves. Optic nerve exploration showed thinning and abnormal pink color. Visual acuity and field improved substantially in postoperative period [2, 6]. In the present era, the surgical exploration of OCA for diagnosis is uncommon. The histopathological findings can be summarized in three headings, namely, (a) arachnoid thickening and adhesions, (b) collections or exudates, and (c) optic nerve and chiasm atrophy. Behari et al. [18] described similar gross pathological findings in their study on sellar and suprasellar tuberculomas. The histology showed areas of caseation with Langerhans giant cells, epitheloid granuloma, lymphocytes, and plasma cells in 50% cases.

The differential diagnosis comprises suprasellar meningioma, pituitary adenoma, craniopharyngioma, glioma of the chiasm, and suprasellar aneurysm. Other etiologies causing OCA are enumerated in Table 22.2.

22.6 Treatment of Optochiasmatic Tuberculosis

Both medical and surgical managements of optochiasmatic TB are well described in literature as case reports and series. The outline for management of a case of optochiasmatic TB is shown in Fig. 22.4.

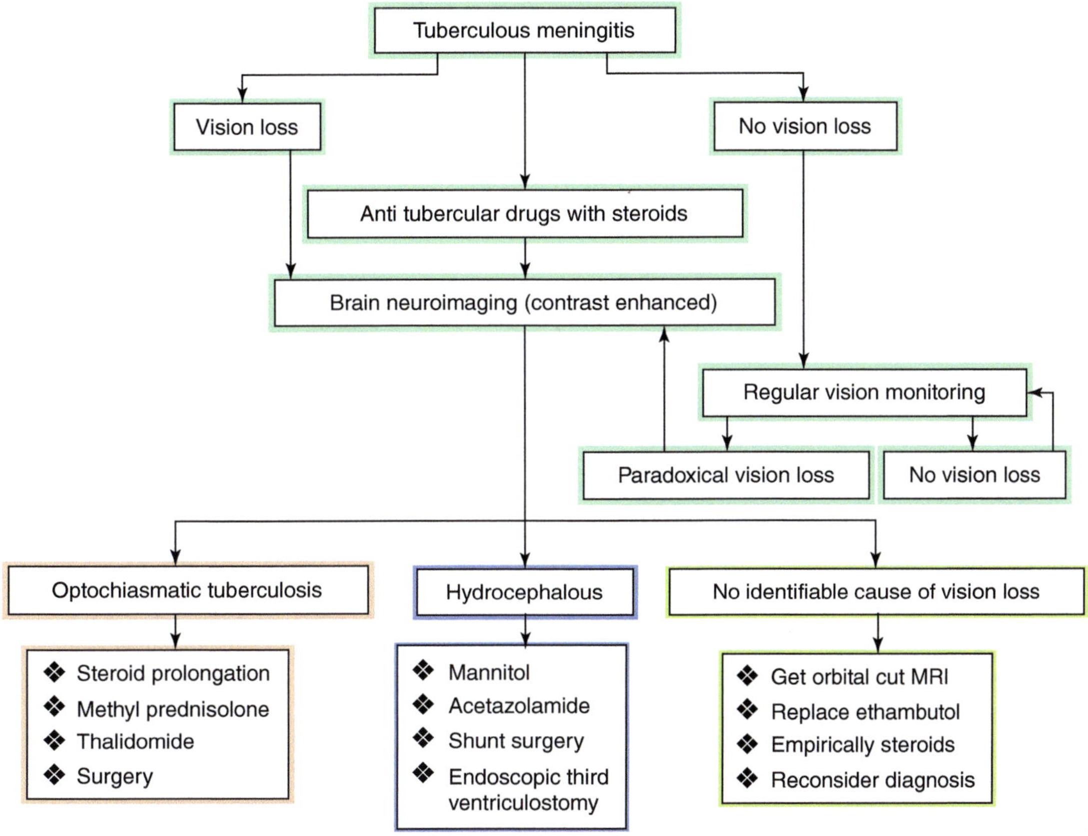

Fig. 22.4 Management algorithm for optochiasmatic tuberculosis

22.6.1 Medical Management

Various medical therapies along with anti-TB therapy have been administered to patients on a case-to-case basis with mixed results.

22.6.1.1 Anti-TB Treatment

Anti-TB treatment for OCA and OCT is not different from treatment protocol for CNS TB. WHO recommends use of streptomycin (STR) in place of ethambutol (EMB) in TBM [102]. This replacement is even more important in cases with visual loss as EMB leads to optic as well as retrobulbar neuritis.

Similar visual involvement may occur in OCA, and thus EMB administration often delays early recognition of this condition. The duration of anti-TB treatment administration in OCA and OCT is controversial and contrary to 12 months of therapy in TBM [102]; the treatment is often prolonged in such cases sometimes even more than 2 years.

22.6.1.2 Corticosteroids

Mortality was high before the advent of STR and para-aminosalicylic sodium (PAS) but dropped to around 50% with the availability of these medications. Further efforts were made to improve outcome by using streptokinase and surgery. Complications related to exudates and its relationship to poor outcome lead to the use of corticosteroid as an adjuvant therapy as early as during the 1950s. Anti-inflammatory and immunomodulatory role of corticosteroid reduces undesirable effects of host factors. In a study by Shane et al. [103] in 1956, survival improved to 92% with usage of corticosteroids along with antimicrobials. Earlier debates regarding decreased penetration of drugs and suppressed host immunity with use of corticosteroids eventually ceased. More and more studies advocated its routine use in children and adults [104–107]. Ultimately, a Cochrane review in 2008 clearly showed benefits of corticosteroids in reducing deaths and severe disabling neurological deficits.

In cases with optochiasmatic involvement, corticosteroids have been used either as dexamethasone or as a pulse therapy of methylprednisolone [9, 12, 31]. In most cases, beneficial effects were seen with this adjuvant therapy, and visual outcome was good. A prospective study evaluating effects of this adjuvant therapy in OCA is lacking.

22.6.1.3 Thalidomide

Thalidomide use as hypnotics soon landed into controversy due to phocomelia in about 10,000 newborns. The drug was withdrawn completely within 5 years. It took many years to establish its role as an immunomodulator in other diseases (erythema nodosum leprosum and multiple myeloma) [108]. With better understanding of pathophysiology of TBM, role of TNF-α, interleukins, and cytokines became established. Less than expected benefits of corticosteroid prompted a search for other drugs. The role of thalidomide in inhibiting TNF-α production prompted its use in TBM. In an animal study [109], thalidomide showed better outcome and protective effects on rabbit infected with mycobacterium. It also reduced TNF-α levels in blood and CSF in a dose-dependent manner. This was followed by an open-label pilot study by Schoeman et al. [110] in children with TBM. In enrolled 15 patients, CSF levels of TNF-α decreased, basal exudates decreased at 1 month, infarcts reduced, and hydrocephalus could be managed medically only. This study inspired the authors to go for a randomized controlled trial, which was stopped prematurely due to greater side effects and unexpected deaths in thalidomide arm [111]. Later on, Tsenova et al. [112] showed promising effects of IMiD3 (a thalidomide analogue) on experimental rabbit models of TBM. It resulted in reduced CSF levels of TNF-α, reduced CSF leukocytosis, and lesser pathological effects on the brain. This drug was well tolerated and free from teratogenic effects too. Initial results of thalidomide use in stage II and III showed improvement with decreased exudates and complications. Optochiasmatic involvement is a result of increased basal exudates. In 2004, Roberts et al. [27] reported two cases of CNS tuberculomas with one being disseminated TB with OCT. Despite drug compliance and steroids, her vision deteriorated due to enlarging OCT. The institution of thalidomide at a twice daily dosing (50 mg) for more than a year showed promising results and improvement in vision. The radiological resolution was also dramatic. In 2006, Schoeman et al. [113] reported four cases responsive to thalidomide. One of these patients developed visual loss while on treatment for TBM. Thalidomide was started when the patient deteriorated despite anti-TB treatment and steroids. The clinical and visual improvement was dramatic with vision recovering from perception of light (PL) to right eye (RE) (6/24) and left eye (LE) (6/5). In 2009, Stefan et al. [20] reported another such case. The reported child was suffering from acute lymphoblastic leukemia, which was under remission, but developed TBM with OCA. Thalidomide administration improved vision from absent PL to RE (FC) and LE (6/30). In 2010, Schoeman et al. [114] again showed the usefulness of thalidomide in four cases of TBM with OCA. All the cases except one regained 6/6 vision and excellent radiological improvement.

Thus, this literature review supports the utility of thalidomide as a suitable adjuvant to anti-TB treatment and steroids in cases with OCA. Randomized controlled trials are required to substantially prove its role in a robust scientific manner.

22.6.1.4 Streptokinase

The need of adjuvant therapy was soon recognized after less promising effect of STR. Cathie et al. [115] and Lorber et al. [116] used streptokinase to decrease the fibrinous exudates and prevent complications associated with CSF passage blocks. Soon it was noticed that the effect of intrathecal streptokinase was minimal and associated with side effects [117]. Further availability of PAS and isoniazid (INH) lead to improved survival and thus terminated the use of streptokinase.

22.6.1.5 Hyaluronidase

In 1956, Owens et al. [118] studied and published their study on intrathecal effects of hyaluronidase in rhesus monkeys. The nontoxic tolerable effects paved the way for future usage. In 1979 and 1980, Gourie et al. showed its beneficial effect in both spinal and cranial arachnoiditis [119, 120]. Though isolated case reports of hyaluronidase use in hydrocephalus were mentioned earlier in the literature, this series was the largest of such sort. The use of hyaluronidase in OCA was also established in this study with good results. Out of seven patients with visual loss, three showed good improvement with administration of intrathecal hyaluronidase. A lack of further studies and clinical use questions its utility at present times.

22.6.1.6 Interferon and Infliximab

Though other adjuvants like interferon-γ [121] and infliximab [122] have been used in complicated cases of TBM, its use in OCA has not been reported.

22.6.2 Surgical Management

Surgery in TBM is required in selected cases of hydrocephalus, TB abscess, and tuberculoma. Nowadays, surgical intervention for OCA is rare, but previously, surgery was common in such cases. Balado et al. [2] reported the first case of postsurgical visual improvement in an OCA. In a study by Dickmann et al. [123], out of 47 operated OCA cases, only 19 could be followed, in which visual improvement or stabilization occurred in 37% (7/19) cases. Though TB etiology was suspected and was one of the differential diagnoses of OCA, it was not until 1951 when the first case of tubercular OCA was published. In 1951, Yuhl et al. [6] reported the first case of TB OCA with visual involvement, which was operated but death could not be averted owing to disseminated TB status. Surgical intervention for TB OCA decreased with time due to better anti-TB drugs. The visual involvement still occurs, largely as a paradoxical phenomenon and less commonly as a presentation of TBM. In a case series of eight patients, Navarro et al. [34] showed full visual recovery in all cases of TB OCA after the microsurgical release of adhesions around optochiasmatic region preceded by the ventriculoperitoneal shunt. In a recent study by Behari et al. [18], operative interventions were done in eight cases of sellar and suprasellar tuberculoma with basal exudates and arachnoiditis. The postoperative result showed visual improvement in four of five cases with visual involvement.

Evidence from case reports and case series definitely shows the good visual outcome of surgical interventions, but a randomized controlled trial is needed [124]. Till then surgery can be performed on a case-to-case basis depending upon drug response, visual involvement, and the amount of OCA and perichiasmal tuberculomas.

22.7 Prognosis

CNS TB is considered the severest form of extrapulmonary TB. The morbidity and mortality are greatest in stage III patients. In a study by Sharma et al. [16], poor prognosis was significantly higher in patients with cranial nerve deficits. Higher CSF protein is associated with hydrocephalus leading to a relatively poor outcome [125].

The visual prognosis depends upon the baseline presence of basal exudates, papilledema, OCA or OCT, and severely raised CSF proteins [88]. In a study by Anuradha et al. [93], stroke was significantly associated with stage III and visual loss. Raut et al. [61] showed hydrocephalus to be higher in patients with cranial nerve deficits, papilledema, basal exudates, and visual impairment.

In the summarized table (see Table 22.1), a total of 122 reported cases of OCA and OCT were described. No outcome details were available for 37 patients. Out of 85 patients with available outcome data, 68 patients showed improvement in vision, 14 patients showed no improvement, and death occurred in only three cases. Thus this review of cases of OCA and OCT shows good outcome with appropriate and timely treatment.

22.8 Future Research

As vision is the most important of all the special sense of body, preservation of its function is of utmost importance. Early recognition and reliable predictors of its affection is required. Greater role of CSF biomarkers like cytokines and interleukins may be evaluated in future studies.

Regular imaging follow-up may detect OCA at an earlier stage. Low threshold for repeat imaging in cases with visual involvement may detect the paradoxical development of OCA and OCT.

Further, guidelines for steroid dosage and duration and institution of other drugs like thalidomide, interferon, and infliximab are required. A guideline regarding timing and approach of surgical intervention is the need of the hour.

References

1. Global tuberculosis report. In: World Health Organization. http://www.who.int/tb/publications/global_report/en/. Accessed 21 Jun 2016
2. Balado M, Satanowsky P (1930) Tratamiento quirúrgico de la atrofia de la papila. Archivos de Oftalmología Hispano-Americanos 30(358):558
3. Bruetsch WL (1948) Etiology of optochiasmatic arachnoiditis. Arch Neurol Psychiatry 59:215–228
4. Bruetsch WL (1947) Surgical treatment of syphilitic primary atrophy of the optic nerves (syphilitic optochiasmatic arachnoiditis). Arch Ophthalmol 38: 735–754
5. Heuer GJ, Vail DT (1931) Chronic cisternal arachnoiditis producing symptoms of involvement of the optic nerves and chiasm. Arch Ophthalmol 5:334
6. Yuhl ET, Rand CW (1951) Tuberculous opticochiasmatic arachnoiditis: report of a case. J Neurosurg 8:441–443
7. Idrizaj A (2015) Paradoxical growth of optochiasmatic tuberculoma during the treatment of tuberculous meningitis. Anglisticum J (IJLLIS) 3:181–185
8. Ahmetgjekajz I, Kabashi-Muqaj S, Lascu LC, Bondari S, Bondari A (2014) Paradoxical growth of optochiasmatic tuberculoma during the treatment of tuberculous meningitis. Curr Health Sci J 40:225–227
9. Nema N, Verma A, Singh K, Mehar V (2014) Management of paradoxical response in pediatric tubercular meningitis with methylprednisolone. Middle East Afr J Ophthalmol 21:189
10. Verma R, Gupta M, Chaudhari TS (2014) Neurogenic vision loss: causes and outcome. An experience from a tertiary center in Northern India. J Neurosci Rural Pract 5:340–348
11. Verma R, Patil TB, Lalla R (2014) Tuberculous optochiasmatic arachnoiditis. J Glob Infect 6:89
12. Joseph M, Mendonca TM, Vasu U, Nithyanandam S, Mathew T (2013) Paradoxical growth of presumed optochiasmatic tuberculomas following medical therapy. JAMA Ophthalmol 131:1463–1467
13. Verma R, Chaudhari TS (2013). Unusual fundus examination findings in tuberculous meningitis. BMJ case reports. 8;bcr2012008138
14. Lima MA, Aversa A, Maranhão-Filho P, Lima GA, Curi A, Schmaltz CA, Santanna FM (2012) Optochiasmatic tuberculoma as the sole manifestation of late recurrent tuberculosis. Rev Inst Med trop S Paulo 54:229–230
15. Wani N, Khan N, Kosar T, Qayum A (2010) Optochiasmatic tuberculomas: a vision threatening paradoxical response in tuberculous meningitis. Turk Neurosurg 22:246–249
16. Sharma P, Garg RK, Verma R, Singh MK, Shukla R (2011) Incidence, predictors and prognostic value of cranial nerve involvement in patients with tuberculous meningitis: a retrospective evaluation. Eur J Intern Med 22:289–295
17. Sinha MK, Garg RK, Anuradha HK, Agarwal A, Singh MK, Verma R, Shukla R (2010) Vision impairment in tuberculous meningitis: predictors and prognosis. J Neurol Sci 290:27–32
18. Behari S, Shinghal U, Jain M, Jaiswal AK, Wadwekar V, Das KB, Jha S (2009) Clinicoradiological presentation, management options and a review of sellar and suprasellar tuberculomas. J Clin Neurosci 16:1560–1566
19. Ghosh AK, Agrawal A, Singhal S (2009) Diagnosis: tubercular optochiasmatic arachnoiditis. Iran J Radiol 6:101–102
20. Stefan DC, Andronikou S, Freeman N, Schoeman J (2009) Recovery of vision after adjuvant thalidomide in a child with tuberculous meningitis and acute lymphoblastic leukemia. J Child Neurol 24:166–169
21. Yeh S, Cunningham MA, Patronas N, Foroozan R (2009) Optic neuropathy and perichiasmal tuberculomas associated with mycobacterium tuberculosis meningitis in pregnancy. Can J Ophthalmol 44:713–715
22. Aliyu SH, Ganesan D, Enoch DA, Watts C, Lever AM (2007) Tuberculous meningitis and hydrocephalus treated successfully with a combination of immunomodulation and cerebrospinal fluid diversion. Infect Dis J Pak 16:22–24

23. Sunbul M, Leblebicioglu H, Turan D, Esen S, Onder A, Ozaras R, Ozturk R (2007) Permanent visual loss despite appropriate therapy in tuberculous meningitis. South Med J 100:228–229
24. Meyer S, Struffert T, Gottschling S (2006) Tuberculous meningitis. Lancet 367:1682
25. Tsai MH, Huang YC, Lin TY (2004) Development of tuberculoma during therapy presenting as hemianopsia. Pediatr Neurol 31:360–363
26. do Souto AA, Fonseca AL, Gadelha M, Donangelo I, Chimelli L, Domingues FS (2003) Optic pathways tuberculoma mimicking glioma: case report. Surg Neurol 60:349–353
27. Roberts MT, Mendelson M, Meyer P, Carmichael A, Lever AM (2003) The use of thalidomide in the treatment of intracranial tuberculomas in adults: two case reports. J Infect 47:251–255
28. Sharma K, Pradhan S, Varma A, Rathi B (2003) Irreversible blindness due to multiple tuberculomas in the suprasellar cistern. J Neuroophthalmol 23:211–212
29. Sodhi PK, Grover SB, Singh D, Gulati P (2001) Diagnosis of optochiasmatic tuberculosis revealed by computed tomography and magnetic resonance imaging. Ann Ophthalmol 33:252–256
30. Silverman IE, Liu GT, Bilaniuk LT, Volpe NJ, Galetta SL (1995) Tuberculous meningitis with blindness and perichiasmal involvement on MRI. Pediatr Neurol 12:65–67
31. Poon WS, Ahuja A, Li AK (1993) Optochiasmatic tuberculoma causing progressive visual failure: when has medical treatment failed? Postgrad Med J 69:147–149
32. Teoh R, Poon W, Humphries MJ, O'Mahony G (1988) Suprasellar tuberculoma developing during treatment of tuberculous meningitis requiring urgent surgical decompression. J Neurol 235:321–322
33. Kingsley DP, Hendrickse WA, Kendall BE, Swash M, Singh V (1987) Tuberculous meningitis: role of CT in management and prognosis. J Neurol Neurosurg Psychiatry 50:30–36
34. Navarro IM, Peralta VH, Leon JA, Varela EA, Cahrera JM (1981) Tuberculous optochiasmatic arachnoiditis. Neurosurgery 9:654–660
35. Iraci G, Giordano R, Gerosa M, Pardatscher K, Tomazzoli L (1980) Tuberculoma of the anterior optic pathways: case report. J Neurosurg 52:129–133
36. Scott RM, Sonntag VK, Wilcox LM, Adelman LS, Rockel TH (1977) Visual loss from optochiasmatic arachnoiditis after tuberculous meningitis: case report. J Neurosurg 46:524–526
37. Coyle JT (1969) Chiasmatic arachnoiditis: a case report and review. Am J Ophthalmol 68:345–349
38. Kidd D (2010) The optic chiasm. Handb Clin Neurol 102:185–203
39. Rios JC, Galper MW, Naidich TP (2012) Ventricles and intracranial subarachnoid spaces. In: Naidich TP, Castillo M, Cha S, Smirniotopoulos JG (eds) Imaging of the brain. Elsevier Health Sciences, Philadelphia, pp 245–271
40. Garg RK (2010) Tuberculous meningitis. Acta Neurol Scand 122:75–90
41. Kim DK, Park SN, Park KH, Yeo SW (2014) A case of direct intracranial extension of tuberculous otitis media. Ear Nose Throat J 93:68–74
42. Dando SJ, Mackay-Sim A, Norton R, Currie BJ, John JA, Ekberg JA, Batzloff M, Ulett GC, Beacham IR (2014) Pathogens penetrating the central nervous system: infection pathways and the cellular and molecular mechanisms of invasion. Clin Microbiol Rev 27:691–726
43. Donald PR, Schaaf HS, Schoeman JF (2005) Tuberculous meningitis and miliary tuberculosis: the rich focus revisited. J Infect 50:193–195
44. Thwaites G (2013) The pathophysiology of tuberculosis meningitis. In: Christodoulides M (ed) Meningitis: cellular and molecular basis, vol 26. CAB International, Wallingford/Oxfordshire, pp 153–167
45. Thwaites GE, van Toorn R, Schoeman J (2013) Tuberculous meningitis: more questions, still too few answers. Lancet Neurol 12:999–1010
46. Hosseini H, Tourbah A (1999) Sarcoid related optochiasmatic arachnoiditis: favourable outcome confirmed with MRI. J Neurol Neurosurg Psychiatry 67:690
47. Carpinteri R, Patelli I, Casanueva FF, Giustina A (2009) Inflammatory and granulomatous expansive lesions of the pituitary. Best Pract Res Clin Endocrinol Metab 23:639–650
48. Dhanwal DK, Vyas A, Sharma A, Saxena A (2010) Hypothalamic pituitary abnormalities in tubercular meningitis at the time of diagnosis. Pituitary 13:304–310
49. Dastur DK, Lalitha VS, Udani PM, Parekh US (1970) The brain and meninges in tuberculous meningitis-gross pathology in 100 cases and pathogenesis. Neurol India 18:86–100
50. Afghani B, Lieberman JM (1994) Paradoxical enlargement or development of intracranial tuberculomas during therapy: case report and review. Clin Infect Dis 19:1092–1099
51. Akhaddar A, El Hassani MY, Chakir N, Jiddane M (2001) Optochiasmatic tuberculoma: complication of tuberculous meningitis. Report of a case and review of the literature. J Neuroradiol 28:137–142
52. Teoh R, Humphries MJ, O'Mahony GA (1987) Symptomatic intracranial tuberculoma developing during treatment of tuberculosis: a report of 10 patients and review of the literature. Q J Med 63:449–460
53. Green JA, Chau TT, Farrar JJ, Friedland JS, Thwaites GE (2011) CNS infection, CSF matrix metalloproteinase concentrations, and clinical/laboratory features. Neurology 76:577–579
54. Green JA, Elkington PT, Pennington CJ, Roncaroli F, Dholakia S, Moores RC, Bullen A, Porter JC, Agranoff D, Edwards DR, Friedland JS (2010) Mycobacterium tuberculosis upregulates microglial matrix metalloproteinase-1 and-3 expression and secretion via NF-κB– and activator protein-1–dependent monocyte networks. J Immunol 184:6492–6503

55. Rai D, Garg RK, Mahdi AA, Jain A, Verma R, Tripathi AK, Singh MK, Malhotra HS, Singh GP, Ahmad MK (2014) Cerebrospinal fluid cytokines and matrix metalloproteinases in human immunodeficiency seropositive and seronegative patients of tuberculous meningitis. Ann Indian Acad Neurol 17:171–178
56. Sinha HP, Modi M, Prabhakar S, Singh P (2015) Do cytokines correlate with disease activity in tuberculous meningitis? Neurology Asia 20:243–250
57. Yadav A, Chaudhary C, Keshavan AH, Agarwal A, Verma S, Prasad KN, Rathore RK, Trivedi R, Gupta RK (2010) Correlation of CSF proinflammatory cytokines with MRI in tuberculous meningitis. Acad Radiol 17:194–200
58. Chiang SS, Khan FA, Milstein MB, Tolman AW, Benedetti A, Starke JR, Becerra MC (2014) Treatment outcomes of childhood tuberculous meningitis: a systematic review and meta-analysis. Lancet Infect Dis 14:947–957
59. Christensen AS, Andersen AB, Thomsen VO, Andersen PH, Johansen IS (2011) Tuberculous meningitis in Denmark: a review of 50 cases. BMC Infect Dis 11:47
60. Pehlivanoglu F, Yasar KK, Sengoz G (2012) Tuberculous meningitis in adults: a review of 160 cases. Scientific World Journal 2012:1–6
61. Raut T, Garg RK, Jain A, Verma R, Singh MK, Malhotra HS, Kohli N, Parihar A (2013) Hydrocephalus in tuberculous meningitis: Incidence, its predictive factors and impact on the prognosis. J Infect 66:330–337
62. van Well GT, Paes BF, Terwee CB, Springer P, Roord JJ, Donald PR, van Furth AM, Schoeman JF (2009) Twenty years of pediatric tuberculous meningitis: a retrospective cohort study in the western cape of South Africa. Pediatrics 123:e1–e8
63. Mistr S, Chavis PS (2006) Treatment of neuro-ophthalmologic manifestations of tuberculosis. Curr Treat Options Neurol 8:53–67
64. Davis EJ, Rathinam SR, Okada AA, Tow SL, Petrushkin H, Graham EM, Chee SP, Guex-Crosier Y, Jakob E, Tugal-Tutkun I, Cunningham ET Jr (2012) Clinical spectrum of tuberculous optic neuropathy. J Ophthalmic Inflamm Infect 2:183–189
65. Madge SN, Prabhakaran VC, Shome D, Kim U, Honavar S, Selva D (2008) Orbital tuberculosis: a review of the literature. Orbit 27:267–277
66. Mooney AJ (1956) Some ocular sequelae of tuberculous meningitis: a preliminary survey, 1953–54. Am J Ophthalmol 41:753–768
67. Fernandes M, Vemuganti GK, Pasricha G, Bansal AK, Sangwan VS (2003) Unilateral tuberculous conjunctivitis with tarsal necrosis. Arch Ophthalmol 121:1475–1478
68. Whitford J, Hansman D (1977) Primary tuberculosis of the conjunctiva. Med J Aust 1:486–487
69. Sen DK (1980) Tuberculosis of the orbit and lacrimal gland: a clinical study of 14 cases. J Pediatr Ophthalmol Strabismus 17:232–238
70. Myers TD, Smith JR, Lauer AK, Rosenbaum JT (2002) Iris nodules associated with infectious uveitis. Br J Ophthalmol 86:969–974
71. Seward DN (1973) Tuberculoma of the ciliary body. Med J Aust 1:297
72. Tabbara KF (2005) Ocular tuberculosis: anterior segment. Int Ophthalmol Clin 45:57–69
73. Nanda M, Pflugfelder SC, Holland S (1989) Mycobacterium tuberculosis scleritis. Am J Ophthalmol 108:736–737
74. Massaro D, Katz S, Sachs M (1964) Choroidal tubercles: a clue to hematogenous tuberculosis. Ann Intern Med 60:231–241
75. Gupta V, Gupta A, Arora S, Bambery P, Dogra MR, Agarwal A (2003) Presumed tubercular serpiginous like choroiditis: clinical presentations and management. Ophthalmology 110:1744–1749
76. Mansour AM (1998) Optic disk tubercle. J Neuroophthalmol 18:201–203
77. Chawla R, Garg S, Venkatesh P, Kashyap S, Tewari HK (2004) Case report of tuberculous panophthalmitis. Med Sci Monit 10:CS57–CS59
78. Malhotra HS, Garg RK, Gupta A, Saxena S, Majumdar A, Jain A (2012) An unusual cause of visual impairment in tuberculous meningitis. J Neurol Sci 318:174–177
79. Stechschulte SU, Kim RY, Cunningham ET (1999) Tuberculous neuroretinitis. J Neuroophthalmol 19: 201–204
80. Moldow B, La Cour M (2003) Eales' disease in Inuit: report of four cases. Acta Ophthalmol Scand 81:304–308
81. Hartmann E (1945) Optochiasmic arachnoiditis. Arch Ophthalmol 33:68–77
82. Werring DJ, Marsden CD (1999) Visual hallucinations and palinopsia due to an occipital lobe tuberculoma. J Neurol Neurosurg Psychiatry 66:684
83. Verma BM, Srivastava SK, Srivastava JR (1981) Ocular menifestations of tubercular meningitis and their prognostic value in children. Indian J Ophthalmol 29:301–302
84. Lana-Peixoto MA, Bambirra EA, Pittella JE (1980) Optic nerve tuberculoma: a case report. Arch Neurol 37:186–187
85. Schlernitzauer DA, Hodges FJ, Bagan M (1971) Tuberculoma of the left optic nerve and chiasm. Arch Ophthalmol 85:75–78
86. Monga PK, Dhaliwal U (2009) Paradoxical reaction in tubercular meningitis resulting in involvement of optic radiation. Indian J Ophthalmol 57:139–141
87. Aaron S, Mathew V, Anupriya A, Sunithi M, Maya T, Goel M, Alexander M (2010) Tuberculous optochiasmatic arachnoiditis. Neurol India 58:732–735
88. Sinha MK, Garg RK, Anuradha HK, Agarwal A, Parihar A, Mandhani PA (2010) Paradoxical vision loss associated with optochiasmatic tuberculoma in tuberculous meningitis: a report of 8 patients. J Infect 60:458–466
89. Brancusi F, Farrar J, Heemskerk D (2012) Tuberculous meningitis in adults: a review of a decade of developments focusing on prognostic factors for outcome. Future Microbiol 7:1101–1116

90. Garg RK, Paliwal V, Malhotra HS (2011) Tuberculous optochiasmatic arachnoiditis: a devastating form of tuberculous meningitis. Expert Rev Anti Infect Ther 9:719–729
91. Iraci G, Galligioni F, Gerosa M, Secchi AG, Fiore D, Zampieri P, Rigobello L, Tomazzoli L, Pardatscher K, Marin G, Scattolin R (1979) Opto-chiasmatic arachnoiditis: a review of traditional neuroradiological diagnosis (82 cases, 1951–1976). Acta Neurochir 48:151–176
92. Andronikou S, Smith B, Hatherhill M, Douis H, Wilmshurst J (2004) Definitive neuroradiological diagnostic features of tuberculous meningitis in children. Pediatr Radiol 34:876–885
93. Anuradha HK, Garg RK, Agarwal A, Sinha MK, Verma R, Singh MK, Shukla R (2010) Predictors of stroke in patients of tuberculous meningitis and its effect on the outcome. QJM 103:671–678
94. Vail D (1939) Syphilitic opticochiasmatic arachnoiditis. Am J Ophthalmol 22:505–517
95. Bollack J, David M, Puech P, Société française d'ophtalmologie (1937) Les Arachnoïdites optochiasmatiques: étude ophtalmologique et neurochirurgicale. Masson & Cie, Paris
96. Maruki C, Nakano H, Shimoji T, Maeda M, Ishii S (1988) Loss of vision due to cryptococcal optochiasmatic arachnoiditis and optocurative surgical exploration. Neurol Med Chir (Tokyo) 28:695–697
97. Iraci G, Pellone M, Scuccimarra A, Fiore D (1976) Posttraumatic optochiasmatic arachnoiditis. Ann Ophthalmol 8:1313–1328
98. Tang RA, Grotta JC, Lee KF, Lee YE (1983) Chiasmal syndrome in sarcoidosis. Arch Ophthalmol 101:1069–1073
99. Bell RA, Robertson DM, Rosen DA, Kerr AW (1975) Optochiasmatic arachnoiditis in multiple sclerosis. Arch Ophthalmol 93:191–193
100. Gruber H, Pendl G (1980) Paraneoplastic optochiasmatic arachnoiditis (author's transl). Klin Monbl Augenheilkd 177:380–383
101. Carreras EM, Lyons CJ, Cochrane DD (2014) Delayed visual loss from optochiasmatic arachnoiditis after resection of craniopharyngioma: case report. J Neurosurg Pediatr 13:520–524
102. World Health Organization (2010) Treatment of tuberculosis: guidelines. World Health Organization, Geneva
103. Shane SJ, Copp SE, Krzyski TK (1956) Tuberculous meningitis: combined corticosteroid and antimicrobial therapy. Can Med Assoc J 75:631
104. Buonsenso D, Serranti D, Valentini P (2010) Management of central nervous system tuberculosis in children: light and shade. Eur Rev Med Pharmacol Sci 14:845–853
105. Green JA, Tran CT, Farrar JJ, Nguyen MT, Nguyen PH, Dinh SX, Ho ND, Ly CV, Tran HT, Friedland JS, Thwaites GE (2009) Dexamethasone, cerebrospinal fluid matrix metalloproteinase concentrations and clinical outcomes in tuberculous meningitis. PLoS One 4:e7277
106. Shah I, Meshram L (2014) High dose versus low dose steroids in children with tuberculous meningitis. J Clin Neurosci 21:761–764
107. Thwaites GE, Bang ND, Dung NH, Quy HT, Oanh DT, Thoa NT, Hien NQ, Thuc NT, Hai NN, Lan NT, Lan NN (2004) Dexamethasone for the treatment of tuberculous meningitis in adolescents and adults. N Engl J Med 351:1741–1751
108. Corral LG, Kaplan G (1999) Immunomodulation by thalidomide and thalidomide analogues. Ann Rheum Dis 58:i107–i113
109. Tsenova L, Sokol K, Victoria HF, Kaplan G (1998) A combination of thalidomide plus antibiotics protects rabbits from mycobacterial meningitis-associated death. J Infect Dis 177:1563–1572
110. Schoeman JF, Springer P, Ravenscroft A, Donald PR, Bekker LG, van Rensburg AJ, Hanekom WA, Haslett PA, Kaplan G (2000) Adjunctive thalidomide therapy of childhood tuberculous meningitis: possible anti-inflammatory role. J Child Neurol 15:497–503
111. Schoeman JF, Springer P, van Rensburg AJ, Swanevelder S, Hanekom WA, Haslett PA, Kaplan G (2004) Adjunctive thalidomide therapy for childhood tuberculous meningitis: results of a randomized study. J Child Neurol 19:250–257
112. Tsenova L, Mangaliso B, Muller G, Chen Y, Freedman VH, Stirling D, Kaplan G (2002) Use of IMiD3, a thalidomide analog, as an adjunct to therapy for experimental tuberculous meningitis. Antimicrob Agents Chemother 46:1887–1895
113. Schoeman JF, Fieggen G, Seller N, Mendelson M, Hartzenberg B (2006) Intractable intracranial tuberculous infection responsive to thalidomide: report of four cases. J Child Neurol 21:301–308
114. Schoeman JF, Andronikou S, Stefan DC, Freeman N, van Toorn R (2010) Tuberculous meningitis-related optic neuritis: recovery of vision with thalidomide in 4 consecutive cases. J Child Neurol 25:822–828
115. Cathie IA, MacFarlane JC (1950) Adjuvants to streptomycin in treating tuberculous meningitis in children. Lancet 256:784–789
116. Lorber J (1964) Fibrinolytic agents in the treatment of tuberculous meningitis. J Clin Pathol 17:353–354
117. Fletcher AP (1954) Intrathecal fibrinolysis with streptokinase in tuberculous meningitis. J Clin Invest 33:69
118. Owens G, Clark SL (1956) Some effects of injections of hyaluronidase into the subarachnoid space of experimental animals. J Neurosurg 13:223–229
119. Gourie-Devi M, Satishchandra P (1991) Hyaluronidase as an adjuvant in the management of tuberculous spinal arachnoiditis. J Neurol Sci 102:105–111
120. Gourie-Devi M, Satish P (1980) Hyaluronidase as an adjuvant in the treatment of cranial arachnoiditis (hydrocephalus and optochiasmatic arachnoiditis) complicating tuberculous meningitis. Acta Neurol Scand 62:368–381

121. Lee JY, Yim JJ, Yoon BW (2012) Adjuvant interferon-γ treatment in two cases of refractory tuberculosis of the brain. Clin Neurol Neurosurg 114:732–734
122. Blackmore TK, Manning L, Taylor WJ, Wallis RS (2008) Therapeutic use of infliximab in tuberculosis to control severe paradoxical reaction of the brain and lymph nodes. Clin Infect Dis 47:e83–e85
123. Dickmann GH, Cramer FK, Kaplan AD (1951) Opto-chiasmatic arachnoiditis: surgical treatment and results. J Neurosurg 8:355–359
124. Marcus AO, Demakas JJ, Ross AH, Duick DS, Crowell RM (1986) Optochiasmatic arachnoiditis with treatment by surgical lysis of adhesions, corticosteroids, and cyclophosphamide: report of a case. Neurosurgery 19:101–103
125. Hsu PC, Yang CC, Ye JJ, Huang PY, Chiang PC, Lee MH (2010) Prognostic factors of tuberculous meningitis in adults: a 6-year retrospective study at a tertiary hospital in northern Taiwan. J Microbiol Immunol Infect 43:111–118
126. Kalkan A, Serhatlioglu S, Ozden M, Denk A, Demirdag K, Yilmaz T, Kilic SS (2006) Paradoxically developed optochiasmatic tuberculoma and tuberculous lymphadenitis: a case report with 18-month follow up by MRI. Southern medical journal 99:388–393
127. Purvin V, Herr GJ, De Myer W (1988) Chiasmal neuritis as a complication of Epstein-Barr virus infection. Archives of neurology 45:458–460

Peripheral Neuropathy Due to Tuberculosis

23

Bhushan Malhari Warpe

Contents

Abbreviations

AFB	Acid fast bacilli
CBC	Complete blood count
CD	Cluster of differentiation
CNS	Central nervous system
CT	Computed tomography
EMB	Ethambutol
EMG	Electromyography
FNAC	Fine-needle aspiration cytology
GAN	Greater auricular nerve
GBS	Guillain-Barré syndrome
H&E	Hematoxylin and Eosin
HIV	Human immunodeficiency virus
IENFD	Intraepidermal nerve fiber density
INH	Isoniazid
MRI	Magnetic resonance imaging
NCS	Nerve conduction study
PN	Peripheral neuropathy
PNS	Peripheral nervous system
PZA	Pyrazinamide
RIF	Rifampicin
STR	Streptomycin
TB	Tuberculosis
TSH	Thyroid-stimulating hormone
USG	Ultrasonography
ZN	Ziehl-Neelsen

B.M. Warpe, MBBS, MD, DNB (Pathology)
Department of Pathology, B.K.L. Walawalkar Rural Medical College, Shreekshetra Dervan, Kasarwadi, At post-Sawarde, Chiplun, District-Ratnagiri, 415606, Maharashtra, India
e-mail: bhushan.warpe@gmail.com

M. Turgut et al. (eds.), *Tuberculosis of the Central Nervous System*,
DOI 10.1007/978-3-319-50712-5_23

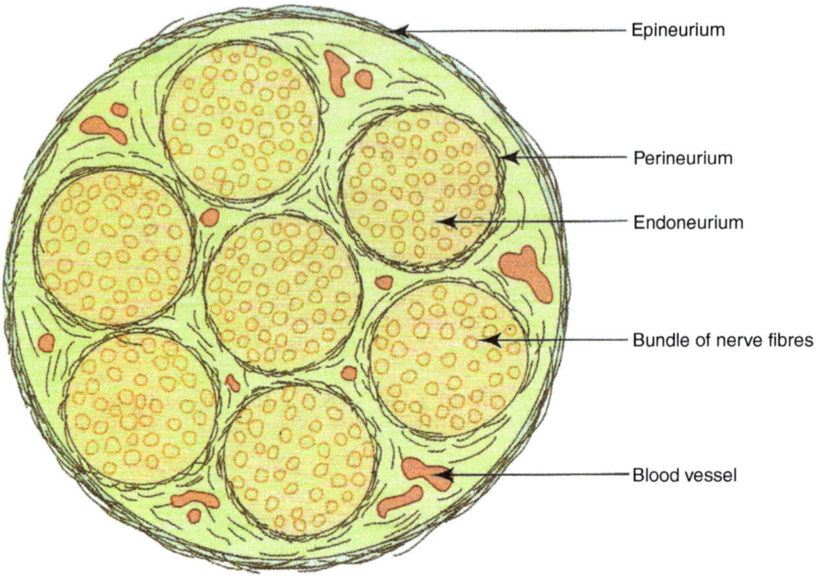

Fig. 23.1 Normal histology – pictorial representation: transverse cut section of a peripheral nerve

23.1 Introduction

Tuberculosis (TB) is a disease with exuberant body tissues being involved and can show unexpected ways of clinical presentation, especially in developing countries wherein it is rampant. The primary involvement of peripheral nerves must be considered as peripheral neuropathy (PN) due to TB may not be always iatrogenic [1–4]. Retrospectively, an expected good outcome to anti-TB therapy confirms the diagnosis of TB [1–4]. High degree of suspicion in such TB cases is required with unexpected ways of presentation. Prompt diagnosis and timely inception of anti-TB therapy can help prevent complications like PN and, thus, avoid unwanted surgeries in such patients.

23.2 Histology of Normal Peripheral Nerve

Each peripheral nerve (spinal or cranial) is made of bundles of nerve fibers (axons) which may be nonmyelinated axons and/or myelinated axons. The axons which are myelinated are surrounded by a multilayered myelin sheath. The Schwann cells cover the nerve fibers, and each Schwann cell contains one myelinated fiber or several nonmyelinated fibers [5].

The bundles are held together by connective tissue which provides structural support as well as nutritional support by carrying blood vessels to nerve fibers. The connective tissue framework is well appreciated in cross section of a nerve, where the following structures can be observed (Fig. 23.1) [5]:

Epineurium: dense connective tissue surrounding the entire nerve

Perineurium: a sleeve of flattened specialized epithelial cells surrounding the bundles of nerve fibers

Endoneurium: loose connective tissue composed of reticular fibers supporting individual nerve fibers

23.3 Peripheral Neuropathy

23.3.1 Introduction to Peripheral Neuropathy

The disease or harm affecting the peripheral nerves, which curtails the normal functions of organs/glands or other health aspects like locomotion, which is related to the type of nerve affected, is called PN. The systemic diseases like leprosy and diabetes, deficiency of vitamins, drugs like chemotherapeutic agents, radiation treatment, trauma, extreme alcoholism, impaired immune system, celiac disease, or infections caused by viruses are common etiologies of PN.

- PN is of two types: genetic (present since birth) or idiopathic (unknown cause) [6, 7].
  - PN can also be classified as follows [6–8]:
    1. PN wherein just one nerve is involved is called "mononeuropathy."
    2. PN affecting multiple or numerous nerves in almost the same areas on both the body sides is called "symmetrical polyneuropathy" or simply "polyneuropathy."
    3. PN is called as "mononeuritis multiplex," "multifocal mononeuropathy," or "multiple mononeuropathy," when two or more discrete nerves in different areas of the body are involved.
  - PN can also be classified as:

1. Acute PN (an acute neuropathy with sudden occurrence, fast progression, and slow resolution). Acute neuropathies need prompt diagnosis.
2. Chronic PN (a chronic state wherein clinical symptoms of neuropathy occur and progress slowly).

Sensory nerves that carry body sensations to organs/tissues, motor nerves which facilitate muscle activity, and autonomic nervous system which helps facilitate heart rate, temperature of the body, and respiration can be involved by PN. Simultaneously, more than one type of nerve can be involved by PN.

PN affecting the motor nerves can cause body cramps, twitching of muscles, muscle atrophy, and degeneration of tissues like bones/skin/hair/nails. Also weakened muscles, faulty body balance/posture, and incoordination are the result of PN affecting the motor nerves.

Sensory neuropathy results in loss of touch/vibration/position sense causing improper coordination, impaired sensitivity to change in temperature, tingling, and burning sensation of the body with pain sensation even on non-painful light touch stimuli called allodynia.

PN affecting autonomic nervous system causes varied symptoms, based on the type of glands/organs which are involved, but commonly seen are improper control of urinary bladder, altered blood pressure or heart rate, and decreased normal capacity to sweat [6–8].

23.3.2 Signs and Symptoms of Peripheral Neuropathy

The expected normal functions of peripheral nerves are affected by diseases or improper functioning of the respective nerves. The signs and symptoms are different based on the type of the nerve fiber that is affected.

PN affecting the sensory nerve function commonly includes the following:

- Functional loss or "negative" symptoms: impaired gait and body balance and numbness of limbs
- Functional gain or "positive" symptoms: pricking kind of pain, itching, tingling sensation, and crawling sensation [9]

PN affecting the motor nerve function commonly includes the following:

- Functional loss or "negative" symptoms: muscle loss, body weakness, easy fatigability, and gait problems
- Functional gain or "positive" symptoms: muscle cramps and twitching of muscles [10]

Generally in nerve length-dependent PN, abnormal altered sensation and pain occur symmetrically and usually affect the ends of long nerves such as those at distal ends of lower limbs. Also important to note is the fact that sensory signs and symptoms due to PN usually precede motor signs and symptoms such as muscle weakness [11]. PN affecting "nerves of the autonomic nervous system" causes symptoms like micturition difficulty, standing posture induced whirling sensation, hard stools, and xerostomia [10].

23.3.3 Diagnosis of Peripheral Neuropathy

When a patient presents with clinical signs and symptoms such as pricking pain sensation and limb weakness, PN must be taken into consideration. On ruling out CNS lesions by appropriate investigations like CT brain or MRI brain, the diagnosis of PN must be favored based on clinical/family history, lab investigations, and detailed checkup [11]. The patients who have generalized neuropathies generally have loss of distal motor/sensory neural functions, although patients with peripheral nerve lesions may apparently appear normal.

There are inflammatory neuropathies like GBS which cause proximal weakness, while in mononeuropathies, there are focal sensory/motor disturbances. Typically, in PN, ankle jerk reflex is absent [11].

The physical exam of the patient must be done. One must look out for feet ulcerations apart from absent deep ankle reflex.

When large nerve fiber-related PN occurs, the physical examination reveals reduced sensation of light touch/vibration sense. Reduced sensation to vibration sense is elicited by tuning fork test using a 128-Hz tuning fork. Other advanced tests like EMG and NCS can help examine the large myelinated nerve fiber function [11].

The PN due to autonomic nervous system dysfunction tends to affect the tiny thin and non-myelinated nerve fibers, and such affection causes small-fiber PN. Sweat test and tilt-table tests can be used to diagnose PN due to small nerve fiber involvement. A skin biopsy of 3 mm thickness from calf muscle is taken to measure the skin intraepidermal nerve fiber density (IENFD), that is, the nerve density in the outer skin layer (epidermis) is measured [9]. The decreased small nerve fibers in the epidermis help in diagnosing the condition of small-fiber PN.

Laboratory work-ups include CBC, vitamin B12 assays, levels of thyroid-stimulating hormone (TSH), metabolic work-up to screen for diabetes and prediabetes, and serum immunofixation test to test for antibodies present in blood [10].

23.3.4 Causes of Peripheral Neuropathy

The causes of PN are broadly narrated as follows:

- Genetic disorders: Charcot-Marie-Tooth disease [12], hereditary neuropathy with increased chances of pressure palsy, and Friedreich's ataxia.
- Toxic causes: drugs overdose (statins, phenytoin, vincristine, metronidazole, nitrofurantoin), ethyl alcohol [13, 14], organic herbicides, organic/heavy metals, and excess vitamin B6 intake. Long-term linezolid treatment can also cause PN.
- Adverse outcome of fluoroquinolones: associated with irreversible neuropathy [15].
- Metabolic and endocrine disorders: liver failure, porphyria, amyloidosis, hypothyroidism, diabetes mellitus [16], and chronic renal failure.
- Vitamin deficiency conditions: vitamin B1 (thiamine), vitamin B12 (methylcobalamin), vitamin E, and vitamin A.
- Inflammatory diseases: SLE, GBS, multiple sclerosis, leprosy, Sjögren's syndrome, Lyme disease, babesiosis, and sarcoidosis [17].
- Traumatic conditions: projectile injuries (including gunshot injuries), strokes, prolonged blood flow occlusion, cutting, compression, pinching, and lightning strikes.
- Agent Orange exposure [18].
- Chemotherapy-induced PN [19].
- Other causes: electric shock injury, HIV [20], radiation therapy, malignant conditions, shingles, and TB [1–4].

23.4 Peripheral Neuropathy Due to Tuberculosis

23.4.1 Introduction to Tuberculosis-Related Peripheral Neuropathy

One out of three individuals in the world is affected by TB. It is a leading cause of human morbidity and mortality which mostly present with cervical lymphadenopathy [21]. TB, a disease caused by *Mycobacterium tuberculosis*, is an infectious disease that continues to be a significant health problem in a developing country like India [22].

Early diagnosis for strategic management requires high index of clinical suspicion and systematic patient work-up. The usual diagnostic methods employed worldwide are histopathology, smear microscopy/fine-needle aspiration cytology (FNAC), and mycobacterial culture on biopsy [22].

TB is a chronic granulomatous disease. Granuloma is a collection of epithelioid cells. Granulomatous inflammation in histopathology means central caseation necrosis surrounded by epithelioid cells, Langhans giant cells, foreign-body giant cells, and peripheral rim of lymphocytes which are surrounded by fibroblastic proliferation.

Lymphadenitis with granulomas can be seen in numerous conditions like sarcoidosis, lymphomas, carcinoma, sarcoma, fungal infections, toxoplasmosis, cat-scratch disease, inflammatory bowel diseases, collagen-vascular disorders, and reticuloendothelial system-related disorders. Ziehl-Neelsen (ZN) stain in FNAC and its modified version of Fite-Faraco stain for tissue/biopsy help highlight the acid-fast bacilli (AFB) in such cases. However, little is known about primary involvement of PN due to TB [22].

TB neuropathy has been reported in optic nerve, cranial nerve II, but very few reports exist on TB-related PN [23–25]. PN is a unique and unusual presentation of TB. Important differential diagnoses of the TB-related PN are sarcoidosis, leprosy, external jugular vein thrombosis, and lymphadenitis (specific/nonspecific). PN due to TB is under-reported due to lack of awareness because leprosy comes first to mind rather than TB.

The cause of PN associated with TB is controversial. The possible etiologies include toxic reactions of anti-TB therapy, especially with rifampicin (RIF), pyrazinamide (PZA), isoniazid (INH) and ethambutol (EMB). Also direct invasion of nerves, immune-mediated damage and neuropathy, vasculitic and compressive neuropathy, and meningitic reaction are possible causes [1–5].

23.4.2 Tuberculosis-Related Peripheral Neuropathy: Reported Manuscripts

23.4.2.1 Tuberculosis Affecting Sural Nerve

Orrell et al. (2002) reported the first case of peripheral nerve/right sural nerve granuloma in a TB patient of African origin, living in England [1]. The patient was a 23-year-old gentleman who had pricking sensation in his soles that propagated to his toes. His condition worsened in a month of follow-up with bilateral foot drop, numb toes, and weakened ankles. Further after three months, the patient noticed right-sided cervical lymphadenopathy and a liver mass. Various clinical neurological tests and lab tests were conducted. EMG revealed lower limb involvement of distal sensory and motor axonal polyneuropathy.

Neck lymph node biopsy revealed many large caseating TB granuloma with modified ZN stain contributory for AFB. The biopsy of the sural nerve conducted to assess the inflammatory/vasculitic component to neuropathy revealed noncaseating TB-related granuloma with inflammation and without giant cells. ZN stain was not contributory for AFB in the sural nerve. There was marked immunostaining for CD-4 T-lymphocytes and also for CD-68 cells in the area of granuloma which is a macrophage-monocyte marker. The lymphocytes were also sparsely immunostained with CD-8. They started the patient on anti-TB therapy, and patient's peripheral nerve condition improved significantly later on follow-up-based clinical tests.

This patient's report described the rare caseating TB granulomas in the right sural nerve with subsequent TB lymphadenopathy. The TB-related PN was seen before anti-TB therapy was started. The delayed hypersensitivity reaction without specific indication of PN mechanism was suggested as the pathological explanation for the patient's problem.

This case infers that cervical TB lymphadenopathy may clinically present after TB-related PN. Starting the patient on anti-TB therapy is the ultimate remedy for such cases. Biopsy of sural nerve was instrumental for diagnosis of TB-related PN. Systematic work-up leads to best management in such cases.

23.4.2.2 Tuberculosis Affecting Phrenic Nerve in Children

In a South African-based, case series study by Goussard et al. (2009), pediatric phrenic nerve palsy was related to be associated with confirmed cases of intrathoracic TB [4]. In this case series of eight cases, pediatric phrenic nerve palsy was associated with phrenic nerve infiltration after TB lymphadenitis. TB lymphadenitis was confirmed by culture studies, and *Mycobacterium tuberculosis* was the bacteria cultured in all of the eight cases.

Elevated diaphragm on chest X-ray along with left upper lobe consolidation was seen in all the eight cases studied. Chest fluoroscopy studies helped confirm the phrenic nerve palsy. On CT-chest study, left-sided hilar and paratracheal lymph glands were enlarged along with right-sided mediastinal displacement.

Two out of the eight pediatric cases had complication of respiratory failure requiring intensive respiratory support. Five out of the eight pediatric cases continued to remain symptomatic after anti-TB therapy for which corticosteroids were supplemented in the first month on their respective admission. In all five cases, diaphragmatic plication was done.

On proper follow-up, two out of the eight pediatric cases had repeated respiratory tract infections due to underlying lung damage, while the remaining six were found to be asymptomatic.

In conclusion, in cases of pediatric TB, look for chest or other CNS complaints. CT-chest and chest X-ray can show mediastinal shift and diaphragmatic changes related to phrenic nerve palsy. Phrenic nerve palsy is confirmed on fluoroscopy.

23.4.2.3 Tuberculosis Affecting Peripheral Nerves of Both Lower Limbs

Naha et al. (2011) illustrated the need to keep high degree of clinical suspicion for TB in mind, in patients with unexplained PN when associated with systemic symptoms of TB. They also inferred that the disseminated TB cases can present unusually with associated breast lump with positive AFB in breast lump FNAC along with sputum AFB smear positivity [26].

A 25-year-old human immunodeficiency virus (HIV) sero-negative housewife from Karnataka, India, came with complaint of burning sensation in both feet for previous 15 months. She had weight loss and fever for six months. She also had a palpable left breast lump from 30 days.

On physical examination, allodynia and hyperesthesia were noted over the lower extremities. Sensory neuropathy was confirmed by NCS. Chronic axonopathy was diagnosed on nerve biopsy study. Palpable left breast lump aspirate and sputum were positive for AFB.

Patient was a case of disseminated TB with bilateral distal lower limb PN (exact nerve not quoted in this literature but may be sural nerve was involved bilaterally). The disseminated TB patient responded well to anti-TB therapy, later with subsequent disappearance of tingling sensation and other systemic symptoms.

In conclusion, disseminated TB may have unusual presentation and needs proper work-up as complaints of PN may follow other clinical signs and symptoms like chest complaints, lymphadenopathy, weight loss, low-grade fever, and even unusual breast lump due to TB. With disseminated TB, HIV testing is a must due to frequent association with TB.

23.4.2.4 Tuberculosis Affecting Median Nerve

Poulose et al. (2011) reported a TB case affecting the median nerve in Kerala, India [27]. A 21-year-old female patient presented with slow-growing, left forearm swelling on volar aspect of 10-week duration, extending into the wrist measuring around 5 cm × 2 cm. Marked tingling sensation was seen along the distribution course of the left median nerve. There were no distal neurological deficits.

The local ultrasonography (USG) of the swelling had revealed features suggestive of chronic tenosynovitis. Local MRI was done which showed raised uptake in STIR and TIW images with altered signal along the course of the median nerve reaching up to carpal tunnel. On preoperative exploration, median nerve was thickened, and there was left median nerve which was inseparable from the soft tissue swelling (Fig. 23.2). With these intraoperative findings, peripheral nerve tumor like schwannoma/neurofibroma became the operative diagnosis; however, the affected nerve was not resected.

On cutting the affected median nerve longitudinally, on operation table, the findings noted were of thickened nerve sheaths with granular material within it. The granular material within the nerve substance was sent for histopathology. The surgeons planned for second definite surgery after histopathology report. Biopsy revealed features of caseating chronic granulomatous lesion consistent with diagnosis of peripheral nerve TB. They suggested that it must be due to direct infiltration of median nerve by TB bacilli. The patient responded well to anti-TB therapy, and there was subsequent disappearance of tingling sensation and other symptoms. The TB-related PN was before anti-TB therapy was started and it subsided with this therapy.

In conclusion, intra-operative alertness is required with high degree of suspicion and biopsy rather than nerve resection is important here in such cases, since hateful surgery is a total waste.

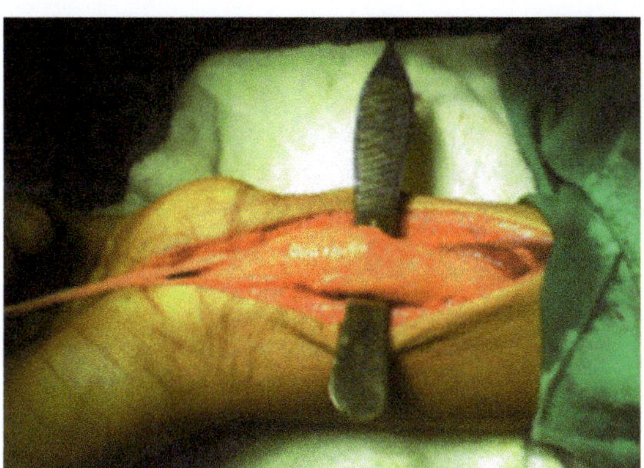

Fig. 23.2 Preoperative findings – thickened median nerve of left upper limb

23.4.2.5 TB Affecting Greater Auricular Nerve (GAN): First Reported Case

In 2014, I came across a single, discrete cervical nerve affected by TB after TB lymphadenitis, which is the first case with TB-related PN involving a cervical based peripheral nerve [2]. In our patient, the neuropathy preceded the anti-TB therapy. The primary involvement of peripheral nerves must be considered as PN due to TB may not be always iatrogenic.

A 69-year-old female presented with left-sided neck swelling since 13 months and pain over the swelling since one week. She also complained of progressive weight loss for the last six months. On examination, a single, 9 × 2 × 1 cm firm, tender, tubular swelling was noted over the left side of the neck. The chest X-ray and neck X-ray were normal. Neck USG report was suspicious of thrombosed retromandibular vein, and non-contrast computed tomography (CT) of the neck was indicative of thrombosis of the left external jugular vein. CT chest revealed no specific finding like lung consolidation, pleural effusion, or malignancy. USG abdomen and CT abdomen performed for the presence of lymphadenopathy or any other mass lesion revealed mild hepatomegaly with no evidence of primary malignancy.

With the suspicion of a cervical vascular lesion, FNAC study of the swelling was not performed. Based on the clinical and radiological findings, this patient was operated under general anesthesia. The excised mass from the left side of the neck was sent for histopathological study (Fig. 23.3). On gross examination, the specimen consisted of a single cord-like tubular tissue of size 9 × 2 × 0.5 cm, with an irregular mass adhered to its center with minute yellowish, 2–3 mm-sized tiny nodules on the external surface.

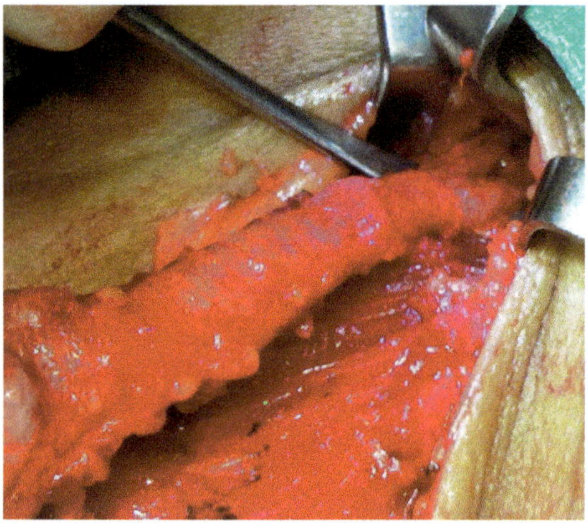

Fig. 23.3 The dissected cord-like structure with minute 2–3 mm nodules on the external surface

On hematoxylin and eosin (H&E) staining, caseating epithelioid cell granulomas were identified in the lymph nodes, the nerve substance, and the surrounding tissue. Special stains for AFB performed on the lymph node and the nerve were negative. With characteristic microscopic features, the final impression given was TB lymphadenitis with perineuritis and nerve granuloma (Fig. 23.4). TB specialists started the patient on anti-TB therapy based on the histopathological report and their clinical suspicion.

During follow-up at three months, local examination revealed no pain or residual swelling in the neck, and the patient responded well to anti-TB therapy. On follow-up at six months, the patient had no recurrent swelling and had regained the lost body weight with a sense of well-being. However, because of nerve resection, she developed postoperative sensory deficit over the region supplied by greater auricular nerve (GAN), i.e., the skin present over the parotid gland, both the aural surfaces and the corresponding mastoid process.

In conclusion, neck swelling can present with GAN-related neural pain rather than palpable TB

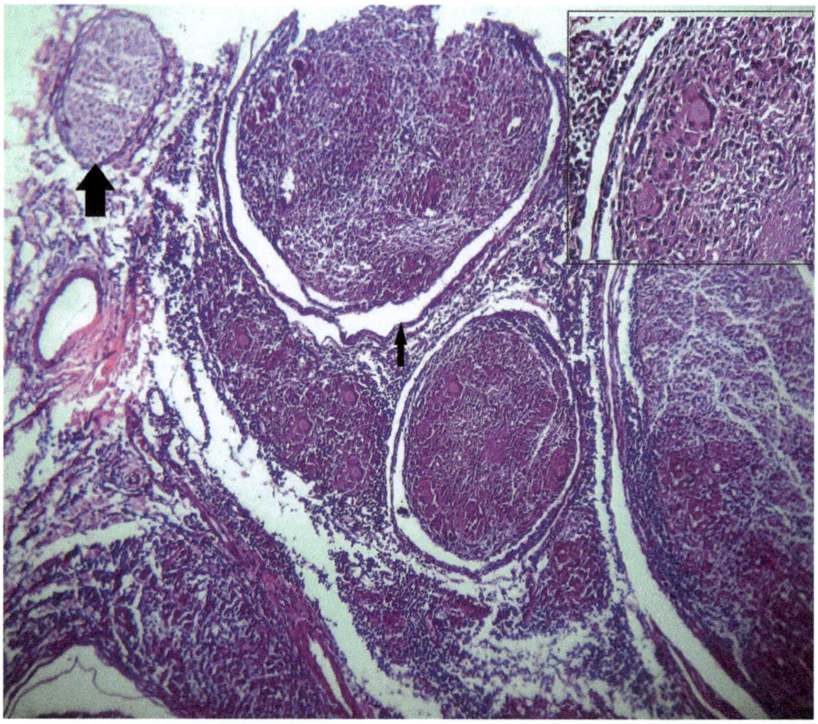

Fig. 23.4 Caseating granulomas in the nerve fascicles and surrounding lymphoid tissue [hematoxylin and eosin (H&E), ×100], *thin arrow* denotes perineurium, while *thick arrow* shows uninvolved nerve fascicle. *Inset* (H&E, 400) – granuloma with Langhans giant cell inside the nerve substance proper

lymphadenopathy and without any findings suggestive of TB or other granulomatous lesion somewhere else in the body. Lack of preoperative documentation of the evidence of TB can be a problem in such cases. Wrong work-up or diagnosis like CT-diagnosed neck vascular lesion can make doctors apprehensive of advising FNAC or biopsy. Here patient had preoperative examination followed by nerve resection or excisional biopsy after ruling out the vascular lesion on the operation table. The resected GAN, neural tissue revealed TB granulomas within the neural substance and within the surrounding lymph nodes. The patient had responded well to anti-TB therapy, but due to GAN resection, the patient had sensory deficit locally over the area supplied by GAN. Ideally, CT neck should have been reported twice with a senior radiologist's opinion in such a case. In this case, after alleged minute regional cervical lymphadenopathy, GAN got involved after perilymphadenitis.

23.4.2.6 Tuberculosis Affecting Greater Auricular Nerve (GAN): Second Reported Case

In 2015, Chaurasia et al. from Varanasi, Uttar Pradesh, India, reported the second case of GAN/cervical nerve involvement in a 30-year-old man [28]. Clinically the patient had a tubular shaped swelling in the right side of the neck, which proved to be TB neuritis involving GAN, pathologically. This patient had tubular, cord-like, subcutaneous tender lump in the right side of the neck measuring 4 × 1.2 cm along with same sided reddish discoloration of the cheek, which was involved along the distribution/supply of anterior and posterior branches of GAN. It had caused impaired pain and temperature sensations on corresponding area. Clinically leprous neuritis and external jugular vein thrombosis were the differentials that were thought.

USG neck report suggested it as superficial GAN/nerve thickening. Then multidrug therapy for leprosy was given to patient without clinical improvement. The USG neck ruled out possibility of any vein thrombosis. FNAC advised from the neck lump was diagnostic as patient was not willing for a biopsy. FNAC from the cervical nerve revealed tuberculous caseating granuloma, with positive AFB on ZN staining. The patient showed good response on anti-TB therapy.

In conclusion, in this case, no response to multidrug therapy for leprosy, FNAC smear showing caseating epithelioid cell granuloma, and positive AFB stain on ZN staining helped diagnose the case. Here without biopsy, FNAC and good response to anti-TB therapy retrospectively helped confirm the diagnosis of TB-related GAN involvement.

23.4.3 Tuberculosis-Related Peripheral Neuropathy: Associated Findings and Discussion

Lymphadenitis is the most frequent presentation of extrapulmonary TB. Cervical lymph nodes are the commonest lymph nodes to get involved and present as a neck mass [29, 30]. However, cervical nerve involvement associated with cervical lymphadenitis is rarely quoted in literature. True infectious diseases of peripheral nerves are rare. PN commonly occurs following exanthematous fevers and as a complication of various acute bacterial infections [31, 32].

One of the commonest causes of PN is leprosy. In lepromatous leprosy, there is peripheral nerve infiltration by lepra bacilli along with inflammatory cells and fibroblastic growth resulting in fusiform enlargement of the affected nerves. The peripheral nerve involvement in tuberculoid leprosy is due to acute neuritis [33].

Neuropathy in patients with TB was in the past mostly related to chronic alcoholism, malnutrition, anti-TB therapy [34], and meningitis-related radiculopathy [31, 34].

In TB, cellular response comprises of macrophages and lymphocytes (TH_1). The accumulated macrophages transform to epithelioid histiocytes by interferon gamma, secreted by TH_1 lymphocytic cells and characterized by granulomatous response of TB [33]. It is unknown as to how the caseating neural granulomas are related to the symptoms and signs of PN. Possible etiologies include vascular effect or nerve compressive effect or cytokine-mediated nerve damage and subsequent PN.

Peripheral nerves can be directly affected by TB. PN can be due to pressure effects on peripheral nerves and toxic neural damage caused by TB exudative fluid [34]. PN is a unique and unusual presentation of TB and is attributed to compression by vertebral collapse or cold abscess according to Naha et al. [26]. They have concluded that advanced studies are required to understand the neurotoxicity-based mechanism in TB and thus pinpoint the exact mediators. Nerve involvement secondary to regional TB lymphadenitis is reported by Goussard et al. [4]. They have published a case series involving eight pediatric cases of phrenic nerve palsy caused by TB lymphadenitis and its subsequent phrenic nerve infiltration. According to them, nerve compression by inflammatory granulomatous tissue is responsible for PN.

TB neuritis occurring after starting anti-TB therapy has been studied, especially by INH and EMB drugs [35, 36]. INH has propensity to combine with pyridoxine (vitamin B6) causing the deficiency of the latter. This results in pyridoxine deficiency-related neuropathy that is prevented by coadministration of pyridoxine with INH during anti-TB therapy. Neuropathies are known to occur with EMB and streptomycin (STR) combination. Retrobulbar toxic neuropathy is caused by EMB drug which has propensity to cause distal sensory PN, which is more often reversible. STR is vestibulotoxic but does not cause PN [36].

The association of TB with GBS is not clearly known. There are very few reports of these two conditions coexisting in a single patient [32]. In HIV, *Mycobacterium avium*-intracellulare has been isolated as a causative factor of HIV-related PN [37]. Lana-Peixoto et al. (1980) described isolated caseating tuberculous granulomata involving the optic nerve in a TB patient [38].

Rarely, PN can be a manifestation seen with sarcoidosis. Epineural noncaseating granulomas may be elicited. Sarcoidosis and TB may coexist rarely, that is, after steroid therapy for sarcoidosis, TB can occur [39]. The proper anti-TB therapy response may make doubtful associated condition of sarcoidosis as unlikely in TB neuritis patients [40].

23.4.4 TB-Related Peripheral Neuropathy: Treatment

The treatment of PN is related to treating the underlying etiology on finding out the same on prompt basis. Blood sugar estimation tests are must if PN is due to diabetes or in Pre-diabetes. Strict control of blood sugar levels can better the outcome of PN in prediabetes. Intravenous immunoglobulin or steroids can significantly better the PN caused by immune-mediated nerve damage/diseases. PN caused by dietary deficiencies can be treated with systematic supplementation.

This means that most of the treatment modalities in PN are symptomatic modalities. Similarly, in cases of PN due to TB, the patients are started on proper dosage of anti-TB therapy which are the four main drugs of RIF, PZA, EMB, and INH supplemented with pyridoxine to circumvent the INH-related pyridoxine deficiency.

23.4.5 Tuberculosis-Related Peripheral Neuropathy: Inference

TB neuritis involving peripheral nerve is rare even though TB is a disease with widespread body tissue involvement. TB can show many unusual modes of presentation with unusual sites. High grade of suspicion on the part of specialists and tissue diagnosis through biopsy rather than FNAC becomes imperative in such unusual cases. Proper response to anti-TB therapy helps in retrospectively diagnosing TB in such cases. No known definitive evidence of PN must be evident before inception of anti-TB therapy. The primary involvement of peripheral nerves must be considered as PN due to TB may not be always iatrogenic and it needs further advanced case studies in a larger population preferably in the developing countries.

Conclusion

TB is a common problem worldwide, more so in the developing world, which is a known chronic infection associated with caseating granulomatous inflammation. TB affects many body tissues with unexpected sites of presentation like the peripheral nerves causing PN. PN due to TB is underreported due to lack of awareness because leprosy comes first to mind rather than TB whenever there is PN. Nevertheless PN is a common term of clinicians, but primary PN due to TB, excluding those caused by anti-TB therapy, is uncommon. The primary involvement of peripheral nerves must be considered as PN due to TB may not be always iatrogenic. Proper response to anti-TB therapy helps in retrospectively diagnosing TB in such cases. A high clinical suspicion must be borne in mind while dealing with suspected TB cases showing unusual clinical presentation. Prompt diagnosis, perfect effective treatment by anti-TB therapy, and systematic case follow-up can help avert TB-related PN and, thus, avoid unwanted surgeries in patients, thus making this world a better, healthy world to live and let live.

References

1. Orrell RW, King RHM, Bowler JV, Ginsberg L (2002) Peripheral nerve granuloma in a patient with tuberculosis. J Neurol Neurosurg Psychiatry 73:769–772
2. Warpe BM, Poflee SV, Pande NP, Shrikhande AV (2014) Tuberculous neuritis: a rare sequel of a common disease. Indian J Pathol Microbiol 57:69–71
3. Chaurasia RN, Kumar A, Jaiswal S (2013) Entrapment neuropathy secondary to tubercular abscess: uncommon presentation of a common disease. Ann Indian Acad Neurol 16:597–598
4. Goussard P, Gie RP, Kling S, Andronikou S, Janson JT, Roussouw GJ (2009) Phrenic nerve palsy in children associated with confirmed intrathoracic tuberculosis: diagnosis and clinical course. Pediatr Pulmonol 44:345–350
5. Gunasegaran JP (2010) Nervous system. In: Gunasegaran JP (ed) Textbook of histology and a practical guide, vol 2. Elsevier, Haryana, pp 147–163
6. Hughes RAC (2002) Clinical review: peripheral neuropathy. BMJ 324:466
7. Torpy JM, Kincaid JL, Glass RM (2010) Patient page: peripheral neuropathy. JAMA 303:1556
8. Peripheral Neuropathy Fact Sheet (2014) National Institute of Neurological Disorders and Stroke (NINDS). NIH Publication No 15-4853
9. Cioroiu CM, Brannagan TM (2014) Peripheral neuropathy. Curr Geriatr Rep 3:83–90
10. Azhary H, Farooq MU, Bhanushali M, Majid A, Kassab MY (2010) Peripheral neuropathy: differential diagnosis and management. Am Fam Physician 81:887–892
11. Watson JC, Dyck JPB (2015) Peripheral neuropathy: a practical approach to diagnosis and symptom management. Mayo Clin Proc 90:940–951
12. Gabriel JM, Erne B, Pareyson D, Sghirlanzoni A, Taroni F, Steck AJ (1997) Gene dosage effects in hereditary peripheral neuropathy. Expression of peripheral myelin protein 22 in Charcot-Marie-Tooth disease type 1A and hereditary neuropathy with liability to pressure palsies nerve biopsies. Neurology 49:1635–1640
13. Gaist D, Jeppesen U, Andersen M, Garcia Rodriguez LA, Hallas J, Sindrup SH (2002) Statins and risk of polyneuropathy: a case-control study. Neurology 58:1333–1337
14. Corrao G, Zambon A, Bertu L, Botteri E, Leoni O, Contiero P (2004) Lipid lowering drugs prescription and the risk of peripheral neuropathy: an exploratory case-control study using automated databases. J Epidemiol Community Health 58:1047–1051
15. Cohen JS (2001) Peripheral neuropathy associated with fluoroquinolones. Ann Pharmacother 35:1540–1547
16. Kiziltan ME, Akalin MA, Sahin R, Uluduz D (2007) Peripheral neuropathy in patients with diabetes mellitus presenting as Bell's palsy. Neurosci Lett 427:138–141
17. Heck AW, Phillips LH 2nd (1989) Sarcoidosis and the nervous system. Neurol Clin 7:641–654
18. Stellman JM, Stellman SD, Christian R, Weber T, Tomasallo C (2003) The extent and patterns of usage of Agent Orange and other herbicides in Vietnam. Nature 422:681–687
19. Wilkes G (2007) Peripheral neuropathy related to chemotherapy. Semin Oncol Nurs 23:162–173
20. Gonzalez-Duarte A, Cikurel K, Simpson DM (2007) Managing HIV peripheral neuropathy. Curr HIV/AIDS Rep 4:114–118
21. World Health Organization Fact Sheet N104. Tuberculosis (2010) The WHO website http://www.who.int/mediacentre/factsheets/fs104/en/index.html. Accessed 3 June 2010
22. Sarwar A, Haque AU, Aftab S, Mustafa M, Moatasim A, Siddique S (2004) Spectrum of morphological changes in tuberculous lymphadenitis. Int J Pathol 2:85–89
23. Amin NH, Hitam WHW, Yunus R, Shatriah I (2012) Isolated optic neuritis secondary to presumed tuberculosis in an immunocompetent child. Med J Malays 67:102–104
24. Jaafar J, Hitam WHW, Noor RJAM (2012 Jul) Bilateral atypical optic neuritis associated with tuberculosis in an immunocompetent patient. Asian Pac J Trop Biomed 2(7):586–588
25. Raghibi A, Hitam WHW, Noor RJAM, Embong Z (2012) Optic perineuritis secondary to tuberculosis: a

rare case presentation. Asian Pac J Trop Biomed 2:S1206–S1208
26. Naha K, Dasari MJ, Prabhu M (2011) Tubercular neuritis: a new manifestation of an ancient disease. Australasian Med J 4:674–676
27. Poulose SP, Sugath S, Gopalkrishnan KC (2011) Tuberculosis affecting the median nerve. Kerala J Orthop 24:43–45
28. Chaurasia RN, Jaiswal S, Mishra VN, Joshi D (2015) Greater auricular nerve tuberculosis: an unusual presentation of a common disease. Open J Clin Med Case Rep 1:1–6
29. Sharma SK, Mohan A (2004) Extrapulmonary tuberculosis. Indian J Med Res 120(4):316–353
30. Cavanagh JB (1979) The peripheral nervous system. In: Symmers WSC (ed) Systemic pathology, vol 2 . Churchill Livingstone, New York, pp 2296–2348Thirty-eight Authors
31. Peiris JB, Wikramasinghe HR, Chandrashekhar MA (1974) Tuberculous polyradiculitis. BMJ 4:107
32. Vyravanathan S, Senanayake N (1983) Guillain-Barre syndrome associated with tuberculosis. Postgrad Med J 59:516–517
33. Said G (2001) Leprous neuropathy. In: Mendell JR, Kissel JT, Cornblath DR (eds) Diagnosis and management of peripheral nerve disorders. Oxford University Press, Oxford, pp 551–564
34. McAdam AJ, Sharpe AH (2010) Infectious diseases. In: Kumar V, Abbas AK, Fausto N, Aster JC (eds) Pathological basis of disease, vol 8. WB Saunders, Philadelphia, pp 331–398
35. Mebrotra MP, Pursnani ML, Patney NL, Tandon RK, Jain RK (1982) Tuberculous meningitis: its neurological complications with special reference to their prognostic significance. J Assoc Physicians India 30:869
36. Tugwell P, James SL (1972) Peripheral neuropathy with ethambutol. Postgrad Med J 48:667–670
37. Erdem S, Kissl JT, Mendell JR (2001) Toxic neuropathies: drugs, metals, and alcohol. In: Mendell JR, Kissel JT, Cornblath DR (eds) Diagnosis and management of peripheral nerve disorders. Oxford University Press, Oxford, pp 297–343
38. Wrozlek MA, Rao C, Kozlowski PB, Sher JH (1989) Muscle and nerve involvement in AIDS patient with disseminated Mycobacterium intracellulare infection. Muscle Nerve 12:247–249
39. Lana-Peixoto MA, Bambirra EA, Pittella JE (1980) Optic nerve tuberculoma. Arch Neurol 37:186–187
40. Litinsky I, Elkayam O, Flusser G, Segal R, Yaron M, Caspi D (2002) Sarcoidosis: TB or not TB? Ann Rheum Dis 61:385–386

Imaging Findings of Tuberculosis of the Cranial and Peripheral Nerves

24

Mudit Gupta, Jitender Saini,
and Rakesh Kumar Gupta

Contents

M. Gupta, DNB
Department of Radiology, Safdarjung Hospital,
New Delhi, India
e-mail: muditdr@gmail.com

J. Saini, MD, DM
Neuroimaging & Interventional Radiology, National
Institute of Mental Health and Neuro Science,
Bengaluru, India
e-mail: jsaini76@gmail.com

R.K. Gupta, MD (✉)
Department of Radiology and Imaging, Fortis
Memorial Research Institute, Gurgaon,
Haryana, India
e-mail: rakeshree1@gmail.com

Abbreviations

AFB	Acid fast bacilli
CN	Cranial nerve
CNS	Central nervous system
CSF	Cerebrospinal fluid
DR	Drug resistant
EMB	Ethambutol
EON	Ethambutol-induced optic neuropathy
ICP	Intracranial pressure
IL	Interleukin
INH	Isoniazid
LETM	Longitudinally extensive transverse myelitis
MDR	Multidrug resistant
MRI	Magnetic resonance imaging
NAT2	N-acetyltransferase type 2
OCA	Optochiasmatic arachnoiditis
OM	Otitis media
PCR	Polymerase chain reaction
PN	Peripheral neuropathy
SNHL	Sensorineural hearing loss
TB	Tuberculosis
TBM	Tuberculous meningitis
TOM	Tubercular otitis media

24.1 Introduction

Cranial and peripheral nerve involvement in TB of CNS is commonly observed in the clinical practice. The involvement of these structures

M. Turgut et al. (eds.), *Tuberculosis of the Central Nervous System*,
DOI 10.1007/978-3-319-50712-5_24

may be due to its primary involvement by the disease or may be involved as a part of disease process involving the brain and meninges. Isolated cranial nerve (CN) palsies are often ascribed to lesions of the respective nerves along its extra-axial courses. Imaging features have been described as a part of the meningitis which involves the brain, or it may primarily involve the meninges of the lower spinal cord and is referred to as arachnoiditis. In this chapter, we will focus on cranial and peripheral nerve involvement due to *Mycobacterium tuberculosis*.

CN involvement is seen in 17–70% of patients and occurs in the background of diffuse leptomeningeal TB. Impairment has been attributed to ischemia or entrapment of the nerves in basal exudates [1, 2].

24.2 Cranial Nerves

24.2.1 Optic Nerve (II) and Optic Chiasma

Impairment of vision is one of the distressing complications of TBM, and it affects 27–32% patients in adult population and higher incidence of 43–72% in pediatric population [3–5]. It has been commonly ascribed to optochiasmatic arachnoiditis (OCA) and optochiasmatic granuloma and rarely due to optic chiasm compression by dilated third ventricle, choroid tubercle, optic disk granuloma, ethambutol (EMB) toxicity, and occipital infarct [3, 6, 7].

Inflammatory changes with exudates in the leptomeninges around the optic chiasm and the optic nerves are referred to as OCA. This may result in decrease in the visual acuity with variable progression to partial or total blindness. It may be found in other conditions like rheumatoid arthritis, sarcoidosis, Epstein-Barr viral infection, besides TBM. OCA causes 41% of visual impairment in TBM, and mechanisms include optic atrophy owing to pressure and/or traction on the optic nerve or perichiasmal inflammatory process with superimposed vascular insult to the optic pathway [8–10]. OCA on MRI appears as diffusely thickened and homogenously enhancing optic nerve and chiasm (Fig. 24.1) [11]. Optic perineuritis typically shows a distinctive pattern of enhancement around the optic nerve ("tramtrack" on axial and "doughnut" on coronal views) [12]. Associated intraparenchymal tuberculomas can help in clinching the diagnosis [13]. These findings in baseline MRI have been found to predict blindness at 6 months [8].

Raised CSF protein content is a known risk factor [8]. Higher CSF concentration of IL6 is associated with significant neurological deficit [14]. Aaron et al. demonstrated questionable change with therapy, suggesting the need to prevent this complication [15].

Early recognition may be useful, as the vision does not deteriorate further on starting

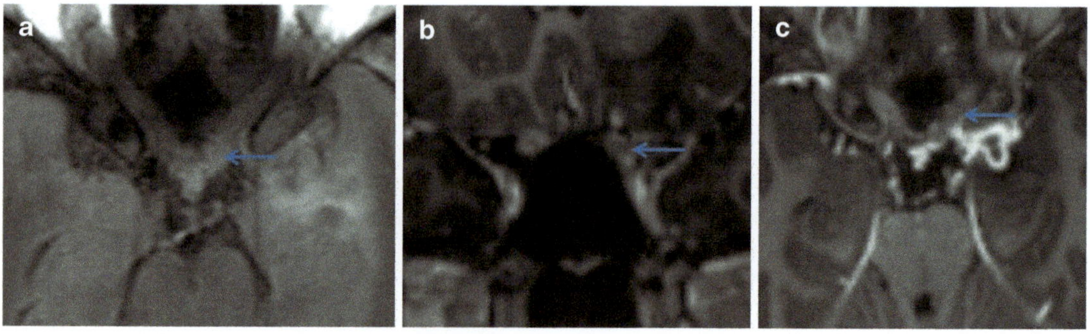

Fig. 24.1 A 23-year-old male presents with insidious-onset left-sided hemianopia. Axial FLAIR (**a**), post-contrast T1-weighted fat-suppressed coronal (**b**) and axial (**c**) images at level of suprasellar cistern show left-sided optochiasmatic arachnoiditis (*arrow*)

treatment. Patient survival and neurological outcome in patients with TBM is known to improve with corticosteroid treatment, which act by reducing the harmful effects of pro-inflammatory molecules released following destruction of *M. tuberculosis*. The clinical improvement with corticosteroid treatment is also attributed to reduction in cerebral edema and/or vasculitis [16].

Development of visual loss during TBM treatment may be related to drug toxicity and/or arachnoiditis, besides involvement of the anterior optic pathway by tuberculomas. The optochiasmatic region may rarely be involved by paradoxical development of tuberculomas during anti-TB therapy [17]. Differential diagnosis of multiple ring-enhancing lesions due to tuberculomas on MRI includes neurocysticercosis, pyogenic abscesses, metastasis, and toxoplasmosis [18, 19]. Paradoxical development of tuberculomas is treated by continuation of anti-TB therapy as usual with addition of systemic corticosteroids that overcomes the host body inflammatory response to the breakdown products of *M. tuberculosis* [8, 20]. MRI helps in exact localization of tuberculoma with respect to the optic nerve and chiasm (Fig. 24.2). This helps in surgical decompression planning of optochiasmatic tuberculomas which are causing significant visual deterioration. Orbital TB may also present as orbital apex syndrome [21–23]. Imaging can demonstrate ring-enhancing lesions of intra-conal compartment.

EMB is part of the four drug regimen used for treatment of TB of CNS and is a contributory factor in EMB-induced optic neuropathy (EON) with an incidence of 1.5%. The risk for development of EON gets higher with decrease in renal function and higher daily dose of EMB [24]. Neuroimaging of chiasm is usually normal; however, MRI may show increased T2 signal within the optic chiasm without restricted diffusion [25, 26].

Visual function improves in about one-third of these patients after discontinuation of treatment [27]. Patients with optic disk pallor may not improve during follow-up, and this finding may be a sign of a poor prognosis.

Literature has documented an incubation period varying from 15 days to 2 years following commencement of EMB treatment to the onset of EON [28]. EMB toxicity affects the small size papillomacular bundle axons, and optic disk pallor develops months after the fibers are lost.

24.2.2 Oculomotor (III), Trochlear (IV), and Abducens (VI) Nerves

Due to the long course these CNs follow inside the cranium, compressive lesions and microvascular ischemia in TBM may cause palsy to these CNs [29]. Other causes include vasculitis, tuberculoma situated in the midbrain region,

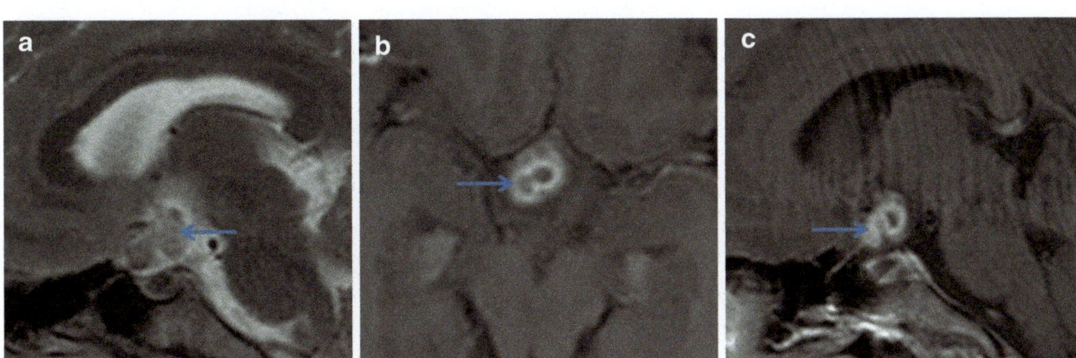

Fig. 24.2 Optochiasmatic tuberculomas in a young female. Mid sagittal T2WI (**a**), post-contrast T1-weighted fat-suppressed axial (**b**), and midsagittal (**c**) images show rim-enhancing multiple tuberculomas around the optic chiasma (*arrow*)

sellar and suprasellar tubercular lesions, and cavernous sinus lesions [30].

TBM is a rare but not unusual cause of oculomotor palsy [31, 32]. Typical findings on MRI are neural thickening, increased T2 intensity, and post-contrast enhancement, particularly of the proximal segment [33]. TBM may present with isolated third CN palsy, which responds well to four-drug anti-TB therapy and intravenous corticosteroids; however, delayed diagnosis and management may result in poor prognosis [34, 35].

Sixth nerve is the commonest CN involved in TBM followed by oculomotor and trochlear nerves [6, 31, 32, 36]. Abducens palsy may also be secondary to increased ICP. Altiparmak et al. published a proven case of TBM presenting with vertical diplopia [29]. The symptoms resolved a month of initiating anti-TB therapy [35].

Brainstem tuberculomas in isolation are rare and account for 2.5–8% of the total intracranial tuberculomas [37]. Sharma et al. presented cases of ophthalmoplegia due to brainstem tuberculoma presenting as rim-enhancing lesions [38].

Pituitary TB may present a diagnostic dilemma because it is hard to differentiate a pituitary adenoma from pituitary tuberculoma. MRI is ideal to establish the differential diagnosis. The thickened pituitary stalk on contrast MRI may be helpful in the differentiation of sellar/suprasellar TB from pituitary adenomas [39, 40]. Dulce and colleagues have shown cases of sellar tuberculomas presenting with CN palsies and endocrinopathies [41].

Several case reports concluded that intracranial tuberculomas in the cavernous sinus can mimic a neoplasm or other inflammatory pathologies like sarcoidosis and fungal infections. High index of suspicion should be maintained in the presence of risk factors. These lesions shows intense homogeneous enhancement and appear hypointense on T2-weighted imaging. The presence of other coexisting lesions may support the diagnosis [42]. In the absence of negative bacteriological studies, the diagnosis is usually accepted on the basis of pathological results of the lesion [43, 44]. However, a presumptive treatment with anti-TB drugs may result in favorable outcome and may avert the need for a surgery [45].

24.2.3 Trigeminal Nerve (V)

Trigeminal nerve is the largest CN [46]. Disease involving this nerve may cause sudden and severe pain within its distribution, typically the maxillary or mandibular branches [47]. Neuropathy may present along the entire course of the nerve, from its origin in brainstem to its peripheral branches. The common causes are tortuous vessels in prepontine cistern, brainstem lesions, and meningitis, the latter of which may show enhancement in vicinity of root entry zone (Fig. 24.3) [48, 49].

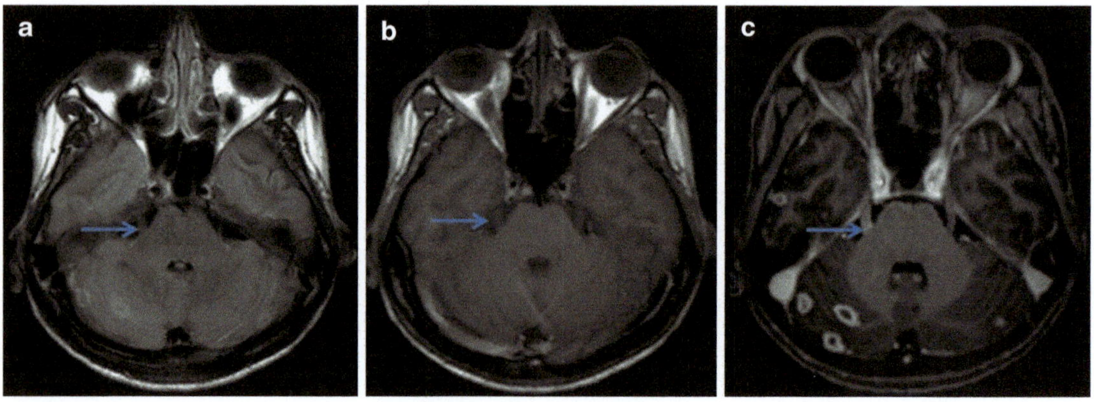

Fig. 24.3 A 28-year-old male presented with right facial pain while on treatment for multiple tuberculomas. Axial FLAIR (**a**), T1WI (**b**), and post-contrast T1-weighted fat-suppressed (**c**) images show altered signal intensity and perineural enhancement of the right trigeminal nerve (*arrow*)

TB may involve the nerve at the Meckel's cave or cavernous sinus, and the disease process may extend into the infratemporal fossa along the course of mandibular nerve causing expansion of the foramen ovale and destruction of the adjacent bone [50–52]. Direct compression on the trigeminal nerve by a venous varix secondary to TBM-induced superior sagittal sinus thrombosis has also been reported [53, 54].

24.2.4 Facial Nerve (VII)

Different types of clinical presentations secondary to brain stem tuberculoma have been reported in literature and include one and a half syndrome, glaucoma mimic, unilateral paralysis of saccades, Millard-Gubler syndrome, isolated bilateral ptosis, horizontal gaze palsy, myokymia, facial contracture, and Foville's syndrome [55, 56].

Facial nerve palsy may be associated with TOM. It is a rare cause of chronic suppurative infection (0.05–0.9%) of the middle ear [57]. Peripheral facial palsy has been found to be present in 9.6% of patients of TOM, which is higher than in patients with suppurative OM [58]. Imaging findings may mimic a tumor causing facial nerve dysfunction [33]. Response rates are favorable with surgical decompression and anti-TB therapy [59].

24.2.5 Vestibulocochlear Nerve (VIII)

Literature shows a higher incidence of conductive hearing loss than SNHL with TBM [58, 60]. Kuan et al. studied the autopsy specimen of the temporal bone of a patient with SNHL following TBM [61]. They found invasion of the labyrinth by TB disease through the internal acoustic canal and induced a retrocochlear pattern of SNHL. There appeared to be significant degeneration of the organ of Corti and the loss of most spiral ganglion cells and cochlear nerve fibers, particularly the basal turn, and of sensory cells of all cristae and maculae. MRI shows T2-hyperintensities of bilateral mastoids and middle ears, inflammatory changes in the petrous apices, and extensive pachymeningeal thickening along the temporal convexities [62].

Stach et al. presented a case of sudden SNHL secondary to tuberculoma involving the root entry zone of the VIIIth CN. MRI localized the lesion at the cerebellopontine angle [63].

Ototoxic hearing loss is also common in patients of MDR-TB treated with aminoglycosides [64, 65]. The injectable drugs are known to selectively destroy the basal hair cells of the basilar membrane that sense the higher frequencies [66].

24.2.6 Glossopharyngeal (IX), Vagus (X), and Spinal Accessory (XI) Nerves

Hoarseness itself is not a common manifestation of pulmonary TB but may present when the granulomatous inflammation involves recurrent laryngeal nerves in the mediastinum [67]. Richardus et al. reported a case of IX and XI CN palsy presenting with torticollis and deviation of the uvula. MRI depicted nasopharyngeal mass involving the craniovertebral junction [62].

24.2.7 Hypoglossal (XII)

TB spondylitis is a common disease of the spine especially in developing countries. Nearly 1% of all cases of spinal TB involve craniocervical junction. Hypoglossal nerve palsy is not an uncommon neurological finding (Fig. 24.4); however, isolated involvement of the hypoglossal nerve is rare and is restricted to case reports or small case series. Craniocervical junction TB is a common cause of hypoglossal nerve involvement [68–70]. The radiological evidence of cord compression may not always correlate with clinical presentation as the neurological deficits are also due to instability besides cervicomedullary compression [71].

24.3 Spinal and Peripheral Nerves

During experimental evolution of TB in mice, *M. tuberculosis* sequester in the lungs within a few hours, followed by redistribution during the following days [72]. This explains why anti-TB

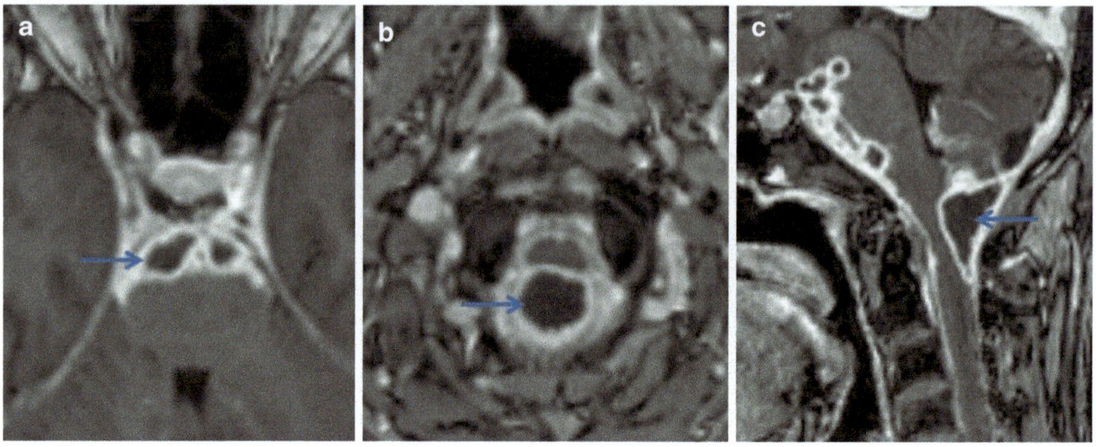

Fig. 24.4 A 50-year-old man presented with TBM with multiple CN involvement while on treatment. Axial post-contrast T1-weighted fat-suppressed images at the level of upper pons (**a**), medulla (**b**), and midsagittal section at level of cervico-vertebral junction (**c**) show rim-enhancing TB arachnoiditis with CSF loculation (*arrows*) trapping the bilateral third and hypoglossal nerves

therapy is able to have full effect on a sensitive germ before *M. tuberculosis* reaches the nerves. When they do, they can be detected in the peri-neural and Schwann cells, autonomic ganglia, and histiocytes. Lesions of the neurons are caused by the compression which these formations exert.

24.3.1 Peripheral Neuropathy

Peripheral neuropathy (PN) is a condition which may affect sensory, motor, or autonomic nerves, compromising the relay of information from different parts of the body. It is anticipated that as many as 500 million people in the world suffer from PN, and the problem is commonly seen among individuals with TB [73, 74]. All patients with TB should undergo routine evaluation for PN at each clinical encounter [75].

For most patients with TB, the cause of PN will be multifactorial, resulting from the disease itself [76] or type IV hypersensitivity reaction [77], common comorbid conditions [78, 79], and the medications used to bring about cure [80, 81].

Isoniazid (INH) is one of the medications most commonly associated with PN [82], with incidence up to 10% [83]. The drug's mechanism of action against *M. tuberculosis* leads to depletion of pyridoxine (vitamin B6), which results in neurotoxicity [84]. NAT2 is crucial for metabolization and inactivation of INH [85]. Molecular screening of patients for variants of NAT2 might be useful for the clinical prediction and preclusion of INH-induced polyneuropathy [86].

Studies have reported 13–17% incidence of PN for patients with DR-TB [87]. Most cases have been attributed to prolonged administration of second-line drugs, including cycloserine, ethionamide, fluoroquinolones, clofazimine, and linezolid [88–91]. Therefore, it is important that, whenever possible, treatment for DR-TB be based on drug-susceptibility testing with a goal of maximizing effectiveness while limiting toxicity [75]. Management should focus on halting damage to the nerve, although care should be taken not to compromise the TB regimen and alleviating symptoms [75].

Cervicothoracic TB osteomyelitis and resultant paraspinal abscess has been known to cause brachial plexus neuropathy [92]. Abscess around the brachial plexus may result in brachial plexopathy, and its decompression along with anti-TB therapy may cure such patients (Fig. 24.5).

24.3.2 Radiculomyelitis

The term TB radiculomyelitis was coined by Wadia and Dastur, which includes spinal cord complications of TBM, arachnoiditis, and spinal

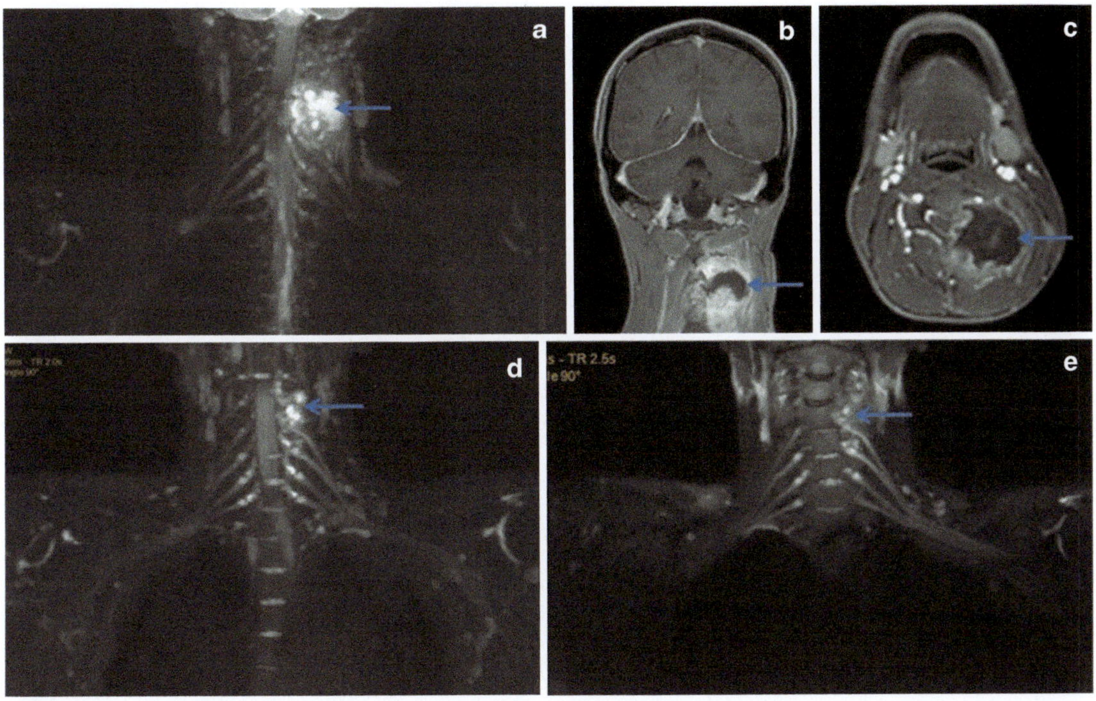

Fig. 24.5 A 35-year-old man presented with left-sided root pain. Coronal fat-suppressed T2-weighted image (**a**) shows large T2 hyperintense area around left fourth and fifth spinal nerve root and trunk. Coronal (**b**) and axial (**c**) post-contrast T1-weighted fat-suppressed images show rim-enhancing cervical abscess in the corresponding region (*arrows*). The abscess was drained which cultured *Mycobacterium tuberculosis*. Coronal fat-suppressed T2-weighted images (**d**, **e**) on follow-up study at 6 months show small residual disease with normally visible nerve roots (*arrow*)

tuberculoma [93, 94]. Recent literature has documented a high incidence of spinal and/or radicular syndrome in patients of TBM to the tune of 23–76% [95–97]. Although anti-TB therapy has decreased the mortality due to TBM significantly, it has failed to decrease complications such as spinal arachnoiditis [96].

The proposed pathological mechanisms are hematogenous spread of *M. tuberculosis* to the parenchyma and meninges of spinal cord, gravitation of exudate to the lumbosacral region, and, rarely, by direct extension from vertebral TB [93]. The subarachnoid space between the spinal duramater and the leptomeninges may be filled with thick gelatinous exudate, and it encases the spinal cord and nerve roots (Fig. 24.6). The most common MRI findings are spinal meningeal enhancement, lumbosacral arachnoiditis, and thoracic myelitis; less commonly, CSF loculations, tuberculoma, and syrinx [95].

TB myelitis is an important cause of paraparesis in Indian setting [98]. It may be confused with other forms of viral myeloradiculopathies; however, elevated CSF protein, reduction of sugar, predominantly lymphocytic cell count, and the presence of AFB should confirm the diagnosis [95]. PCR for *M. tuberculosis* in CSF is considered a specific diagnostic test [99]. Most spinal cord lesions appear hyperintense on T2 and iso- or hypointense on T1-weighted imaging [100]. Post-contrast imaging reveals loculation and obliteration of the subarachnoid space along with linear intradural enhancement [101].

Cord atrophy, cavitation, and/or the presence of syrinx on MRI may be linked with poor outcome [100]. The basis of acute syringomyelia in TBM has been attributed to thrombosis and endarteritis of the spinal cord vessels leading to subsequent myelomalacia [102]. There is no known medical treatment for this complication [103]. MRI is the modality of choice of detecting

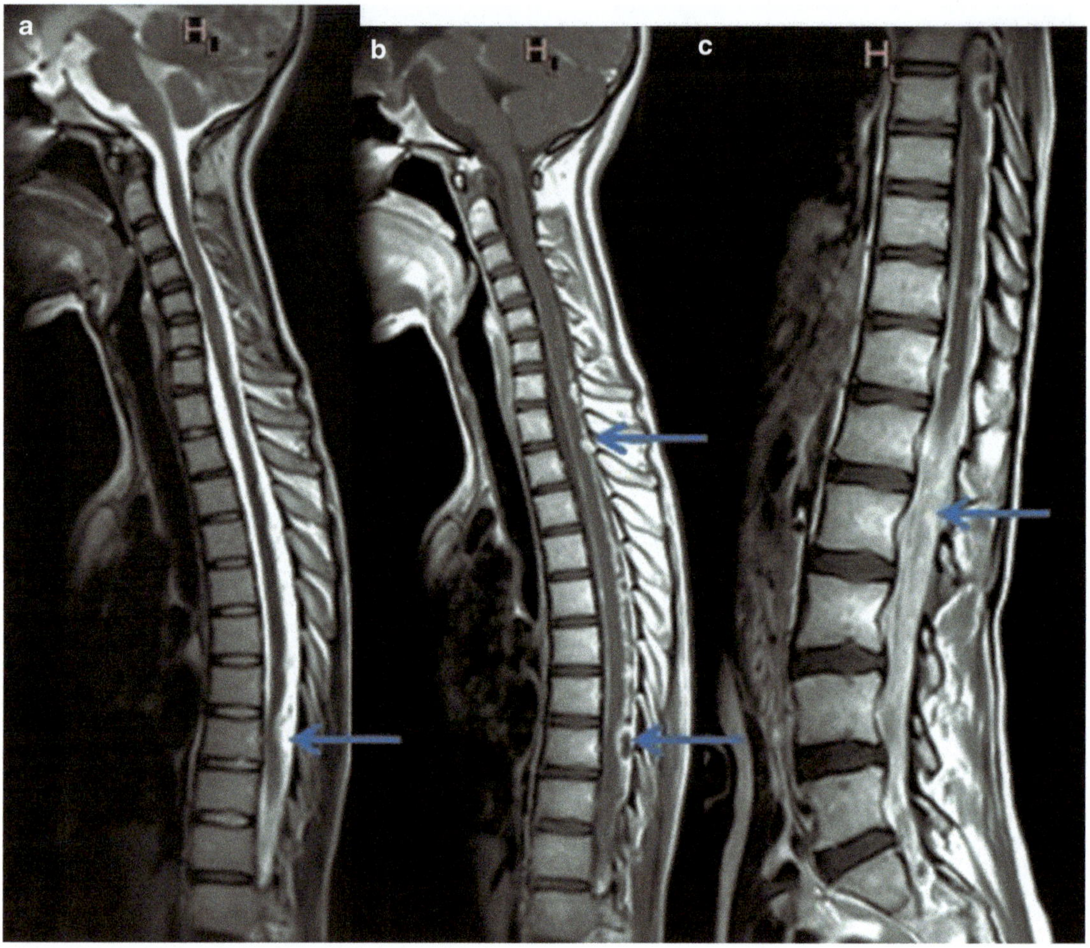

Fig. 24.6 A 34-year-old man presented with lower motor neuron palsy on treatment for TB. Midsagittal T2WI of cervicodorsal spine (**a**) and post-contrast T1-weighted fat-suppressed images of cervicodorsal spine (**b**) and dorsolumbar spine (**c**) show rim-enhancing as well as diffusely enhancing TB arachnoiditis (*arrows*) trapping lumbosacral spinal roots

TB-related myelopathy as it provides greater details of pathological changes within and around the spinal cord such as syrinx formation and arachnoiditis [104].

LETM is characterized by contiguous immune-mediated inflammatory lesion of spinal cord extending to three or more spinal cord segments [105]. TB is an uncommon cause of LETM [106]. MRI shows contiguous long segment intramedullary lesion, which appears isointense on T1-weighted and hyperintense on T2-weighted imaging with cord expansion. There might be coexisting brain tuberculomas. An abnormal activation of the immune system against the spinal cord is thought to be the main etiologic mechanism [107]. A timely identification and treatment of this entity with corticosteroids is essential to prevent irreversible damage and morbidity [108].

Conclusion

We conclude that cranial and peripheral nerve involvement in TB is not uncommon and may be affected by the disease or may be drug induced [109] and should be treated as per the cause of its involvement.

References

1. Uysal G, Köse G, Güven A, Diren B (2001) Magnetic resonance imaging in diagnosis of childhood central nervous system tuberculosis. Infection 38:148–153
2. Sharma P, Garg RK, Verma R, Singh MK, Shukla R (2011) Incidence, predictors and prognostic value of cranial nerve involvement in patients with tuberculous meningitis: a retrospective evaluation. Eur J Intern Med 22:289–295
3. Misra UK, Kalita J, Srivastava M, Mandal SK (1996) Prognosis of tuberculous meningitis: a multivariate analysis. J Neurol Sci 137:57–61
4. Kalra V, Ghose S (1985) Optic nerve involvement in tuberculous meningitis. Indian Pediatr 22:783–785
5. Amitava AK, Alarm S, Hussain R (2001) Neuro-ophthalmic features in pediatric tubercular meningoencephalitis. J Pediatr Ophthalmol Strabismus 38:229–234
6. Berger JR (1994) Tuberculous meningitis. Curr Opin Neurol 7:191–200
7. Padhi TR, Basu S, Das T, Samal B (2011) Optic disc tuberculoma in a patient with miliary tuberculosis. Ocul Immunol Inflamm 19:67–68
8. Sinha MK, Garg RK, Anuradha HK, Agarwal A, Parihar A, Mandhani PA (2010) Paradoxical vision loss associated with optochiasmatic tuberculoma in tuberculous meningitis: a report of 8 patients. J Infect 60:458–466
9. Mooney AJ (1956) Some ocular sequelae of tuberculous meningitis; a preliminary survey, 1953-54. Am J Ophthalmol 41:753–768
10. Silverman IE, Liu GT, Bilaniuk LT, Volpe NJ, Galetta SL (1995) Tuberculous meningitis with blindness and perichiasmal involvement on MRI. Pediatr Neurol 12:65–67
11. Raghibi A, Wan Hitam WH, Noor RAM, Embong Z (2012) Optic perineuritis secondary to tuberculosis: a rare case presentation. Asian Pac J Trop Biomed 2:S1206–S1208
12. Purvin V, Kawasaki A, Jacobson DM (2001) Optic perineuritis: clinical and radiographic features. Arch Ophthalmol 119:1299–1306
13. Sivadasan A, Alexander M, Mathew V, Mani S, Patil AKB (2013) Radiological evolution and delayed resolution of an optic nerve tuberculoma: challenges in diagnosis and treatment. Ann Indian Acad Neurol 16:114–117
14. Simmons CP, Thwaites GE, Quyen NTH, Torok E, Hoang DM, Chau TTH, Mai PP, Lan NT, Dung NH, Quy HT, Bang ND, Hien TT, Farrar J (2006) Pretreatment intracerebral and peripheral blood immune responses in Vietnamese adults with tuberculous meningitis: diagnostic value and relationship to disease severity and outcome. J Immunol 176:2007–2014
15. Anupriya A, Sunithi M, Maya T, Goel M, Alexander M, Aaron S, Mathew V (2010) Tuberculous optochiasmatic arachnoiditis. Neurol India 58:732–735
16. Garg RK, Paliwal V, Malhotra HS (2011) Tuberculous optochiasmatic arachnoiditis: a devastating form of tuberculous meningitis. Expert Rev Anti-Infect Ther 9:719–729
17. Ahmetgjekaj I, Kabashi-Muçaj S, Lascu LC, Bondari S, Bondari A (2014) Paradoxical growth of optochiasmatic tuberculoma during the treatment of tuberculous meningitis. Curr Health Sci J 40:225–227
18. Trivedi R, Saksena S, Gupta RK (2009) Magnetic resonance imaging in central nervous system tuberculosis. Indian J Radiol Imaging 19:256–265
19. Gupta RK, Kathuria MK, Pradhan S (1999) Magnetization transfer MR imaging in CNS tuberculosis. AJNR Am J Neuroradiol 20:867–875
20. Monga PK, Dhaliwal U (2009) Paradoxical reaction in tubercular meningitis resulting in involvement of optic radiation. Indian J Ophthalmol 57:139–141
21. Sharma K, Pradhan S, Varma A, Rathi B (2003) Irreversible blindness due to multiple tuberculomas in the suprasellar cistern. J Neuroophthalmol 23:211–212
22. Banait S, Jain J, Parihar PH, Karwassara V (2012) Orbital tuberculosis manifesting as proptosis in an immunocompromised host. Indian J Sex Transm Dis 33:128–130
23. Hughes EH, Petrushkin H, Sibtain NA, Stanford MR, Plant GT, Graham EM (2008) Tuberculous orbital apex syndromes. Br J Ophthalmol 92:1511–1517
24. Lee EJ, Kim S-J, Choung HK, Kim JH, Yu YS (2008) Incidence and clinical features of ethambutol-induced optic neuropathy in Korea. J Neuroophthalmol 28:269–277
25. Kho RC, Al-Obailan M, Arnold AC (2011) Bitemporal visual field defects in ethambutol-induced optic neuropathy. J Neuroophthalmol 31:121–126
26. Osaguona VB, Sharpe JA, Awaji SA, Farb RI, Sundaram ANE (2014) Optic chiasm involvement on MRI with ethambutol-induced bitemporal hemianopia. J Neuroophthalmol 34:155–158
27. Kumar A, Sandramouli S, Verma L, Tewari HK, Khosla PK (1993) Ocular ethambutol toxicity: is it reversible? J Clin Neuroophthalmol 13:15–17
28. Choi SY, Hwang JM (1997) Optic neuropathy associated with ethambutol in Koreans. Korean J Ophthalmol 11:106–110
29. Altiparmak UE, Ersoz I, Kutlu G, Yagci R, Inan L, Duman S (2008) Isolated trochlear nerve palsy in a patient with tuberculous meningitis: short report. Neuroophthalmology 32:17–19
30. Shukla S, Trivedi A, Singh K, Sharma V (2010) Pituitary tuberculoma. J Neurosci Rural Pract 1:30–31
31. Daif A, Obeid T, Yaqub B, AbdulJabbar M (1992) Unusual presentation of tuberculous meningitis. Clin Neurol Neurosurg 94:1–5
32. Kumar MP, Vivekanand U, Umakanth S (2014) A study of etiology and prognosis of oculomotor nerve paralysis. Edorium J Neurol 2014:1–8

33. Sanei Taheri M, Karimi MA, Haghighatkhah H, Pourghorban R, Samadian M, Delavar Kasmaei H (2015) Central nervous system tuberculosis: an imaging-focused review of a reemerging disease. Radiol Res Pract 2015:202806
34. Chakrabarti S, Pan K (2014) Isolated oculomotor nerve palsy as initial presentation of tuberculous meningitis. Natl J Integ Res Med 5:136–138
35. Moon S, Son J, Chang W (2008) A case of oculomotor nerve palsy and choroidal tuberculous granuloma associated with tuberculous meningoencephalitis. Korean J Ophthalmol 22:201–204
36. Thwaites GE, van Toorn R, Schoeman J (2013) Tuberculous meningitis: more questions, still too few answers. Lancet Neurol 12:999–1010
37. Kumar R, Jain R, Kaur A, Chhabra DK (2000) Brain stem tuberculosis in children. Br J Neurosurg 14:356–361
38. Sharma K, Kanaujia V, Jaiswal S, Jain A, Kumar S, Srivastava AK, Jaiswal AK (2012) Brain stem tuberculoma presenting with isolated ocular motility abnormality: a series of two cases and review of literature. Oman J Ophthalmol 5:61–63
39. Sinha S, Singh AK, Tatke M, Singh D (2000) Hypophyseal tuberculoma: direct radiosurgery is contraindicated for a lesion with a thickened pituitary stalk: case report. Neurosurgery 46:735–738
40. Pereira J, Vaz R, Carvalho D, Cruz C (1995) Thickening of the pituitary stalk: a finding suggestive of intrasellar tuberculoma? Case report. Neurosurgery 36:1013–1015
41. Bonifacio-Delgadillo D, Aburto-Murrieta Y, Salinas-Lara C, Sotelo J, Montes-Mojarro I, Garcia-Marquez A (2014) Clinical presentation and magnetic resonance findings in sellar tuberculomas. Case Rep Med 2014:961913
42. Morgado C, Ruivo N (2005) Imaging meningo-encephalic tuberculosis. Eur J Radiol 55:188–192
43. Grayeli AB, Redondo A, Salama J, Rey A (1998) Tuberculoma of the cavernous sinus: case report. Neurosurgery 42:179–181
44. Jaimovich SG, Thea VC, Guevara M, Gardella JL (2013) Cavernous sinus tuberculoma mimicking a neoplasm: case report, literature review, and diagnostic and treatment suggestions for tuberculomas in rare locations. Surg Neurol Int 4:158
45. Rebai R, Boudawara MZ, Bahloul K, Chabchoub I, Chaari S, Boudawara T, Ben Mansour H (2001) Cavernous sinus tuberculoma: diagnostic difficulties in a personal case. Surg Neurol 55:372–375
46. Sanders RD (2010) The trigeminal (V) and facial (VII) cranial nerves: head and face sensation and movement. Psychiatry 7:13–16
47. Bennetto L, Patel NK, Fuller G (2007) Trigeminal neuralgia and its management. BMJ 334:201–205
48. Hashmi MA, Guha G, Saha B (2010) Trigeminal neuralgia in an HIV patient. J Global Infect Dis 2:65–66
49. Sens MA, Higer HP (1991) MRI of trigeminal neuralgia: initial clinical results in patients with vascular compression of the trigeminal nerve. Neurosurg Rev 14:69–73
50. Kesavadas C, Somasundaram S, Rao RM, Radhakrishnan VV (2007) Meckel's cave tuberculoma with unusual infratemporal extension. J Neuroimaging 17:264–268
51. Goel A, Nadkarni T, Desai AP (1999) Tuberculoma in the Meckel's cave: a case report. Neurol India 47:238–240
52. Gilbert T, Chidiac C, Bonnefoy M, Ferry T (2015) Tuberculosis of the cavum revealed by acute facial pain. BMJ Case Rep. doi:10.1136/bcr-2015-211294
53. Tsimiklis CA, Gragnaniello C, Abou-Hamden A (2014) Venous sinus thrombosis secondary to tuberculous meningitis: a novel cause of trigeminal neuralgia. BMJ Case Rep 2014:pii: bcr2014207238
54. Sharma C, Kumawat B, Tripathi G, Dixit S (2008) Isolated sensory trigeminal neuropathy- a rare clinical presentation of brain stem tuberculoma. Case report. Intern J Neurol 11:5
55. Gautam VKS (2014) Brainstem tuberculoma presenting as stroke. Int J Med 2:68–70
56. Sharif M, More V, Purandare S (2010) Brainstem tuberculoma – presenting as Millard Gubler syndrome. Indian J Pediatr 77:707
57. Vaamonde P, Castro C, García-Soto N, Labella T, Lozano A (2004) Tuberculous otitis media: a significant diagnostic challenge. Otolaryngol Head Neck Surg 130:759–766
58. Cho Y-S, Lee H-S, Kim S-W, Chung K-H, Lee D-K, Koh W-J, Kim MG (2006) Tuberculous otitis media: a clinical and radiologic analysis of 52 patients. Laryngoscope 116:921–927
59. Karkera GV, Shah DD (2006) Silent mastoiditis-tuberculous aetiology presenting as facial nerve palsy. Indian J Otolaryngol Head Neck Surg 58:108–110
60. Vernon M (1967) Tuberculous meningitis and deafness. J Speech Hear Disord 32:177–181
61. Kuan C-C, Kaga K, Tsuzuku T (2007) Tuberculous meningitis-induced unilateral sensorineural hearing loss: a temporal bone study. Acta Otolaryngol 127:553–557
62. Richardus RA, Jansen JC, Steens SCA, Arend SM (2011) Two immigrants with tuberculosis of the ear, nose, and throat region with skull base and cranial nerve involvement. Case Rep Med 2011:675807
63. Stach BA, Westerberg BD, Roberson JB Jr (1998) Auditory disorder in central nervous system miliary tuberculosis: case report. J Am Acad Audiol 9:305–310
64. Harris T, Bardien S, Schaaf HS, Petersen L, De Jong G, Fagan JJ (2012) Aminoglycoside-induced hearing loss in HIV-positive and HIV-negative multidrug-resistant tuberculosis patients. S Afr Med J 102:363–366

65. Thomas JAB (1950) The toxic effect of streptomycin on the VIII cranial nerve. Proc R Soc Med 43:1107–1109
66. Selimoglu E (2007) Aminoglycoside-induced ototoxicity. Curr Pharm Des 13:119–126
67. Yew WW, Chau CH, Lee J, Wong PC, Leung CK (2001) Hoarseness due to recurrent laryngeal nerve palsy from intrathoracic mycobacteriosis. Int J Tuberc Lung Dis 5:1074–1075
68. Ebadi H, Fathi D (2012) Unilateral hypoglossal nerve palsy: as the only presentation of tuberculosis. Acta Med Iran 50:717–720
69. Richards IM, White AM, O'Sullivan MM, Jessop JD, Williams BD (1989) Unilateral palsy of the hypoglossal nerve in a patient with tuberculosis of the first cervical vertebra. Br J Rheumatol 28:540–542
70. Warwick-Brown NP (1984) Cranial nerve palsies following tuberculosis. J Laryngol Otol 98:217–219
71. Mohindra S, Gupta SK, Mohindra S, Gupta R (2006) Unusual presentations of craniovertebral junction tuberculosis: a report of 2 cases and literature review. Surg Neurol 66:94–99
72. Mauss H (1971) Effect of isoniazid on the evolution of the pulmonary lesions in tuberculosis in mice. Pathol Biol 19:743–750
73. Marks DJB, Dheda K, Dawson R, Ainslie G, Miller RF (2009) Adverse events to antituberculosis therapy: influence of HIV and antiretroviral drugs. Int J STD AIDS 20:339–345
74. Kass JS, Shandera WX (2010) Nervous system effects of antituberculosis therapy. CNS Drugs 24:655–667
75. Mafukidze AT, Calnan M, Furin J (2016) Peripheral neuropathy in persons with tuberculosis. J Clin Tuberc Other Mycobact Dis 2:5–11
76. Warpe BM, Poflee SV, Pande NP, Shrikhande AV (2014) Tuberculous neuritis: a rare sequel of a common disease. Indian J Pathol Microbiol 57:69–71
77. Orrell RW, King RHM, Bowler JV, Ginsberg L (2002) Peripheral nerve granuloma in a patient with tuberculosis. J Neurol Neurosurg Psychiatry 73:769–771
78. Dai L, Mahajan SD, Guo C, Zhang T, Wang W, Li T, Jiang T, Wu H, Li N (2014) Spectrum of central nervous system disorders in hospitalized HIV/AIDS patients (2009–2011) at a major HIV/AIDS referral center in Beijing, China. J Neurol Sci 342:88–92
79. Dooley KE, Chaisson RE (2009) Tuberculosis and diabetes mellitus: convergence of two epidemics. Lancet Infect Dis 9:737–746
80. Blain PG, Lane R (1998) Neurological disorders. In: Davies's textbook of adverse drug reactions. Chapman and Hall Medical, London, p 585
81. Ghavanini AA, Kimpinski K (2014) Revisiting the evidence for neuropathy caused by pyridoxine deficiency and excess. J Clin Neuromuscul Dis 16:25–31
82. Vilholm OJ, Christensen AA, Zedan AH, Itani M (2014) Drug-induced peripheral neuropathy. Basic Clin Pharmacol Toxicol 115:185–192
83. Zilber LA, Bajdakova ZL, Gardasjan AN, Konovalov NV, Bunina TL, Barabadze EM (1963) The prevention and treatment of isoniazid toxicity in the therapy of pulmonary tuberculosis. Bull World Health Organ 29:457–481
84. Sanfeliu C, Wright JM, Kim SU (1999) Neurotoxicity of isoniazid and its metabolites in cultures of mouse dorsal root ganglion neurons and hybrid neuronal cell line. Neurotoxicology 20:935–944
85. Evans DA, Manley KA, McKusick VA (1960) Genetic control of isoniazid metabolism in man. Br Med J 2:485–491
86. Stettner M, Steinberger D, Hartmann CJ, Pabst T, Konta L, Hartung HP, Kieseier BC (2015) Isoniazid-induced polyneuropathy in a tuberculosis patient – implication for individual risk stratification with genotyping? Brain Behav 5:e00326
87. Furin JJ, Mitnick CD, Shin SS, Bayona J, Becerra MC, Singler JM, Alcantara F, Castañieda C, Sanchez E, Acha J, Farmer PE, Kim JY (2001) Occurrence of serious adverse effects in patients receiving community-based therapy for multidrug-resistant tuberculosis. Int J Tuberc Lung Dis 5:648–655
88. Mukherjee JS, Rich ML, Socci AR, Joseph JK, Virú FA, Shin SS, Furin JJ, Becerra MC, Barry DJ, Kim JY, Bayona J, Farmer P, Smith Fawzi MC, Seung KJ (2004) Programmes and principles in treatment of multidrug-resistant tuberculosis. Lancet 363:474–481
89. Shin SS, Hyson AM, Castañeda C, Sánchez E, Alcántara F, Mitnick CD, Fawzi MC, Bayona J, Farmer PE, Kim JY, Furin JJ (2003) Peripheral neuropathy associated with treatment for multidrug-resistant tuberculosis. Int J Tuberc Lung Dis 7:347–353
90. Roongruangpitayakul C, Chuchottaworn C (2013) Outcomes of MDR/XDR-TB patients treated with linezolid: experience in Thailand. J Med Assoc Thail 96:1273–1282
91. Cholo MC, Steel HC, Fourie PB, Germishuizen WA, Anderson R (2012) Clofazimine: current status and future prospects. J Antimicrob Chemother 67:290–298
92. Aycıcek A, Eser O, Sezer M, Degırmencı B (2009) A neck mass with brachial plexus injury: Pott's disease. Am J Otolaryngol 30:350–352
93. Wadia NH, Dastur DK (1969) Spinal meningitides with radiculo-myelopathy. 1. Clinical and radiological features. J Neurol Sci 8:239–260
94. Dastur D, Wadia NH (1969) Spinal meningitides with radiculo-myelopathy. 2. Pathology and pathogenesis. J Neurol Sci 8:261–297
95. Gupta R, Garg RK, Jain A, Malhotra HS, Verma R, Sharma PK (2015) Spinal cord and spinal nerve root involvement (myeloradiculopathy) in tuberculous meningitis. Medicine 94:e404

96. Kakar A, Madan VS, Prakash V (1997) Syringomyelia – a complication of meningitis – case report. Spinal Cord 35:629–631
97. Kotil K, Alan MS, Bilge T (2007) Medical management of Pott disease in the thoracic and lumbar spine: a prospective clinical study. J Neurosurg Spine 6:222–228
98. Mishra A, Kanwar RS, Santanu B, Kumar A, Dudeja RK, Jain AK, Agarwal AK (2004) Acute granulomatous (tubercular) myelitis. J Indian Acad Clin Med 5: Available from: http://medind.nic.in/jac/t00/i2/jact00i2p182.pdf
99. Haldar S, Sharma N, Gupta VK, Tyagi JS (2009) Efficient diagnosis of tuberculous meningitis by detection of Mycobacterium tuberculosis DNA in cerebrospinal fluid filtrates using PCR. J Med Microbiol 58:616–624
100. Wasay M, Arif H, Khealani B, Ahsan H (2006) Neuroimaging of tuberculous myelitis: analysis of ten cases and review of literature. J Neuroimaging 16:197–205
101. Hernández-Albújar S, Arribas JR, Royo A, González-García JJ, Peña JM, Vázquez JJ (2000) Tuberculous radiculomyelitis complicating tuberculous meningitis: case report and review. Clin Infect Dis 30:915–921
102. Garg RK, Malhotra HS, Kumar N (2014) Paradoxical reaction in HIV negative tuberculous meningitis. J Neurol Sci 340:26–36
103. Ramanathan SR, Ahluwalia T (2010) Rare complication: acute syringomyelia due to tuberculoma and tubercular meningitis. J Neurosci Rural Pract 1:123–125
104. Kaynar MY, Koçer N, Gençosmanoğlu BE, Hanci M (2000) Syringomyelia – as a late complication of tuberculous meningitis. Acta Neurochir 142:935–938
105. West TW (2013) Transverse myelitis-a review of the presentation, diagnosis, and initial management. Discov Med 16:167–177
106. Jain RS, Kumar S, Tejwani S (2015) A rare association of tuberculous longitudinally extensive transverse myelitis (LETM) with brain tuberculoma. Springerplus 4:476
107. Putruele AM, Legarreta CG, Limongi L, Rossi SE (2005) Tuberculous transverse myelitis: case report and review of the literature. Clin Pulm Med 12:46
108. Geri G, Passeron A, Heym B, Arlet J-B, Pouchot J, Capron L, Ranque B (2013) Paradoxical reactions during treatment of tuberculosis with extrapulmonary manifestations in HIV-negative patients. Infection 41:537–543
109. Stavros K, Simpson DM (2014) Understanding the etiology and management of HIV-associated peripheral neuropathy. Curr HIV/AIDS Rep 11:195–201

Part V

Laboratory Studies in Neuro-Tuberculosis

Traditional and New Laboratory Procedures

25

Güliz U. Güleç and Ahmet T. Turgut

Contents

G.U. Güleç, MD (✉)
Deparment of Infectious Diseases, Adnan Menderes University School of Medicine, Aydın, Turkey
e-mail: gulizuyar@yahoo.com

A.T. Turgut, MD
Department of Radiology, Hacettepe University School of Medicine, Ankara, Turkey
e-mail: ahmettuncayturgut@yahoo.com

Abbreviations

ADA	Adenosine deaminase
AFB	Acid-fast bacillus
BCG	Bacille Calmette-Guerin
CNS	Central nervous system
CSF	Cerebrospinal fluid
ELISA	Enzyme-linked immunosorbent assay
ELISpot	Enzyme-linked immunospot assay
ESAT-6	Early secretory antigenic target-6
HIV	Human immunodeficiency virus
IFN-γ	Interferon-γ
IGRA	Interferon gamma release assay
IL	Interleukin
LAM	Lipoarabinomannan
LJ	Lowenstein-Jensen
MC	Mononuclear cell
MGIT	Mycobacterial growth indicator tube
MODS	Mycobacterial observation drug suscep tibility
NAA	Nucleic acid amplification
PCR	Polymerase chain reaction
PPD	Purified protein derivative
TB	Tuberculosis
TBM	Tuberculous meningitis
TNF	Tumor necrosis factor
TST	Tuberculin skin test
WHO	World Health Organization

M. Turgut et al. (eds.), *Tuberculosis of the Central Nervous System*,
DOI 10.1007/978-3-319-50712-5_25

25.1 Introduction

Tuberculosis (TB) can spread to almost every organ, and clinical manifestation depends on localization of the infection [1]. Central nervous system (CNS) involvement develops in nearly 1% of infected persons. Of the various presentations of TB of CNS, tuberculous meningitis (TBM) is the most common (70–80%) followed by tuberculoma and abscess [2, 3]. The clinical picture is different in children and in adults. In children, disseminated forms and the risk of progression to severe forms are reported with higher incidence [4].

TB is one of the leading opportunistic infection in people living with *human immunodeficiency virus* (HIV) and transplant recipients. HIV infection notably increases the risk for acquisition, progression, morbidity, and mortality of TB [5]. Extrapulmonary manifestations especially CNS involvement are five times more likely in HIV-positive individuals [5]. In 2014, there were an estimated 9.6 million people to have fallen ill with TB, and 12% of these were HIV positive. Worldwide TB killed 1.5 million people annually (1.1 million HIV negative and 0.4 million HIV positive) [6].

M. tuberculosis is a nonspore-forming, nonmotile aerobic bacillus with a cell wall rich in high-molecular-weight lipids. The slow-growing bacillus needs 15–20 h for generation time and 3–8 weeks for visible growth on solid media [7]. The knowledge-related *M. tuberculosis* genotype is that genotype influences disease phenotype and that interaction between host and bacterial genotypes and the development of TB is present [8].

The inhaled bacilli colonize alveolar macrophages and may spread to local lymph nodes and bloodstream. As a rule, it generally involves the lungs, but it has also some extrapulmonary systemic manifestations like intraocular involvement (Fig. 25.1). Importantly, the blood-brain barrier protects the CNS from the circulatory system. Despite the integrity of this barrier, some microorganisms can cross the barrier to cause TBM or encephalitis [9]. A caseous granuloma termed as "Rich focus" develops in the meninges.

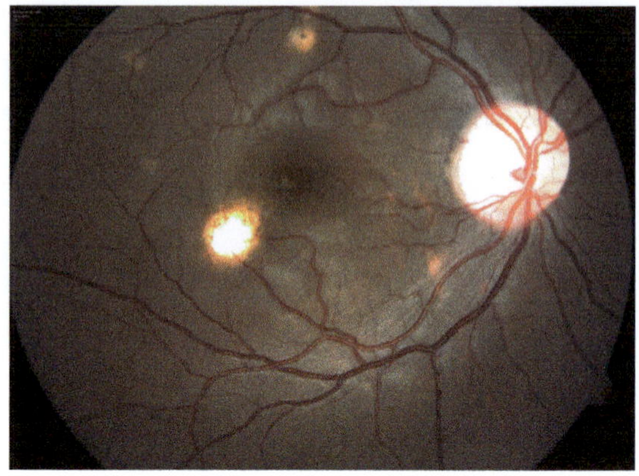

Fig. 25.1 Fundus photograph of a patient with tuberculous meningitis depicting polymorphic, yellowish, relatively discrete lesions suggestive of choroid tubercles (Courtesy of RK Garg, MD)

Rupture of a Rich focus into the subarachnoid space initiates a powerful inflammatory T cell response. Alterations in cytokine levels in patients can influence the immune system functions and hereby the signs, symptoms, and sequelae of TB of CNS [8, 10].

Early identification of TB of CNS is important and crucial for the accomplishment of treatment. Diagnosis is still problematic despite many advances in techniques [4]. Structural properties of microorganism and immune response of the host compose the main idea of laboratory tests. In this chapter we aimed to review the traditional and new laboratory procedures for TB of CNS.

25.2 Microbiological Analysis

If the clinical presentation is suggestive of TB of CNS, cerebrospinal fluid (CSF) specimens should be collected, transported, and processed urgently. Routine analyses (cell counts and differential, protein and glucose level) and microbiologic tests for bacteria, fungi, and *M. tuberculosis* should be done [11, 12]. Definitive diagnosis of TB of CNS depends on detection of tuberculous bacilli in the CSF either by smear microscopy or by culture. It should be kept in mind that atypical CSF findings may be obtained in HIV-coinfected individuals [11, 12].

Table 25.1 Traditional staining techniques for mycobacteria

Method	Carbol fuchsin method		Fluorochrome method	
Process	*Ziehl-Neelsen* a fixed smear covered with carbol fuchsin is heated, rinsed, decolorized with acid alcohol, and counterstained with methylene blue	*Kinyoun* is modified to make heating unnecessary	*Auramine O*	*Auramine rhodamine*
Properties	The organisms appear as slightly bent, beaded rods 2–4 µm long and 0.2–5 µm wide		Dyes specifically bind to the cell wall of *Mycobacteria* and the counterstaining with potassium permanganate prevents nonspecific fluorescence	

25.2.1 Cytological Examination

The CSF profile of TB of CNS is not specific for TB and mimics both infectious and noninfectious CNS diseases [11]. The characteristic analysis of CSF in TB of CNS shows a moderate pleocytosis with lymphocytic predominance, moderately elevated protein levels, and low glucose levels (hypoglycorrhachia) [13, 14]. Total white blood cell in CSF range between 100 and 500 cells/µl with mononuclear lymphocytic predominance, protein levels range between 100 and 500 mg/dl, and glucose levels are usually less than 45 mg/dl [15].

In a series of 160 adult cases of TB of CNS in Turkey found lymphocyte domination in 65%, high protein levels in 72% of the cases. CSF/serum glucose ratio was <0.6 and < 0.3 in 95% and 55% of the cases [16].

25.2.2 Smear Microscopy

Mycobacterial cell wall due to the presence of large amount of lipoidal material is resistant to decolorizing agent. The term acid-fast bacillus (AFB) is practically synonymous with mycobacteria, although *Nocardia* and some other organisms can be acid fast [7]. Any biologic fluid or material can be examined directly (e.g., pleural fluid, CSF, urine, gastric lavage fluid), although thin fluids are best examined after sedimentation by centrifugation [7].

Traditional staining technique using Ziehl-Neelsen, Kinyoun, or auramine-rhodamine is a rapid and practical method with low-cost and high predictive value. (Table 25.1). Nevertheless, the sensitivity of CSF staining techniques is generally <20% [13]. CSF sample volume, duration of slide examination, and the technical expertise of laboratory personnel are important factors [17, 18]. Sensitivity can reach up to 60% when used larger CSF volumes although it is difficult to obtain this especially from children [17, 18]. One of the reasons of low detection rate is that intracellular *M. tuberculosis* can hardly be stained by acid-fast dyes. So techniques to reveal the presence of intracellular and extracellular *M. tuberculosis* were developed. A modified staining method Ziehl-Neelsen combined with cytospin and Triton X-100 can reveal AFB within the immune cells using of only 0.5 ml CSF specimen, and the detection rate of extracellular AFB was significantly improved as well [19].

25.2.3 Culture Techniques

The growth of *M. tuberculosis* in culture is the gold standard. Culture techniques allow drug susceptibility testing which can influence drug selection and prognosis [13]. Normally sterile tissues or fluids such as CSF do not require decontamination, as some loss of mycobacterial viability does occur. But these specimens can be concentrated and the sediment is used for culture [7, 20].

A variety of solid and liquid media are available for the culture of mycobacteria:

- Solid egg based: Lowenstein-Jensen (LJ)
- Solid agar based: Middlebrook 7H11
- Liquid broth: Middlebrook 7H12

The macroscopic and microscopic growth of mycobacteria may vary with the type of media. Liquid broth cultures require shorter incubation times (1–3 weeks) as compared to solid media (3–8 weeks). Nevertheless, solid media allow examination of colony morphology, detection of mixed cultures, and quantification of growth. For these reasons, it is rational to use liquid and solid media in conjunction to ensure recovery [7].

Culture positivity rates were reported between 25% and 75%, but results are only available after 2–6 weeks of incubation, and negative results cannot be used to exclude a TB diagnosis [17, 21].

Commercial automated liquid broth systems greatly facilitate mycobacterial culture (Table 25.2). They monitor mycobacterial growth by detection of carbon dioxide production or oxygen consumption through radiometric, fluorometric, or colorimetric indicators [7, 20, 22]. They have been shown to be more efficient than LJ culture in the diagnosis of TBM [22].

Mycobacterial observation drug susceptibility (MODS) technique has been found to be more sensitive than CSF smear and more rapid than conventional TB culture (with a median time to positivity of 6 days) and useful for the detection of drug resistance in a number of studies [8, 20].

Thakur et al. reported that the recovery rate of automated BACTEC mycobacterial growth indicator tube (MGIT) 960 system was higher (27.4%) than LJ media (10.9%) [23]. The mean time of detection in MGIT and LJ media for *M. tuberculosis* were 18 days and 38 days, respectively [23].

A multicenter study from Turkey confirmed that the automated culture system was superior to LJ culture for the diagnosis of TBM [12]. Concordant use of two-culture system provided significant benefit over using them singly. In addition, both of the culture systems were found to be significantly better than molecular methods (81.8%, 72.7%, and 57.3%, respectively) [12].

25.3 Molecular Analysis

Molecular-based techniques such as nucleic acid amplification (NAA) tests have become important because of time-consuming traditional methods. These techniques demonstrate the presence of nucleic acid of tubercle bacilli in clinical specimens such as CSF. The typical NAA method is the polymerase chain reaction (PCR) assay [24]. Real-time PCR, isothermal strand displacement, or transcription-mediated amplification and ligase chain reaction are the alternative tests [8].

NAA tests are categorized as commercial or in-house. Several commercially available NAA tests such as the Amplicor *M. tuberculosis* tests (Roche Molecular Systems, Branchburg, NJ, USA) and the amplified *M. tuberculosis* direct test (MTD; Gen-Probe Inc., San Diego, CA, USA) have been developed for the rapid diagnosis of TB [25, 26]. The superiority of NAA tests is the rapidity so that the results can be obtained about 3–6 h from receipt of specimen [25]. NAA

Table 25.2 Commercial liquid culture systems

System	Properties		
BACTEC MGIT (Becton Dickinson Microbiology Systems, Sparks, MD)	Fluorometric method	Detects growth in 1–3 weeks	
MODS	CSF pellet inoculated into a microtiter plate	Uses Middlebrook 7H9 broth culture	Direct drug susceptibility testing in liquid culture
BACTEC 460 TB system (Becton-Dickinson, Towson, MD)	Radiometric method	A selective liquid media, containing C14-labeled palmitic acid	

tests can detect fewer than 10 bacilli in clinical specimens or cultures [8]. Nevertheless, the presence of small number of microorganisms and inhibitor substances in the CSF hinder applying NAA techniques to the rapid diagnosis of TB of CNS [24, 25].

The validity of NAA tests has been extensively studied since the early 1990s and has shown that the specificity is high but sensitivity is variable [8, 25]. Sensitivity is highest in smear-positive respiratory samples and lower in smear-negative and in extrapulmonary samples. Thus, a negative result does not rule out the diagnosis of TB of CNS [8].

In a study of Christie et al., 20 atypical cases with TB of CNS manifested as encephalitis were identified [27]. Of the cases, all had a positive CSF culture, but only 4 of 17 (24%) were CSF PCR positive, and none had a positive smear [27].

In a study from Pakistan, which is a country with high TB incidence, a total of 766 clinical samples including 76 CSF were analyzed for the clinical utility of *M. tuberculosis* PCR. The positivity rate for CSF specimens was 42.1% [28].

Nevertheless, a systematic review and meta-analysis of 14 studies showed that commercial NAA test for diagnosis of TBM had a high specificity (98%, 95% CI 97–99%), but a low sensitivity when compared with culture (56%, 95% CI 46–66%) [25].

The Xpert MTB/RIF test (Cepheid CA, USA) is a commercial NAA test that uses real-time PCR to determine *M. tuberculosis* and identify rifampin resistance [29]. Manual DNA extraction is not required because of the cartridge-based form, and the closed system diminishes the risk for cross-contamination [21]. As the initial diagnostic test for CSF specimens in suspected TBM patients, World Health Organization (WHO) recommends the use of this test rather than conventional microscopy and culture [6, 29].

Several studies have reported successful use of the Xpert MTB/RIF test on extrapulmonary samples, with sensitivities of upon 80% and specificity reaching 100% [15, 16, 21, 25, 30]. However, the number of CSF samples in these studies was low [21]. Tortoli et al. evaluated the performance of the Xpert system on different extrapulmonary specimens in a country with low TB incidence [31]. Overall sensitivity and specificity were 81.3 and 99.8% [31]. In 204 South-African patients, of whom 87% were HIV infected, overall sensitivity and specificity of Xpert MTB/RIF were 62% (48%–75%) and 95% (87%–99%), respectively [30]. A significant increase in the sensitivity and specificity was shown in some studies when a large volume of centrifuged CSF pellet was used [21, 30].

The diagnostic accuracy of in-house PCR tests is poorly defined because of the wide variability in sensitivity and specificity [25].

For comparison of PCR, microscopy, and culture, a cohort study was designed. CSF samples of 230 adult patients with suspected meningitis are evaluated by using in-house real-time PCR targeting IS6110, ZN staining, and liquid and solid media for culture. TBM was diagnosed in 207 patients, 17.9% of them was HIV infected. PCR had a high positivity rate (68%) among both HIV-infected and noninfected patients, higher than microscopy (11%), and solid (36%) and liquid (44%) media [32].

In another study, 178 specimens including 25 CSF were evaluated for IS6110-targeted PCR as compared to LJ culture for the diagnosis of extrapulmonary TB [1]. Nine of 25 CSF samples were PCR positive, but 3 positive PCR in non-TBM were considered as false positive result [1].

The diagnostic accuracy of the combination of NAA tests was assessed in a study among children. GenoType®MTBDRplus and Xpert MTB/RIF assays, microscopy and culture were performed on 101 CSF samples. Although improvement in sensitivity was obtained with the combination of culture and NAA tests, they cannot serve as a rule-out test [33].

25.4 Immunoserological and Biochemical Tests

25.4.1 Antigen Detection Tests

M. tuberculosis adapts to its environment by altering its transcriptional responses. So for the diagnosis of several forms of extrapulmonary TB, the optimum antigens or antigen combinations may vary [34]. The antigens that will be used for antigen detection tests should have some properties; indeed antigen should be specific to *M. tuberculosis*: (1) common expression by in vivo bacteria, (2) being in the extracellular environment, and (3) resistant to degradation by the host inflammatory processes [34].

Nowadays, it is believed that antigen detection is more sensitive than antibody detection. The early phase of TB infection, corticosteroid therapy, or immune deficient status may result false negativity for antibody detection tests. And they cannot distinguish acute or latent infection [35]. For developing and simplifying of antigen detection tests, many efforts have been made, but their prognostic power still remains poor. Tests that detect multiple antigens compared to that detect single antigens may yield higher sensitivities [34].

Early secreted antigen target-6 (ESAT-6) is an *M. tuberculosis*-specific, early secreted, and low-molecular-weight protein [36]. It is recognized by specific (IFN)-γ-secreting T cells. These T cells present much more in patients with an active infection, and the numbers of them are significantly higher in the CSF than in the peripheral blood. Therefore, ESAT-6-induced specific IFN-γ responses can be useful in diagnosis of TB of CNS [35].

Intracellular mycobacteria were investigated by ESAT-6 immunocytochemical stain using rabbit anti-ESAT-6 polyclonal antibody in a study [36]. After counterstaining with methylene blue, visualization of yellow-brown granules in the cytoplasm under light microscopy was defined as positive result [36]. The sensitivity of ESAT-6 immunostain was 75.1% [36]. But limitation of the test was relatively high number of false positive results [36]. Song et al. reported quantitative detection of ESAT-6 in CSF using indirect enzyme-linked immunosorbent assays (ELISA) protocol [35].

Lipoarabinomannan (LAM) is a *M. tuberculosis* cell wall component, has immunoregulatory and anti-inflammatory effects, and serves as a virulence factor of mycobacteria [17]. A LAM-ELISA test (Clearview®TB ELISA, Inverness Medical Innovations, MA, USA) has been developed [17, 29]. The sensitivity and specificity of the test were reported as 64–69% and 62–65% for diagnosis of culture- or PCR-positive TBM. Higher sensitivity and specificity were noted in HIV-infected patients with CD4 cell counts below 100 cells/ mm^3 [29].

In a meta-analysis including 21 extrapulmonary TB study, five studies targeting LAM, ESAT-6, Ag85 complex, and the 65-kDa antigen in CSF provided the highest sensitivity (87%; 95% CI, 61–98%), but low specificity (84%; 95% CI, 60–95%) [34].

25.4.2 Tuberculin Skin Test (TST)

A purified protein derivative (PPD) from *M. tuberculosis* has long been used as skin test. TST provides evidence of previous TB infection and lacks diagnostic specificity in bacille Calmette-Guerin (BCG)-vaccinated individuals [35]. The factors that influence TST reactivity after BCG vaccination are the strain, dose, and number of BCG vaccine used, the technique of and age at vaccination, nutritional/health status, the time interval between vaccination and TST, and the number of intervening tuberculin tests [37]. The diagnostic benefit of TST for TB of CNS varies from 10% to 50% [13, 35, 37].

25.4.3 Interferon Gamma Release Assays (IGRAs)

IGRAs are in vitro tests that are based on IFN-γ release after T cell stimulation by antigens. The two commercially available IGRAs are (1) the QuantiFERON TB-GOLD In-Tube (QFT-G-IT) (Cellestis Ltd., Carnegie, Australia) which uses ELISA to measure the concentration of IFN-γ and (2) T-SPOT.TB test (Oxford Immunotec, Abingdon, UK) which measures the number of IFN-γ-producing cells, after incubation of whole blood or peripheral blood mononuclear cell

(MC) with *M. tuberculosis* antigens [38]. These tests indicate recent or remote exposure to *M. tuberculosis* of symptom-free individuals but cannot accurately distinguish active TB from latent TB infection. So the clinical use of IGRAs is limited in intermediate to high endemicity regions [13, 39].

IFN-γ can be easily induced in peripheral blood monocytes or whole blood. However, because of the low number and short half-life of T cells, detection of them in CSF is difficult in TBM patients. The sensitivity and specificity of *M. tuberculosis*-specific antigen detection directly in CSF vary between 35–95% and 95–100%, respectively [39]. The enzyme-linked immunospot assay (ELISpot) detects IFN-γ-secreting T cells specific for ESAT-6 and CFP (Culture Filtrate Protein)-10. In a small prospective clinical study, sensitivity and specificity of ELISpot in CSF were 90% and 100%. They suggest that it could be a useful tool for rapid diagnosis of TBM [40].

Moreover, *M. tuberculosis*-specific T cells are compartmentalized more to the infected sites than to the circulating blood. Kim et al. evaluated the usefulness of peripheral blood MC and CSF-MC-based ELISpot assays for the diagnosis of active TB [41]. The sensitivity of the peripheral blood MC ELISpot was 91% and 63%, respectively. CSF-MC ELISpot's sensitivity and specificity were 75% and 75%, respectively [41]. They demonstrated that the ratio of CSF to peripheral blood MC ELISpot results can distinguish between active and latent TB with a specificity of 100% [41].

25.4.4 Cytokines and Chemokines

Cytokines and chemokines are small protein molecules that have important role in the pathogenesis of TB. They regulate immunological responses by stimulating wide range of inflammatory cells. The impact of cytokines on different cell types could be different [38].

Their diagnostic and prognostic potential have been established in many studies. IFN-γ, tumor necrosis factor (TNF)-α, and interleukin (IL)-12 are the main cytokines. Other elevated chemokines include IL-8 (CXCL-8), MCP (monocyte chemoattractant protein/CCL-2)-1, MCP-3 (CCL-7), MCP-5 (CCL-12), RANTES (regulated on activation normal T cell expressed and secreted) (CCL-5), MIP (macrophage inflammatory protein/CCL-3)-1-α, MIP-1-β (CCL-4), MIP-2 (CXCL-2), and IP-10 (IFN-γ-inducible protein/CXCL-10) [38].

In a study of children aged 3 months–13 years, CSF and serum samples of 56 TBM and 55 non-TBM patients were assessed for 28 soluble mediators [10]. The CSF concentrations of IL13, VEGF (vascular endothelial growth factor), and cathelicidin LL-37 were significantly elevated ($p < .05$), and the concentration of IL17 was lower in the TBM patients group compared to patients with viral and bacterial meningitis [10]. The serum concentrations of IL17, cathelicidin LL-37, IFN-γ, and bFGF were significantly elevated in TBM group ($p < .05$) [10].

In another study, the levels of 26 cytokines and chemokines in plasma, pleural fluid, and CSF were examined by Luminex liquid array-based multiplexed immunoassays [42]. In plasma MIG (monokine induced by IFN-γ), G-CSF and notably IP-10 levels were significantly increased in active TB [42]. In CSF, MIG and IP-10 showed promising diagnostic values in distinguishing TBM and non-TBM [42].

25.4.5 Adenosine Deaminase (ADA)

ADA is an enzyme related with purine metabolism. It is considered to be a marker of cellular immunity because of its association with maturation of monocytes, macrophages, and T lymphocytes. An increase in ADA levels is observed in CSF of TBM patients. The sensitivity and specificity of ADA in CSF range from 60–90% and 80–90%, respectively. The cutoff values used in various studies ranged from >5.0 to >15 IU/l. The role of ADA measurement in differentiation TBM from other types of meningitis is conflicting in several studies. It also seems a not useful diagnostic tool in HIV-infected TBM patients [14, 15, 43].

It is simple, inexpensive, and rapid test. Disadvantage of the test is no standardized cutoff levels for the TBM diagnosis have been established. Nevertheless, multicenter studies are needed for standardization of the test. Maybe it can be used as a supportive diagnostic test for TBM [14, 15, 43].

25.4.6 Tuberculostearic Acid

Tuberculostearic acid is a fatty acid component of the *M. tuberculosis* cell wall. Its measurement in CSF of TBM patient via gas chromatography showed high sensitivity and specificity in limited studies. Nevertheless, expensive equipment and complexity of sample preparation protocol has limited the clinical use of this technique [14, 15].

Conclusion

Rapid and definitive diagnosis and starting anti-TB chemotherapy quickly are the most important factors for prognosis of this devastating illness. The definitive diagnosis of TB of CNS relies on the isolation of *M. tuberculosis* from CSF. But traditional staining has very low sensitivity, and culture usually takes weeks and is relatively insensitive. Molecular methods are rapid, but show variable sensitivity and should not be used to exclude the diagnosis of TB of CNS. Also they cannot be performed in all clinical laboratories because of requirement for technical equipment and personnel. The clinical use of the immunoserological tests is limited in intermediate to high endemicity regions because it cannot distinguish active TB from latent TB. The reports about biomarkers are controversial. The search should focus on convenient marker. Unfortunately, there is no established diagnostic method that is capable of rapid detection with high sensitivity and specificity. Studies are still ongoing for improving traditional diagnostic methods. Combining traditional and new methods will be beneficial for rapid detection.

References

1. Makeshkumar V, Madhavan R, Narayanan S (2014) Polymerase chain reaction targeting insertion sequence for the diagnosis of extrapulmonary tuberculosis. Indian J Med Res 139:161–166
2. Mahale RR, Meht A, Uchil S (2015) Estimation of cerebrospinal fluid cortisol level in tuberculous meningitis. J Neurosci Rural Pract 6:541–544
3. Miftode EG, Dorneanu OS, Leca DA, Juganariu G, Teodor A, Hurmuzache M, Nastase EV, Anton-Paduraru DT (2015) Tuberculous meningitis in children and adults: a 10-year retrospective comparative analysis. PLoS One 10:e01133477
4. Hajia M, Amirzargar AA, Nazari M, Davodi NR, Zarandi MK (2015) A five years study of tuberculous meningitis in Iran. Iran J Pathol 10:290–294
5. Nelson CA, Zunt JR (2011) Tuberculosis of the central nervous system in immunocompromised patients: HIV infection and solid organ transplant recipients. Clin Infect Dis 53:915–926
6. WHO (2015) Global tuberculosis report 2015, 20th edn. World Health Organization, Geneva
7. Fitzgerald DW, Sterling TR, Haas DW (2010) Mycobacterium tuberculosis. In: Mandell GL, Bennett JE, Dolin R (eds) Principles and practice of infectious diseases, 7th edn. Churchill Livingstone, Philadelphia, pp 3129–3163
8. Török ME (2015) Tuberculous meningitis: advances in diagnosis and treatment. Br Med Bull 113:117–131
9. Be NA, Kim KS, Bishai WR, Jain SK (2009) Pathogenesis of central nervous system tuberculosis. Curr Mol Med 9:94–99
10. Visser DH, Solomons RS, Ronacher K, van Well GT, Heymans MW, Walzl G, Chegou NN, Schoeman JF, van Furth AM (2015) Host immune response to tuberculous meningitis. Clin Infect Dis 60:177–187
11. Chin JH (2014) Tuberculous meningitis. Neurol Clin Pract 4:199–205
12. Erdem H, Ozturk-Engin D, Elaldi N, Gulsun S, Sengoz G, Crisan A, Johansen IS, Inan A, Nechifor M, Al-Mahdawi A, Civljak R, Ozguler M, Savic B, Ceran N, Cacopardo B, Inal AS, Namiduru M, Dayan S, Kayabas U, Parlak E, Khalifa A, Kursun E, Sipahi OR, Yemisen M, Akbulut A, Bitirgen M, Dulovic O, Kandemir B, Luca C, Parlak M, Stahl JP, Pehlivanoglu F, Simeon S, Ulu-Kilic A, Yasar K, Yilmaz G, Yilmaz E, Beovic B, Catroux M, Lakatos B, Sunbul M, Oncul O, Alabay S, Sahin-Horasan E, Kose S, Shehata G, Andre K, Alp A, Cosic G, Gul HC, Karakas A, Chadapaud S, Hansmann Y, Harxhi A, Kirova V, Masse-Chabredier I, Oncu S, Sener A, Tekin R, Deveci O, Karabay O, Agalar C (2014) The microbiological diagnosis of tuberculous meningitis: results of Haydarpasa-1 study. Clin Microbiol Infect 20:O600–O608
13. Cherian A, Thomas SV (2011) Central nervous system tuberculosis. Afr Health Sci 11:116–127

14. Rock RB, Olin M, Baker CA, Molitor TW, Peterson PK (2008) Central nervous system tuberculosis: pathogenesis and clinical aspects. Clin Microbiol Rev 21:243–261
15. Philip N, William T, John DV (2015) Diagnosis of tuberculous meningitis: challenges and promises. Malays J Pathol 37:1–9
16. Pehlivanoglu F, Kart Yasar K, Sengoz G (2012) Tuberculous meningitis in adults: a review of 160 cases. Scientific World Journal 2012:169028
17. Brancusi F, Farrar J, Heemskerk D (2012) Tuberculous meningitis in adults: a review of a decade of developments focusing on prognostic factors for outcome. Future Microbiol 7:1101–1116
18. Marx GE, Chan ED (2011) Tuberculous meningitis: diagnosis and treatment overview. Tuberc Res Treat 2011:798764
19. Chen P, Shi M, Feng G-D, Liu J-Y, Wang B-J, Shi X-D, Ma L, Liu X-D, Yang Y-N, Dai W, Liu T-T, He Y, Li J-G, Hao X-K, Zhao G (2012) A highly efficient Ziehl-Neelsen stain: identifying de novo intracellular *Mycobacterium tuberculosis* and improving detection of extracellular *M. tuberculosis* in cerebrospinal fluid. J Clin Microbiol 50:1166–1170
20. Caws M, Dang TM, Torok E, Campbell J, Do DA, Tran TH, Nguyen VC, Nguyen TC, Farrar J (2007) Evaluation of the MODS culture technique for the diagnosis of tuberculous meningitis. PLoS One 2:e1173
21. Nhu NT, Heemskerk D, do DA T, TTH C, NTH M, HDT N, PPL L, Minh Ha DT, Merson L, Van Thinh TT, Day J, Chau NV, Wolbers M, Farrar J, Caws M (2014) Evaluation of GeneXpertw MTB/RIF for diagnosis of tuberculous meningitis. J Clin Microbiol 52:226–233
22. Venkataswamy MM, Rafi W, Nagarathna S, Ravi V, Chandramuki A (2007) Comparative evaluation of bactec 460tb system and lowenstein-jensen medium for the isolation of *M. tuberculosis* from cerebrospinal fluid samples of tuberculous meningitis patients. Indian J Med Microbiol 25:236–240
23. Thakur R, Goyal R, Sarma S (2010) Laboratory diagnosis of tuberculous meningitis – is there a scope for further improvement? J Lab Physicians 2:21–24
24. Takahashi T, Tamura M, Takasu T (2012) The PCR-based diagnosis of central nervous system tuberculosis: up to date. Tuberc Res Treat 2012:831292
25. Pai M, Flores LL, Pai N, Hubbard A, Riley LW, Colford JM (2003) Diagnostic accuracy of nucleic acid amplification tests for tuberculous meningitis: a systematic review and meta-analysis. Lancet Infect Dis 3:633–643
26. Centers for Disease Control and Prevention (2009) Updated guidelines for the use of nucleic acid amplification tests in the diagnosis of tuberculosis. MMWR Morb Mortal Wkly Rep 58:7–10
27. Christie LJ, Loeffler AM, Honarmand S, Flood JM, Baxter R, Jacobson S, Alexander R, Glaser CA (2008) Diagnostic challenges of central nervous system tuberculosis. Emerg Infect Dis 14:1473–1475
28. Amin I, Idrees M, Awan Z, Shahid M, Afzal S, Hussain A (2011) PCR could be a method of choice for identification of both pulmonary and extrapulmonary tuberculosis. BMC Res Notes 4:332
29. Cox JA, Lukande RL, Kalungi S, Van Marck E, Lammens M, Van de Vijver K, Kambugu A, Nelson AM, Colebunders R, Manabe YC (2015) Accuracy of lipoarabinomannan and Xpert MTB/RIF testing in cerebrospinal fluid to diagnose tuberculous meningitis in an autopsy cohort of HIV-infected adults. J Clin Microbiol 53:2667–2673
30. Patel VB, Theron G, Lenders L, Matinyena B, Connolly C, Singh R, Coovadia Y, Ndung'u T, Dheda K (2013) Diagnostic accuracy of quantitative PCR (Xpert MTB/RIF) for tuberculous meningitis in a high burden setting: a prospective study. PLoS Med 10:e1001536
31. Tortoli E, Russo C, Piersimoni C, Mazzola E, Monte PD, Pascarella M, Borroni E, Mondo A, Piana F, Scarparo C, Coltella L, Lombardi G, Cirillo DM (2012) Clinical validation of Xpert MTB/RIF for the diagnosis of extra-pulmonary tuberculosis. Eur Respir J 40:442–447
32. Chaidir L, Ganiem AR, van der Zanden A, Muhsinin S, Kusumaningrum T, Kusumadewi I, van der Ven A, Alisjahbana B, Parwati I, van Crevel R (2012) Comparison of real time IS6110-PCR, microscopy, and culture for diagnosis of tuberculous meningitis in a cohort of adult patients in Indonesia. PLoS One 7:e52001
33. Solomons RS, Visser DH, Friedrich SO, Diacon AH, Hoek GP, Marais BJ, Schoeman JF, van Furth AM (2015) Improved diagnosis of childhood tuberculous meningitis using more than one nucleic acid amplification test. Int J Tuberc Lung Dis 19:74–80
34. Flores LL, Steingart KR, Dendukuri N, Schiller I, Minion J, Pai M, Ramsay A, Henry M, Laal S (2011) Systematic review and meta-analysis of antigen detection tests for the diagnosis of tuberculosis. Clin Vaccine Immunol 18:1616–1627
35. Song F, Sun X, Wang X, Nai Y, Liu Z (2014) Early diagnosis of tuberculous meningitis by an indirect ELISA protocol based on the detection of the antigen ESAT-6 in cerebrospinal fluid. Ir J Med Sci 183:85–88
36. Feng G, Shi M, Ma L, Chen P, Wang B, Zhang M, Chang X, Su X, Yang Y, Fan X, Dai W, Liu T, He Y, Bian T, Duan L, Li J, Hao X, Liu J, Xue X, Song Y, Wu H, Niu G, Zhang L, Han C, Lin H, Lin Z, Liu J, Jian J, Zhang J, Tian Y, Zhou B, Wang J, Xue C, Han X, Wang J, Wang S, Thwaites G, Zhao G (2014) Tuberculous meningitis. Am J Resp Crit Care 189:475–781
37. Joos TJ, Miller WC, Murdoch DM (2006) Tuberculin reactivity in bacilli Calmette- Guerin vaccinated populations: a compilation of international data. Int J Tuberc Lung Dis 10:883–891
38. Mihret A, Abebe M (2013) Cytokines and chemokines as biomarkers of tuberculosis. J Mycobac Dis 3:128

39. Qin L, Zhang L, Zhang Y, Shi X, Zhang Y, Liu X (2015) Diagnostic value of T-cell interferon-γ release assays on cerebrospinal fluid for tuberculous meningitis. PLoS One 10:e0141814
40. Thomas MM, Hinks TS, Raghuraman S, Ramalingam N, Ernst M, Nau R, Lange C, Kösters K, Gnanamuthu C, John GT, Marshall B, Lalvani A (2008) Rapid diagnosis of Mycobacterium tuberculosis meningitis by enumeration of cerebrospinal fluid antigen-specific T-cells. Int J Tuberc Lung Dis 12:651–657
41. Kim S, Chu K, Choi S, Song K, Kim H, Kim N, Park S, Yoon B, Oh M, Choe K (2008) Diagnosis of central nervous system tuberculosis by T-cell-based assays on peripheral blood and cerebrospinal fluid mononuclear cells. Clin Vaccine Immunol 15:1356–1362
42. Yang Q, Cai Y, Zhao W, Wu F, Zhang M, Luo K, Zhang Y, Liu H, Zhou B, Kornfeld H, Chen X (2014) IP-10 and MIG are compartmentalized at the site of disease during pleural and meningeal tuberculosis and are decreased after antituberculosis treatment. Clin Vaccine Immunol 21:635–1644
43. Karsen H, Koruk ST, Karahocagil MK, Calisir C, Baran FC (2011) Comparative analysis of cerebrospinal fluid adenosine deaminase activity in meningitis. Swiss Med Wkly 141:w13214

Methods of Microbiological Confirmation in Tuberculous Meningitis

26

Amita Jain

Contents

A. Jain, MD
Department of Microbiology, King George's Medical University, Lucknow, UP, India
e-mail: amita602002@yahoo.com

Abbreviations

ADA	Adenosine deaminase activity
AFB	Acid-fast bacilli
CNS	Central nervous system
CRI	Colourimetric redox indicator
CSF	Cerebrospinal fluid
DNA	Deoxyribonucleic acid
DST	Drug susceptibility testing
ELISA	Enzyme-linked immunosorbent assay
FRET	Fluorescence resonance energy transfer
HIV	Human immunodeficiency virus
IGRA	Interferon gamma release assays
kDA	Kilodalton
LED	Fluorescent light-emitting diode
LJ	Lowenstein–Jensen
LPA	Line probe assay
MDR	Multidrug resistance
MGIT	Mycobacterium growth indicator tube
MODS	Microscopic observation drug susceptibility
MTBC	*Mycobacterium tuberculosis* complex
NAATs	Nucleic acid amplification tests
NRA	Nitrate reductase assay
NTM	Non-tuberculous mycobacteria
PCR	Polymerase chain reaction
REMA	Resazurin microtitre assay
TB	Tuberculosis
TBM	Tuberculous meningitis
WHO	World Health Organization
XDR	Extensively drug resistance
ZN	Ziehl–Neelsen

M. Turgut et al. (eds.), *Tuberculosis of the Central Nervous System*,
DOI 10.1007/978-3-319-50712-5_26

26.1 Introduction

Tuberculous meningitis (TBM) is the most lethal form of extra-pulmonary tuberculosis (TB) that accounts for about 5% of all extra-pulmonary TB. Delayed diagnosis of TBM is universally associated with poor treatment outcome [1], and studies from developing as well as developed countries have reported high fatality rates (>40%) [2]. Because of non-specific clinical features and the deadly consequences of a missed diagnosis, accurate, early confirmation of diagnosis is an essential component in the management of TBM. Unfortunately, many tests used for laboratory confirmation of TB, even today, are antique with compromised sensitivity and specificity. Moreover, methods used for laboratory confirmation of TBM and other forms of extra-pulmonary TB are not different from those used for laboratory confirmation of pulmonary TB, except that the diagnostic indices of these tests may vary according to clinical presentation.

The World Health Organization (WHO) has promoted evaluation and development of many newer and existing technologies, most of them for pulmonary TB. Based on available evaluation till date, a comprehensive WHO recommended list of tests is available (Table 26.1). Some of these tests can diagnose the disease along with detection of drug resistance, while others can only diagnose the presence or absence of *M. tuberculosis*. In this chapter, we will discuss the available methods for laboratory confirmation of TBM.

26.2 Specimen

Laboratory confirmation of TBM is best made with cerebrospinal fluid (CSF) [4]. CSF specimen is collected by lumber puncture, at the time of hospital admission before starting the antibiotics, and submitted to the laboratory, without delay. The diagnostic yield of CSF microscopy and culture for *M. tuberculosis* increases with the volume of CSF submitted, and repeat lumbar puncture should be performed if the diagnosis remains uncertain. The safe volume of CSF which can be collected at different age groups is described by Thwaites [4] (Table 26.2). Desired

Table 26.1 An overview of progress in the development and evaluation of TB diagnostics

Technologies endorsed by WHO
Molecular technologies
Xpert MTB/RIF[a]
Line probe assays (for smear-positive specimens or culture isolates)
Microscopy
Ziehl–Neelsen and fluorescence microscopy methods[a]
Culture-based technologies
Commercial liquid culture systems and rapid speciation[a]
Non-commercial culture and drug susceptibility testing methods[a]
Evaluated by WHO and not recommended
Commercial serodiagnostics (all manufacturers)
Interferon gamma release assays for the detection of active TB (all settings)
Evaluated by WHO but not yet endorsed due to insufficient evidence
Molecular technologies
TB LAMP, Eiken, Japan
GenoType MTBDRsl, Hain Lifescience, Germany
On the market but evidence for use not yet submitted to WHO for evaluation
Molecular technologies
ICubate System, ICubate, USA
TB drug resistance array, CapitalBio, China
EasyNAT TB Diagnostic kit, Ustar Biotechnologies, China
Truelab/Truenat MTB, Molbio/bigtec Diagnostics, India
Nonmolecular technologies
Alere Determine TB-LAM, Alere, USA
Technologies in early development in early phase of development
Volatile organic compounds
BreathLink, Menssana Research, USA
Prototype breathanalyzer device, Next Dimensions Technology, USA
Molecular technologies
Alere Q, Alere, USA
B-SMART, LabCorp, USA
Genedrive MTB/RIF ID, PRIMA, UK
LATE-PCR, Brandeis University, USA
GeneXpert XDR cartridge, Cepheid, USA
TruArray MDR 78, Akkoni, USA
INFINITIMIB Assay, AutoGenomics, USA
Culture-based technologies
BNP Middlebrook, NanoLogix, USA
MDR-XDR TB Color Test, FIND, Switzerland/Imperial College, UK
TREK Sensititre MYCOTB MIC plate, Trek Diagnostic Systems/Thermo Fisher Scientific, USA
Other technologies
TB Rapid Screen (Global BioDiagnostics, USA)
TBDx, Signature Mapping Medical Sciences, USA

Adapted from WHO [3]

[a]Approved by WHO for use in diagnosis of EPTB including TBM

Table 26.2 Estimates of safe recommended CSF volume taken at lumbar puncture for different age groups

Patient population	Safe CSF volume to take at lumber puncture (ml)
Adult	15–17
Adolescent	12–17
Young child	10–15
Infant	6–9
Term neonate	2–4

Adapted from Thwaites et al. [4]

CSF volume varies from case to case; however, since it is an invasive sample whatever volume is available, it should not be rejected and submitted to the laboratory for investigations.

For diagnostic purposes, sputum sample should also be collected for an AFB smear and culture, even from cases without respiratory symptoms. At least two consecutive sputum specimens should be examined. Approximately 60% of children with TBM have radiological evidence of pulmonary TB [5].

26.3 Examination of the Cerebrospinal Fluid

Examination of the CSF is essential and typically reveals a moderate pleocytosis (leucocytosis) (10–1000 × 10^3 cells/ml, mostly lymphocytes), raised protein (0.5–3.0 g/l) and CSF/plasma glucose <50% [6]. These values can be useful in initial screening and differentiating from bacterial meningitis (Table 26.3); however, differentiation from viral and cryptococcal meningitis may be difficult [7]. Atypical CSF findings are well described in immunosuppressed patients; CSF can be acellular or contain a predominance of neutrophils [8, 9]. Atypical CSF findings have been repeatedly described in children with TBM as well [10]. The values may change with duration of illness in an untreated patient [10] (Table 26.4).

26.4 Microscopy

The most common method for diagnosing TBM worldwide remains smear microscopy which was developed more than 100 years ago.

Table 26.3 Values of CSF parameters in TBM and bacterial meningitis

Marker	Tuberculous meningitis	Acute bacterial meningitis	*P* value
CSF cells (per μL)	120 (0–1640)	4000 (40–22,400)	<0.001
CSF neutrophils (%)	15 (0–100)	100 (50–100)	<0.001
CSF/blood glucose	0.33(0.04–0.50)	0.19(0.00–0.50)	<0.001
CSF protein (mg/dL)	146 (20–1000	313(32–1000)	<0.001

Adapted from Vibha et al. [11]

Demonstration of acid-fast bacilli (AFB) in CSF may be crucial for the rapid diagnosis of TBM; hence, every effort should be made to demonstrate AFB. Literature suggests that they can be seen in up to 80% of adult cases but in only 15–20% of children. Positive CSF smear and culture is independently associated with large volumes (>6 ml) of CSF submitted for examination; repeated lumbar punctures and CSF examination also increase diagnostic yield [12, 13]. A simple modification to the CSF Ziehl–Neelsen (ZN) stain improves its diagnostic performance. Using cytospin to prepare a monolayer of CSF white cells on a slide, and permeabilizing the cells with TritonX-100 before and during the ZN stain, helps in visualization of AFB by light microscopy in 82.9% of patients with TBM. Intracellular bacteria can be seen in 87.8% of positive specimens [14].

For demonstration of AFB in smear, either conventional ZN light microscopy or light-emitting diode (LED) fluorescence microscopy is used (Fig. 26.1). LED microscopy is more sensitive than ZN microscopy and has qualitative, operational and cost advantages. In 2009, WHO recommended that LED microscopy be phased in as an alternative for ZN microscopy [25]. LEDs provide a relatively inexpensive light source attachments (a LED light), requiring less power than conventional fluorescence microscopes, and can run on batteries. LED bulbs have a long half-life and do not release toxic products, if broken. The diagnostic accuracy of LED microscopy is comparable to that of conventional fluorescence

Table 26.4 Values of CSF parameters in TBM

Tests	Performance	WHO endorsement	Remark	# of references
CSF smear examination for AFB	Can detect up to 80% case in adults and 15–20% in children. Specificity is 100%	YES	Can be improved by using Larger CSF volumes Repeated sampling LED microscope Centrifugation	[12–15]
Culture on solid (LJ) media	Can detect 1/3 of cases only	YES	Major concerns Poor sensitivity Long turn-around time	[16]
Culture on Liquid Media (MGIT)	More sensitive than culture on LJ approximately by 10%	YES	More prone for contamination Significant biohazard	[17, 18]
In-house NAAT	Specificity 95–100%, sensitivity 40–60%	NO	Sensitivity improved by Multiplexing Nested PCR Concentration of CSF Use of real-time platform	[6, 19–22]
Commercial NAAT	Sensitivity 56%, specificity 98%	NO	Standardization difficult due to Inadequate standardization of laboratory techniques Use of highly variable reference standards	[23]
Xpert MTB/RIF	Sensitivity 80.5%, specificity 98.7%	YES	Better to rule in a case than ruling out Best results on centrifuged CSF	[24]

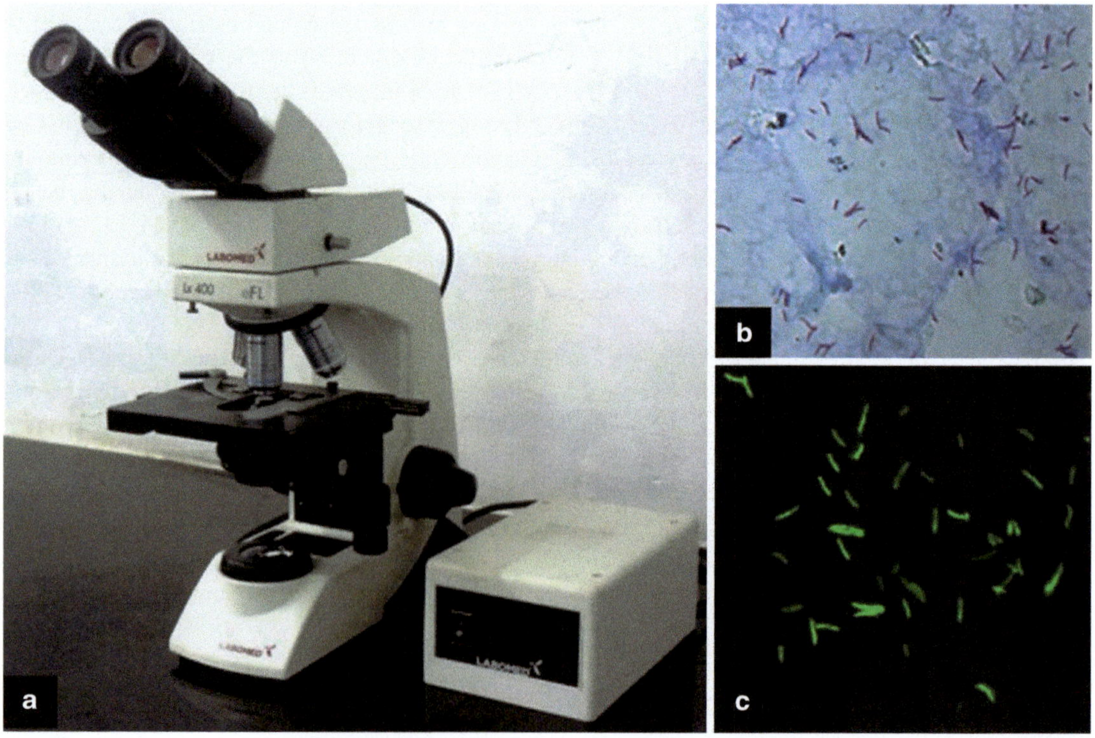

Fig. 26.1 Microscopic examination of clinical sample. (**a**) Fluorescent LED microscope; (**b**) acid-fast bacilli in Ziehl–Neelsen-stained slide (under 1000× magnification and in *bright light*); (**c**) acid-fast bacilli in auramine-stained slide (under 400× magnification and in *fluorescent light*)

microscopy and is better than that of ZN microscopy (by an average of 10%) [15].

Microscopy is simple and inexpensive and allows rapid detection. It is suitable even for peripheral-level laboratories and can be done safely in a laboratory that has implemented only a low level of biosafety measures. However, microscopy for AFB cannot distinguish *Mycobacterium tuberculosis* complex (MTBC) from non-tuberculous mycobacteria (NTM), viable from nonviable organisms and drug-susceptible strains from drug-resistant strains [25].

26.5 Culture and Species Identification

Culture of *M. tuberculosis* from CSF is regarded as the most definitive diagnosis, although this is rarely attained, as TBM is a paucibacillary disease. TBM can be confirmed in only ~1/3 of clinically suspected cases using culture methods [26]. Moreover, mycobacterial culture may take up to 42 days and has limited sensitivity (<50%) compared to clinical diagnostic criteria [5, 16].

Mycobacteria can be cultured in specific solid media like Lowenstein–Jensen (LJ) or liquid media like Mycobacterial Growth Indicator Tube (MGIT®) (Figs. 26.2 and 26.3). Bacterial growth can be identified visually as on LJ media (i.e. by identifying specific characteristics) or by automated detection of its metabolism as seen in MGIT. Liquid culture methods are more sensitive than LJ culture [17]. All positive mycobacterial cultures must be tested to identify MTBC [25]. Differentiation of the members of MTBC is necessary for the treatment of individual patients, which can be achieved using either phenotypic [27] or genotypic methods [28]. The use of rapid immunochromatographic assays to identify cultured isolates is recommended because they provide results in 15 min [29].

Solid culture methods are less expensive than liquid media, but the results are almost always delayed because of the slow growth of mycobacteria. Liquid culture increases the culture yield by approximately 10% over solid media, and automated systems like MGIT® reduce the diagnostic delay to days rather than weeks. However, liquid systems are more prone to contamination and mandate appropriate additional biosafety measures [29].

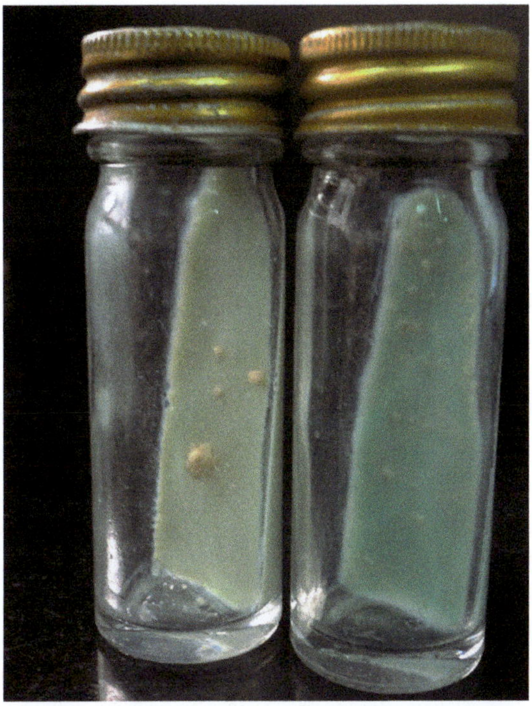

Fig. 26.2 Positive *Mycobacterium tuberculosis* growth on Lowenstein–Jensen (*LJ*) media slants

Culture and identification of *M. tuberculosis* provide a definitive diagnosis and also provide the necessary isolates for conventional DST. However, culture is complex, expensive, time taking and requiring huge laboratory infrastructure. Culture also requires specific laboratory equipment, skilled technicians and appropriate biosafety measures [25].

26.6 Drug Susceptibility Testing

There are no authentic estimates available on prevalence of drug-resistant extra-pulmonary TB, but sparse information mostly derived either from retrospective cohort studies or TB surveillance data is available from different parts of the world. The drug resistance among cases of TBM has been reported increasingly in many countries

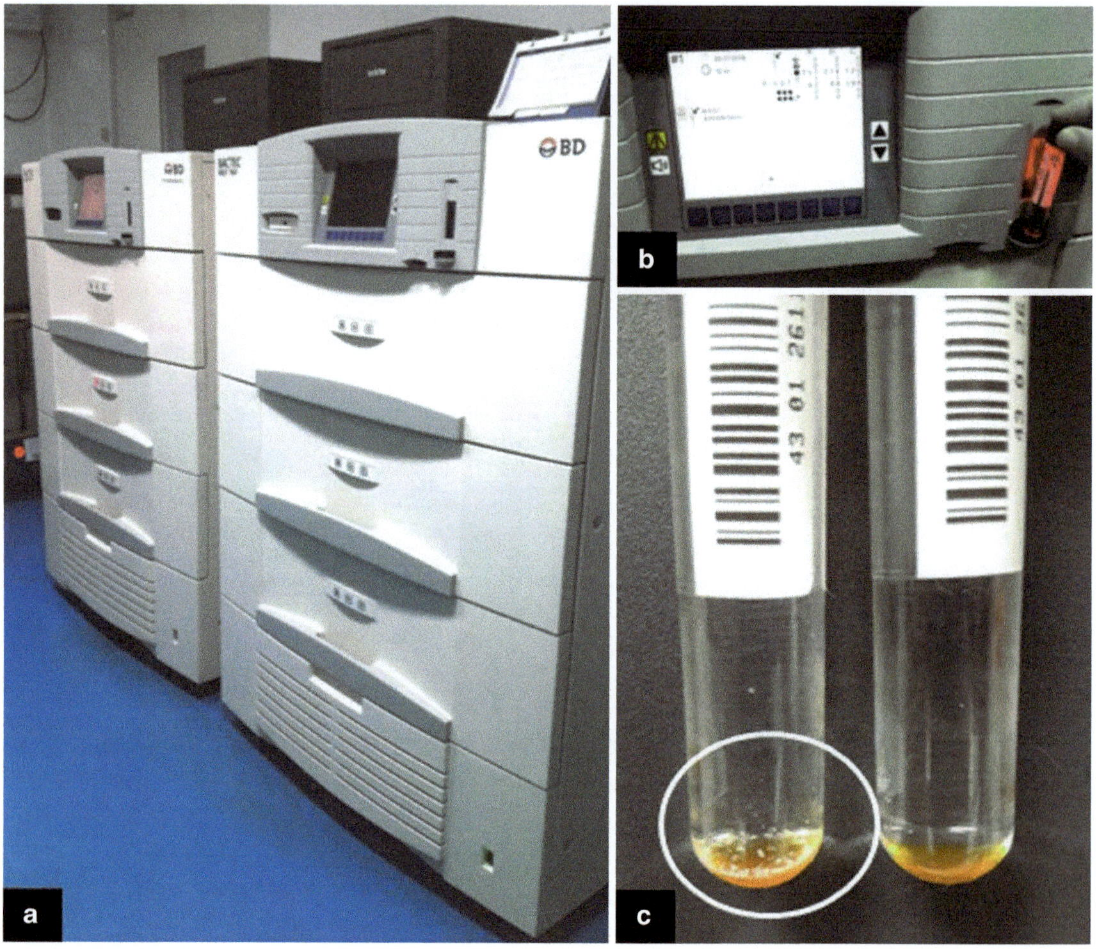

Fig. 26.3 Isolation of *Mycobacterium tuberculosis* by semi-automated liquid culture system. (**a**) BACTEC MGIT 960 machine (Beckton, Dickson, Sparks, Md.); (**b**) Scanning and incubation of liquid culture tube (inoculated with sample) into the machine; (**c**) Positive *M. tuberculosis* growth in liquid medium (*encircled*)

[18, 30–32]. The possibility of XDR strains in extra-pulmonary site has also been reported from India [18]. Studies from different countries have compared the drug resistance profiles of *M. tuberculosis* isolates recovered from pulmonary and extra-pulmonary sites and showed negative association of extra-pulmonary TB with drug resistance [33]. As per data accrued from different countries, the prevalence of MDR may vary from 1% to 69% of total of extra-pulmonary TB cases [33, 34].

Different methods are available for detection of drug resistance in *M. tuberculosis*. Nonmolecular DST methods take longer to provide results and are suitable for use in laboratories with appropriate infrastructure (particularly biosafety precautions). Phenotypic methods involve culturing *M. tuberculosis* in the presence of anti-TB agents. Interpretation is done by the presence of growth (which indicates resistance) or inhibition of growth (which indicates susceptibility). Both solid and liquid media have been extensively validated for DST. Liquid culture systems for DST take as little as 10 days to conclude the results, compared with the 28–42 days needed for conventional solid media [29]. Genotypic methods are based on looking for specific molecular mutations associated with resistance against individual anti-TB agents. Line probe assays (LPAs) have been adopted by many countries for rapid first-line DST (to rifampicin and isoniazid) on smear-positive specimens or cultures. The use of LPA on smear-negative and extra-pulmonary TB samples is not recommended; however, this can be used on isolates from extra-pulmonary TB samples. WHO recommends the use of Xpert MTB/RIF even in AFB-negative and extra-pulmonary TB samples including CSF [35].

26.7 Nonconventional Methods for Drug Susceptibility Testing

Nonconventional methods of culture and DST are less expensive than commercially available liquid culture methods but are prone to errors due to lack of standardization and local variations in the methods. WHO-evaluated methods include the microscopic observation drug susceptibility (MODS) assay, the colourimetric redox indicator (CRI) methods and the nitrate reductase assay (NRA) [36]. NRA is based on ability of *M. tuberculosis* to reduce nitrate to nitrite. The reduction can be detected by using specific reagents which produce colour change [37, 38]. MODS assay relies on microscopic detection of cording growth that is characteristic of *M. tuberculosis* [39]. CRI method or resazurin microtitre assay (REMA) is based on oxidation–reduction of resazurin dye [40]. All these three methods are rapid, easy to perform, inexpensive and recommended by WHO since 2011 [41].

26.7.1 Microscopic Observation Drug Susceptibility Method

A novel culture method using a broth culture medium has been designed for use in resource-poor settings. It is used for both diagnosis and DST. For detection of *M. tuberculosis*, in cases of TBM, MODS showed a low sensitivity but the susceptibility data matched with that of 1% proportion method [42]. One of the studies reported positive and negative predictive values for MODS as 100% and 71.3%, respectively, for HIV-infected patients and 100% and 69.8% for HIV-negative patients of TBM. [43]. It is much cheaper than the use of commercial liquid culture media and incorporates drug susceptibility testing in the initial culture phase, allowing rapid detection of drug-resistant isolates [39]. Evaluation of MODS for detection of drug resistance in pulmonary TB showed high sensitivity (92.7%) and specificity (98%) for detection of rifampicin resistance [41]. It has been shown to have superior sensitivity to solid LJ culture media with a substantially reduced (median 7 day) time to positivity. It has also been shown to be superior or equivalent to commercial broth culture systems in terms of yield and time to positivity [44].

26.7.2 Colourimetric Redox Indicator Method

A coloured indicator like resazurin is added to liquid culture medium on a microtitre plate after culturing *M. tuberculosis* strains in the presence of anti-TB agents, in vitro. Resistance is detected by a change in the colour of the indicator, which is proportional to the number of viable mycobacteria in the medium. Recently, resazurin, a non-proprietary product, has been identified as the main component of Alamar blue. No expensive equipment is needed for conducting REMA; however, biosafety issues remain [41]. The method is slower than conventional DST methods using commercial liquid culture and molecular LPAs [45].

26.7.3 Nitrate Reductase Assay

NRA is a highly sensitive and specific method for detection of resistance to all first-line anti-TB drugs except ethambutol [41]. NRA is performed in solid LJ medium used routinely for the diagnosis of TB in conventional diagnostic laboratories. Laboratories do not have to change to another new media as it is performed in the same solid medium, which is routinely used, reducing the risk of production of aerosols [46]. No specialized or additional equipment is required.

26.8 Nucleic Acid Amplification Tests

26.8.1 Conventional Method

For the diagnosis of TBM, the detection of MTBC DNA in CSF samples using PCR has been widely performed as more rapid, sensitive and specific diagnostic method. The results of PCR studies in the CSF have shown high specificity (95–100%) with limited sensitivity (40–60%) [8, 47, 48] meaning thereby that nucleic acid amplification tests (NAATs) can confirm a diagnosis of TBM, but cannot rule it out [4]. Several variations in the PCR methodologies have been attempted to improve the sensitivity and specificity of the test. Various mycobacterial gene targets, such as insertion sequence (*IS*)*6110*; *IS1081*; *16S* rRNA DNA; *devR* (transcriptional regulator, Rv3133c); 65 kDa (heat shock protein 65, *hsp65*; Rv0440), MPB-64/MPT-64 (mycobacterial protein from species tuberculosis, *mpb64*; Rv1980c), 38 kDa (phosphate-binding lipoprotein, *pstS1*; Rv0934) and MTP-40 (membrane-associated phospolipase C1; Rv2351c) proteins; *TRC4* (conserved repetitive element), IA9110; *GCRS* (guanine–cytosine-rich repetitive sequence); *fbp*, encoding fibronectin-binding protein B (30 kDa, Ag85B protein; Rv1886c); *hupB*, encoding histone-like DNA-binding protein (Rv2986c); and *dnaJ*, encoding chaperone protein (Rv0352), have been used for NAAT [19, 49–55]. Of all the above targets, mpb64 and *IS*6110 were found to be best performing targets, and multiplexing both the targets improved sensitivity and specificity [19]. Nested PCR which is another variation tried to improve the diagnostic sensitivity and specificity [20]. Immunomagnetic enrichment of the CSF sample has also led to improved sensitivity [21]. In 2003, a systematic review evaluated the test accuracy of NAATs in the diagnosis of TBM [23]. Summary accuracy measures of 35 studies with in-house NAATs could not be determined due to heterogeneity of the tests. Reasons for heterogeneity included (1) inadequate standardization of laboratory techniques, (2) the use of highly variable reference standards and (3) small patient numbers with limited statistical power [2, 56].

26.8.2 Commercial Method

Commercially available nucleic acid amplification kits, such as the Gen-Probe amplified direct test [57], and its modification [58] and other PCR kits such as the Cobas Amplicor [59, 60] have demonstrated higher sensitivities ranging from 60% to 83% and specificity of 100%. According to a meta-analysis of studies reported before 2002, commercial NAATs were 56% sensitive (95% CI 46–66) and 98% specific (97–99) [23]. These values were pooled result of the 14 studies with commercial NAATs. According to another meta-analysis published in 2014, pooled estimates of diagnostic accuracy of newer commercial NAAT's diagnostic accuracy measured against a cerebrospinal fluid *M. tuberculosis* culture-positive gold standard were sensitivity 0.64, specificity 0.98 and diagnostic odds ratio 64.0. Heterogeneity was limited; P value = 0.147 and I2 = 33.85% [60].

Available data suggest that sensitivity of NAAT might be improved by real-time PCR [60–65]. The use of real-time PCR and product detection by fluorescence using FRET (fluorescence resonance energy transfer) probes or SYBR green has been tried for detection of mycobacteria by several groups [66, 67]. Quantitative nested real-time PCR assays were also tried [61]. Real-time detection has a higher sensitivity compared to conventional methodology. By assaying CSF filtrates rather than sediments, sensitivity can be further improved although these findings need to be confirmed [63].

In spite of attempts at improving sensitivity using PCR, attempts have generally not been fruitful by these in-house commercial, conventional or real-time PCR tests. Requirement for simultaneous testing of rifampicin resistance using multiple target genes was also felt, more so by high endemic countries. PCR platforms are generally located in reference laboratories, require technical expertise, are expensive and are prone to contamination and therefore are not suitable for use by lower level of laboratories. Although NAATs promise a rapid, definitive diagnosis of TBM, the performance of first-generation NAATs is suboptimal and variable. None of these in-house or commercial assays are endorsed by WHO.

26.8.3 XPERT MTB/RIF

More recently, a closed PCR system, Xpert MTB/RIF (Cepheid, Sunnyvale, CA, USA), has been developed (Fig. 26.4). The Xpert MTB/RIF assay uses real-time PCR and has sensitivity and specificity values equivalent to those from in vitro CSF culture and its susceptibility to rifampicin, and results are available within 2 h [68]. Xpert MTB/RIF requires minimal training to operate, is a potentially point-of-care test and has good accuracy in smear-negative pulmonary TB [69, 70], extra-pulmonary TB including TBM [71] and HIV with TB [72]. It is economical than culture and has become available as a frontline diagnostic in several high-burden countries [68]. One study reported that the assay was nearly 12 times more sensitive than microscopy for the diagnosis of TBM, but the cost of processing one Xpert MTB/RIF test was 82 times higher than the cost of microscopy [73]. The addition of vortexing step to sample processing increases sensitivity for confirmed TBM by 20% (*P*_0.04) [71]. A meta-analysis [74] of studies reported up to October, 2011, estimated that Xpert MTB/RIF is more sensitive compared with culture for the diagnosis of extra-pulmonary TB. Another meta-analysis of 18 studies involving 4461 samples showed that Xpert sensitivity differed substantially between sample types. In cerebrospinal fluid, Xpert pooled sensitivity was 80.5% (95% CI 59.0–92.2%) and specificity was 98.7% against culture. Based on this systematic review, the World Health Organization now recommends Xpert over conventional tests for diagnosis of TB including *M. tuberculosis* [24].

The Xpert MTB/RIF test correctly identified more positive TBM in patients infected with HIV living in areas where there are high levels of TB infection cases than the other tests used to diagnose TBM, within 24 h of first seeing a patient. However, the test accuracy was best when the CSF sample was centrifuged at high speed [75]. The Xpert MTB/RIF test is useful in determining that a patient has TBM. It is not useful in determining that a patient does not have TBM [76].

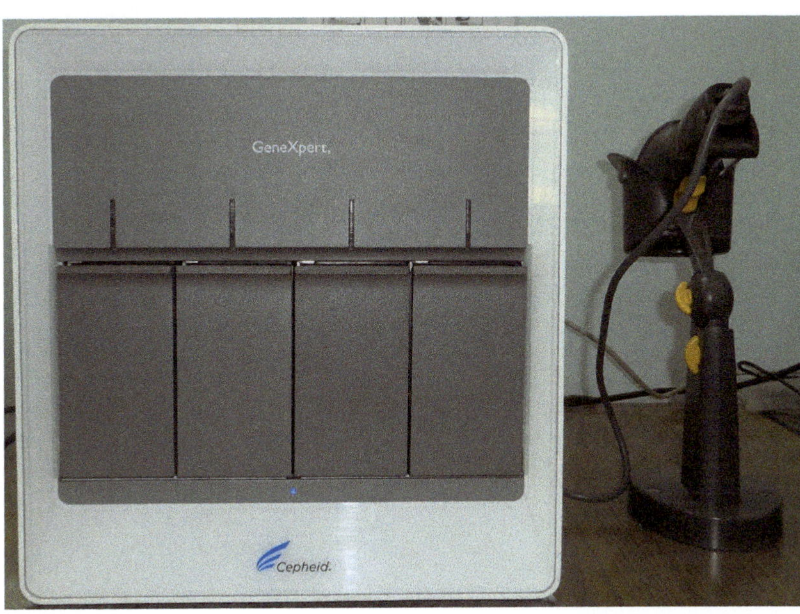

Fig. 26.4 Xpert MTB/RIF machine, a model for processing of four samples simultaneously

26.9 Adenosine Deaminase Method

ADA is considered an indicator for the cell-mediated immunologic reaction. It is found mainly in T lymphocytes [76]. ADA has been considered as a marker of cell-mediated immunity and may reflect host-defensive mechanisms. ADA is an enzyme that degrades adenosine into inosine and ammonia. ADA activity in pleural fluids, peritoneal fluids and pericardial fluids is a useful indicator of tuberculous infection [77–80]. The role of CSF ADA activity has been evaluated for the early diagnosis of TBM. Piras and Gakis [81] have suggested increased CSF ADA activity as a diagnostic marker for TBM. Following their lead, many previous studies have suggested that CSF ADA activity could be used as a method for differentiating TBM from non-TBM [82–84]. Many studies have been published signifying the diagnostic value of CSF ADA; there are no reports of standardized ADA cut-off values and serum ADA activity for diagnosing TBM [82]. The role of ADA in diagnosing TBM is not validated in a large-scale study. CSF ADA levels depend on the patient's immune status, sample size, racial differences and age. Hence, CSF ADA activity should be interpreted with caution in light of the patient's condition [85].

26.10 Interferon Gamma Release Assays

Interferon gamma release assays (IGRA) are validated and discarded for use in diagnosis of any form of TB including TBM under any setting, by WHO [3]. Commercially, two IGRA tests are available: Quanti-FERON-TB Gold [QFT-G] and an enzyme-linked immune spot assay (T-SPOT TB). Quanti-FERON-TB Gold In-Tube (QFT-G-IT) test uses enzyme-linked immunosorbent assay (ELISA) technique to measure cell-mediated immunity in response to proteins specific for *M. tuberculosis* complex [86]. The sensitivity and specificity of the test vary markedly, and it has been demonstrated that both whole blood and CSF QFT-G-IT have low sensitivity and specificity in diagnosing TBM and had no prognostic value [87]. Some studies have reported that CSF lymphocytes die rapidly when stimulated with *M. tuberculosis*-specific antigens *ex vivo* and the test fails [88].

Conclusion

Available tests for microbiological confirmation of TBM are still suboptimal. Xpert MTB/RIF is a good point-of-care test with limited sensitivity. Cost is a limiting factor for resource-poor countries where most of the cases are. Even today, holding on to strong clinical suspicion and early initiation of treatment will render best treatment outcome. There is a serious need for a more sensitive, specific and economical point-of-care test for laboratory confirmation of TBM, to facilitate better case management.

References

1. Hopewell PC (1994) Overview of clinical tuberculosis. In: Bloom BR (ed) Tuberculosis pathogenesis, protection, and control. ASM Press, Washington, DC, pp 25–46
2. Thwaites GE, Caws M, Chau TT, Dung NT, Campbell JI, Phu NH, Hien TT, White NJ, Farrar JJ (2004) Comparison of conventional bacteriology with nucleic acid amplification (amplified mycobacterium direct test) for diagnosis of tuberculous meningitis before and after inception of antituberculosis chemotherapy. J Clin Microbiol 42:996–1002
3. World Health Organization (2013) Global tuberculosis report 2013. WHO, Geneva
4. Thwaites G, Fisher M, Hemingway C, Scott G, Solomon T, Innes J (2009) British Infection Society guidelines for the diagnosis and treatment of tuberculosis of the central nervous system in adults and children. J Infect 59:167e87
5. van Well GT, Paes BF, Terwee CB, Springer P, Roord JJ, Donald PR, van Furth AM, Schoeman JF (2009) Twenty years of pediatric tuberculous meningitis: a retrospective cohort study in the western cape of South Africa. Pediatrics 123:e1–e8
6. Thwaites G (2013) Tuberculous meningitis. Medicine 41:683–685
7. Solari L, Soto A, Agapito JC, Acurio V, Vargas D, Battaglioli T, Accinelli RA, Gotuzzo E, Stuyft PV (2013) The validity of cerebrospinal fluid parameters for the diagnosis of tuberculous meningitis. Int J Infect Dis 17:e1111–e1115

8. Thwaites GE, Tran TH (2005) Tuberculous meningitis: many questions, too few answers. Lancet Neurol 4:160–170
9. Torok ME, Chau TT, Mai PP, Phong ND, Dung NT, Chuong LV, Lee SJ, Caws M, de Jong MD, Hien TT, Farrar JJ (2008) Clinical and microbiological features of HIV-associated tuberculous meningitis in Vietnamese adults. PLoS One 3:e1772
10. Starke JR (1999) Tuberculosis of the central nervous system in children. Semin Pediatr Neurol 6:318–331
11. Vibha D, Bhatia R, Prasad K, Srivastava MP, Tripathi M, Kumar G, Singh MB (2012) Validation of diagnostic algorithm to differentiate between tuberculous meningitis and acute bacterial meningitis. Clin Neurol Neurosurg 114:639–644
12. Stewart SM (1953) The bacteriological diagnosis of tuberculous meningitis. J Clin Pathol 6:241–242
13. Kennedy DH, Fallon RJ (1979) Tuberculous meningitis. JAMA 241:264–268
14. Feng GD, Shi M, Ma L, Chen P, Wang BJ, Zhang M, Chang XL, Su XC, Yang YN, Fan XH, Dai W, Liu TT, He Y, Bian T, Duan LX, Li JG, Hao XK, Liu JY, Xue X, Song YZ, Wu HQ, Niu GQ, Zhang L, Han CJ, Lin H, Lin ZH, Liu JJ, Jian Q, Zhang JS, Tian Y, Zhou BY, Wang J, Xue CH, Han XF, Wang JF, Wang SL, Thwaites GE, Zhao G (2014) Diagnostic accuracy of intracellular mycobacterium tuberculosis detection for tuberculous meningitis. Am J Respir Crit Care Med 189:475–481
15. World Health Organization (2011) Fluorescent light-emitting diode (LED) microscopy for diagnosis of tuberculosis: policy statement. World Health Organization, Geneva
16. Hosoglu S, Geyik MF, Balik I, Aygen B, Erol S, Aygencel TG, Mert A, Saltoglu N, Dokmetas I, Felek S, Sunbul M, Irmak H, Aydin K, Kokoglu OF, Ucmak H, Altindis M, Loeb M (2002) Predictors of outcome in patients with tuberculous meningitis. Int J Tuberc Lung Dis 6:64–70
17. Hooker JA, Muhindi DW, Amayo EO, Mc'ligeyo SO, Bhatt KM, Odhiambo JA (2003) Diagnostic utility of cerebrospinal fluid studies in patients with clinically suspected tuberculous meningitis. Int J Tuberc Lung Dis 7:787–796
18. Balaji V, Daley P, Anand AA, Sudarsanam T, Michael JS, Sahni RD, Chordia P, George IA, Thomas K, Ganesh A (2010) Risk factors for MDR and XDR-TB in a tertiary referral hospital in India. PLoS One 5:e9527
19. Raj A, Singh N, Gupta KB, Chaudhary D, Yadav A, Chaudhary A, Agarwal K, Varma-Basil M, Prasad R, Khuller GK, Mehta PK (2016) Comparative evaluation of several gene targets for designing a multiplex-PCR for an early diagnosis of extrapulmonary tuberculosis. Yonsei Med J 57:88–96
20. Scarpellini P, Cinque SR, Delfanti F, Gianotti N, Terreni MR, Vago L, Lazzarin A (1995) Nested polymerase chain reaction for diagnosis and monitoring treatment response in AIDS patients with tuberculous meningitis. AIDS 9:895–900
21. Mazurek GH, Reddy V, Murphy D, Ansari T (1996) Detection of *Mycobacterium tuberculosis* in cerebrospinal fluid following immunomagnetic enrichment. J Clin Microbiol 34:450–453
22. Shankar P, Manjunath N, Mohan KK, Prasad K, Behari M, Ahuja GK (1991) Rapid diagnosis of tuberculous meningitis by polymerase chain reaction. Lancet 337:5–7
23. Pai M, Flores LL, Pai N, Hubbard A, Riley LW, Colford JM (2003) Diagnostic accuracy of nucleic acid amplification tests for tuberculous meningitis: a systematic review and meta-analysis. Lancet Infect Dis 3:633–643
24. Denkinger CM, Schumacher SG, Boehme CC, Dendukuri N, Pai M, Steingart KR (2014) Xpert MTB/RIF assay for the diagnosis of extrapulmonary tuberculosis: a systematic review and meta-analysis. Eur Respir J 44:435–446
25. World Health Organization (2015) Implementing tuberculosis diagnostics: policy framework. WHO, Geneva
26. Thwaites G, Chau TT, Mai NT, Drobniewski F, McAdam K, Farrar J (2000) Tuberculous meningitis. J Neurol Neurosurg Psychiatry 68:289–299
27. Niemann S, Richter E, Rüsch-Gerdes S (2000) Differentiation among members of the Mycobacterium tuberculosis complex by molecular and biochemical features: evidence for two pyrazinamide-susceptible subtypes of *M. bovis*. J Clin Microbiol 38:152–157
28. Parsons LM, Brosch R, Cole ST, Somoskövi Á, Loder A, Bretzel G, Van Soolingen D, Hale YM, Salfinger M (2002) Rapid and simple approach for identification of *Mycobacterium tuberculosis* complex isolates by PCR-based genomic deletion analysis. J Clin Microbiol 40:2339–2345
29. World Health Organization (2007) Use of liquid TB culture and drug susceptibility testing (DST) in low and medium income settings. WHO, Geneva
30. Baumann MH, Nolan R, Petrini M, Lee YG, Light RW, Schneider E (2007) Pleural tuberculosis in the United States: incidence and drug resistance. Chest 131:1125–1132
31. Robert J, Trystram D, Truffot-Pernot C, Jarlier V (2003) Multidrug-resistant tuberculosis: eight years of surveillance in France. Eur Resp J 22:833–837
32. Lai C-C, Liu W-L, Tan C-K, Huang Y-C, Chung K-P, Lee M-R, Hsueh P-R (2011) Differences in drug resistance profiles of Mycobacterium tuberculosis isolates causing pulmonary and extrapulmonary tuberculosis in a medical centre in Taiwan, 2000–2010. Int J Antimicrob Agents 38:125–129
33. Singh PK, Jain A (2015) Epidemiological perspective of drug resistant extrapulmonary tuberculosis. World J Clin Infect Dis 5:77–85
34. Jain A, Dixit P, Jaiswal I, Garg RK, Kumar R (2012) Drug resistance in mycobacterial isolates from meningitis cases. Pediatr Infect Dis J 31:13–17
35. World Health Organization (2013) Policy update: Xpert MTB/RIF assay for the diagnosis of pulmonary and extrapulmonary TB in adults and children. WHO, Geneva

36. World Health Organization (2011) Noncommercial culture and drug-susceptibility testing methods for screening patients at risk for multidrug-resistant tuberculosis: policy statement. WHO, Geneva
37. Shikama M, Ferro e Silva R, Villela G, Sato D, Martins M, Giampaglia C, da Silva R, Ferro e Silva P, da Silva Telles M, Martin A (2009) Multicentre study of nitrate reductase assay for rapid detection of rifampicin-resistant *M. tuberculosis*. Int J Tuberc Lung Dis 13:377–380
38. Angeby KK, Klintz L, Hoffner SE (2002) Rapid and inexpensive drug susceptibility testing of Mycobacterium tuberculosis with a nitrate reductase assay. J Clin Microbiol 40:553–555
39. Moore DA, Evans CA, Gilman RH, Caviedes L, Coronel J, Vivar A, Sanchez E, Piñedo Y, Saravia JC, Salazar C (2006) Microscopic-observation drug-susceptibility assay for the diagnosis of TB. N Engl J Med 355:1539–1550
40. Palomino JC, Martin A, Camacho M, Guerra H, Swings J, Portaels F (2002) Resazurin microtiter assay plate: simple and inexpensive method for detection of drug resistance in *Mycobacterium tuberculosis*. Antimicrob Agents Chemother 1:2720–2720
41. Dixit P, Singh U, Sharma P, Jain A (2012) Evaluation of nitrate reduction assay, resazurin microtiter assay and microscopic observation drug susceptibility assay for first line antitubercular drug susceptibility testing of clinical isolates of *M. tuberculosis*. J Microbiol Methods 88:122–126
42. Neelakantan S, Jain A, Singh P, Prakash S, Dixit P, Kalyan R, Garg RK, Kumar R, Singh M (2014) Performance of newer and conventional diagnostic methods in detection of drug sensitive and resistant tuberculous meningitis. Asian Pac J Trop Dis 30:S648–S652
43. Nguyen QN, Dang MH, Do AT, Caws M, Torok E, Campbell J, Tran HC, Nguyen VC, Nguyen TC, Farrar J (2008) Routine diagnosis of Tuberculous Meningitis with MODS assay. Int J Infect Dis 31:e319–e320
44. Arias M, Mello FC, Pavón A, Marsico AG, Alvarado-Gálvez C, Rosales S, Pessôa CLC, Pérez M, Andrade MK, Kritski AL (2007) Clinical evaluation of the microscopic-observation drug-susceptibility assay for detection of tuberculosis. Clin Infect Dis 44:674–780
45. Montoro E, Lemus D, Echemendia M, Martin A, Portaels F, Palomino JC (2005) Comparative evaluation of the nitrate reduction assay, the MTT test, and the resazurin microtitre assay for drug susceptibility testing of clinical isolates of *Mycobacterium tuberculosis*. J Antimicrob Chemother 55:500–505
46. Martin A, Panaiotov S, Portaels F, Hoffner S, Palomino JC, Angeby K (2014) The nitrate reductase assay for the rapid detection of isoniazid and rifampicin resistance in *Mycobacterium tuberculosis*: a systematic review and meta-analysis. J Antimicrob Chemother 1:56–64
47. Nguyen LN, Kox LF, Pham LD, Kuijper S, Kolk AH (1996) The potential contribution of the polymerase chain reaction to the diagnosis of tuberculous meningitis. Arch Neurol 53:771–776
48. Caws M, Wilson SM, Clough C, Drobniewski F (2000) Role of IS6110 targeted PCR, biochemical, clinical and immunological criteria for diagnosis of tuberculous meningitis. J Clin Microbiol 38:3150–3155
49. Makeshkumar V, Madhavan R, Narayanan S (2014) Polymerase chain reaction targeting insertion sequence for the diagnosis of extrapulmonary tuberculosis. Indian J Med Res 139:161–166
50. Narayanan S, Parandaman V, Narayanan PR, Venkatesan P, Girish C, Mahadevan S, Rajajee S (2001) Evaluation of PCR using TRC4 and IS6110 primers in detection of tuberculous meningitis. J Clin Microbiol 39:2006–2008
51. Mehta PK, Raj A, Singh N, Khuller GK (2012) Diagnosis of extrapulmonary tuberculosis by PCR. FEMS Immunol Med Microbiol 66:20–36
52. Haldar S, Bose M, Chakrabarti P, Daginawala HF, Harinath BC, Kashyap RS, Kulkarni S, Majumdar A, Prasad HK, Rodrigues C, Srivastava R, Taori GM, Verma-Basil M, Tyagi JS (2011) Improved laboratory diagnosis of tuberculosis – the Indian experience. Tuberculosis 91:414–426
53. Sharma K, Sinha SK, Sharma A, Nada R, Prasad KK, Goyal K, Rana SS, Bhasin DK, Sharma M (2013) Multiplex PCR for rapid diagnosis of gastrointestinal tuberculosis. J Global Infect Dis 5:49–53
54. Sharma K, Gupta N, Sharma A, Singh G, Gupta PK, Rajwanshi A, Varma SC, Sharma M (2013) Multiplex polymerase chain reaction using insertion sequence 6110 (IS6110) and Mycobacterial protein fraction from BCG of Rm 0.64 in electrophoresis target genes for diagnosis of tuberculous lymphadenitis. Indian J Med Microbiol 31:24–28
55. Kashyap RS, Shekhawat SD, Nayak AR, Purohit HJ, Taori GM, Daginawala HF (2013) Diagnosis of tuberculosis infection based on synthetic peptides from *Mycobacterium tuberculosis* antigen 85 complex. Clin Neurol Neurosurg 115:678–683
56. Lang AM, Feris-Iglesias J, Pena C, Sanchez JF, Stockman L, Rys P, Roberts GD, Henry NK, Persing DH, Cockerill FR (1998) Clinical evaluation of Gen-Probe amplified direct test for the detection of Mycobacterium tuberculosis complex organisms in cerebrospinal fluid. J Clin Microbiol 36:2191–2194
57. Cloud JL, Shutt C, Aldous W, Woods G (2004) Evaluation of a modified Gen-Probe amplified direct test for detection of Mycobacterium tuberculosis complex organisms in cerebrospinal fluid. J Clin Microbiol 42:5341–5344
58. Bonington A, Strang JI, Klapper PE, Hood SV, Rubombora W, Penny M, Willers R, Wilkins EG (1998) Use of Roche AMPLICOR *Mycobacterium tuberculosis* PCR in early diagnosis of tuberculous meningitis. J Clin Microbiol 36:1251–1254
59. Bayram A, Celiksoz C, Karsligil T, Balci I (2006) Automatized PCR evaluation of *Mycobacterium*

tuberculosis complex in respiratory and non-respiratory specimens. FEMS Immunol Med Microbiol 46:48–52
60. Solomons RS, van Elsland SL, Visser DH, Hoek KG, Marais BJ, Schoeman JF, van Furth AM (2014) Commercial nucleic acid amplification tests in tuberculous meningitis – a meta-analysis. Diagn Microbiol Infect Dis 78:398–403
61. Takahashi T, Nakayama T (2006) Novel technique of quantitative nested real-time PCR assay for *Mycobacterium tuberculosis* DNA. J Clin Microbiol 44:1029–1039
62. Takahashi T, Tamura M, Asami Y, Kitamura E, Saito K, Suzuki T, Takahashi SN, Matsumoto K, Sawada S, Yokoyama E, Takasu T (2008) Novel "wide range" quantitative nested real-time PCR assay for *Mycobacterium tuberculosis* DNA-development and methodology. J Clin Microbiol 46:1708–1715
63. Haldar S, Sharma N, Gupta VK, Tyagi JS (2009) Efficient diagnosis of tuberculous meningitis by detection of *Mycobacterium tuberculosis* DNA in cerebrospinal fluid filtrates using PCR. J Med Microbiol 58:616–624
64. Chaidir L, Ganiem AR, Vander Zanden A, Muhsinin S, Kusumaningrum T, Kusumadewi I, van der Ven A, Alisjahbana B, Parwati I, van Crevel R (2012) Comparison of real time IS6110-PCR, microscopy, and culture for diagnosis of tuberculous meningitis in a cohort of adult patients in Indonesia. PLoS One 7:e52001
65. Bhigjee AI, Padayachee R, Paruk H, Hallwirth-Pillay KD, Marais S, Connoly C (2007) Diagnosis of tuberculous meningitis: clinical and laboratory parameters. Int J Infect Dis 11:348–354
66. Lachnik J, Ackermann B, Bohrssen A, Maass S, Diephaus C, Puncken A, Stermann M, Bange FC (2002) Rapid cycle PCR and fluorimetry for detection of mycobacteria. J Clin Microbiol 40:3364–3373
67. Heginbothom ML, Magee JT, Flanagan PG (2003) Evaluation of the Idaho Technology Light Cycler PCR for the direct detection of *Mycobacterium tuberculosis* in respiratory specimens. Int J Tuberc Lung Dis 7:78–83
68. Lawn SD, Nicol MP (2011) XpertH MTB/RIF assay: development, evaluation and implementation of a new rapid molecular diagnostic for tuberculosis and rifampicin resistance. Future Microbiol 6:1067–1082
69. Boehme CC, Nabeta P, Hillemann D, Nicol MP, Shenai S, Krapp F, Allen J, Tahirli R, Blakemore R, Rustomjee R, Milovic A (2010) Rapid molecular detection of tuberculosis and rifampin resistance. N Engl J Med 363:1005–1015
70. Bowles EC, Freyee B, van Ingen J, Mulder B, Boeree MJ, van Soolingen D (2011) Xpert MTB/RIF®, a novel automated polymerase chain reaction–based tool for the diagnosis of tuberculosis. Int J Tuberc Lung Dis 15:988–989
71. Nhu NT, Heemskerk D, Chau TT, Mai NT, Nghia HD, Loc PP, Ha DT, Merson L, Van Thinh TT, Day J, van Vinh CN (2014) Evaluation of GeneXpert MTB/RIF for diagnosis of tuberculous meningitis. J Clin Microbiol 52:226–233
72. Theron G, Peter J, van Zyl-Smit R, Mishra H, Streicher E, Murray S, Dawson R, Whitelaw A, Hoelscher M, Sharma S, Pai M (2011) Evaluation of the Xpert MTB/RIF assay for the diagnosis of pulmonary tuberculosis in a high HIV prevalence setting. Am J Respir Crit Care Med 184:132–140
73. Alvarez-Uria G, Azcona JM, Midde M, Naik PK, Reddy S, Reddy R (2012) Rapid diagnosis of pulmonary and extrapulmonary tuberculosis in HIV-infected patients. Comparison of LED fluorescent microscopy and the GeneXpert MTB/RIF assay in a district hospital in India. Tuberc Res Treat 2012:932862
74. Chang K, Lu W, Wang J, Zhang K, Jia S, Li F, Deng S, Chen M (2012) Rapid and effective diagnosis of tuberculosis and rifampicin resistance with Xpert MTB/RIF assay: a meta-analysis. J Infect 64:580–588
75. Patel VB, Theron G, Lenders L, Matinyena B, Connolly C, Singh R, Coovadia Y, Ndung'u T, Dheda K (2013) Diagnostic accuracy of quantitative PCR (Xpert MTB/RIF) for tuberculous, meningitis in a high burden setting: a prospective study. PLoS Med 10:e1001536
76. Pettersson T, Klockars M, Weber TH, Somer H (1991) Diagnostic value of cerebrospinal fluid adenosine deaminase determination. Scand J Infect Dis 23:97–100
77. Ocana I, Martinez-Vazquez JM, Segura RM, Fernandez-De-Sevilla T, Capdevila JA (1983) Adenosine deaminase in pleural fluids. Test for diagnosis of tuberculous pleural effusion. Chest 84:51–53
78. Chen ML, Yu WC, Lam CW, Au KM, Kong FY, Chan AY (2004) Diagnostic value of pleural fluid adenosine deaminase activity in tuberculous pleurisy. Clin Chim Acta 341:101–107
79. Tuon FF, Litvoc MN, Lopes MI (2006) Adenosine deaminase and tuberculous pericarditis – a systematic review with meta-analysis. Acta Trop 99:67–74
80. Voigt MD, Kalvaria I, Trey C, Berman P, Lombard C, Kirsch RE (1989) Diagnostic value of ascites adenosine deaminase in tuberculous peritonitis. Lancet 1:751–754
81. Piras MA, Gakis C (1973) Cerebrospinal fluid adenosine deaminase activity in tuberculous meningitis. Enzyme 14:311–317
82. Chotmongkol V, Teerajetgul Y, Yodwut C (2006) Cerebrospinal fluid adenosine deaminase activity for the diagnosis of tuberculous meningitis in adults. Southeast Asian J Trop Med Public Health 37:948–952
83. Choi SH, Kim YS, Bae IG, Chung JW, Lee MS, Kang JM, Ryu J, Woo JH (2002) The possible role of cerebrospinal fluid adenosine deaminase activity in the diagnosis of tuberculous meningitis in adults. Clin Neurol Neurosurg 31:10–15
84. Moghtaderi A, Niazi A, Alavi-Naini R, Yaghoobi S, Narouie B (2010) Comparative analysis of cerebrospinal fluid adenosine deaminase in tuberculous and non-

tuberculous meningitis. Clin Neurol Neurosurg 112:459–462

85. Choa B-H, Kima BC, Yoona G-J, Choia S-M, Changa J, Leea S-H, Parka M-S, Shinb JH, Kima M-K, Choa K-H (2013) Adenosine deaminase activity in cerebrospinal fluid and serum for the diagnosis of tuberculous meningitis. Clin Neurol Neurosurg 115:1831–1836
86. Mazurek GH, Jereb J, Vernon A, LoBue P, Goldberg S, Castro K (2010) Updated guidelines for using interferon gamma release assays to Detect Mycobacterium tuberculosis Infection d United States, 2010. MMWR Recomm Rep 59:1–25
87. Vidhate MR, Singh MK, Garg RK, Verma R, Shukla R, Goel MM, Makker A, Jain A (2011) Diagnostic and prognostic value of Mycobacterium tuberculosis complex specific interferon gamma release assay in patients with tuberculous meningitis. J Infect 62:400–403
88. Simmons CP, Thwaites GE, Quyen NT, Chau TT, Mai PP, Dung NT, Stepniewska K, White NJ, Hien TT, Farrar J (2005) The clinical benefit of adjunctive dexamethasone in tuberculous meningitis is not associated with measurable attenuation of peripheral or local immune responses. J Immunol 175:579–590

Part VI

Therapy of Tuberculosis of the Nervous System and Its Coverings

Medical Therapy

27

Şule T. Gülen, Mehmet Turgut, Güliz U. Güleç, Ahmet T. Turgut, and Ali Akhaddar

Contents

Ş.T. Gülen, MD (✉)
Department of Chest Diseases, Adnan Menderes University School of Medicine, Aydın, Turkey
e-mail: dr_suletas@yahoo.com.tr

M. Turgut, MD, PhD
Department of Neurosurgery, Adnan Menderes University School of Medicine, Aydın, Turkey
e-mail: drmturgut@yahoo.com

G.U. Güleç, MD
Department of Infectious Diseases, Adnan Menderes University School of Medicine, Aydın, Turkey
e-mail: gulizuyar@yahoo.com

A.T. Turgut, MD
Department of Radiology, Hacettepe University School of Medicine, Ankara, Turkey
e-mail: ahmettuncayturgut@yahoo.com

A. Akhaddar, MD, IFAANS
Department of Neurosurgery, Avicenne Military Hospital of Marrakech. Mohammed V University, Rabat, Morocco
e-mail: akhaddar@hotmail.fr

Abbreviations

CNS	Central nervous system
CSF	Cerebrospinal fluid
EMB	Ethambutol
HIV	Human immunodeficiency virus
INH	Isoniazid
MDR	Multidrug resistant
MIC	Minimum inhibitor concentration
NICE	National Institute for Health and Clinical Excellence
PAS	Para-aminosalicylic acid
PN	Peripheral neuropathy
PZA	Pyrazinamide
RIF	Rifampicin
STR	Streptomycin
TB	Tuberculosis
TBM	Tuberculous meningitis
WHO	World Health Organization
XDR	Extensively drug resistant

M. Turgut et al. (eds.), *Tuberculosis of the Central Nervous System*,
DOI 10.1007/978-3-319-50712-5_27

27.1 Introduction

Central nervous system (CNS) tuberculosis (TB) consists 1% of all TB cases and 5–10% of all extrapulmonary TB cases. TB develops due to primary hematogenous dissemination of TB bacillus from the primary focus located in pulmonary, peribronchial, and peritracheal regions. Miliary dissemination is another way of dissemination. CNS TB includes TB meningitis (TBM), intracranial tuberculomas, TB abscesses, spinal TB, and arachnoiditis (Figs. 27.1 and 27.2). TBM is the most common and serious form of CNS TB [1–3]. The number of clinical studies about CNS TB is less compared to pulmonary TB. There is an ongoing debate about the treatment modalities and the duration [4]. CNS TB is more prevalent among *human immunodeficiency virus* (HIV)-positive and pediatric patient populations. Empirical treatment should be initiated immediately since any delay can lead to mortality and morbidity [1, 2].

In this section anti-TB agents and corticosteroids will be discussed based on literature knowledge.

27.2 Antituberculosis Drugs

Since the late initiation of the treatment can lead to mortality or serious morbidity, empirical treatment should be started immediately after the prediagnosis of CNS TB. The main components in the treatment of CNS TB are the same as in other TB manifestations and can be listed as isoniazid (INH), rifampicin (RIF), pyrazinamide (PZA), ethambutol (EMB), and streptomycin (STR) [1, 3, 5]. In this section, first-line and second-line anti-TB agents will be discussed.

27.2.1 Isoniazid

INH (isonicotinic acid hydrazide) is the most commonly used anti-TB agent. It is the main component of the anti-TB treatment since the efficiency of the agent against TB has been found in 1952 [6]. INH is effective against bacilli that are actively reproducing. INH is used as a single-dose treatment (maximum 300 mg), can be absorbed from gastrointestinal tract near to full concentration, and reaches the peak plasma concentration (2–5 μg/ml) in 1–2 h. This concentration is far

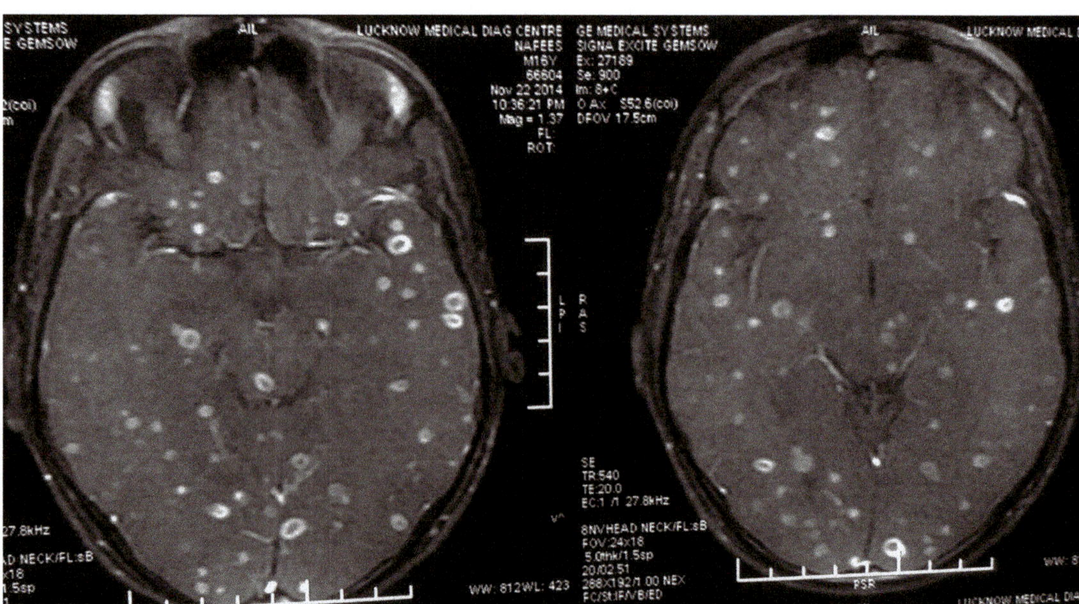

Fig. 27.1 Contrast-enhanced MRI shows miliary tuberculoma of the brain in patient with miliary pulmonary TB (Courtesy of RK Garg)

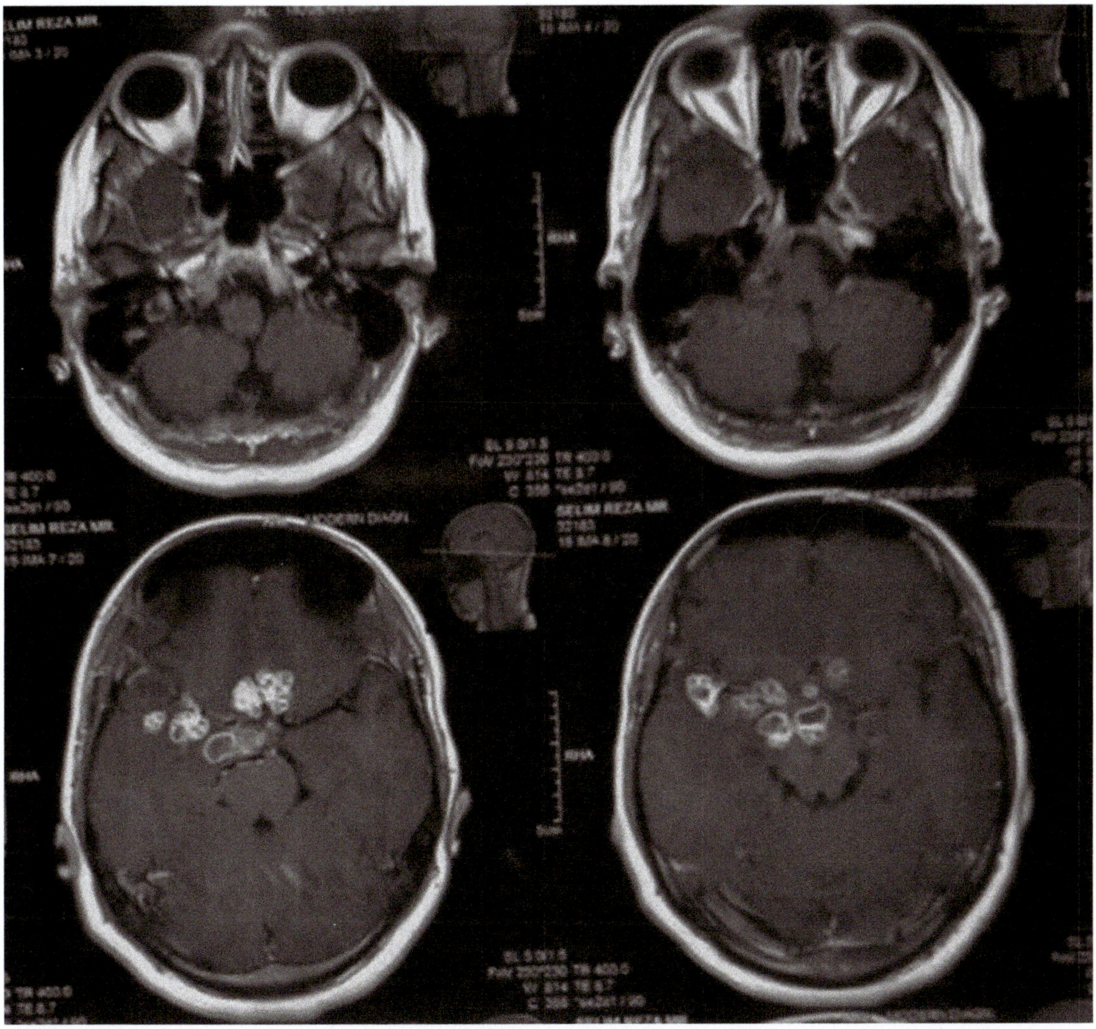

Fig. 27.2 Axial T1-weighted contrast-enhanced MRIs demonstrating multiple tuberculomas in the basal parts of both the cerebral hemispheres and brainstem (Courtesy of FH Chowdhury)

above the minimum inhibitory concentration (MIC) of the drug for TB bacillus. INH can penetrate to all body fluids, cavities, and CNS and reaches the similar levels of concentration [6].

27.2.2 Rifampicin

RIF has been synthesized from *Streptomyces mediterranei* in 1957 and has been used as one of the main components of anti-TB treatment since 1971 [7]. RIF is a bactericidal antibiotic and effective against intracellular, rapidly reproducing bacillus and bacillus with low metabolic activity and slow reproduction. It is rapidly absorbed from the gastrointestinal tract after oral use (maximum 600 mg/day) and reaches to its peak plasma concentration (7–14 μg/ml) within 1. 5–3 h. It can penetrate through the inflamed meninx and reach to the treatment doses in CSF [8, 9].

27.2.3 Pyrazinamide

Although the exact mechanism of action of PZA is not fully understood; it sterilizes the semi-dormant bacillus present in the acidic environment in necrotic caseous lesions [10, 11]. The drug can be absorbed from the gastrointestinal tract after oral use in standard dose. It reaches to its peak plasma concentration (50 μg/ml) 2 h after oral use [12]. PZA can penetrate through the inflamed meninx and can be used in CNS TB [13].

27.2.4 Ethambutol

EMB is a bacteriostatic synthetic anti-TB agent. It inhibits arabinosyltransferase that requires for biosynthesis of arabinogalactan in the cell wall [14]. Seventy five to eighty percent of the drug is absorbed after oral use and reaches to peak plasma concentration in 2–3 h. It penetrates to all body tissues but cannot penetrate into CNS. The CSF concentration of the agent is in between 10% and 50% of the plasma concentration even in the presence of meninx inflammation [15].

27.2.5 Streptomycin

STR is a bactericidal antibiotic which inhibits the protein synthesis by binding to 30s subunit of the bacterial ribosome irreversibly and can be used intramuscularly [16]. It can penetrate to extracellular fluid but cannot penetrate to intracellular compartment. The blood-brain barrier penetration is very low even in the presence of TBM [17]. Among patients in a high-incidence country, the relatively high resistance rate to STR limits its usage. Kanamycin, amikacin, or capreomycin can be used instead of STR [18].

27.2.6 Fluoroquinolones

Moxifloxacin, gatifloxacin, and levofloxacin are the most effective agents among fluoroquinolones. These agents can be used in the treatment of multiple drug-resistant (MDR) TB and in the prophylaxis of patients who had a contact with a MDR TB patient [19, 20]. Since the use of EMB is contraindicated in CNS TB, fluoroquinolones are the fourth most effective agent in CNS TB. These drugs are contraindicated in pregnant and breast-feeding women [21].

27.2.7 Ethionamide and Prothionamide

These bacteriostatic agents are the second choice in the treatment of MDR TB. Thionamides can only be orally used and their gastrointestinal absorption is very well. It can rapidly penetrate to all tissues, and CSF concentration is very near to plasma concentration even without meninx inflammation [16].

27.2.8 Cycloserine

Cycloserine is the second-line therapy in the treatment of MDR TB. It can be used in the presence of hepatotoxicity since it is non-hepatotoxic. It can be rapidly absorbed from the gastrointestinal tract near fully. It can only be used orally and penetrates to all tissues. CSF concentration of the agent is near to its plasma concentration [15].

27.3 Penetration of Antituberculosis Agents into Cerebrospinal Fluid

The CSF penetration of the anti-TB agents is very crucial in the treatment of CNS TB. CSF penetration of INH, RIF, and PZA is quite well. INH can penetrate to CSF in adequate levels in the entity of meningeal inflammation. The CSF concentration is in between 20% and 90% of plasma concentration and 10–15 times higher than MIC of TB bacillus. CSF concentration of RIF can reach to 20–30% of plasma concentration in the entity of meningeal inflammation. EMB and STR are not found in the CSF in the lack of meninx inflammation but can reach to 10–50% of the plasma concentration in the presence of meninx inflammation. CSF penetration of PZA, ethionamide, and cycloserine is adequate [22–24]. Also fluoroquinolones have excellent CSF penetration [25].

In conclusion, a great majority of the first-line anti-TB chemotherapeutical agents can penetrate to CSF, and the CSF concentrations of these agents are increased in the presence of meninx inflammation. Therefore, intrathecal treatment is not routinely used in treatment of CNS TB.

27.4 Treatment Modalities and Duration

There is not a consensus about the treatment modality and the duration of the treatment against CNS TB. According to American Thoracic Society/Centers for Disease Control and Prevention/Infectious Diseases Society of America, the duration of the treatment should be 9–12 months. It is recommended to use the combination of INH, RIF, PZA, and EMB for 2 months and to continue the treatment with INH and RIF for 7–10 months [18]. In the guideline of World Health Organization (WHO) published in 2010, the duration of the treatment was indicated as 9 months, and it was also stated that a shorter treatment for 6 months similar to pulmonary TB can also be used [26]. In the guideline of National Institute for Health and Clinical Excellence (NICE) published in 2011, it was stated that there is not enough evidence in order to decrease the duration of the treatment and the treatment should be continued for 12 months [27]. The duration can be different in patients with neurological deficit or HIV [18, 26, 27].

Although the treatment modalities are different than each other, we can divide it into two as initiation and maintenance treatments. In the initiation treatment, it is aimed to eradicate the rapidly reproducing bacillus with bactericidal activity. Discontinuation of the treatment can lead to drug resistance and failure of the treatment. INH, RIF, and PZA should be started in the initiation therapy since these are bactericidal antibiotics and can penetrate to CSF in adequate levels. STR or EMB can be added as the fourth agent [5, 28]. The maintenance treatment lasts for 7–10 months, and combination of INH and RIF is used in the maintenance treatment [18, 26–28]. In children with TBM, an initial four-drug regimen of INH, RIF, PZA, and ethionamide or an aminoglycoside is recommended [18].

The treatment modalities have been changed since the invention of new anti-TB agents during the last 50 years. The first ever treatment combination was para-aminosalicylic acid (PAS), INH, and STR, and the duration of the treatment was 24 months. EMB replaced PAS in the mid-1960s, and the duration was decreased to 18 months. RIF was invented in the late 1960s, and the duration was decreased to 9–12 months with the 95% of success rate. The treatment has been using orally since the introduction of PZA in the early 1980s, and the duration was decreased to 6–8 months. The relapse rate was decreased to 8% from 22% with the use of PZA and to 3% with the use of RIF [1, 29].

The combination of 2 months of INH, RIF, PZA, and EMB initiation therapy and 4–6 months of INH and RIF maintenance therapy has been using since 1980s [26]. The 6 months and 8 months of total treatment modalities have been compared in the multicenter studies, and the 6 months of therapy was found to be more successful [22, 30]. However in the guideline of NICE published in 2011, it was stated that these studies were not adequate or reliable and the treatment should be continued for 12 months, and it can be prolonged up to 18 months in patients who cannot tolerate the PZA treatment [27].

INH, RIF, and PZA should be included in all treatment modalities of CNS TB since these agents are bactericidal and penetrate to CSF in adequate levels. All agents should be used as a single-dose oral treatment (STR can be used by intramuscular injection) [26]. The pharmacological doses of the agents are summarized in the Table 27.1.

Table 27.1 Anti-TB agents used in the treatment of CNS TB and doses

Name	Daily dose (mg/kg/day) (pediatric patients)	Daily dose (mg/kg/day) (adult)	Maximum daily dose (mg)	Duration (months)
Isoniazid	5–15	5	300	6–12
Rifampicin	10–20	10	600	6–12
Pyrazinamide	15–20	15	1000	2
Ethambutol	15–25	15	1500	2
Streptomycin	15–20	15	1000	2

27.5 Treatment-Related Complications

27.5.1 Peripheral Neuropathy

Peripheral neuropathy (PN) is one of the most common complications of INH. INH leads to PN by altering the metabolism of pyridoxine (vitamin B6) which is a neurotransmitter of CNS. Pyridoxine prophylaxis is advised in patients with malnutrition, HIV, renal failure, and epilepsy. The proposed dose of pyridoxine is 25 mg/day. The dose can be increased to 100–300 mg/day in the presence of serious neurologic adverse effects [15, 31].

27.5.2 Hepatotoxicity

RIF and INH have a potential of hepatotoxicity. The risk is significantly increased in patients with HIV, viral hepatitis, and alcoholism. Other factors related with the hepatotoxicity are underlying hepatic disease, hepatotoxic drug use, and postpartum period [32, 33]. RIF can lead to asymptomatic hyperbilirubinemia, and the hepatitis is in the form of cholestasis [34]. PRZ-related hepatitis is rarely seen with standard doses. Addition of PRZ to the combination of INH and RIF is not related with a significant increase in the hepatotoxicity. Isolated transaminase elevation is more common in this combination [16]. Transaminase level should be monitored in patients with the hepatotoxicity risk [32]. Although there are conflicting opinions about the approach to these patients, the treatment should be stopped in the presence of three- to fivefold bilirubin increase, nausea, vomiting, and jaundice. A non-hepatotoxic agent such as EMB or STR can be started, and a fluoroquinolone (i.e., moxifloxacin) can be added. Since RIF and INH are the two most important agents in the treatment of CNS TB, plasma transaminase levels should be monitored closely and added to the treatment when the plasma transaminase level decreases to normal levels [32, 35].

27.5.3 Nephrotoxicity

PRZ and EMB are eliminated from the kidney, and dose adjustment should be made in patients with a creatinine clearance level below 30 ml/min. Dose adjustment is also recommended in aminoglycoside or cycloserine using patients with low creatinine clearance [36].

27.5.4 Optic Neuritis

Optic neuritis is defined as optical nerve damage manifested as decreased visual acuity and red/green dyschromatopsia developed in one or both eyes due to EMB use. The incidence is increased in patients with renal failure or patients using higher doses of EMB. EMB should be stopped and excluded from the treatment in the presence of optic neuritis development. Routine use of EMB in pediatric patients is not advised since visual acuity cannot be evaluated in these patients [15, 32].

27.6 Role of Corticosteroids

The subject about the role of corticosteroids in TB treatment is controversial. Corticosteroids prevent tissue damage and decreases the symptoms by decreasing the inflammatory cytokine secretion [25]. CNS and pericardial TB are the subtypes that corticosteroid use is indicated. There are several studies indicating that corticosteroid use decreases the mortality and morbidity risk in CNS TB. The mortality risk was found to be decreased especially in pediatric population with the use of corticosteroids. Although controlled studies are necessary about the use of corticosteroids in HIV-positive patients, initial adjunctive corticosteroid therapy is advised for the treatment of CNS TB in all HIV-negative patients [18, 27, 37, 38]. The dose and the route are also controversial about the steroid use. Parenteral (intravenous) 0.3–0.4 mg/kg/day dexamethasone can be initiated and used for 6–8 weeks with decreasing doses. Methylprednisolone (1 mg/kg/day) or another oral corticosteroid can also be initiated, and the dose can be decreased according to the clinical status of the patient. Intrathecal administration of the corticosteroids is not recommended [25, 32, 38].

27.7 Resistance to Antituberculosis Therapy

The emergence of resistant TB forms, which are difficult to treat, is a major global health problem [39]. MDR-TB is outlined as resistance to at least RIF and INH. An additional resistance to any fluoroquinolone and second-line injectable agent (amikacin, kanamycin, or capreomycin) to MDR-TB is defined extensively drug-resistant (XDR) TB [39, 40]. MDR-TB should be considered if there is a history of prior TB treatment, contact with a patient with MDR-TB, or inadequate clinical response to first-line therapy [40, 41]. Mortality among MDR-TBM cases is very high [24, 41]. Mostly, the treatment of MDR-TBM is endured in the treatment of MDR pulmonary TB [41]. Whereas resistance to INH, one of the most valuable first-line anti-TB agents for TBM, can affect the prognosis of TBM treatment more than that of pulmonary TB [42].

The management of TBM with MDR strains is best guided by drug susceptibility testing results and the CSF penetration properties of anti-TB drugs. A regimen with at least five effective anti-TB drugs for condensed phase is recommended by WHO [20]. The MDR-TB regimen should include PZA, a fluoroquinolone, a second-line injectable agent, and two of ethionamide (or prothionamide), cycloserine (or terizidone), linezolid, and clofazimine [20]. A total length of treatment period of 20 months, including a condensed phase of 8 months, is proposed for most patients. But the period may be revised according to patient's response to therapy [20].

The lack of effective and well-tolerated medications and adverse drug reactions complicate the treatment of MDR-TB of CNS. Patients should be treated by physicians experienced in this field [40].

Conclusion

CNS TB is a dangerous disease with a high mortality and morbidity risk requiring long-term treatment. Although there is an ongoing debate about the treatment modalities and the duration, the most important factor affecting the success rate of the treatment is the early initiation of therapy. Future studies are necessary in order to reveal the efficacy of short-term treatment with combination of the four agents. Treatment duration was indicated as 9–12 months. Use of corticosteroids in HIV-negative patients and pediatric patients can decrease the mortality and risk of neurological morbidity development. Resistance to anti-TB therapy is a special issue that must be managed properly. Rapid and accurate diagnosis, choosing a regimen including most appropriate drug for CSF penetration, have become more important for MDR-TB of CNS.

References

1. Cherian A, Thomas SV (2011) Central nervous system tuberculosis. Afr Health Sci 11:116–127
2. Golden MP, Vikram HR (2005) Extrapulmonary tuberculosis: an overview. Am Fam Physician 72:1761–1768
3. Thwaites GE, Chau TT, Stepniewska K, Phu NH, Chuong LV, Sinh DX, White NJ, Parry CM, Farrar JJ (2002) Diagnosis of adult tuberculous meningitis by use of clinical and laboratory features. Lancet 360:1287–1292
4. Garg RK (1999) Tuberculosis of the central nervous system. Postgrad Med J 75:133–140
5. Wiles CM (2005) The meningitis. In: Walton J (ed) Brain's disease of the nervous system, Oxford, vol 4, pp 160–170
6. Zhang Y (2004) Isoniazid. In: Rom WN, Garay SM (eds) Tuberculosis, 2nd edn. Lippincott Williams & Wilkins, Philadelphia, pp 739–758
7. Iseman MD (2002) Tuberkuloz kemoterapisi, doğrudan gözetimli tedavi dahil. (in Turkish). In: Iseman MD (ed) Klinisyenler icin Tuberkuloz Kılavuzu (in Turkish) (trans: Özkara Ş). Nobel Tıp Kitabevleri, İstanbul, pp 271–321
8. Vernon AA (2004) Rifamycin antibiotics, with a focus on newer agents. In: Rom WN, Garay SM (eds) Tuberculosis, 2nd edn. Lippincott Williams & Wilkins, Philadelphia, pp 759–771
9. Telenti A, Imboden P, Marchesi F, Matter L, Schopfer K, Bodmer T, Lowrie D, Colston MJ, Cole S (1993)

Detection of RIF-resistant mutations in *Mycobacterium tuberculosis*. Lancet 341:647–651
10. Girling DJ (1984) The role of pyrazinamide in primary chemotherapy for pulmonary tuberculosis. Tubercle 65:1–4
11. Heifets LB, Lindholm-Levy PJ (1990) Is pyrazinamide bactericidal against *Mycobacterium tuberculosis?* Am Rev Respir Dis 141:250–252
12. Conte JE, Golden JA, Duncan S, McKenna E, Zurlinden E (1999) Intrapulmonary concentrations of pyrazinamide. Antimicrob Agents Chemother 43:1329–1333
13. Ellard GA, Humphries MJ, Gabriel M, Teoh R (1987) Penetration of pyrazinamide into the cerebrospinal fluid in tuberculous meningitis. Br Med J 294:284–285
14. Yakrus MA, Driscoll J, McAlister A, Sikes D, Hartline D, Metchock B, Starks AM (2016) Molecular and growth-based drug susceptibility testing of *Mycobacterium tuberculosis* complex for ethambutol resistance in the United States. Tuberc Res Treat 2016:3404860
15. American Thoracic Society/Centers for Disease Control and Prevention/ Infectious Diseases Society of America (2003) Treatment of tuberculosis. Am J Respir Crit Care Med 167:603–662
16. Chan ED, Chatterjee D, Iseman MD, Heifets LB (2004) Pyrazinamide, ethambutol, ethionamide, and aminoglycosides. In: Rom WM, Garay SM (eds) Tuberculosis, 2nd edn. Lippincott Williams & Wilkins, Philadelphia, pp 773–789
17. Heifets LB, Lindholm-Levy PJ (1989) Comparison of bactericidal activities of streptomycin, amikacin, kanamycin, and capreomycin against *M. avium* and *M. tuberculosis*. Antimicrob Agents Chemother 33:1298–1301
18. Nahid P, Dorman SE, Alipanah N, Barry PM, Brozek JL, Cattamanchi A, Chaisson LH, Chaisson RE, Daley CL, Grzemska M, Higashi JM, Ho CS, Hopewell PA, Keshavjee SA, Lienhardt C, Menzies R, Merrifield C, Narita M, O'brien R, Peloquin CA, Raftery A, Saukkonen J, Schaaf HS, Sotgiu G, Starke JR, Migliori GB, Vernon A (2016) Official American Thoracic Society/Centers for Disease Control and Prevention/ Infectious Diseases Society of America clinical practice guidelines: treatment of drug-susceptible tuberculosis. Clin Infect Dis 63(7):e147–e195. doi:10.1093/cid/ciw376
19. Moadebi S, Harder CK, Fitzgerald MJ, Elwood KR, Marra F (2007) Fluoroquinolones for the treatment of pulmonary tuberculosis. Drugs 67:2077–2099
20. World Health Organization (2016) WHO treatment guidelines for drug resistant tuberculosis, 2016 update. WHO/HTM/TB/2016.04
21. Mehlhorn AJ, Brown DA (2007) Safety concerns with fluoroquinolones. Ann Pharmacother 41:1859–1866
22. Donald PR, Gent WL, Seifart HI, Lamprecht JH, Parkin DP (1992) Cerebrospinal fluid isoniazid concentrations in children with tuberculous meningitis: the influence of dosage and acetylation status. Pediatrics 89:247–250
23. Ellard GA, Humphries MJ, Allen BW (1993) Cerebrospinal fluid drug concentrations and the treatment of tuberculous meningitis. Am Rev Resp Dis 148:650–655
24. Thwaites GE, Lan NT, Dung NH, Quy HT, Oanh DT, Thoa NT, Hien NQ, Thuc NT, Hai NN, Bang ND, Lan NN, Duc NH, Tuan VN, Hiep CH, Chau TT, Mai PP, Dung NT, Stepniewska K, White NJ, Hien TT, Farrar JJ (2005) Effect of antituberculosis drug resistance on response to treatment and outcome in adults with tuberculous meningitis. J Infect Dis 192:79–88
25. Marx GE, Chan E (2011) Tuberculous meningitis: diagnosis and treatment overview. Tuberc Res Treat 2011:798764
26. World Health Organization (2010) Treatment of tuberculosis: guidelines, 4th edn. World Health Organization, Geneva WHO/HTM/TB/2009.420
27. National Institute for Health and Clinical Excellence (2011) Tuberculosis. NICE Clinical Guidelines, No. 117
28. Pickering LK, Baker CJ, Long SS, JA MM (2006) Tuberculosis. In: Red book: 2006 report of the Committee on Infectious Diseases, 27th edn. American Academy of Pediatrics, Elk Grove Village, pp 678–698
29. Fox W, Ellard GA, Mitchison DA (1993) Studies on the treatment of tuberculosis undertaken by the British Medical Research Council tuberculosis units, 1946–1986. Int J Tuberc Lung Dis 3(10 Suppl 2):231–279
30. Jindani A, Nunn AJ, Enarson DA (2004) Two 8 month regimens of chemotherapy for treatment of newly diagnosed pulmonary tuberculosis: international multicentre randomised trial. Lancet 364(9441):1244–1251
31. Snider DE Jr (1980) Pyridoxine supplementation during INH therapy. Tubercle 61:191–196
32. Hagan G, Nathani N (2013) Clinical review: tuberculosis on the intensive care unit. Crit Care 17:240
33. Salpeter S (1993) Fatal INH-induced hepatitis: its risk during chemoprophylaxis. West J Med 159:560–564
34. Sanders WEJ (1976) Rifampin. Ann Intern Med 85:82–86
35. Saukkonen JJ, Cohn DL, Jasmer RM, Schenker S, Jereb JA, Nolan CM, Peloquin CA, Gordin FM, Nunes D, Strader DB, Bernardo J, Venkataramanan R, Sterling TR (2006) An official ATS statement: hepatotoxicity of antituberculosis therapy. Am J Respir Crit Care Med 174:935–952
36. Milburn H, Ashman N, Davies P, Doffman S, Drobniewski F, Khoo S, Ormerod P, Ostermann M, Snelson C (2010) Guidelines for the prevention and management of Mycobacterium tuberculosis infection and disease in adult patients with chronic kidney disease. Thorax 65:557–570
37. Thwaites G, Fisher M, Hemingway C, Scott G, Solomon T, Innes J (2009) British Infection Society guidelines for the diagnosis and treatment of tubercu-

losis of the central nervous system in adults and children. J Infect 59:167–187
38. Thwaites GE, Nguyen DB, Nguyen HD, Hoang TQ, Do TT, Nguyen TC, Nguyen QH, Nguyen TT, Nguyen NH, Nguyen TN, Nguyen NL, Nguyen HD, Vu NT, Cao HH, Tran TH, Pham PM, Nguyen TD, Stepniewska K, White NG, Tran TH, Farrar JJ (2004) Dexamethasone for the treatment of tuberculous meningitis in adolescents and adults. N Engl J Med 351:1741–1751
39. Sagonda T, Mupfumi L, Manzou R, Makamure B, Tshabalala M, Gwanzura L, Mason P, Mutetwa R (2014) Prevalence of extensively drug resistant tuberculosis among archived multidrug resistant tuberculosis isolates in Zimbabwe. Tuberc Res Treat 2014:349141
40. Wang YT, Chee CB, Hsu LY, Jagadesan R, Kaw GJ, Kong PM, Lew YJ, Lim CS, Lim TT, Lu KF, Ooi PL, Sng LH, Thoon KC (2016) Ministry of health clinical practice guidelines: prevention, diagnosis and management of tuberculosis. Singapore Med J 57(3):118–124
41. Rock RB, Olin M, Baker CA, Molitor TW, Peterson PK (2008) Central nervous system tuberculosis: pathogenesis and clinical aspects. Clin Microbiol Rev 21:243–261
42. Senbayrak S, Ozkutuk N, Erdem H, Johansen IS, Civljak R, Inal AS, Kayabas U, Kursun E, Elaldi N, Savic B, Simeon S, Yilmaz E, Dulovic O, Ozturk-Engin D, Ceran N, Lakatos B, Sipahi OR, Sunbul M, Yemisen M, Alabay S, Beovic B, Ulu-Kilic A, Cag Y, Catroux M, Inan A, Dragovac G, Deveci O, Tekin R, Gul HC, Sengoz G, Andre K, Harxhi A, Hansmann Y, Oncu S, Kose S, Oncul O, Parlak E, Sener A, Yilmaz G, Savasci U, Vahaboglu H (2015) Antituberculosis drug resistance patterns in adults with tuberculous meningitis: results of haydarpasa-iv study. Ann Clin Microbiol Antimicrob 14:47

Surgical Therapy of Tuberculosis of the Nervous System and Its Coverings

28

Walter A. Hall, Ahmet T. Turgut, and Mehmet Turgut

Contents

W.A. Hall, MD (✉)
Department of Neurosurgery, SUNY Upstate Medical University, Syracuse, New York 13210, USA
e-mail: hallw@upstate.edu

A.T. Turgut, MD
Department of Neurosurgery, Adnan Menderes University School of Medicine, Aydın, Turkey

Department of Radiology, Hacettepe University School of Medicine, Ankara, Turkey
e-mail: ahmettuncayturgut@yahoo.com

M. Turgut, MD, PhD
Department of Neurosurgery, Adnan Menderes University School of Medicine, Aydın, Turkey
e-mail: ahmettuncayturgut@yahoo.com

Abbreviations

AIDS	Acquired immunodeficiency syndrome
CEPs	Cartilage end plates
CNS	Central nervous system
CRP	C-reactive protein
CSF	Cerebrospinal fluid
CT	Computed tomography
EA	Epidural abscess
EMB	Ethambutol
ESR	Erythrocyte sedimentation rate
FLAIR	Fluid-attenuated inversion recovery
HASTE	Half-Fourier acquisition single-shot turbo spin-echo
HIV	Human immunodeficiency virus
IICP	Increased intracranial pressure
ioMRI	Intraoperative MRI
MRI	Magnetic resonance imaging
PCR	Polymerase chain reaction
PPD	Purified protein derivative
PZA	Pyrazinamide
RIF	Rifampin
SE	Subdural empyema
SM	Streptomycin
SWI	Susceptibility-weighted imaging
TB	Tuberculosis
TBA	Tuberculous brain abscess
TBM	Tuberculous meningitis
TST	Tuberculin skin test
WBC	White blood cell

M. Turgut et al. (eds.), *Tuberculosis of the Central Nervous System*,
DOI 10.1007/978-3-319-50712-5_28

28.1 Introduction

There are a number of factors that will influence the development of an intracranial infection: the virulence of the offending organism, the integrity of the immune system of the host, the microbiological inoculum size, and whether immunosuppression is present, either inherent or medication related. The likelihood of a central nervous system (CNS) infection developing is also influenced by the prolongation of survival in cancer patients and whether an organ transplant is present. Detecting an intracranial infection and following the therapeutic response are now possible due to the availability of computed tomography (CT) and magnetic resonance imaging (MRI). The ability to sample remote areas of the brain suspected to harbor infection can now be accomplished using neuronavigation and intraoperative MRI (ioMRI) guidance [1]. The availability of new antimicrobial agents with better penetration of the CNS and reduced systemic toxicity has improved our ability to treat some CNS infections that were previously uniformly fatal, such as tuberculosis (TB). The prompt identification of the causative organism combined with surgical decompression of neural elements can result in improved clinical outcomes. The infectious etiologies of TB that can affect the brain and require surgical intervention are epidural abscess (EA), subdural empyema (SE), and tuberculous brain abscess (TBA). Spinal infectious involvement is usually limited to the vertebral column or the epidural space.

28.2 Patient Selection

The clinical manifestations of TB that involves the CNS include diffuse exudative leptomeningitis, serous tuberculous meningitis (TBM), EA, SE, TBA, and intraspinal abscess where concurrent TBM and TBA affect 10–50% of patients [2]. The symptomatology associated with TB of the CNS includes headaches, lethargy, coma, weight loss, meningismus, hemiparesis, seizures, and fever and can be seen in all age groups in endemic areas [2]. The hematogenous spread of TB to the brain from a pulmonary source occurs in 10–15% of patients in developing regions of the world [3].

Underlying predisposing conditions that can lead to the development of TB of the CNS include acquired immunodeficiency syndrome (AIDS), diabetes mellitus, pregnancy, intravenous drug use, immigration, homelessness, population overcrowding, and immunosuppression associated with advanced age, alcoholism, chemotherapy, and organ transplantation [2–4]. The rate of reactivation of latent TB in patients with human immunodeficiency virus (HIV) infection is 3–12 times higher than in patients without HIV infection [5]. Approximately 20–36% of HIV patients develop TB of CNS usually in the form of meningitis in the presence of disseminated disease [5]. Neurological manifestations occur in more than 12% of TB cases with immune reconstitution inflammatory syndrome that occurs after the initiation of highly active antiretroviral therapy [5]. Kidney and lung transplant recipients are particularly susceptible to TB infection with 10–25% developing TBA [5].

The prognosis for patients with SE is related to the extent of the infection, the level of consciousness, and whether there was a delay in diagnosis before initiating treatment [2, 6]. The mortality rate from SE is higher with burr hole drainage than with craniotomy which could be due to the medical condition of the patient which necessitated their treatment with burr holes. SE has a morbidity rate of 26% and a mortality rate of 12% [7]. TB of the CNS of the brain usually carries a poor prognosis although 40% in coma made a full recovery [4]. A miliary pattern of the disease in the brain carries a poor prognosis [2].

In recent years, the resurgence of TB has been associated with a concomitant rise in spinal TB known as Pott's disease in Southeast Asia and Africa and many countries of Middle East and Eastern Europe including Turkey [8–11]. Although the disc space can become infected with atypical TB, the vertebral bodies are more likely to be involved. TB spinal osteomyelitis is seen in at-risk populations such as those with HIV infection. One single vertebral level is usually involved in spinal TB, but multiple levels can be affected in 20% [8].

Spinal EA due to *Mycobacterium tuberculosis* is common in Asia and Africa and is becoming more common in North America. Because of the high incidence of HIV infection in Russia, eastern and central Africa, and India, *M. tuberculosis* is highly prevalent. Crowded living conditions, malnutrition, and the emergence of resistant strains of TB can lead to the propagation of the disease. The bone and joints are affected in 3–5% of patients with TB in contrast to 60% of patients with coexisting HIV infection [12]. The spine is involved in half of those TB patients with bone involvement. The thoracolumbar spine is the most commonly involved location due to either hematogenous spread or by direct extension from a pulmonary source. The clinical course for spinal TB is more indolent than most other spinal infections and results in spinal deformity development more often [12]. The posterior elements of the vertebral body are more commonly involved in spinal TB than in other spinal infections producing deformity more often. Paraspinal abscess is common with liquid pus in the early stages that lead to caseous material with bony necrosis, ligamentous disruption, and spinal deformity in later stages [12]. In chronic infection, a fibrous reaction occurs that improves but does not completely restore spinal stability.

28.3 Preoperative Testing

As with most intracranial infections, the peripheral white blood cell (WBC) count is elevated in EA, SE, and TBA. Blood cultures may be positive in SE and TBA. In TBA, the peripheral WBC count is elevated in 60–70%, and the erythrocyte sedimentation rate (ESR) is increased in up to 90% of cases [2, 6]. The ESR and C-reactive protein (CRP) levels are elevated in EA, SE, and TBA, and these markers can be used to diagnose the presence of an infection and to follow the response of that infection to treatment. The WBC, ESR, and CRP counts are usually elevated in vertebral osteomyelitis. The ESR and CRP levels can be elevated after surgery with the ESR level reaching a peak at postoperative day 5 and remaining elevated for weeks, whereas the CRP level is maximal at 2 days and returns to normal after 5–14 days [8]. The fact that the CRP is normal before the ESR makes the test more useful for diagnosing late infections. In patients suspected to have spinal infection, blood cultures should be drawn before antibiotics are started to maximize the diagnostic yield of identifying the responsible organism. Ideally, the blood cultures should be drawn from three different sites at different times.

The cerebrospinal fluid (CSF) profile for patients with TBM will demonstrate a lymphocytic pleocytosis and a low glucose level. Culturing the CSF for *M. tuberculosis* has a sensitivity of 18–83%, and the results are often delayed for weeks [13, 14]. Due to the increasing prevalence of drug-resistant strains of the organism, it is essential that antibiotic susceptibility testing be performed on the isolates. Analysis of the CSF using the polymerase chain reaction (PCR) can diagnose TBM, although the test has not been standardized [13, 14]. A positive purified protein derivative (PPD) test or gamma interferon release assay can be used to diagnose latent TB, but both tests lack the sensitivity and specificity to support or exclude the diagnosis of meningitis [13]. In areas where TB is endemic, spondylitis can occur by hematogenous dissemination. In patients suspected to have TB spondylitis, a tuberculin skin test (TST) should be performed [8].

Although rarely obtained today, plain cranial x-rays can demonstrate sinusitis, mastoiditis, or osteomyelitis. Plain spine radiographs are not very sensitive or specific for diagnosing vertebral osteomyelitis. Erosion of the vertebral cartilage end plates (CEPs) or rarefaction of the vertebral body can take weeks to develop with collapse or fracture of the body representing a late development [8]. In particular, CT is the best study for evaluating bony involvement of TB, cranium (Fig. 28.1) or spine, called Pott's disease (Fig. 28.2), and it is essential for preoperative

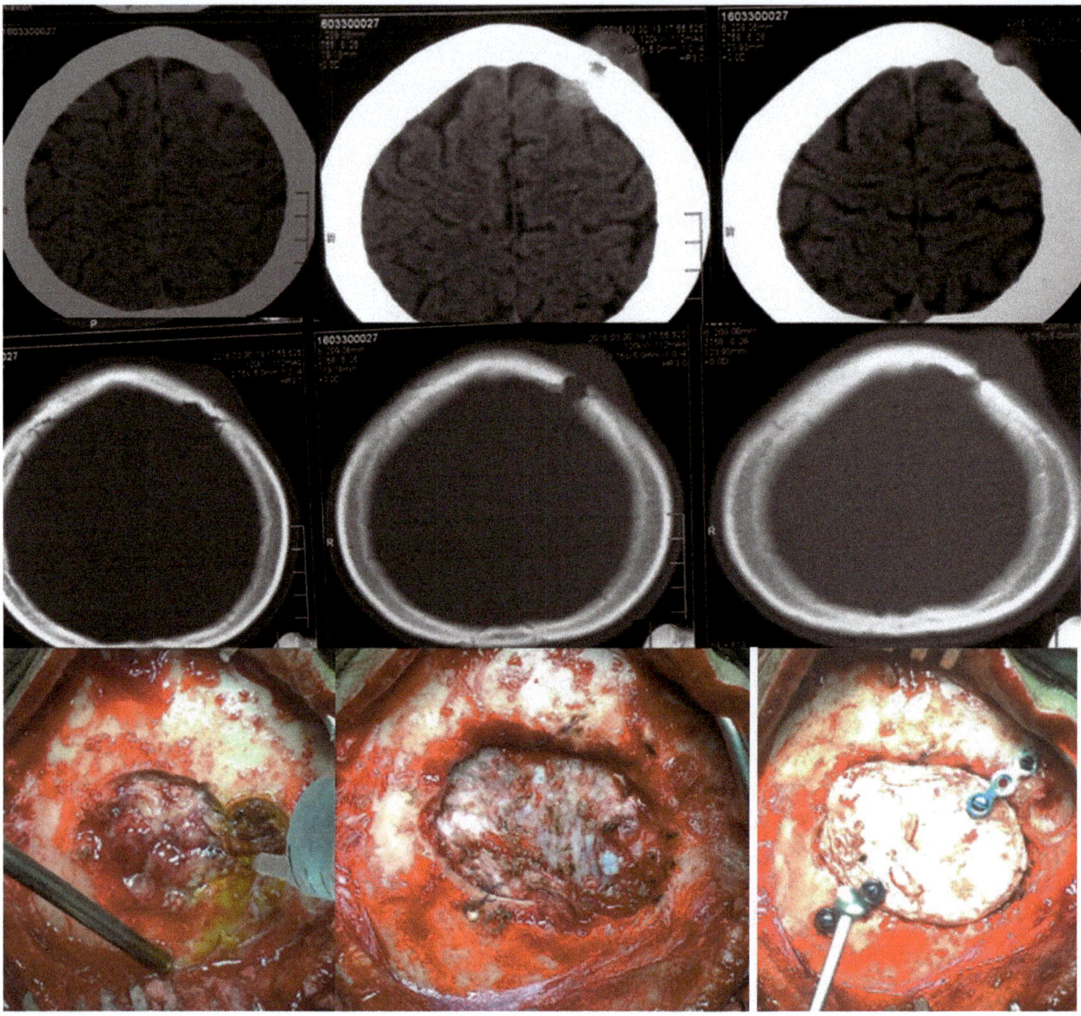

Fig. 28.1 CT of the cranium showing a TB lesion located left frontal bone with extension to the scalp and extradural space. Note that intraoperative pictures illustrating cranial defect area in the left frontal region (Courtesy of FH Chowdhury)

planning if surgical fixation of the vertebral column is indicated [8]. The administration of intravenous contrast can demonstrate enhancement in the face of an infected disc or bone in the presence of an abscess. Those enhancing areas seen on CT can represent targets for CT-guided biopsy or aspiration that may lead to the identification of the causative organism. Although not as sensitive or specific for detecting spinal infection as MRI, CT is usually adequate in patients unable to have MRI due to the presence of implanted devices or when they are morbidly obese. Myelography is rarely used because of its invasive nature and the potential to seed the CSF in the presence of infection leading to the development of TBM.

Radiologically, an enhanced MRI is probably the most reliable imaging modality for diagnosing vertebral column infections. For discitis, MRI has a sensitivity and specificity of over 90%, and in vertebral osteomyelitis, the sensitivity is 96% and the specificity is 93% [8]. Intravenous contrast will demonstrate inflammation of the vertebral CEPs and abscess formation (Fig. 28.2). Destruction of the CEPs, vertebral body collapse, and kyphotic deformities are late findings seen in vertebral column infection [8].

Cerebral tuberculomas enhance intensely after contrast administration on CT and MRI and are often surrounded by significant cerebral edema [4]. Two-thirds of patients have multiple lesions on CT or MRI that are located in the cerebral hemispheres, although the brainstem and cerebellum can also be involved (Figs. 28.3, 28.4, and 28.5) [15]. Additional findings that can be present on the CT scan in TB of the CNS are hydrocephalus, calcification, mass effect, midline shift, and cortical and subcortical infarction (Fig. 28.6) [2, 15]. A calcified granulomatous reaction involving the basal meninges can also be seen on CT of the head [13]. In some cases, simultaneous involvement of the cerebral hemispheres and the spinal column, called Pott's disease, in same patient may be observed (Fig. 28.7).

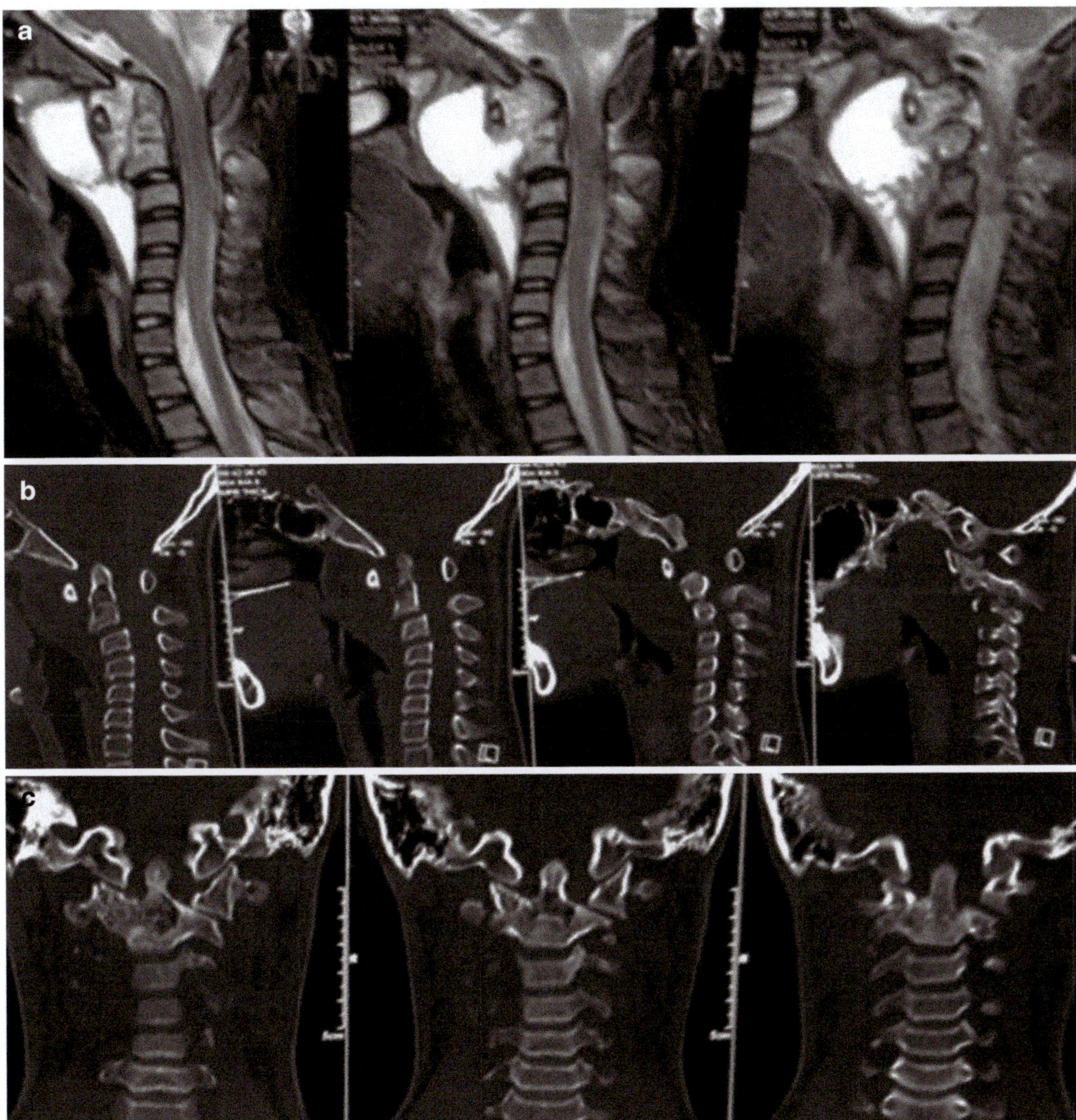

Fig. 28.2 Preoperative parasagittal T1- and T2-weighted MRIs (**a**), parasagittal (**b**) and coronal (**c**) CT sections of a patient with craniovertebral junction TB with instability as well as pre- (**d**) and postoperative (**f**), and x-rays of the same patient. Note that an operative figure demonstrating posterior spinal fusion material (**e**) (Courtesy of FH Chowdhury)

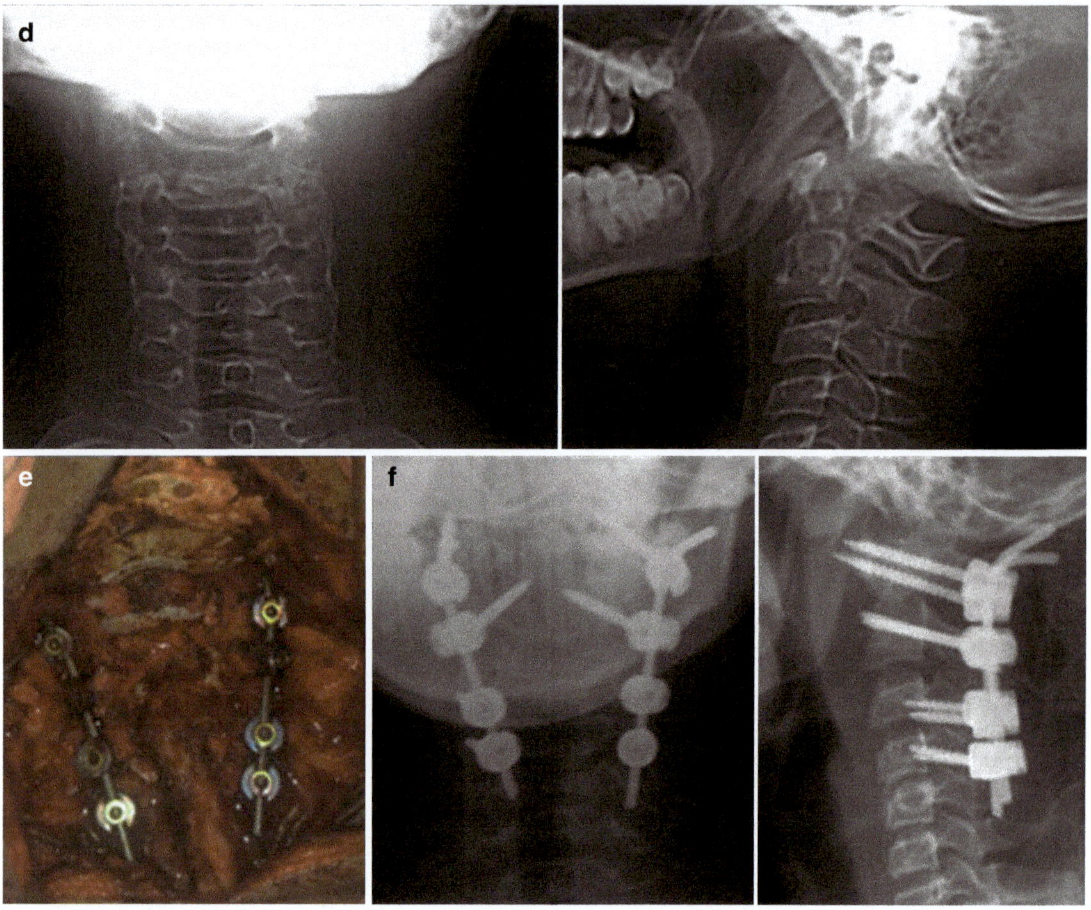

Fig. 28.2 (continued)

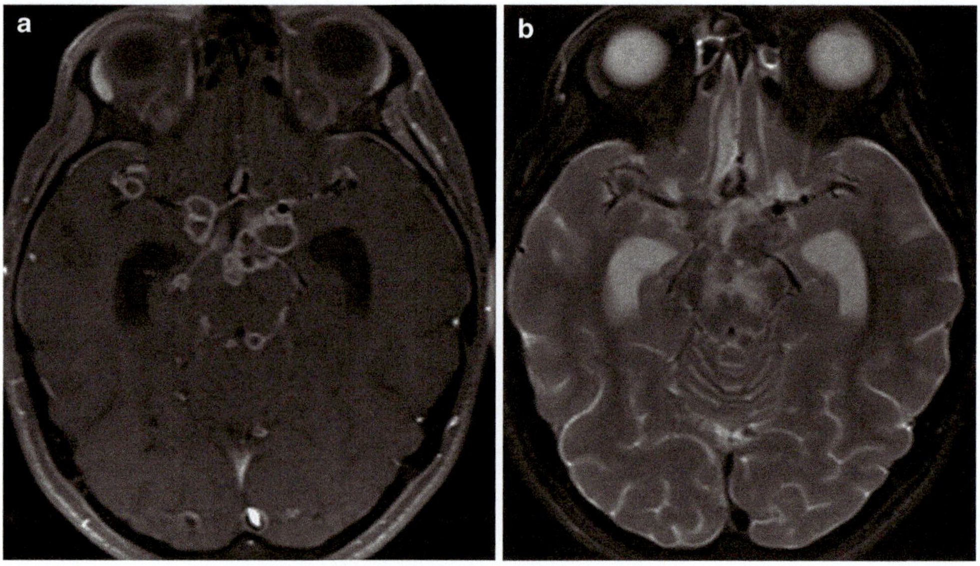

Fig. 28.3 MRI of a 34-year-old female patient, who presented with headache and epileptic seizure, demonstrates the presence of tuberculous meningitis (TBM) affecting basal cistern as well as enhancing multiple TB granulomas in mesencephalon in axial T1 (**a**)- and T2 (**b**)-weighted images (Courtesy of E Kalkan)

MRI of a cerebral tuberculoma will most commonly show a hypointense or isointense center with a hyperintense rim on T2-weighted or fluid-attenuated inversion recovery (FLAIR) scans (Figs. 28.3, 28.4, and 28.8) [2, 15]. Cerebral angiography and CT angiography can be used to diagnose infectious intracranial aneurysms due to *M. tuberculosis*. In some cases, it may be complicated with TBA with parameningeal collection and venous thrombosis, in addition to intra-axial tuberculomas (Fig. 28.4).

28.4 Medical Management

Once the diagnosis of TBM is suspected, antibiotic therapy should begin immediately because of the high morbidity and mortality rates without treatment. Once the diagnosis of TB of the CNS is made either by brain biopsy or via craniotomy, anti-TB chemotherapy in the form of isoniazid (INH), rifampin (RIF), pyrazinamide (PZA), and either ethambutol (EMB) or streptomycin (SM) should be administered for 12–18 months [2]. The combination can be altered once the results of the antibiotic susceptibility testing are known. When EMB and/or PZA were used to treat tuberculoma, resolution was seen in 18.2% after 9 months and in 54% after 24 months [16]. The rate of tuberculoma resolution was not influenced by the number of lesions, corticosteroid administration, prior anti-TB treatment, or symptom duration prior to presentation, although larger lesions took longer to resolve than did smaller ones [16]. In TBM, adjuvant corticosteroid administration has been shown to decrease neurologic sequelae and improve survival [14].

The reasons to treat a cerebral tuberculoma medically include a location deep within the brain or in an area with eloquent neurological function, the inability of the patient to have general anesthesia because of medical comorbidities, the presence of concurrent TBM or ventriculitis, the presence of multiple lesions (Figs. 28.3, 28.4, 28.5, 28.6, 28.7, and 28.8), or when the placement of a shunt is necessary because of the presence of hydrocephalus that could become infected if the TBA is treated surgically [2, 6]. In general, the maximum diameter of the lesions that are treated medically should not exceed 2.5 cm. A major disadvantage to medical management alone is the potential that the intracerebral process being treated does not represent TB, but is actually a hematoma, neoplasm, or cerebral infarct.

In spontaneous spinal infections, the administration of antibiotic therapy tailored to treat the causative organism is the mainstay of treatment with surgery usually reserved for select indications such as neurologic impairment or spinal instability. Medical treatment is usually successful for the majority of patients with TB vertebral osteomyelitis [8]. Postoperative osteomyelitis is treated with a combination of surgical debridement and appropriate antibiotic therapy.

The initial antibiotic regimen for treatment of spinal TB is a combination of four drugs for 2 months: INH, RIF, EMB, and PZA. Subsequently, the antibiotic coverage is reduced to INH and RIF for a 6–12-month course of treatment. Due to the emergence of multidrug-resistant TB, antibiotic susceptibility testing of the isolate is essential. The patient's response to treatment should be monitored closely with a lack of symptomatic improvement, continued elevation of the CRP after 4 weeks of therapy, and persistent fevers suggesting that the treatment has failed [8]. Medical treatment alone can lead to a solid spinal fusion in 65–79% of TB cases [8].

In spontaneous spinal infections, the administration of antibiotic therapy tailored to treat the causative organism is the mainstay of treatment with surgery usually reserved for select indications such as neurologic impairment or spinal instability. Medical treatment is usually successful for the majority of patients with TB vertebral osteomyelitis (Figs. 28.7 and 28.9) [8]. Postoperative osteomyelitis is treated with a combination of surgical debridement and appropriate antibiotic therapy.

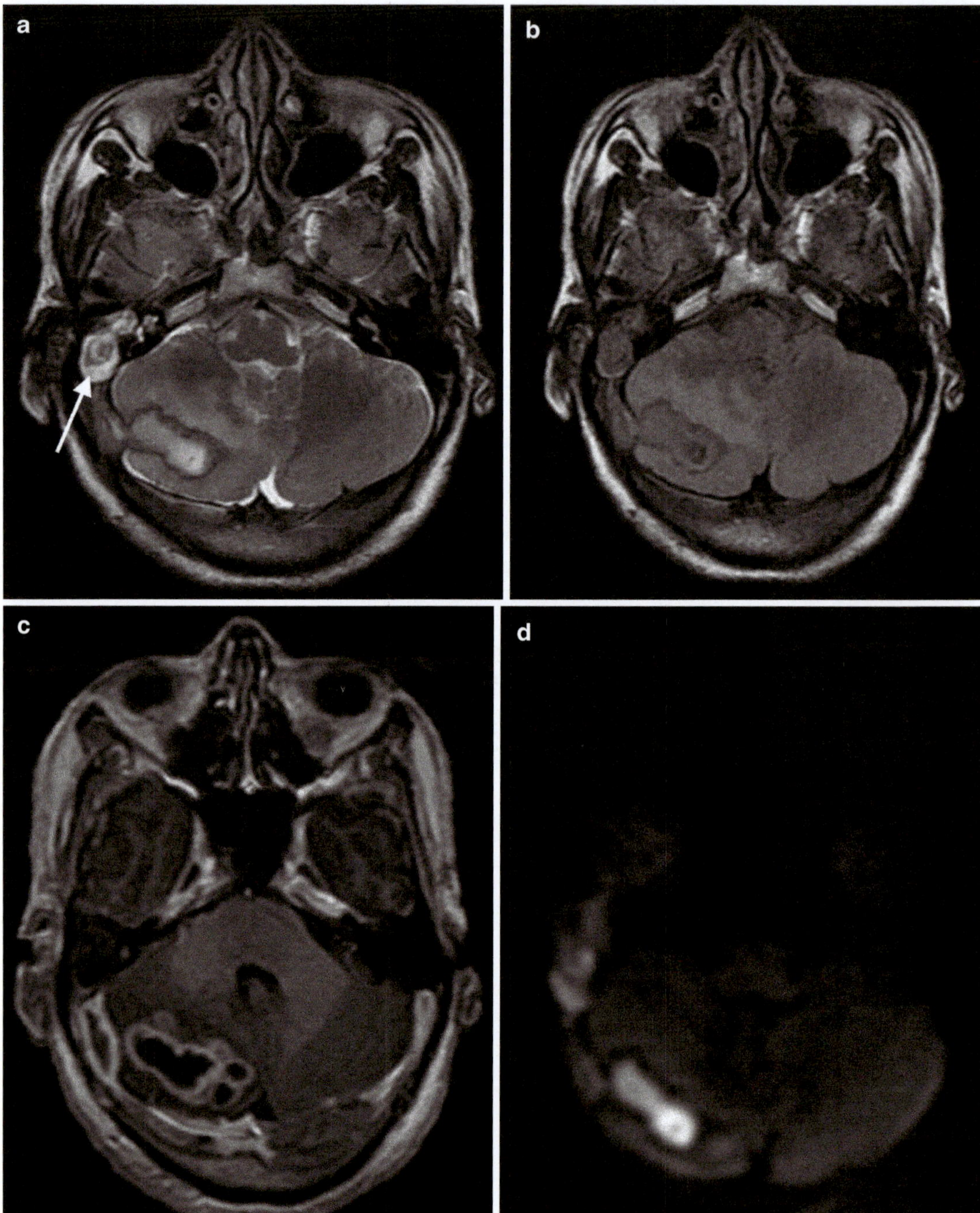

Fig. 28.4 MRI of the brain showing a right cerebellar conglomerate lesion which is hyperintense on T2W (**a**) and iso- to hypointense on T2-FLAIR (**b**) with an evidence of parameningeal collection on T1-gadolinium-contrast sequence (**c**). Restriction on DWI is evident (**d**). Thrombosis of right jugular bulb can be noted (*arrow*, **a**). The findings are suggestive of a TB abscess with parameningeal collection and venous thrombosis (Courtesy of RK Garg)

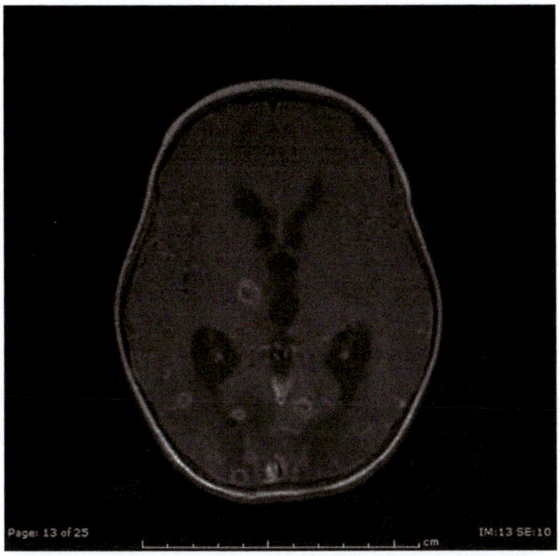

Fig. 28.5 Axial T1-weighted contrast-enhanced MRI of the brain in a 5-year-old male that presented with seizures showing multiple intracranial tuberculomas

28.5 Surgical Tricks

Intracranial surgical procedures to treat EA, SE, and TBA can be both diagnostic and therapeutic. The successful drainage of intracranial suppuration is dependent on the viscosity of the collection and on its location. When surgically approaching deep-seated or eloquent brain locations, neuronavigation-guided needle aspiration may be necessary. Depending on the viscosity of the presumed fluid collection, it may not be possible to aspirate the material, and antibiotic treatment alone may be required. For this same reason, insertion of a drainage catheter in order to instill antimicrobial agents is often ineffective due to inadequate penetration.

28.5.1 Surgical Aspiration

If the suppurative collection can be aspirated, this approach has several advantages that include the ability to use local anesthesia to perform the procedure; increased intracranial pressure (IICP) may be quickly relieved; the presence of infection is verified; the infection location is confirmed; the causative organism may be isolated; and whether the TBA is encapsulated is determined [2, 6]. Unfortunately aspiration has several disadvantages that include the possibility of rupture of TBA contents into the ventricular system resulting in ventriculitis or their spillage into the subarachnoid space causing meningitis. In the presence of a mature abscess, the potential to need a repeat aspiration procedure of the TBA is quite high.

28.5.2 Repair of Cranial Defects

Burr hole evacuation of EA is often ineffective due to the thick nature of the purulent material, and a formal craniotomy for evacuation may be necessary. If osteomyelitis involving the bone is present, the involved portion of the bone should be debrided with a drill or just removed with the ensuing cranial defect being covered by titanium mesh. If the cranial defect is large and cannot be adequately covered with titanium mesh, a delayed cranioplasty may be necessary after the infection has resolved. Synthetic materials such as PEEK (polyether ether ketone) can be used to cover cranial defects after the infection has been adequately treated. The cranioplasty is secured in place with titanium plates and screws. When treating EA, the dura mater should not be breached unless a SE is strongly suspected.

28.5.3 Craniotomy for Drainage

The majority of patients with SE receive surgical treatment. Craniotomy for drainage of SE is the preferred treatment due to improved clinical outcomes and lower rates of neurological morbidity and repeat surgery [17]. When the SE is the result of TBM in children, medically fragile patients, and has a parafalcine infection location, burr hole drainage can be used for treatment [17]. The burr hole drainage needs to be repeated or followed by a craniotomy in 20% of patients [2, 6].

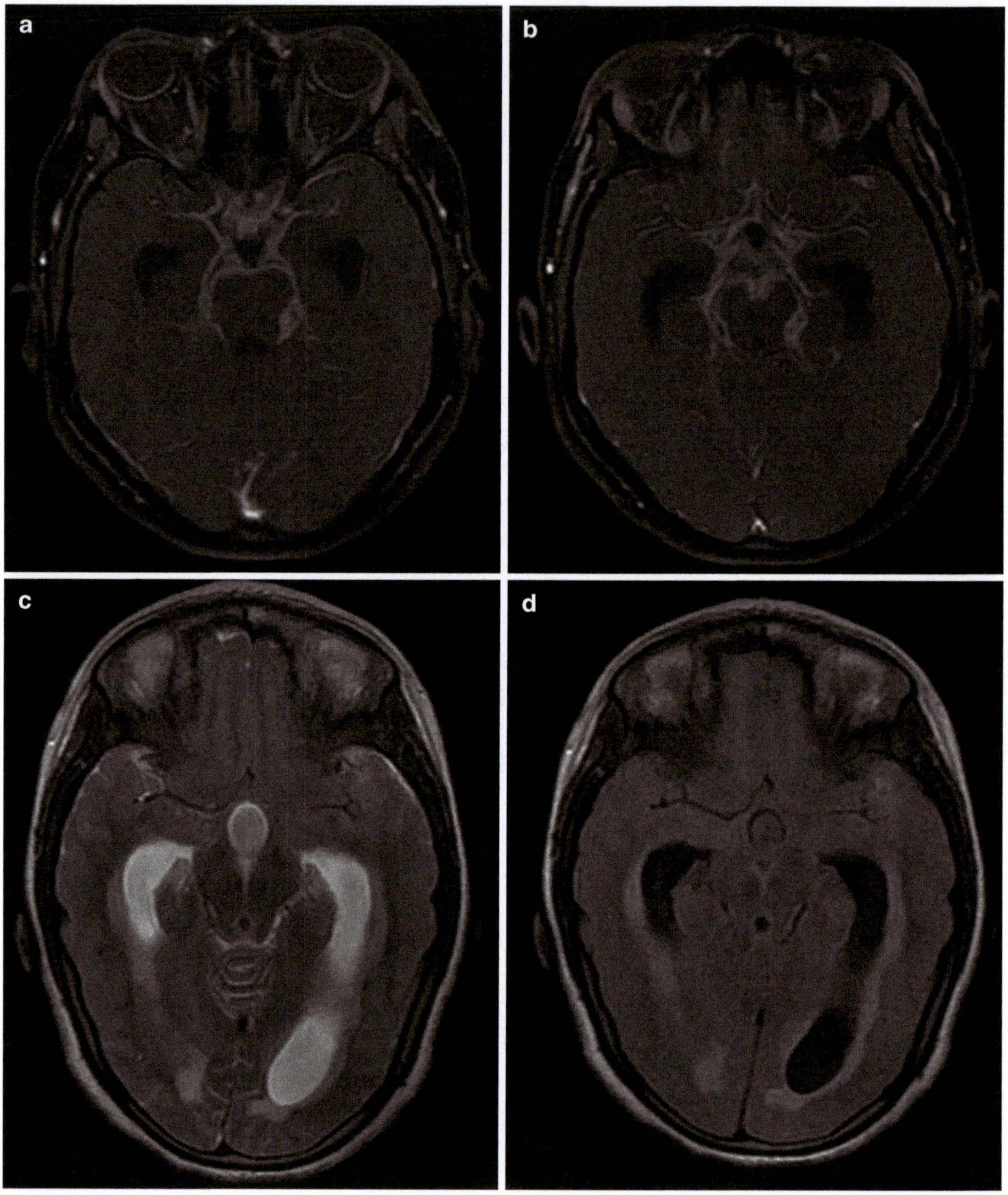

Fig. 28.6 MRI of the brain in a patient with TBM shows gadolinium enhancement of optic nerve sheath, optic chiasma, pituitary and paracavernous areas, perimesencephalic cistern, and middle cerebral artery fissures (**a**, **b**) suggestive of dense exudates and suggestion of TB opto-chiasmatic arachnoiditis. T2W image (**c**) shows enlarged temporal horns of lateral ventricles and an enlarged third ventricle along with suggestion of periventricular oozing on T2-FLAIR sequence (**d**) suggestive of hydrocephalus (Courtesy of RK Garg)

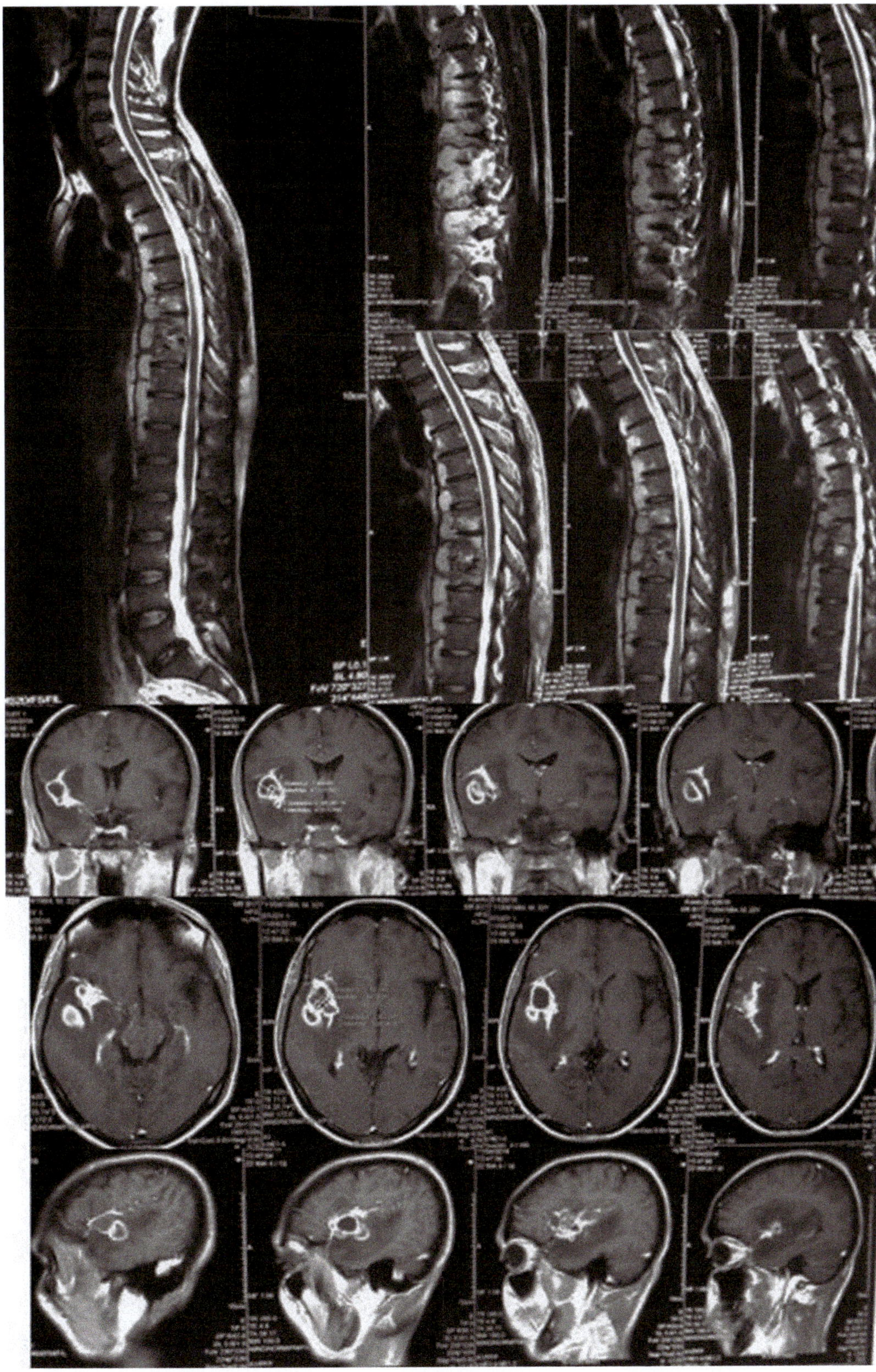

Fig. 28.7 MRI of the brain and spine demonstrates simultaneous TB lesions located right sylvian fissure and Th7–Th9 vertebrae in same patient (Courtesy of FH Chowdhury)

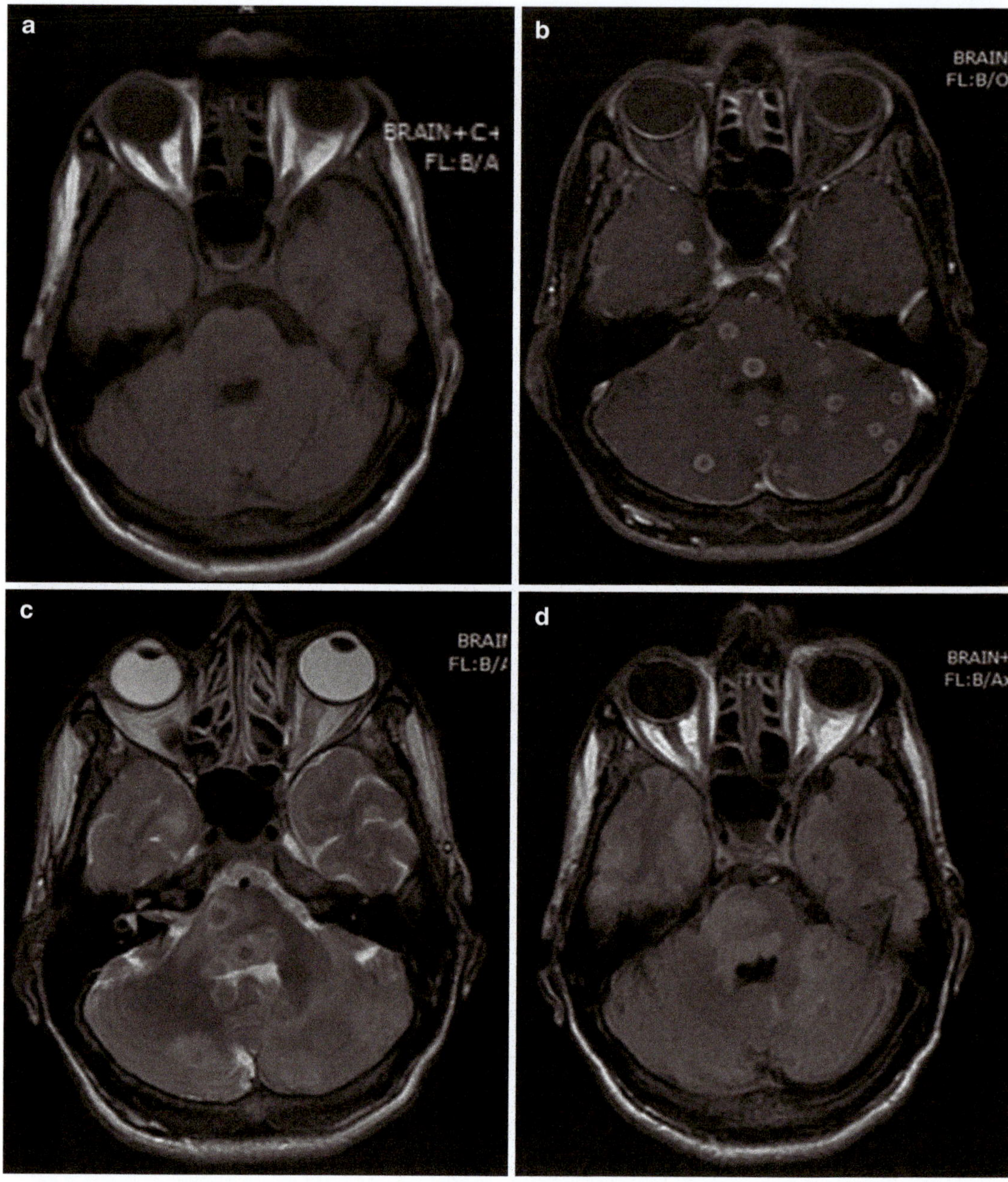

Fig. 28.8 MRI of the brain showing multiple cerebellar, pontine, and right temporal hypointense lesions on T1W image (**a**), which enhance on T1-gadolinium-contrast sequence (**b**), in a patient with miliary TB. The lesions are iso- to hypointense with perilesional edema on T2W (**c**) and T2-FLAIR (**d**) sequences and must be differentiated from other causes of ring-enhancing lesions (Courtesy of RK Garg)

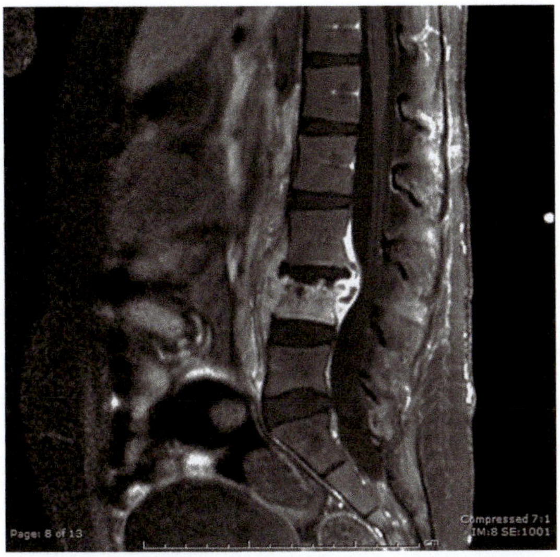

Fig. 28.9 Sagittal T1-weighted contrast-enhanced MRI of the lumbar spine in a 27-year-old female that presented with low back pain demonstrating TB osteomyelitis of the L4 vertebral body

28.5.4 Craniotomy for Resection of Tuberculoma

A TBA or tuberculoma is a granulomatous inflammatory process that can mimic a neoplasm and require a brain biopsy for diagnosis. The pathological findings that confirm the diagnosis are caseous necrosis surrounded by Langhans giant cells and epithelioid histiocytes, with bacilli rarely being demonstrated on acid-fast staining [2]. Unfortunately, stereotactic biopsy of tuberculomas is difficult often due to their small size, and a conclusive diagnosis is only made in 28% of cases [18]. The rate of diagnosis was comparable when either the enhancing rim or the center of the lesion was sampled [18]. Surgical resection of the tuberculoma was reserved for those patients with IICP, the potential for visual loss, or in the face of an enlarging lesion despite the administration of appropriate anti-TB chemotherapy [2, 18]. In the presence of hydrocephalus, CSF diversion is usually necessary.

28.5.5 Surgery of TBA

The surgical management of TBA can be both diagnostic and therapeutic. The two primary surgical techniques that can be utilized to treat TBA are aspiration or excision. Aspiration of the tuberculoma has been described previously, and the open removal of lesions can be considered for cerebellar lesions, multiloculated lesions, surgically accessible lesions not responding to medical therapy, and large lesions causing significant mass effect [2, 6]. Deep or multiple lesions, or those in the cerebritis stage, are best treated medically or via aspiration.

28.5.6 Use of Intraoperative MRI Guidance

In recent years, 1.5 Tesla ioMRI guidance has been used successfully to aspirate or excise TBA. The main advantage to using ioMRI guidance is to confirm the successful drainage or removal of the TBA at the time of surgery. During ioMRI-guided procedures, general anesthesia is used for patient comfort because of the length of the surgery and to prevent the inadvertent displacement of the biopsy needle during aspiration procedures. After general anesthesia is administered, preoperative imaging is performed to localize the craniotomy site using MRI-visible markers placed on the scalp. After this baseline imaging is obtained, the scalp is prepped, and sterilely wrapped surface coils are placed on opposite sides of the head. The incision is made at a location representing the shortest distance to the purulent collection. A burr hole is made, and the disposable Navigus Frameless Passive Biopsy System (Medtronic, Inc., Minneapolis, MN) is secured to the skull. The patient is moved into the magnet, and a novel targeting method known as prospective stereotaxis is employed to determine a safe and accurate pathway to the TBA [19, 20]. This alignment process takes 5–10 min to complete. After the trajectory is determined through the rotation of an MRI-visible alignment stem such that the target will be accessible in two planes, the biopsy needle is passed in a stepwise fashion via a guide tube through the brain. Once the biopsy needle is introduced into the TBA, gentle aspiration is performed until a slight degree of resistance is encountered. The MRI is

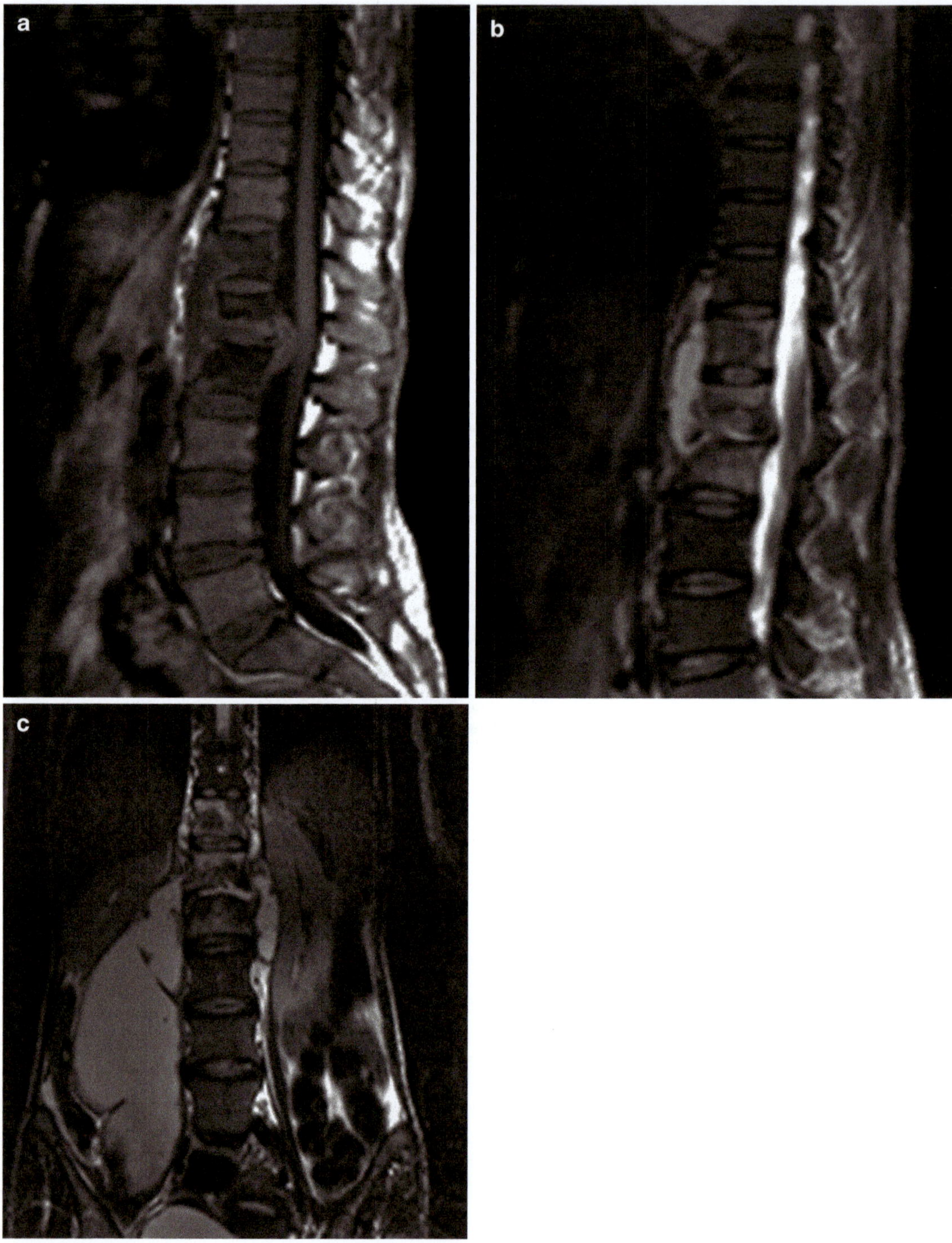

Fig. 28.10 Spinal MRI in T1 weighted (**a**), T2 weighted (**b**), and coronal (**c**) views showing a L1–L2 Pott's disease associated with a right huge psoas abscess (Courtesy of M Benzagmout, MD)

now repeated to determine the amount of pus that has been withdrawn, whether the TBA capsule has collapsed, and to confirm that there is no evidence of intraoperative hemorrhage. After the imaging is complete, the trajectory guide is removed from the skull, the wound is irrigated with antibiotic solution, a collagen sponge is placed over the brain, and a titanium cover is placed over the burr hole to restore the normal skull contour. The galea and skin are closed with absorbable sutures, and the patient is transported to the recovery room for extubation.

Removing a TBA not responding to antimicrobial therapy can also be performed with ioMRI guidance. The procedure for resecting a TBA has some similarities to the aspiration procedure. The patient is induced prior to applying a carbon fiber Malcolm-Rand head holder (Elekta, Decatur, GA) that allows for repeat imaging in the same plane during the surgery. The craniotomy is often performed through one radiofrequency surface coil after the TBA has been localized with MRI-visible markers. Intravenous contrast administration is reserved until the TBA has been removed to prevent leakage into edematous brain parenchyma which makes the interpretation of the ioMRI problematic. T2-weighted MRI such as turbo FLAIR and ultrafast half-Fourier acquisition single-shot turbo spin-echo (HASTE) sequences are used in the TBA. In addition to HASTE sequences, susceptibility-weighted imaging (SWI) is useful for excluding the presence of blood in the operative field at the end of the procedure.

The craniotomy used to remove the TBA is usually smaller than those performed in the main operating room because of the precise preoperative localization. The craniotomy is performed outside the 5 gauss line with standard surgical instruments. Although MRI can be repeated at any point during the surgery, there are usually three times when imaging is performed that are to localize the cranial opening, to confirm removal of the TBA, and to assure the absence of intraoperative hemorrhage. Each imaging update requires no more than 10–15 min, and the surgical instrumentation is removed from the operative field before the patient is moved into the magnet. A primary advantage of using ioMRI is the ability of the surgeon to compensate for the "brain shift" that occurs once CSF has been evacuated when the dura mater is incised, particularly for superficial lesions.

Operating entirely within the magnetic field is possible when it is anticipated that multiple imaging updates will be necessary during the procedure. In this situation all surgical instrumentation from the scalpel to the cranial drill must be MRI compatible. In these cases, the patient is advanced through the magnet to the opposite side in order to perform the surgery. When imaging is needed, the patient is advanced back to the isocenter of the magnet. Placing the clear plastic sterile drape low on the flared opening of the magnet allows for the transport of the patient to the isocenter and for the continual visualization of the surgical site. MRI-compatible bipolar cautery and a titanium pituitary rongeur are utilized to remove the TBA. A liquid crystal display monitor adjacent to the magnet allows the surgeon to visually confirm the absence of the TBA before closing. The craniotomy is closed in the routine fashion with the bone flap being secured in place with a titanium plating system. SWI scans confirm the absence of a hematoma prior to patient transport to the recovery room for extubation.

28.5.7 Surgery for Pott's Disease

Surgical treatment of spinal infection is indicated for diagnosing the responsible organism if less invasive diagnostic methods have been unsuccessful, debridement of infected tissue, drainage of abscesses that have failed to respond to adequate antibiotic treatment, stabilization of the spine, kyphotic deformity correction, sepsis, intractable pain, and compression of the spinal cord (Figs. 28.2, 28.10, and 28.11) or nerve roots causing severe or worsening neurological deficits [8]. Early surgical treatment of kyphosis

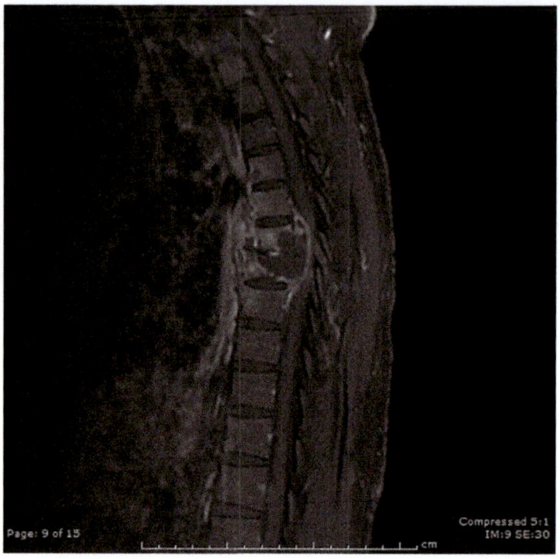

Fig. 28.11 Sagittal T1-weighted contrast-enhanced MRI of the thoracic spine in a 26-year-old male that presented with lower extremity weakness. The epidural collection was drained and the culture grew *Mycobacterium tuberculosis*

in TB osteomyelitis should be considered for patients at risk for progression of the deformity. Risk factors for deformity progression include a kyphotic angle of more than 30°, loss of more than 1.5 times the vertebral body height, radiographic instability, involvement of more than 3 vertebral bodies, involvement of anterior and posterior elements, and disease onset in the immature spine [8]. Surgical treatment of TB spinal EA is useful in the presence of spinal instability or pronounced deformity and when there is progressive neurological impairment such as paraplegia due to spinal cord compression [8, 12]. The role of drainage of extraspinal collections or debridement of involved bone in helping to clear infection remains unclear [12]. However in confirmed spinal instability, pronounced deformity, and neurological deficit, surgical treatment is indicated [12].

In patients suspected to have spinal infection, if blood cultures do not demonstrate an organism on culture after 48 h, a CT-guided percutaneous biopsy of the involved vertebral body or disc is warranted. The sampled tissue should be sent for culture, and the histopathology should be evaluated for granulomas and acid-fast bacilli [8]. If the blood cultures and percutaneous biopsy do not yield a diagnosis, an open biopsy should be performed.

Conclusion

1. Factors that influence to development of an intracranial or spinal infection are the virulence of the causative organism, the integrity of the host immune system, the size of the microbial inoculum, and whether inherent or medication-related immunosuppression is present.
2. Predisposing conditions for the development of CNS TB are acquired immunodeficiency syndrome (AIDS), diabetes mellitus, pregnancy, intravenous drug use, immigration, homelessness, population overcrowding, and immunosuppression associated with advanced age, alcoholism, chemotherapy, and organ transplantation.
3. Preoperative testing should include obtaining a WBC count, ESR, and CRP. These studies can be followed to monitor the patient's response to anti-TB treatment. In patients suspected to have TB spondylitis, a TST should be performed.
4. CT is the best study for evaluating bony involvement due to TB. Enhanced MRI is the most reliable study for diagnosing vertebral column infections due to TB. Intracerebral tuberculomas enhance intensely after contrast administration on CT and MRI.
5. Anti-TB chemotherapy including INH, RIF, PZA, and either EMB or SM should be administered for 12–18 months in cases with TB of the CNS and its coverings.
6. Surgical aspiration of intracerebral collections can be performed to relieve elevated intracranial pressure, localize and confirm the presence of infection, isolate the causative organism, and determine if encapsulation is present. Lesions that are deep, multiple, or in the cerebritis stage are best treated medically or via aspiration.
7. Craniotomy may be indicated to drain TB SE or to diagnose and resect a cerebral

tuberculoma. Resection is reserved for those patients that have increased ICP, have the potential for visual loss, and have enlarging lesions despite appropriate anti-TB treatment. Following medical treatment of TB infection, synthetic materials such as PEEK can be used to cover cranial defects if the cranial bone has TB osteomyelitis.

8. Open surgical treatment of spinal TB infection is indicated for diagnosis when less invasive diagnostic methods have been unsuccessful, to debride infected tissue, to drain abscesses that have not responded to antibiotic therapy, to stabilize the spine, to correct kyphotic deformity, and to relieve compression of the spinal cord or nerve roots causing severe or worsening neurological deficits.

References

1. Hall WA, Liu H, Martin AJ, Pozza CH, Maxwell RE, Truwit CL (2000) Safety, efficacy, and functionality of high-field strength interventional MR imaging for neurosurgery. Neurosurgery 46:632–642
2. Hall WA, Truwit CL (2008) The surgical management of infections involving the cerebrum. Neurosurgery 62:SHC519–SHC531
3. Bayindir C, Mete O, Bilgic B (2006) Retrospective study of 23 pathologically proven cases of central nervous system tuberculomas. Clin Neurol Neurosurg 108:353–357
4. Wasay M, Moolani MK, Zaheer J, Kheleani BA, Smego RA, Sarwari RA (2004) Prognostic indicators in patients with intracranial tuberculoma: a review of 102 cases. J Pak Med Assoc 54:83–87
5. Nissim O, Greenberg G, Cohen ZR, Spiegelmann R (2014) Central nervous system infections in immunocompromised hosts. In: Hall W, Kim P (eds) Neurosurgical infectious diseases. Surgical and nonsurgical management. Thieme, New York, pp 247–268
6. Hall WA (2008) Cerebral infectious processes. In: Loftus CM (ed) Neurosurgical emergencies. Thieme, New York, pp 115–124
7. Nathoo Nadvi SS, van Dellen JR, Gouws E (1999) Intracranial subdural empyema in the era of computed tomography: a review of 699 cases. Neurosurgery 44:529–536
8. Swanson KI, Resnick DK (2014) Vertebral column infections. In: Hall W, Kim P (eds) Neurosurgical infectious diseases. Surgical and nonsurgical management. Thieme, New York, pp 147–162
9. Turgut M (2001) Multifocal extensive spinal tuberculosis (Pott's disease) involving cervical, thoracic and lumbar vertebrae. Br J Neurosurg 15:142–146
10. Turgut M, Özcan OE, Özgen T, Bertan V (1993) Intradural extramedullary tuberculoma of the spinal cord -a case report. Zentralbl Neurochir 54:197–199
11. Turgut M, Özcan OE, Özgen T, Sağlam S, Bertan V, Erbengi A (1989) Tuberculomas of the craniospinal axis. Turk Neurosurg 1:34–38
12. McCutcheon IE (2014) Spinal canal infections. In: Hall W, Kim P (eds) Neurosurgical infectious diseases. Surgical and nonsurgical management. Thieme, New York, pp 163–181
13. Fukuta Y, Byers K (2014) Microbiological diagnosis of central nervous system infections. In: Hall W, Kim P (eds) Neurosurgical infectious diseases. Surgical and nonsurgical management. Thieme, New York, pp 16–29
14. Suryadevara M, Domachowske JB (2014) Meningeal infections. In: Hall W, Kim P (eds) Neurosurgical infectious diseases. Surgical and nonsurgical management. Thieme, New York, pp 107–124
15. Wasay M, Kheleni BA, Moolani MK, Zaheer J, Pui M, Hasan S, Muzaffar S, Bakshi R, Sarawari AR (2003) CT and MRI findings in 100 consecutive patients with intracranial tuberculoma. J Neuroimaging 13:240–247
16. Poonnoose SI, Rajsekhar V (2003) Rate of resolution of histologically verified intracranial tuberculomas. Neurosurgery 53:873–879
17. Nathoo N, Nadvi SS, Gouws E, van Dellen JR (2001) Craniotomy improves outcome for cranial subdural empyemas: computed tomography-era experience with 699 patients. Neurosurgery 49:872–878
18. Mohanty A, Santosh V, Anandh B, Kolluri VR, Vasudev MK, Hegde T, Shankar SK (1999) Diagnostic efficacy of stereotactic biopsies in intracranial tuberculomas. Surg Neurol 52:252–258
19. Hall WA, Truwit CL (2005) Intraoperative MR imaging. Magn Reson Imaging Clin N Am 13:533–543
20. Hall WA, Truwit CL (2005) 1.5 T: spectroscopy-supported brain biopsy. Neurosurg Clin N Am 16:165–172

Hydrocephalus Surgery in Childhood Tuberculous Meningitis with Hydrocephalus

29

Anthony Figaji, Graham Fieggen, and Ursula Rohlwink

Contents

A. Figaji, MD, PhD (✉) • G. Fieggen, MD
U. Rohlwink, PhD
Paediatric Neurosurgery Unit, Division of Neurosurgery, University of Cape Town, Cape Town, South Africa
e-mail: Anthony.Figaji@uct.ac.za; gfieggen@gmail.com; ursulakarin@gmail.com

Abbreviations

CSF	Cerebrospinal fluid
ETV	Endoscopic third ventriculostomy
EVD	External ventricular drain
HIV	Human immunodeficiency virus
ICP	Intracranial pressure
MRI	Magnetic resonance imaging
SIADH	Syndrome of inappropriate antidiuretic hormone
TB	Tuberculosis/tuberculous
TBM	Tuberculous meningitis

29.1 Introduction

Hydrocephalus is common in tuberculous meningitis (TBM) and contributes to poor outcomes [1–4]. But its management is not necessarily as straightforward as hydrocephalus in other conditions. First, managing TBM patients well is not just about hydrocephalus treatment. Effective management must be focused as much on dealing with the other complications of TBM, such as vasculitis, as it is on the hydrocephalus itself. Second, it is not all about placing a shunt or not. If managed well, most patients can be spared lifelong shunt dependency. These are important truths about TBM that are often overlooked.

Unfortunately, we have little evidence to guide our therapies. No standardization exists for the treatment of hydrocephalus due to

M. Turgut et al. (eds.), *Tuberculosis of the Central Nervous System*,
DOI 10.1007/978-3-319-50712-5_29

tuberculosis (TB), and protocols vary widely from center to center. Broadly, these protocols are either selective or nonselective: patients are treated either differentially or uniformly. Even for differentially treated patients, the extent of the selection criteria used varies widely [5–9].

Most centers that see TBM frequently have limited neurosurgical capacity, and where there is capacity, communication between physicians and surgeons is often poor. Clearly, TBM patients with hydrocephalus cannot be effectively managed without neurosurgical assistance. At the same time, good decision-making requires that the surgeon actively consider what is best for the individual patient, whether that be surgery or not. This chapter will discuss what we think these considerations should be.

First, a primer of the most important pathophysiologic aspects of TBM is appropriate. Hydrocephalus occurs in most children with TBM [1, 4]. This is usually communicating (approximately 80% of cases) [1, 4], the cerebrospinal fluid (CSF) being obstructed by exudate at the level of the basal cisterns. But it may also be noncommunicating, that same exudate closing off the fourth ventricular outlet foramina and/or the aqueduct. For us, this distinction is important because it affects the safety of lumbar puncture for diagnosis (and therapy) as well as the options for hydrocephalus treatment.

In addition other pathophysiology is as important. Vasculitis is, indisputably, the most important determinant of poor outcome. Many patients end up with diencephalic or large vessel territory infarcts (Fig. 29.1), and these remain – along with the initial presenting level of consciousness – the strongest predictors of outcome [10–14]. The typical thick, gelatinous exudate that fills the basal cisterns coats the circle of Willis and – very importantly – the small perforating arteries that arise from it, causing inflammation of the vessel walls, intraluminal thrombosis, vasospasm, and external compression (Fig. 29.2) [15, 16].

Hyponatremia is common and probably contributes to brain edema [17–19]. The challenge to management is that many patients are

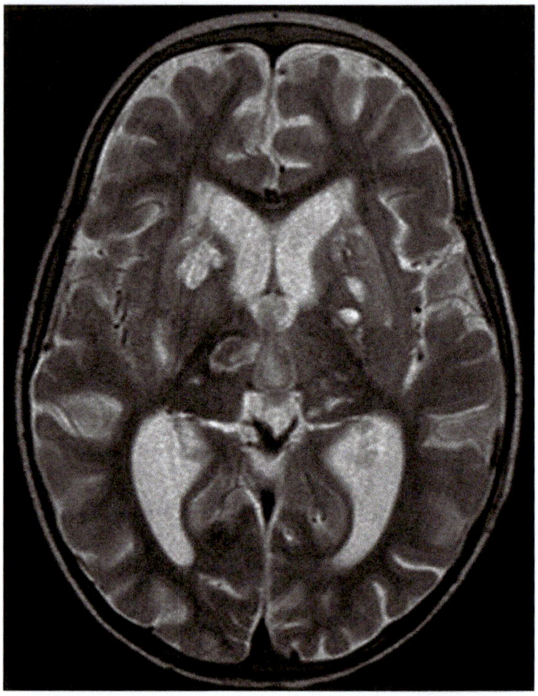

Fig. 29.1 T2-weighted MRI scan of a child with tuberculous meningitis (TBM) showing multiple bilateral infarcts in the basal ganglia and thalami

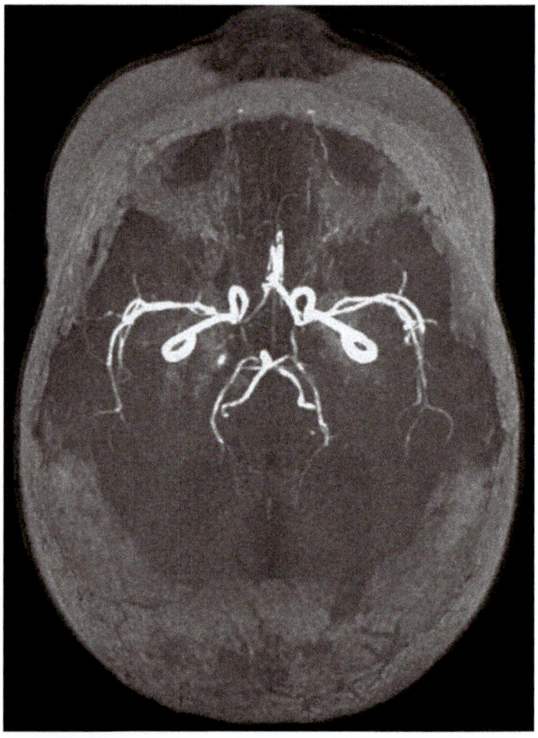

Fig. 29.2 Magnetic resonance angiogram of a child with TBM showing severe involvement of the vessels of the anterior and posterior circulation, with extensive proximal vessel disease and largely absent distal flow

mistreated because the syndrome of inappropriate antidiuretic hormone (SIADH) secretion is presumed incorrectly and fluids are restricted. This is likely a hazardous practice for several reasons: first, an accurate distinction between SIADH and cerebral salt wasting is extremely difficult to make in this clinical situation; second, patients often have a contracted intravascular volume; and third, patients who already have borderline cerebral ischemia will fare even worse if they are rendered hypovolemic through fluid restriction [7, 20].

Seizures, whether clinical or subclinical, may also aggravate brain injury by increasing metabolic demand from a brain already limited in its capacity to provide adequate glucose and oxygen [21, 22]. Spreading depolarization has not been described in TBM, but has been documented in traumatic brain injury and stroke [22], and it would seem reasonable that it occurs also in meningitis, evading our diagnostic methods, but potentially devastating nevertheless. Figure 29.3 demonstrates rhythmic patterns in cerebral dynamics unexplained by conventional monitoring.

While these are important aspects of the disease to remember when considering hydrocephalus treatment, perhaps most important of all is optimal treatment of intracranial pressure (ICP), which may not conform to our standard definitions of what threshold should be targeted. When patients already have compromised cerebral perfusion due to vasculitis, it may well be that any additional ICP may critically narrow the perfusion pressure and so end in stroke. In our experience, brain perfusion is very sensitive to changes in ICP and blood pressure (Fig. 29.4). So the need to control ICP should be clear and therefore also the need to treat hydrocephalus effectively, but the exact approach to accomplish this is not. In absence of clear evidence, centers all over the world have developed different approaches to treat TB hydrocephalus, the most important of which are discussed below.

29.2 Shunt Insertion for All Patients

Some centers uniformly treat TB hydrocephalus with shunt insertion [6, 8, 23–25], believing that selecting patients for various treatments complicates management and does not necessarily improve outcome. Moreover, medical treatment of hydrocephalus and endoscopic

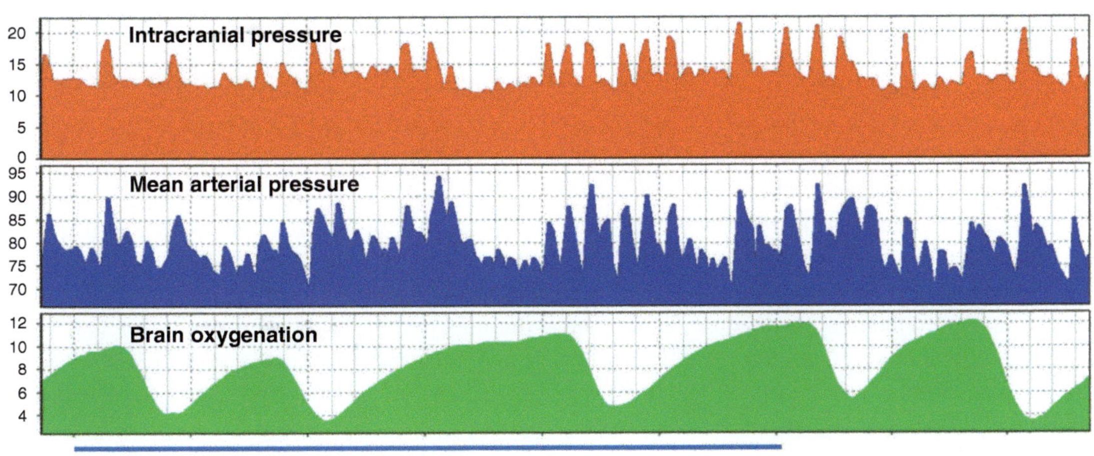

Fig. 29.3 Recorded physiological data of intracranial pressure (ICP), mean arterial pressure, and brain oxygenation (measured by brain oxygen partial pressure monitor) in a patient with TBM. All measurements are in mmHg. The patient was intubated and sedated; continuous electroencephalography did not detect any subclinical seizures. There are brief spikes of ICP and blood pressure not explained by wakefulness of the patient or external stimuli. The rhythmic changes in the brain oxygen appear to be unrelated

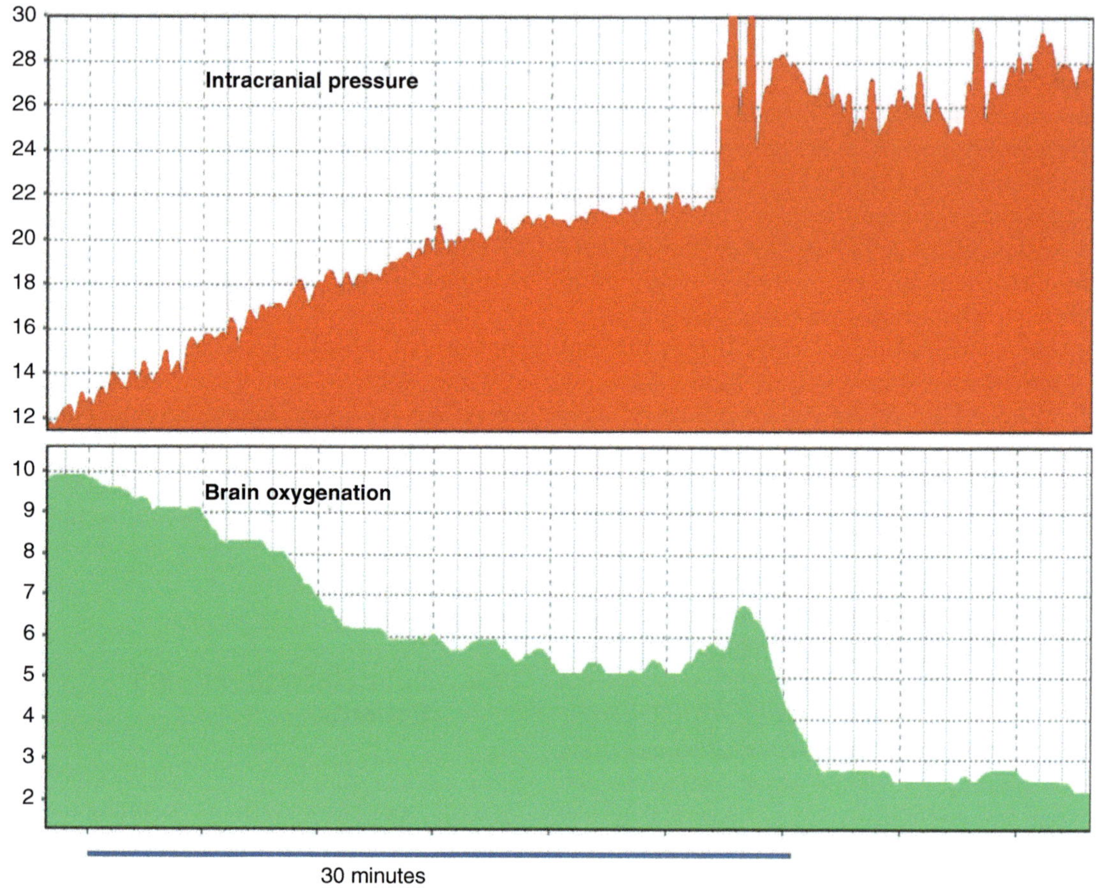

Fig. 29.4 Recording of ICP and brain oxygenation (all measurements in mmHg) demonstrating the decrease of brain oxygenation with progressive increase in ICP. Note that the brain oxygenation starts decreasing well before ICP reaches 20 mmHg. For reference, normal brain oxygen tension is greater than 20 mmHg; levels below 10 mmHg are associated with critical levels of tissue ischemia or hypoxia

third ventriculostomy (ETV) require surveillance and expertise, which may not be available in all centers [26]. While the simplicity and uniformity of this approach may be appealing, the blunt reality is that not all patients need surgery. In fact many, if not most, patients with communicating hydrocephalus can be treated adequately with medical therapy [1, 5, 27], and patients with noncommunicating hydrocephalus may respond to ETV [28, 29]. Therefore, such a nonselective approach, while simple, unnecessarily subjects many patients to lifelong shunt dependency with all the attendant complications thereof.

29.3 External Ventricular Drainage First and then Shunt

A popular approach in many centers is to use an external ventricular drain (EVD) to identify those patients who will benefit from permanent CSF drainage [6, 8, 30]. Patients who improve with temporary drainage then receive a shunt; patients who do not are treated conservatively. The upside of this approach is that shunt surgery is reserved for patients who are most likely to benefit. The downside is that such a temporary test may not select patients adequately: hydrocephalus is only one of the reasons for neurological compromise in TBM patients, and the other mechanisms of neurological compromise are not necessarily irreversible. Patients in the latter group may still improve with good resuscitation, antimicrobials, steroids, and correction of hyponatremia, all of which takes time (and good ICP control), with improvements still possible well beyond the typical EVD trial period. So with this protocol, patients who may yet benefit from hydrocephalus treatment in addition to ongoing medical management may be denied surgery.

29.4 Endoscopic Third Ventriculostomy for All Patients

Since it was first described [29], ETV has become a popular option to treat TB hydrocephalus [9, 31–34]. Indeed, some authors have proposed an ETV in all patients in the hope that some will benefit. This nonselective approach to ETV argues that even patients with communicating hydrocephalus may benefit from ETV, a view that remains highly controversial as most centers still prefer using ETV for patients with suspected noncommunicating hydrocephalus. The results of ETV for communicating hydrocephalus of infectious or post-infectious etiology, especially in young children, are unimpressive. Still, some would argue that even if there is a small chance of success, ETV is worth trying. The problem with this argument is that ETV is a surgical procedure with known complications, which are possibly increased in TBM where the procedure is complicated by the typically thickened third ventricular floor and exudate-filled prepontine cistern [26].

High success rates after ETV for unselected TBM patients have been reported but are difficult to interpret [32, 33, 35]. The resolution of hydrocephalus or lack of recourse to shunt surgery (which is often the proxy measure of success) is difficult to ascribe purely to ETV because most patients have communicating hydrocephalus, which will resolve in more than half of these patients with medical treatment alone. So, many of the patients who are described as ETV success cases may well have not needed any surgery at all.

One study randomized children with TB hydrocephalus to shunt insertion or ETV [36]. Their conclusions appear to be at odds with their results. The authors recommend that long-term outcomes "tilt in favor of ETV" even though the overall success rate was 42% (similar to our previously published results [28]) compared with 68% for shunts. In their opinion, ETV failures tend to occur early, and so there may be some benefit in reserving ETV in the late phase after starting treatment. After ETV, the ventricles were usually still large and then decreased over time. This is not unexpected with ETV, but at the same time, this happens in patients with communicating hydrocephalus who are managed successfully without resorting to any surgery. The study is therefore limited by the lack of comparison to managing communicating hydrocephalus medically. It is also limited methodologically by the small number of patients for a randomized controlled trial; the authors do not state how they calculated what sample size would be sufficient for such a trial. Regardless, it is notable that their success rate for shunt surgery was substantially superior to that of ETV. Long-term follow-up and finer neurocognitive examination would have been helpful – one of the concerns about ETV is that it produces a state of "arrested hydrocephalus" where the ICP may still be greater than normal. If a patient has TBM, with concomitant vasculitis, this would not be ideal.

29.5 Selection Based on Communicating Versus Noncommunicating Hydrocephalus, with Shunting, Endoscopy, and Medical Treatment as Options

At our center, we prefer to distinguish between communicating and noncommunicating hydrocephalus where possible, treating noncommunicating

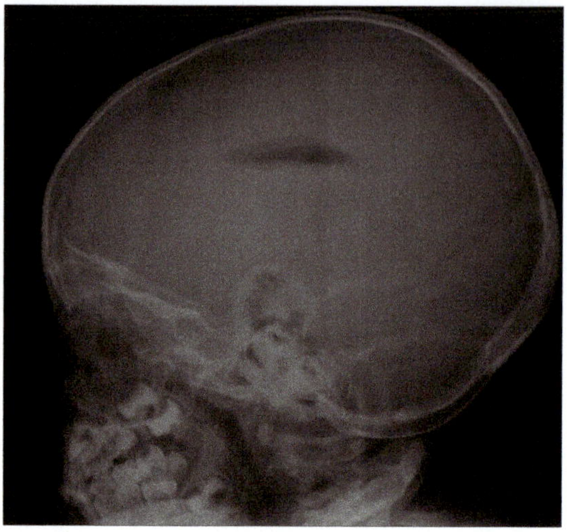

Fig. 29.5 Lateral skull radiograph after a lumbar air encephalogram. The radiograph demonstrates air in the lateral ventricles confirming communicating hydrocephalus

hydrocephalus with surgery (either shunt or ETV) and communicating hydrocephalus with a trial of medical treatment in the first instance while reserving shunt surgery for those who fail this trial [7].

Communicating versus noncommunicating hydrocephalus is determined using air encephalography and/or column testing if there is an EVD in situ, which we have previously described [29, 37]. Briefly, lumbar air encephalography relies on air introduced via a lumbar puncture to rise into the cranium. If the hydrocephalus is communicating, air enters the ventricular system (Fig. 29.5), and if noncommunicating, air enters the subarachnoid space only. Occasionally it is impossible to direct air into the cranium because of spinal subarachnoid disease. If an EVD is present, a column test may be done, in which the opening pressures are compared between the ventricular drain and a lumbar puncture at baseline (using a manometer at both ends) and then again after removal of lumbar CSF.

Most patients have communicating hydrocephalus and so are treated with a trial of medical therapy, which in addition to anti-TB medication and steroids includes the use of acetazolamide and furosemide as well as serial lumbar punctures which we perform daily if the opening pressure is raised and progressively less frequently as the opening pressure reduces [7]. Even though frequent lumbar punctures are inconvenient, experience has shown that it allows safe monitoring and reduction of ICP. Weekly lumbar punctures are an option also described [27], but this potentially allows high ICP to continue unabated for long periods. It is underappreciated how successful judicious medical treatment may be in resolving hydrocephalus (Fig. 29.6).

If a patient presents with severe hydrocephalus and a reduced level of consciousness, we prefer to first place an EVD to reduce ICP immediately and safely. Once this is controlled, we then go about trying to determine whether medical or surgical treatment is optimal. We prefer external ventricular drainage as an initial management in this case because we believe it is safer; it also enables lowering the ICP as much as possible. This may be helpful because cerebral perfusion pressure is narrowed in these patients, not only by increased ICP but also by the vasculitis that usually accompanies the disease, and so patients likely benefit from improved perfusion pressure. Our experience with brain monitoring in these patients suggests that reducing ICP even when in a "normal" range may improve perfusion to the brain, presumably because cerebral blood flow is also limited by vasculitis.

We typically allow for a 3–4-week course of medical therapy for communicating hydrocephalus, based on the work of Schoeman et al. [27]. If this fails to control ICP or if there is evidence of progressive hydrocephalus, patients undergo ventriculoperitoneal shunting. Occasionally, we will insert a shunt before the 3–4-week period has ended if it is clear that ICP remains dangerously elevated despite optimal medical therapy.

Patients with noncommunicating hydrocephalus either undergo ETV or ventriculoperitoneal shunting (Fig. 29.7), depending on whether endoscopic expertise is available at presentation. The advantage of ETV is that a noncommunicating system can be converted to a communicating system, which then can undergo medical therapy to potentially avoid the long-term risks of a shunt. The downside is that these cases are more difficult to do than other causes of hydrocephalus. In particular, the floor is markedly thickened and

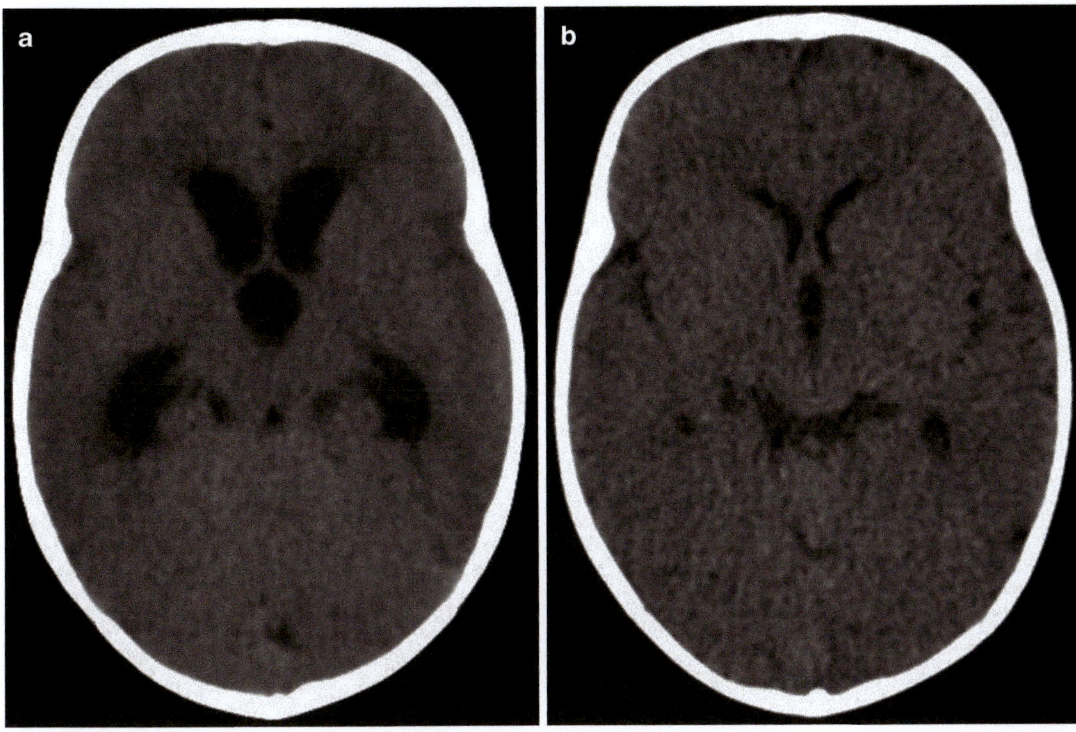

Fig. 29.6 Head CT scans of a child with TB hydrocephalus before and after medical treatment: (**a**) the scan on the *left* shows hydrocephalus at presentation, and (**b**) the scan on the *right* is of the same patient and shows complete resolution of hydrocephalus after medical treatment and control of ICP; no surgery was required

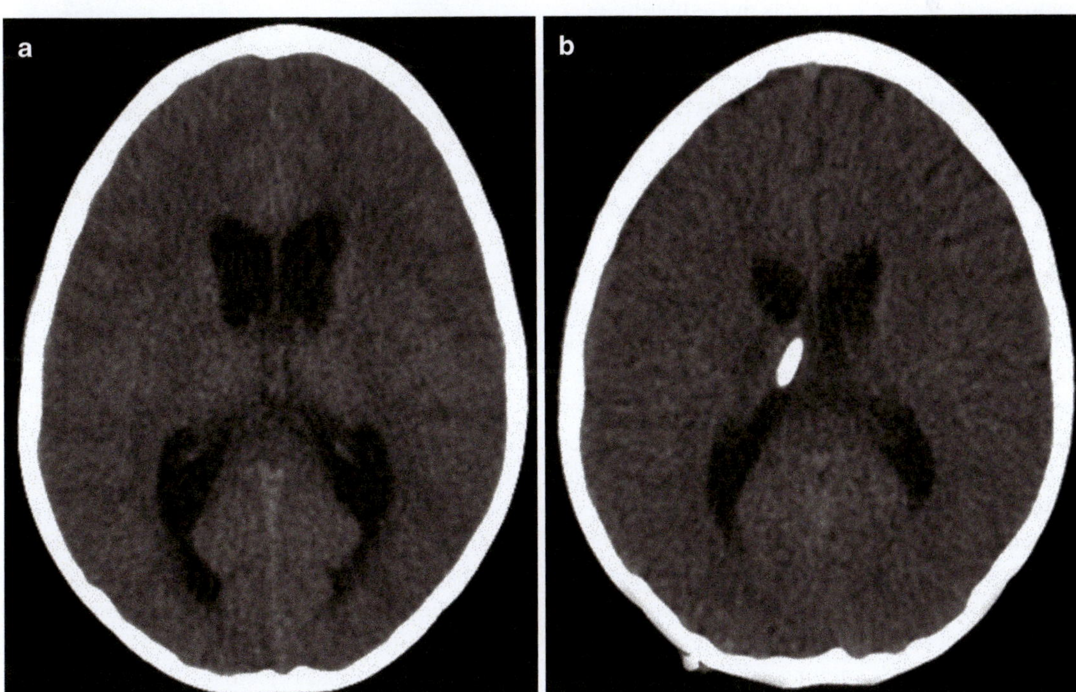

Fig. 29.7 Head CT scans showing TB hydrocephalus (**a**) at presentation, (**b**) with a ventricular shunt in situ

opaque, and the cisternal space is filled with thick gelatinous exudate so typical of TBM. The normal cisternal anatomy is obliterated, which potentially increases the risk of vascular injury and makes confirmation of ETV success challenging [38]. In this situation, a repeat air encephalogram or column test after surgery might demonstrate this newly established communication (at surgery, our bubble sign suggests the same thing – when the stoma is created in the floor of the third ventricle and air bubbles from the previous air encephalogram are encountered then cisternal entry is confirmed). By contrast, shunt insertion is less complicated, but it creates shunt dependency and places the patient at risk of all the well-known long-term complications [5, 25].

Critics of this approach may argue that it is too complicated and subjects the patient to several interventions in the early phase of the disease. Our response is that early aggressive interventions are worthwhile if it maximizes the chance of avoiding infarction and reduces the proportion of patients with lifelong shunt dependency. Where services are inadequate, these can be improved over time if there is enough willpower.

29.6 Additional Considerations

It is worth noting that lumbar subarachnoid disease is not uncommon in TBM patients and may be the reason for failed lumbar punctures and some of the typical characteristics of the CSF [12]. The protein content and viscosity of the lumbar CSF are typically increased in TBM, and in some cases for this reason, lumbar puncture fails to obtain CSF, air encephalography is impossible, and pressure measurement is compromised [12]. If this is suspected, an MRI of the spine should be obtained (Fig. 29.8).

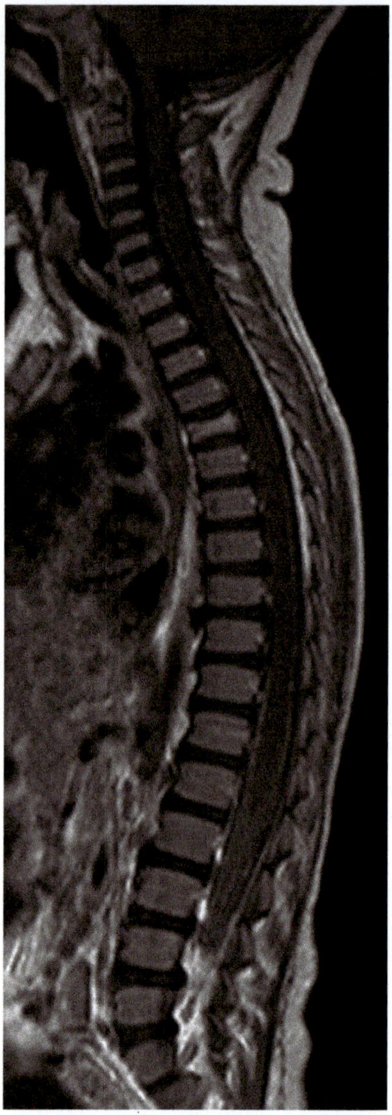

Fig. 29.8 T1-weighted sagittal MRI spine of a child with arachnoiditis of the cord and extensive exudate in the lumbar cistern, obliterating the normal CSF signal

Few studies have examined the treatment of hydrocephalus in HIV-co-infected patients [39, 40]. These are difficult patients to manage because outcomes in general are worse and nihilism often prevails among clinicians treating them. However, some patients who present in a good clinical condition at the outset may have outcomes equal to HIV-negative patients. The general consensus though is that a good outcome is unlikely in patients who present with neurological compromise, in whom shunt surgery may not be of the same benefit. These are data derived from adult studies, which are not directly applicable to children.

Finally, we must remember that hydrocephalus is only part of the treatment of these patients; several other aspects of therapy are as important

[7]. Maintaining perfusion to the brain with careful management of fluid status and correction of hyponatremia (as discussed above) is critical, especially given the high risk of infarction. CSF samples must be sent for GeneXpert and culture to confirm the diagnosis and determine sensitivity, important not only because the diagnosis is often presumptive but also because the incidence of drug resistant TB is rising. In this it should be remembered that the volume of CSF sent affects the likelihood of a positive culture (more CSF is better) [41]. Attention must be paid also to the correct anti-TB drug choice and dosages as well as administration of steroids. Correct use of acetazolamide and furosemide in communicating hydrocephalus is essential, especially because we aim to avoid hypovolemia. Standard chest X-ray and Mantoux testing are part of the routine workup, as is examination of potential contacts. All patients need long-term evaluation for neurocognitive outcomes and may well benefit from rehabilitation therapies.

Conclusion

In summary, there are many unique aspects of TB hydrocephalus and its management that set it apart from the other causes of hydrocephalus. These create a challenge to the treating clinician but also make management interesting. The lack of data informing treatment protocols is an obstacle, but at the same time also creates opportunities to bring greater scientific rigor to the way that we treat our patients. TB is an age old disease. Fortunately, we are still learning new things about it every day.

References

1. Rohlwink UK, Donald K, Gavine B, Padayachy L, Wilmshurst JM, Fieggen GA, Figaji AA (2016) Clinical characteristics and neurodevelopmental outcomes of children with tuberculous meningitis and hydrocephalus. Dev Med Child Neurol 58:461–468
2. Raut T, Garg RK, Jain A, Verma R, Singh MK, Malhotra HS, Kohli N, Parihar A (2013) Hydrocephalus in tuberculous meningitis: Incidence, its predictive factors and impact on the prognosis. J Infect 66:330–337
3. Chan KH, Cheung RT, Fong CY, Tsang KL, Mak W, Ho SL (2003) Clinical relevance of hydrocephalus as a presenting feature of tuberculous meningitis. QJM 96:643–648
4. van Well GT, Paes BF, Terwee CB, Springer P, Roord JJ, Donald PR, van Furth AM, Schoeman JF (2009) Twenty years of pediatric tuberculous meningitis: a retrospective cohort study in the Western Cape of South Africa. Pediatrics 123:e1–e8
5. Lamprecht D, Schoeman J, Donald P, Hartzenberg H (2001) Ventriculoperitoneal shunting in childhood tuberculous meningitis. Br J Neurosurg 15:119–125
6. Palur R, Rajshekhar V, Chandy MJ, Joseph T, Abraham J (1991) Shunt surgery for hydrocephalus in tuberculous meningitis: a long-term follow-up study. J Neurosurg 74:64–69
7. Figaji AA, Fieggen AG (2010) The neurosurgical and acute care management of tuberculous meningitis: evidence and current practice. Tuberculosis (Edinb) 90:393–340
8. Rajshekhar V (2009) Management of hydrocephalus in patients with tuberculous meningitis. Neurol India 57:368–374
9. Rajshekhar V (2015) Surgery for brain tuberculosis: a review. Acta Neurochir 157:1665–1678
10. Andronikou S, Wilmshurst J, Hatherill M, VanToorn R (2006) Distribution of brain infarction in children with tuberculous meningitis and correlation with outcome score at 6 months. Pediatr Radiol 36:1289–1294
11. Springer P, Swanevelder S, van Toorn R, van Rensburg AJ, Schoeman J (2009) Cerebral infarction and neurodevelopmental outcome in childhood tuberculous meningitis. Eur J Paediatr Neurol 13:343–349
12. Rohlwink UK, Kilborn T, Wieselthaler N, Banderker E, Zwane E, Figaji AA (2016) Imaging features of the brain, cerebral vessels and spine in pediatric tuberculous meningitis with associated hydrocephalus. Pediatr Infect Dis J 35(10):e301–e310 (Epub Ahead of Print)
13. Kalita J, Prasad S, Maurya PK, Kumar S, Misra UK (2012) MR angiography in tuberculous meningitis. Acta Radiol 3:324–329
14. Kalita J, Misra UK, Nair PP (2009) Predictors of stroke and its significance in the outcome of tuberculous meningitis. J Stroke Cerebrovasc Dis 18:251–258
15. Lammie GA, Hewlett RH, Schoeman JF, Donald PR (2009) Tuberculous cerebrovascular disease: a review. J Infect 59:156–166
16. Daniel PM (1949) Gross morbid anatomy of the central nervous system of cases of tuberculous meningitis treated with streptomycin. Proc R Soc Med 42:169–174
17. Cotton MF, Donald PR, Schoeman JF, Van Zyl LE, Aalbers C, Lombard CJ (1993) Raised intracranial pressure, the syndrome of inappropriate antidiuretic hormone secretion, and arginine vasopressin in tuberculous meningitis. Childs Nerv Syst 9:10–15; discussion 15–6.
18. Singh BS, Patwari AK, Deb M (1994) Serum sodium and osmolal changes in tuberculous meningitis. Indian Pediatr 31:1345–1350
19. Misra UK, Kalita J, Bhoi SK, Singh RK (2016) A study of hyponatremia in tuberculous meningitis. J Neurol Sci 367:152–157

20. Celik U, Celik T, Tolunay O, Baspinar H, Komur M, Levent F (2015) Cerebral salt wasting in tuberculous meningitis: two cases and review of the literature. Case report. Neuro Endocrinol Lett 36:306–310
21. Parkin M, Hopwood S, Jones DA, Hashemi P, Landolt H, Fabricius M, Lauritzen M, Boutelle MG, Strong AJ (2005) Dynamic changes in brain glucose and lactate in pericontusional areas of the human cerebral cortex, monitored with rapid sampling on-line microdialysis: relationship with depolarisation-like events. J Cereb Blood Flow Metab 25:402–413
22. Lauritzen M, Dreier JP, Fabricius M, Hartings JA, Graf R, Strong AJ (2011) Clinical relevance of cortical spreading depression in neurological disorders: migraine, malignant stroke, subarachnoid and intracranial hemorrhage, and traumatic brain injury. J Cereb Blood Flow Metab 31:17–35
23. Savardekar A, Chatterji D, Singhi S, Mohindra S, Gupta S, Chhabra R (2013) The role of ventriculoperitoneal shunt placement in patients of tubercular meningitis with hydrocephalus in poor neurological grade: a prospective study in the pediatric population and review of literature. Childs Nerv Syst 29:719–725
24. Peng J, Deng X, He F, Omran A, Zhang C, Yin F, Liu J (2012) Role of ventriculoperitoneal shunt surgery in grade IV tubercular meningitis with hydrocephalus. Childs Nerv Syst 28:209–215
25. Sil K, Chatterjee S (2008) Shunting in tuberculous meningitis: a neurosurgeon's nightmare. Childs Nerv Syst 24:1029–1032
26. Figaji AA, Fieggen AG (2013) Endoscopic challenges and applications in tuberculous meningitis. World Neurosurg 79:S24.e9–S24.14
27. Schoeman J, Donald P, van Zyl L, Keet M, Wait J (1991) Tuberculous hydrocephalus: Comparison of different treatments with regard to ICP, ventricular size and clinical outcome. Dev Med Child Neurol 33:396–405
28. Figaji AA, Fieggen AG, Peter JC (2007) Endoscopy for tuberculous hydrocephalus. Childs Nerv Syst 23:79–84
29. Figaji AA, Fieggen AG, Peter JC (2003) Endoscopic third ventriculostomy in tuberculous meningitis. Childs Nerv Syst 19:217–225
30. Agrawal D, Gupta A, Mehta VS (2005) Role of shunt surgery in pediatric tubercular meningitis with hydrocephalus. Indian Pediatr 42:245–250
31. Singh D, Gupta V, Goyal A, Singh H, Sinha S, Singh AK, Kumar S (2003) Endoscopic third ventriculostomy in obstructed hydrocephalus. Neurol India 51:39–42
32. Chugh A, Husain M, Gupta RK, Ojha BK, Chandra A, Rastogi M (2009) Surgical outcome of tuberculous meningitis hydrocephalus treated by endoscopic third ventriculostomy: prognostic factors and postoperative neuroimaging for functional assessment of ventriculostomy. J Neurosurg Pediatr 3:371–377
33. Husain M, Jha DK, Rastogi M, Husain N, Gupta RK (2005) Role of neuroendoscopy in the management of patients with tuberculous meningitis hydrocephalus. Neurosurg Rev 28:278–283
34. Yadav YR, Parihar V, Agrawal M, Bhatele PR (2011) Endoscopic third ventriculostomy in tubercular meningitis with hydrocephalus. Neurol India 59:855–860
35. Singh D, Sachdev V, Singh AK, Sinha S (2005) Endoscopic third ventriculostomy in post-tubercular meningitic hydrocephalus: a preliminary report. Minim Invasive Neurosurg 48:47–52
36. Goyal P, Srivastava C, Ojha BK, Singh SK, Chandra A, Garg RK, Srivastava S (2014) A randomized study of ventriculoperitoneal shunt versus endoscopic third ventriculostomy for the management of tubercular meningitis with hydrocephalus. Childs Nerv Syst 30:851–857
37. Figaji AA, Fieggen AG, Peter JC (2005) Air encephalography for hydrocephalus in the era of neuroendoscopy. Childs Nerv Syst 21:559–565
38. Figaji AA, Fieggen AG (2012) Endoscopic challenges and applications in tuberculous meningitis. World Neurosurg 79(2 Suppl):S24.e9–S24.14
39. Nadvi SS, Nathoo N, Annamalai K, van Dellen JR, Bhigjee AI (2000) Role of cerebrospinal fluid shunting for human immunodeficiency virus-positive patients with tuberculous meningitis and hydrocephalus. Neurosurgery 47:644–649
40. Sharma RM, Pruthi N, Arimappamagan A, Somanna S, Devi BI, Pandey P (2015) Tubercular meningitis with hydrocephalus with HIV co-infection: role of cerebrospinal fluid diversion procedures. J Neurosurg 122:1087–1095
41. Thwaites GE, Caws M, Chau TT, Dung NT, Campbell JI, Phu NH, Hien TT, White NJ, Farrar JJ (2004) Comparison of conventional bacteriology with nucleic acid amplification (amplified mycobacterium direct test) for diagnosis of tuberculous meningitis before and after inception of antituberculosis chemotherapy. J Clin Microbiol 42:996–1002

Role of Endoscopic Third Ventriculostomy in Tuberculous Meningitis with Hydrocephalus

30

Y.R. Yadav, Nishtha Yadav, Vijay Parihar, Shailendra Ratre, and Jitin Bajaj

Contents

Y. Yadav, MCh (✉) • V. Parihar, Mch
S. Ratre, Mch • J. Bajaj, Mch
Department of Neurosurgery, NSCB Medical College
Jabalpur, Madhya Pradesh, 482003, India
e-mail: yadavyr@yahoo.co.in; drvijayparihar@gmail.com; drsratre@gmail.com; bajaj.jitin@gmail.com

N. Yadav, MD
Department of Radiodiagnosis and imaging, All India Institute of Medical Sciences, New Delhi, India
e-mail: nishthayadav@yahoo.com

Abbreviations

CISS	Constructive interference in steady state
CSF	Cerebrospinal fluid
CT	Computed tomography
ETV	Endoscopic third ventriculostomy
EVD	External ventricular drainage
ICP	Intracranial pressure
MR	Magnetic resonance
MRI	Magnetic resonance imaging
PC	Phase contrast
PCR	Polymerase chain reaction
TBM	Tuberculous meningitis

30.1 Introduction

Tuberculous meningitis (TBM) involves infection in the lung, regional lymph nodes, and meninges or brain parenchyma. There is development of subpial or subependymal foci of lesions, called Rich foci, which rupture into the subarachnoid space or ventricle. It continues to remain great public health challenge especially in developing world. TBM remains a diagnostic dilemma. There is a need for high index of clinical suspicion and better diagnostic tests for early detection of disease. Cerebrospinal fluid (CSF) studies for detection of organism or biochemical examination

M. Turgut et al. (eds.), *Tuberculosis of the Central Nervous System*,
DOI 10.1007/978-3-319-50712-5_30

helps in diagnosis. CSF centrifugation optimizes the diagnostic performance [1]. The existence of high density within the basal cisterns in non-contrast computed tomography (CT) and basal enhancement after contrast administration is a good sign for the diagnosis of TBM [2]. Polymerase chain reaction (PCR) can be an efficient method for diagnosis of TBM [3]. Presence of tuberculoma on choroid plexus or ventricle wall, though rare, may help in diagnosis [4].

Hydrocephalus is very common in TBM [5–7]. Early diagnosis of TBM hydrocephalus should be done by early follow-up CT scan (in first 7 days of first CT scan and at 1 month on one's discretion) [8]. Hydrocephalus can be categorized as obstructive, communicating, or due to union of both varieties [9]. Effective and early treatment of hydrocephalus can improve prognosis and decrease incidence of infarct. Shunt procedures and endoscopic third ventriculostomy (ETV) are being used to manage hydrocephalus in TBM. Endoscopic techniques are increasingly used in spine [10–14], cranial [15, 16], and skull base lesions [17–20] in recent times due to the minimally invasive nature, safety, and better outcome. Endoscopic procedures are being used in various types of pathologies such as hematomas [21, 22], congenital lesions [23–25], infective pathologies [26, 27], and tumors [28–30] with encouraging results.

Although role of ETV is controversial in communicating hydrocephalus and in acute phase of disease, its role is established as an alternative to shunt procedures for obstructive hydrocephalus in TBM [31–43]. Comparatively poor results of hydrocephalus due to TBM stress the need for early diagnosis and prompt treatment. Although many factors are related to final outcome, clinical stage of disease at diagnosis and presence of hydrocephalus play an important role in prognosis.

30.2 Indications of Endoscopic Third Ventriculostomy

Although hydrocephalus in early stages of TBM with mild ventriculomegaly may resolve completely in some cases, especially of communicating variety [7], majority of them need some kind of surgery. Modified external ventricular drainage (EVD) and Ommaya reservoir implantation of about 2 weeks can avoid possible complications and long-term indwelling shunt in majority (66%) of patients in early TBM who have mild or moderate hydrocephalus [44, 45].

ETV is indicated in obstructive hydrocephalus in TBM. Although there are reports of ETV being performed in communicating hydrocephalus [35], lumbar peritoneal shunts have been found to be better option in such cases [46, 47]. Selected patients of communicating hydrocephalus with inferior bulging of third ventricle floor or anterior bulging of lamina terminalis can show improvement after ETV. This procedure of ETV not only relieves raised pressure in TBM hydrocephalus (38) but it also helps in making correct diagnosis in suspected cases by detecting tubercles on the wall of the ventricle during surgery. Endoscopy is now treated as the first choice compared to shunt surgery in TBM hydrocephalus especially in chronic stage of disease [40].

Although there was some doubts whether shunt should be done in severe form of TBM hydrocephalus, there are now reports that all patients should be treated with shunts even in poor grades [48–50]. Likewise ETV is also indicated in good as well as in poor grades in TBM as some patients in poor grades could show delayed recovery [36, 39]. Although ETV can be done in the presence of thick exudates and even in patients with prepontine suprasellar tuberculoma especially in expert hands [51], it should be avoided in the acute stage especially in untreated patients [31, 52], because of variable success [5]. ETV in subacute and chronic cases looks to be a rationale for first-line treatment [31, 34, 39, 43, 53].

EVD or Ommaya reservoir after ETV may be useful when there is evidence of doubtful functioning of stoma (poor pulsations at stoma margin, exudates in basal cistern, acute phase of TBM, evidence of intraventricular bleed, multiple shunt failure, poor flow of dye across stoma, and poor disappearance of contrast) or cisternal scarring. Intraoperative decision about shunt surgery is indicated in technically difficult case due to thick and inflamed floor with poor differentiation of anatomy, cisternal scarring, poor pulsations of stoma margin, poor flow of dye across stoma, and delayed clearance of contrast from the basal cisterns.

30.3 Preoperative Workup and Patient Selection

Patients undergoing ETV in TBM hydrocephalus should have sufficiently large lateral or third ventricles and enlarged foramen of Monro to accommodate endoscopic set; otherwise, it could cause injury to ventricle walls or the fornix. It is important to know whether third ventricle floor is thin or thick. Thin third ventricle floor patients are good candidates for ETV, surgery is comparatively simple technically, and the ETV success rate is also good in such cases. Good prepontine space and the absence of basal exudate also favor ETV. There should be sufficient space between brain stem and dorsum sellae and also between basilar artery and dorsum sellae. The distance between midline and posterior communicating artery or third cranial nerve should be known, as small distance predisposes artery or nerve injury during procedure. Presence of large interthalamic adhesions can also create difficulty during the procedure. Although one can observe the presence of any additional membrane such as Liliequist membrane or other membranes after fenestration of third ventricle floor and such membrane can be dealt appropriately intraoperatively, preoperative knowledge prepares surgeon to deal it better. Liliequist membrane if present may be attached to the third nerve, which can risk nerve injury during fenestration. Cistern status is also a critical factor in patient outcome; scarred basal cistern not only adds in the technical difficulty during surgery but also associated with poor outcome.

Patent distal subarachnoid spaces and proper CSF absorption are also necessary for good outcome after ETV. Although it is challenging to measure lumbar outflow resistance preoperatively in a patient requiring ETV, low lumbar outflow resistance suggests good CSF absorption and patent subarachnoid space. Increased outflow resistance could be due to compression of subarachnoid space secondary to dilated ventricle, obliterated subarachnoid space, and/or defective CSF absorption. Although low lumbar outflow resistance generally suggests favorable subarachnoid space, good CSF absorption, and good outcome after ETV, high resistance may not be associated with poor outcome. High resistance could also be due to compression of subarachnoid space secondary to dilated ventricles.

Complex hydrocephalus (combination of both obstructive and communicating hydrocephalus) is quite common in TBM cases [9, 39]. This is due to obliterated basal cisterns or subarachnoid space and/or defective CSF absorption. Cine phase-contrast (PC) magnetic resonance imaging (MRI) can be used for detection of any abnormality in basal cisterns. Detection of early CSF stroke volume in interpeduncular and prepontine cisterns can predict patency of basal cisterns and CSF flow through these cisterns. Good CSF flows in basal cistern alone do not give surety of successful outcome following ETV; distal CSF pathways ahead of the basal cisterns also play crucial role in ETV successfulness [54].

30.4 Surgical Procedure

TBM hydrocephalus is technically demanding to manage endoscopically as compared to other types and needs good skill and training, especially in acute cases [31, 55]. ETV procedure has been depicted elsewhere in our publication [56]. Although semi-sitting position has been described, ETV is generally operated in supine position with head flexed so that the burr hole site is at the uppermost point. Highest site of burr hole averts excessive drainage of CSF and an entrance of air in the ventricles and subdural space, especially in large ventricles. Although ETV can be done free hand without using any telescope holder, use of scope holder is helpful when procedure is prolonged and during introduction and removal of instruments. It can also give rest to the hand, which is holding the assembly. Telescope holder can be tightened or loosened when required. We used holder in a loose knob position during most of the procedure.

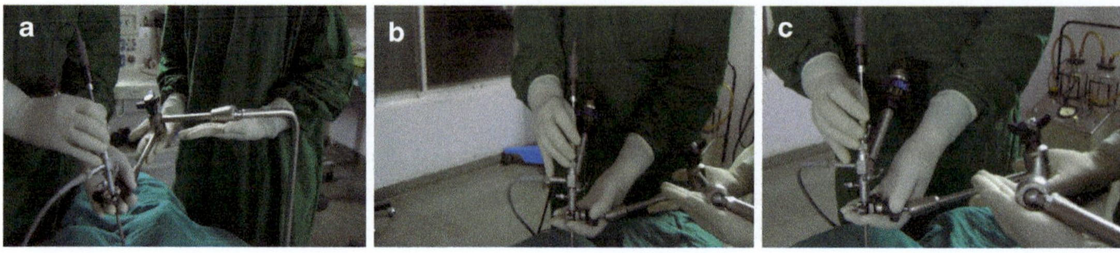

Fig. 30.1 Training lab photographs showing (**a**) assistant supporting joints of telescope holder with loosened knob, which prevents strain on surgeon's hand. It also prevents time loss in loosening or tightening. (**b**) Left hand of surgeon holding endoscope sheath while well-supported right hand being used for surgical maneuver. (**c**) Camera can be supported by body part

Assistant is supporting the holder at tightening knob area and near the joint regions to allow better control and to decrease strain on the hand of the surgeon which is holding endoscope assembly (Fig. 30.1). Excessive drainage of CSF may also precipitate for postoperative subdural hematoma formation. Lateral and third ventricle along with foramen of Monro should be sufficiently large. If there is a slit ventricle secondary to overdrainage in already shunted patient, it is necessary to externalize the shunt to adequately dilate ventricles. Stereotactic guidance along with smaller size of the scope or flexible scope can be used in such patients. Although ETV can be done by flexible scope, we use rigid scope because of better visualization.

A line spanning from interpeduncular cistern and foramen of Monro onto the cranium in preoperative MRI scan accurately determines an exact site of burr hole. Incision just in front to the coronal suture and approximately 2.5–3 cm lateral to the midline on the right side is usually adequate for ETV. Proper direction of brain penetration should be used to reach lateral ventricle at foramen of Monro. Although facility of image guidance can help, marking on the skin near the incision in the direction toward external auditory meatus before patient is draped helps when image guidance facility is not available (Fig. 30.2). Brain cannula is used to perforate ventricle, and then endoscope protected by the sheath is introduced. Peel-away sheath of slightly larger diameter than the endoscope is generally used if the scope does not have sheath. Some systems have sheaths with scope; in such cases peel-away sheath is not required. Peel-away sheath or other sheath avoids lens soiling and brain injury due to repeated scope introduction. It also helps in egress of irrigation fluid and avoids pressure built up. Lactate solution irrigation of normal body temperature implying gravity pressure as against to any pressure procedure is good which avoids any barotraumas to the brain.

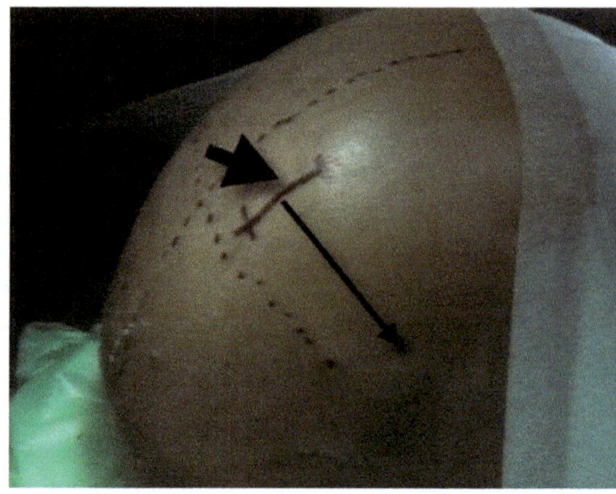

Fig. 30.2 *Thick and short arrow* pointing skin incision. Marking on the skin in the direction toward external auditory meatus (*thin and long arrow*), which guides brain penetration toward foramen of Monro

Telescope is introduced through the foramen of Monro into the third ventricle after identification of junction of thalamostriate vein, septal vein, and choroid plexus. Perforation in the third ventricle floor is made between mammillary bodies and infundibular recess, at the most translucent site. Identification of basilar artery should be done to avoid trauma and hemorrhage during the procedure. Perforation should be done anterior to the basilar artery or its branches. Trajectory in ETV in

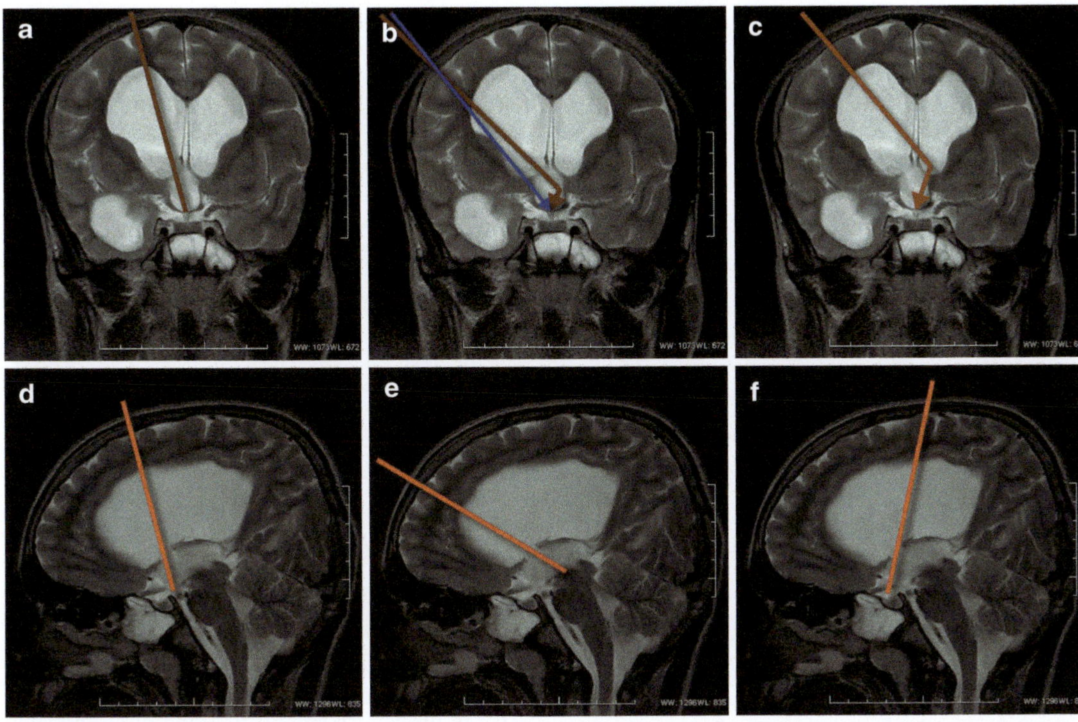

Fig. 30.3 Showing (**a**) correct trajectory in ETV in coronal plane as medial as possible to reach third ventricle floor in midline using rigid scope. (**b**) Wrong lateral trajectory and (**c**) entry through contralateral foramen of Monro risking unilateral and bilateral fornix injury, respectively. (**d**) Correct trajectory in sagittal plane to reach third ventricle floor in between mammillary bodies and infundibular recess. Wrong (**e**) anterior and (**f**) posterior trajectory risking fornix injury

sagittal and coronal plane using rigid scope should be properly planned to avoid fornix injury (Fig. 30.3). Although slow and gentle movement up to about 5 mm has been found to be safe [57], such movements generally should be desisted to avoid fornix injury. If working channel is not opposite to the desired site of interest in the floor of third ventricle, rotation of assembly in desired direction should be done (Fig. 30.4). Microvascular Doppler probe could be effective to see basilar artery and its subdivisions if these structures are not visualized endoscopically. Disciplined probing with the round equipment, if the facility of Doppler is not accessible, can identify position of dorsum sellae. Water-jet dissection approach can be utilized to avoid vascular injury or hemorrhage in thick and opaque third ventricle floor [32, 58]. Fenestration in thin third ventricle floor is just behind the dorsum sellae, and in front of basilar artery while in thick floor, it should be made partly on dorsum sellae and partly just posterior to dorsum sellae. Perforation on the bony part in thick floor prevents stretch of third ventricle wall and related complications. Such stretch in already bulging third ventricle wall can cause third cranial nerve injury apart from bleeding from distant site. Blunt instruments should be used preferably to fenestrate third ventricle floor to prevent vascular injury. Although we do not prefer thermal coagulation especially in thin floor, initial use of low bipolar current helps in making fenestration in thick floor and also to avoid excessive stretch on floor. Original perforation is enlarged to about 5 mm or more size by utilizing Fogarty catheter or ventriculostomy forceps. Liliequist membrane or other membrane can be found in some cases, lying below the third ventricle floor. Such membrane should be perforated under endoscopic control. Septum pellucidum perforation along with ETV could be technically difficult as the proper

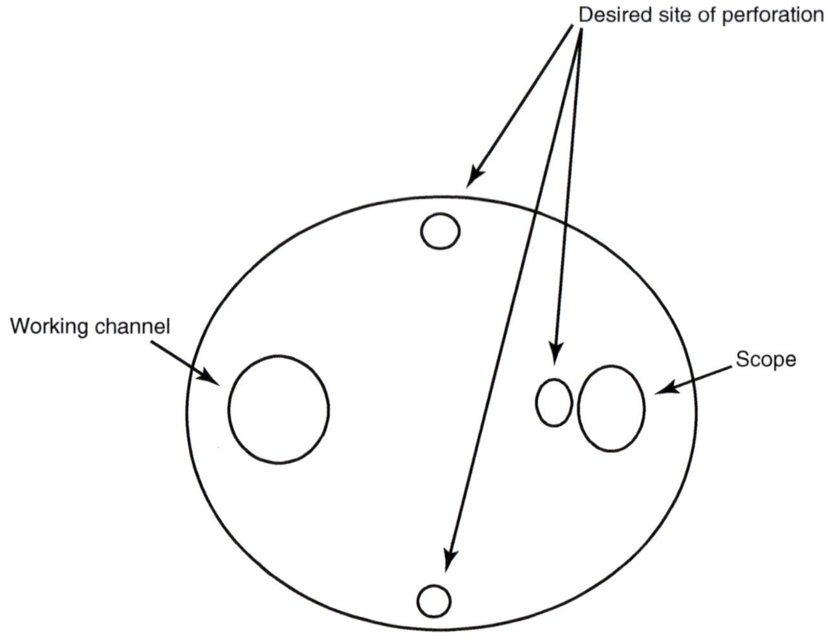

Fig. 30.4 Line diagram showing that if working channel is not opposite to the desired site of perforation in third ventricle floor, clockwise or counterclockwise rotation of assembly in desired direction should be done rather than linear movement to prevent fornix injury

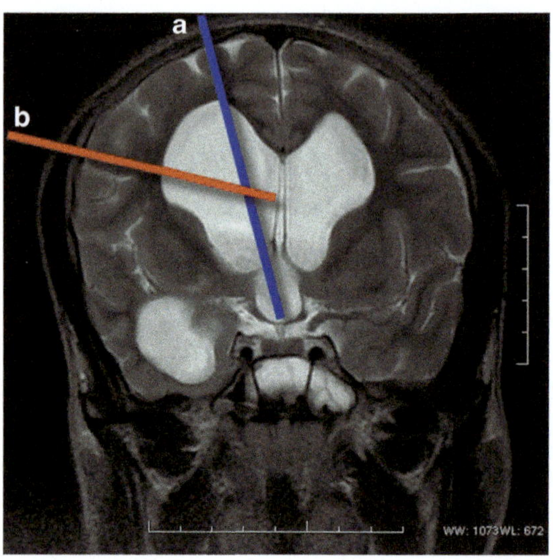

Fig. 30.5 Showing proper trajectory for (**a**) ETV and (**b**) septum perforation is different in coronal plane. It is technically difficult to do both procedures using single trajectory

trajectory for ETV and septum perforation is different in coronal plane (Fig. 30.5). Using gentle bipolar coagulation and grasping forceps with one limb side opening can make ETV and septum perforation possible by single trajectory (Fig. 30.6). All the procedure should be done under constant visualization; if any part of the instrument is not seen, it is either due to very high magnification, scope too close to target area, or when scope and the two limbs of instrument are in straight line. Decreasing magnification, slight withdrawal of scope away from target area, and rotation of instrument in such a way that the scope and the two limbs of instrument make triangular orientation allow proper visualization (Fig. 30.7).

Good pulsations of stoma margin are a good indicator of stoma opening and cisternal status. If there is any doubt about the patency of stoma or basal cisterns after ETV during surgery, an intraoperative evaluation by ventriculo-stomography can provide valuable information [59]. Contrast flow through the stoma and its disappearance from subarachnoid spaces can be observed. Fast disappearance of contrast is a good indicator of stoma and cisternal patency. This simple and effective method can help in verifying the competency of endoscopic approach, thereby helping in taking decision about further management during surgery, such as requirement for shunt if there is slow disappearance of contrast [59, 60].

ETV is likely to be effective if there is favorable anatomy of third ventricle floor, good pulsations of

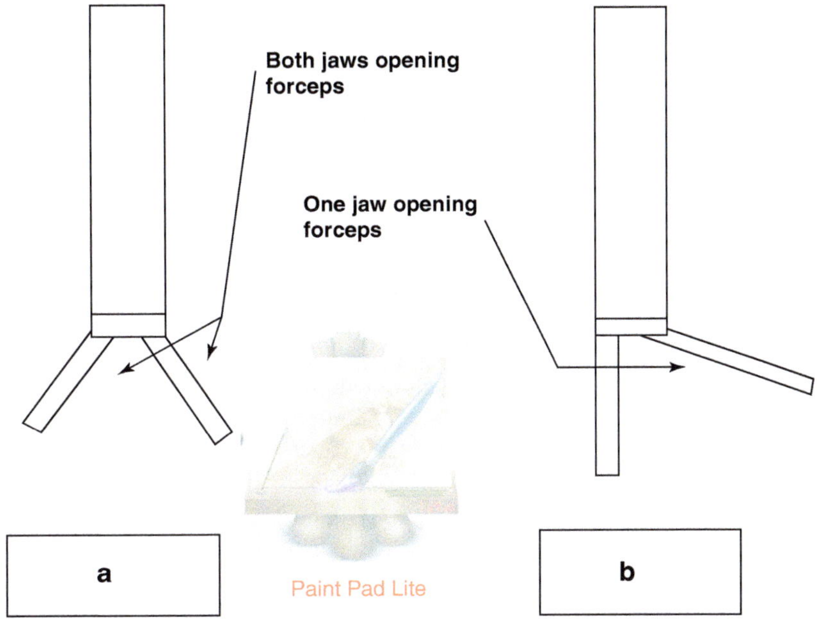

Fig. 30.6 There are generally two types of forceps: (**a**) both limbs opening and (**b**) single limb opening. Technical difficulty using single trajectory for ETV and septum perforation can be overcome by (**b**) one limb side opening forceps, which helps in septum perforation

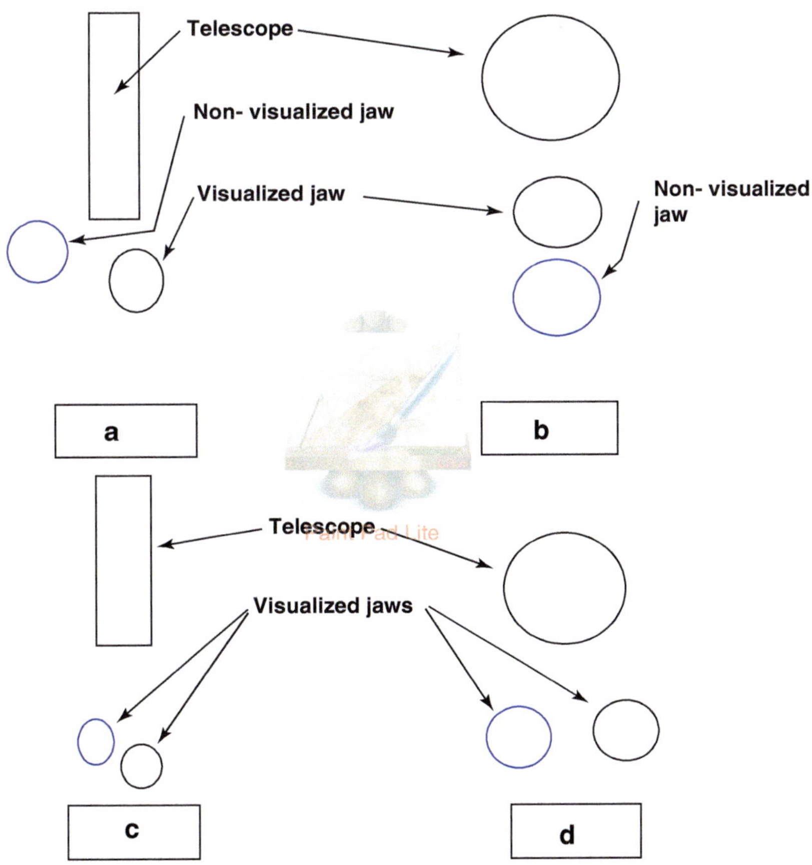

Fig. 30.7 Nonvisualization of instrument is due to very high magnification, (**a**) scope too close to target area, or (**b**) when scope and the two limbs of instrument are in straight line. Decreasing magnification, (**c**) slight withdrawal of scope away from target area, and (**d**) rotation of instrument in such a way that the scope and the two limbs of instrument make triangular orientation allow proper visualization

stoma margins, and good basal cistern without any exudates or scarring. If there is any doubt about stoma or cisternal patency due to not so good stoma pulsations or slow disappearance of dye during intraoperative period, EVD or Ommaya reservoir can be kept which can be used to assess stoma patency in postoperative period. An EVD is also left if there is any small bleeding during procedure. Although some researchers practice use of reservoir routinely, it is useful in certain high-risk patients [61–63] for ETV failure with poor stoma pulsations, patients with repeated shunt malfunctions, cisternal scarring, and acute phase of disease if one opt for ETV. Intraoperative decision of shunt placement can be taken if there is unfavorable third ventricle floor anatomy increasing risk of ETV, other technical difficulties due to thick floor, abnormally enlarged interthalamic adhesions, inflamed floor, poor stoma pulsations, prolonged hold of dye in cistern, etc. (Fig. 30.8).

Choroid plexus coagulation can improve success rate of ETV especially in infants. Any hemorrhage from cortical surface should be stopped by electrocautery. If there is any bleeding from perforation margin, instrument used for fenestration (Fogarty catheter or ventriculostomy forceps) should be used for tamponade effect. It is not desirable to remove that instrument and bring cautery to stop that bleeding point (by the time cautery forceps is brought near the point, visualization of bleeding point may become difficult). Intermittent closure of outflow channel could help in visualization of bleeding point.

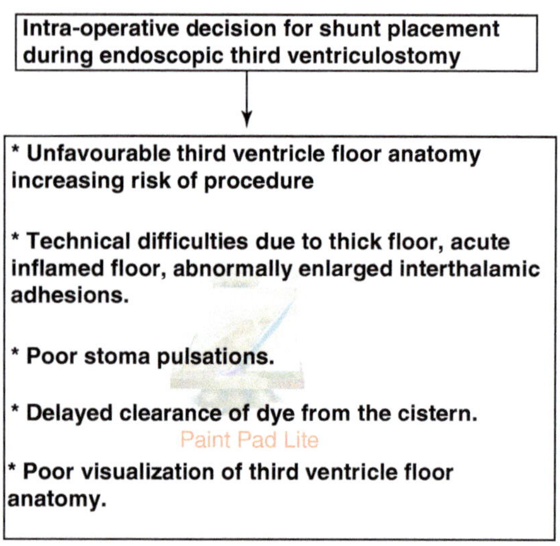

Fig. 30.8 Intraoperative decision of shunt placement can be taken if there is unfavorable third ventricle floor anatomy increasing risk of ETV, other technical difficulties due to thick floor, abnormally enlarged interthalamic adhesions, inflamed floor, poor stoma pulsations, prolonged hold of dye in cistern, poor visualization of third ventricle floor, etc.

ETV after slit ventricle syndrome in TBM hydrocephalus could be challenging. It is difficult to hit small ventricle; the use of small flexible scope, stereotactic guidance using small scope, dilatation of ventricle by exteriorization, and blockage of shunt tube can be used to help ETV procedure. Endoscopic lamina terminalis fenestration as an alternative site of perforation has been described for treatment of hydrocephalus in TBM when the usual site in third ventricle floor is not favorable for perforation [64]. Endoscopic subfrontal approach to the lamina terminalis fenestration has also been described in cadavers by Spena et al. [65].

30.4.1 Results of ETV

Overall, clinical improvement after ETV alone ranges from 58% to 80% in various series [34, 36, 39, 40, 66]. We reported 58% improvement after ETV alone that improved to 80% when lumbar peritoneal shunt was added [39]. Outcome after ETV is superior in without cisternal exudate patients compared to those with exudates [34, 39]. Good nutritional status patients generally have better outcome compared to poor nutritional status patients [39]. ETV is reasonably effective and safe in full-term normal birth weight infants as compared to low birth weight premature infants [39]. Thin and identifiable third ventricle floor patients have better outcome after ETV as compared to thick and opaque floor (Fig. 30.9) [39, 67]. Although age did not make any difference in clinical outcome in most studies [33, 68], adult patients could fair slightly well compared to children [39]. Outcome is superior in better grade compared to patients in poor grade [34, 39].

Majority of patients show early improvement [36, 39]; delayed improvement is also observed. Patients in superior grades generally improve early as compared to poor grade who show delayed

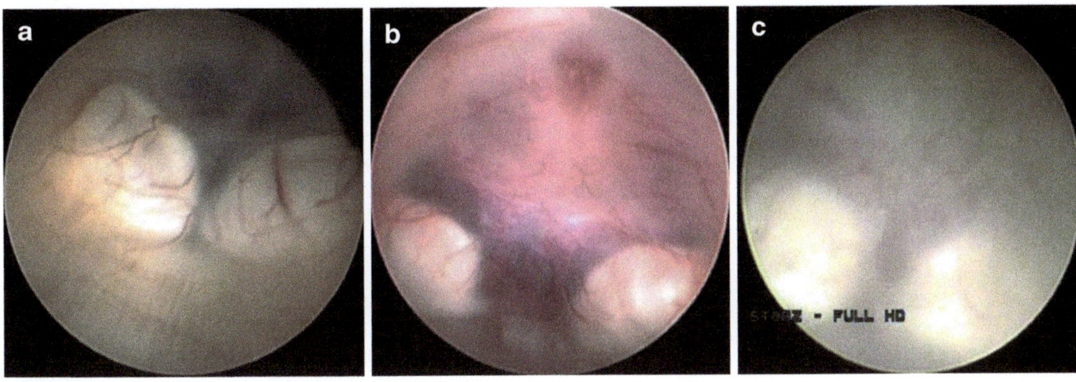

Fig. 30.9 Third ventricle floor can be (**a**) thin (usually in subacute and chronic phase) or (**b**, **c**) thick variety (generally in acute phase or following hemorrhage)

recovery [39]. Outcome after ETV in the chronic phase is superior compared to acute phase [39, 69]. Poor results in acute phase is due to higher incidence of complex hydrocephalus compared to chronic stage [39] which is among significant factor as causes of failure to improve after ETV.

Outcome of ETV in TBM hydrocephalus is poor compared to aqueductal stenosis secondary to congenital cause. The comparatively poor outcome after ETV in TBM compared to aqueductal stenosis is secondary to high prevalence of complex hydrocephalus [9, 39]. The obliteration of CSF pathways and defective absorption of CSF from arachnoid villi can result in persistently elevated intracranial pressure (ICP) in TBM after ETV. Faulty absorption and/or obliteration of CSF pathways in complex hydrocephalus can be temporary or permanent [9]. Most of the patients have temporary defect of absorption, and these patients can be managed by repeated lumbar puncture after ETV before labeling them as failed ETV patients [39, 70]. Repeated lumbar puncture supports by augmenting compliance, improving buffering capacities of the spinal subarachnoid spaces, and decreasing the CSF outflow resistance from the ventricular system. It also promotes reduction in the ventricular volume and allows accelerated permeation of CSF in the intracranial subarachnoid spaces. The chances of complex hydrocephalus in acute phase of disease are more as compared to chronic phase [39]. It is therefore better to do shunt surgery and avoid ETV in acute phase of the disease [31].

The advanced age, neurological status at admission, vaccine status, ischemia, etc. determine prognosis [71]. BCG vaccination might be protective from advance disease as most patients who were vaccinated were seen in early stage of TBM disease [72].

30.4.2 Radiological Outcome

The size of ventricle does not reduce in 3 weeks in about 50% individuals [39]. There may not be any interrelationship between clinical and radiological recovery. Clinical recovery is earlier than the radiological recovery in most patients. In some individuals there may be clinical recovery without any radiological recovery. On the other hand, there may be radiological recovery without any clinical recovery, in few patients, mainly due to associated ischemic infarcts.

30.4.3 Causes of Failure to Improve After ETV and Its Management

There can be many causes of failure to improve after ETV such as block stoma, ischemia, complex hydrocephalus, advanced age, poor neurological status at the time of surgery, etc. (Fig. 30.10). Deterioration after ETV does not always imply that the ETV is not working. Stoma patency does not always suggest that the ETV is efficient

Fig. 30.10 Flow diagram showing various causes of failure to improve after ETV in TBM hydrocephalus and their management

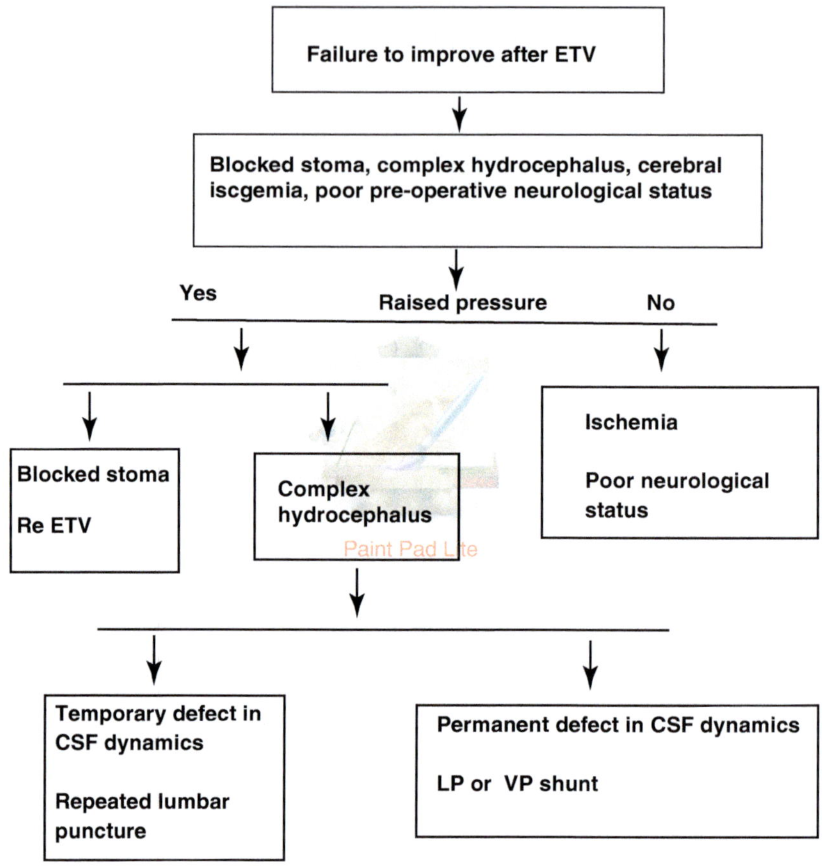

in decreasing ICP. Complex hydrocephalus is one of the significant causes of failure to improve after surgery. Complex hydrocephalus could be due to temporary or permanent defect in the CSF dynamics. Repeated lumbar puncture can manage temporary defect in CSF dynamic abnormality, while lumbar peritoneal shunt could be required when there is a persistently raised ICP even after repeated lumbar puncture. One should be very careful in selecting lumbar peritoneal shunt surgery in TB as there may be associated TB compression at various levels in the spine [73–78]. Repeat ETV is required to treat blocked stoma.

30.4.4 Complications and Its Avoidance

Although endoscopic techniques are having many advantages, procedure could be associated with many limitations. Such complications should be anticipated to improve results [79, 80]. Although ETV procedure is fairly simple, learning curve of the procedure can be improved by microsurgical skills training, practice on cadaver or models, watching expert surgeons, and visiting other departments [81].

ETV technique could be associated with various complications such as hypothermia or disturbance in temperature regulation, intraventricular bleeding, pneumocephalus, bradycardia, fornix injury, hypothalamic injury, cranial nerve injury, failed ETV, endoscopic blind spot, delayed awakening, block stoma, subdural hematoma, intracerebral hemorrhage, CSF leak, chronic subdural hematoma or subdural hygroma, etc. Although rare, mortalities due to fatal hemorrhage have been reported. Details of these complications are described in Table 30.1 and in our earlier publications [79, 80].

Table 30.1 Various complications, avoidance of complications, and its management in endoscopic third ventriculostomy

Complications with their etiologies	Complication avoidance and management
Hypothermia or disturbance in temperature regulation: Small children Exchanges of large amount of irrigation fluid with ventricular cerebrospinal fluid (CSF) Wetting of drapes Hypothalamic injury Use of electrocautery for fenestration of third ventricle floor	Pre-warmed irrigation fluid and blankets Use small amount of irrigation fluid especially in infants Avoid drape wetting by using drainage line connected to outflow channel Midline perforation in third ventricle floor Electrical energy should be avoided
Intraventricular bleeding: Blood might dribble from the burr hole site into lateral ventricle Increased risk in postinfection and hemorrhage patients Excessive and jerky side movements in ventricle Flexible scope removed in curved tip position After incomplete removal or biopsy of intraventricular lesion Wrong entry (too far away from foramen of Monro: anterior or posterior) in the lateral ventricle and then surgeon trying to enter third ventricle by moving the scope Injury to intraventricular bands Repeated insertion of scope without the use of sheath Direct ventricular access by the telescope Use of sharp-edged sheath Injury to interthalamic adhesion	Achieve good hemostasis before penetrating the ventricle and by keeping patties around the sheath Water-jet dissection in opaque and thick floor of third ventricle Removal of flexible scope in a neutral position Peel-away sheath or other sheath should be used to maintain tract to avoid surrounding brain injury if repeated introduction of telescope is required Avoid sharp-edged sheaths Use proper trajectory for lateral ventricle toward external auditory meatus, reenter at a correct site if there is the wrong entry rather than too much movements to enter foramen of Monro Avoid stretching of the floor of third ventricle during perforation, by using initial sharp perforation or electrocautery, in tough third ventricle floor. Hemorrhage from distant vessel could be caused by stretching Hemorrhage and injury to the fornix can be prevented by avoiding significant side movement Proper inspection of underlying vessels before perforation or dilatation can avoid injury to vessels Avoid injury to any vessel during dilatation of stoma when closed ventriculostomy forceps is opened or inflated Fogarty is pulled in third ventricle. Retracting forceps should be partially withdrawn into the third ventricle before it is fully opened. Penetration in floor should be anterior to basilar artery and in midline Using blunt probe for perforation of thin floor Although direct penetration by scope tip should be abstained, angled part of scope should be facing posteriorly to push basilar artery if angled endoscope is used for perforation Use lactated Ringer irrigation for small bleeding It is detrimental to remove ventriculostomy forceps or catheter and to bring bipolar forceps for coagulation, as there is usually a no clear vision by the time the electrocautery forceps is brought in the field Gently keep the same equipment or reinflate catheter on the site of bleeding. Electrocauterization may be undertaken later on if the tamponade effect fails Better visualization of the bleeding point could be helped by intermittent closure of the outflow channel or by forceful irrigation

(continued)

Table 30.1 (continued)

Complications with their etiologies	Complication avoidance and management
	Scope should be kept in the field in severe bleeding, rather than taking it out. Telescope should be positioned in lateral ventricle rather than in third ventricle as even slight movement in the small cavity could produce more hemorrhage. Scope can be withdrawn, but the sheath should be kept in place Remove intraventricular blood before taking out the endoscope assembly Put ventricular drain in residual oozing Liquid can be carefully replaced by equal amount of air, and then bleeding point should be coagulated Rapid conversion to open surgery when hemorrhage is not controlled by any of these procedure
Pneumocephalus: More losing of CSF Wrong burr hole site (not on uppermost point) Nitrous oxide anesthesia	Burr hole at the uppermost site Small dural and brain opening Flushing out air from the irrigation tube, filling the burr hole site with liquid Minimize CSF loss Avoid nitrous oxide
Bradycardia: Raised intracranial pressure (ICP) such as forceful and rapid rate irrigation, blocked outflow channel, and both foramina of Monro are blocked by the scope Too cold fluid irrigation of different osmolarity as compared to plasma Pressure on the hypothalamus by balloon Saline irrigation Stretch on wall of third ventricle	Make sure that outflow is patent and the liquid is flowing out Volume of the cardiac monitor should be turned up, and the noise of the operating room should be low for detection of bradycardia Last action should be reversed when there is bradycardia or asystole Isotonic solution should be used at body temperature Sharp penetration when there is tough floor of third ventricle and initiation of hole in third ventricle by gentle bipolar coagulation Slow and judicious irrigation at a rate of 10 ml/min Avoid pressure by catheter on hypothalamus
Fornix injury: Small size of foramen of Monro Burr hole which is placed anteriorly, posteriorly, or laterally Entrance in contralateral lateral ventricle could injure both fornix Removal of flexible telescope in curved tip position Avoiding direct ventricular tap which extends more than 5–6 cm from the burr hole site Large diameter sheath Misdirected entry in ventricle	Burr hole at proper site Avoid substantial side movements Proper case selection with enlarge foramen of Monro Use of small dimension of scope Increasing size of the foramen of Monro by hydrodissection and decreasing size of the choroid plexus Keep scope tip near the foramen of Monro within lateral ventricle for making an opening in third ventricular floor when foramen is small Flexible scope should be removed in the neutral position Avoiding shifting in third ventricle; rotation can be done to reach targeted object Rotations or slight movement if needed can be done in the lateral ventricle (larger cavity) rather than the third ventricle
Hypothalamic injury: Off midline perforation Wrong site burr hole too lateral, anterior, or posterior compared to correct place Thick third ventricle floor Third ventricle perforation using blunt technique in the thick floor	Midline perforation Correct site of burr hole placement In cases with thick and tough floor, start perforation by either gentle bipolar coagulation or with sharp instrument

Table 30.1 (continued)

Complications with their etiologies	Complication avoidance and management
Cranial nerve injury: Injury to oculomotor and abducens nerve can occur in downward bulging floor and also when penetration is made away from midline. Injuries to nerve can be produced by forcefully shifting an already downward stretched floor Blind introduction of penetrating equipment far below the floor Liliequist membrane attached to third nerve Anomalous anatomy of the third cranial nerve near midline	Position burr hole as medially as possible Midline perforations in third ventricle floor Avoid downward shifting of already stretched floor of third ventricle, by usage of sharp equipment or by making initial perforation with the help of bipolar forceps Opening can be made on the dorsum sellae in thick and tough floor instead of posterior to dorsum Anticipate abnormal anatomy and take corrective steps
Failed ETV: Little space between dorsum sellae and basilar artery Small prepontine space None or poor visualization of third ventricle floor Scarred cistern below floor Upward herniation of the basilar artery and its branch in floor of the ventricle Space-occupying lesion or crowding of posterior fossa structures Large interthalamic adhesion, small foramen of Monro, and a thick third ventricle floor	Proper case selection with sufficient space between dorsum sellae or basilar artery and brain stem Simple selection of case especially in initial learning curve
Endoscopic blind spot: Endoscope can injure structures proximal to its tip (fornix, brain parenchyma, interthalamic adhesion, etc.) when movement is made in third ventricle	Surgeon should train himself to withdraw scope and change direction only under direct visual control Movement of scope in the third ventricle should be avoided; rotation of whole instrument in desired direction can purchase some distance
Delayed awakening: Elevated ICP Anesthesia drugs with prolonged duration of action Hypothermia	Easily titratable short-acting general anesthesia drugs should be elected over long-acting drugs as the surgery may end suddenly Factors causing elevated cranial pressure and hypothermia should be prevented
Block stoma: Inadequate stoma size of less than 5 mm Presence of unappreciated secondary membranes Intraventricular blood Tumor progression toward stoma Postinfective or posthemorrhagic hydrocephalus especially in acute phase	Comparatively larger stoma opening of more than 5 mm Perforation of second membrane present under the third ventricle floor Avoiding ventriculostomy in postinfective and posthemorrhagic lesions and when tumor is present near expected stoma opening Removal of intraventricular bleed
Subdural hematoma: Quick drainage of large amount of CSF Separation of the brain from the dura mater during ventricular access especially when scope is introduced directly without the help of brain cannula Dural or extradural hemorrhage can flow in the subdural space	Avoid faster drainage of large amount of CSF. Replacement of drained fluid by lactated Ringer solution Placing patties by the side of sheath, especially in thin cortical mantle. This also prevents blood entering in subdural space. Controlling all points of bleeding before opening of dura mater Removal or ligation of functioning shunt after ETV Separation of the brain from dura should be prevented by making adequate size of cortical incision and by use of brain cannula for ventricular tap
Intracerebral hemorrhage: Direct puncturing of ventricle by endoscope Overdrainage of ventricular CSF	Use of brain cannula for ventricle puncture rather than direct use of scope Amount of CSF drained should be reduced, packing of the cortical edges, and replenishment of the ventricle Coagulation of bleeding vessel in the tract

(continued)

Table 30.1 (continued)

Complications with their etiologies	Complication avoidance and management
CSF leak: Raised ICP (blocked stoma or complex hydrocephalus) Larger cortical or dural opening, small cortical mantle	Proper management of raised ICP (repeated ventricular tap or lumbar puncture or shunt) Packing of the cortical margin and small dural opening Delayed suture removal Repair of dura in large ventriculomegaly in infants Galeal-pericranial flap
Subdural hygroma: Raised ICP secondary to blocked stoma, due to defective absorption of CSF or faulty permeation Need for Ommaya reservoir after ventriculostomy	Plugging of the cortical margin of ETV trajectory Majority of subdural collections disappear slowly; persistence of collections generally suggest raised pressure secondary to complex hydrocephalus or blockage of stoma Treat cause of raised ICP in persistent collection
Chronic subdural hematoma: Due to overdrained ventricle	Avoid ventricle collapse and expand it before removing the sheath especially in large ventriculomegaly

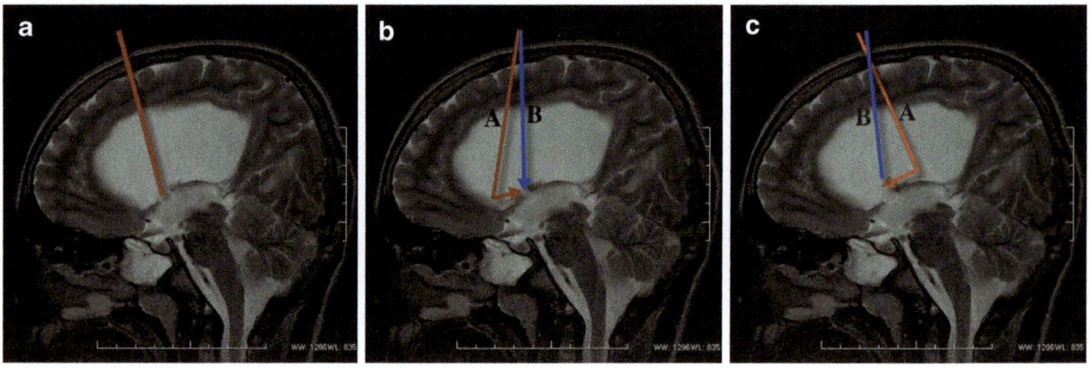

Fig. 30.11 Showing (**a**) proper, (**b**) wrong anterior, and (c) wrong posterior direction of brain penetration to reach foramen of Monro. Brain injury and bleeding from brain parenchyma or ependymal margin can occur if direction of trajectory is not proper and surgeon tries to move from A position of wrong trajectory to B position to reach foramen of Monro

Fornix injury is an important complication in ETV, which should be prevented (Figs. 30.2 and 30.3). Brain injury and bleeding from brain parenchyma or ependymal margin can occur if direction of trajectory toward foramen of Monro is not proper and surgeon tries to enter foramen of Monro by moving the scope (Fig. 30.11). Stroke occurs in about 45% of individuals in TBM both in early and later stage, mainly in the region of basal ganglia. Risk of infarct is high when there is hydrocephalus in TBM [6]. Infarcts are considered to be associated with the involvement of medial striate, thalamotuberal, and thalamostriate arteries that are present in exudates, which are prone to be strained by a coexisting hydrocephalus [82]. Infarct predicts poor outcome at 3 months [83]. Brain ischemia in TBM hydrocephalus is due to vasculitis and raised pressure secondary to hydrocephalus. Ideal management of raised ICP is necessary for improved outcome rather than simply preventing maximum increase in pressure [42].

30.5 Postoperative Imaging and Diagnosis of Stoma Patency

Majority of patients who improve after surgery do not need any investigation. Failure to improve after this surgical procedure can be secondary to the raised ICP (stoma blockage or complex hydrocephalus), vascular compromise, and poor preoperative neurological status. The raised ICP in the early postoperative period could be related to complex hydrocephalus, which could be temporary or permanent.

Decrease in the size of the ventricular edema, decrease of periventricular edema, and widening of subarachnoid space after ETV are indirect evidences of stoma patency. These responses continue during the initial few months after ETV. The decrease in size is more marked in acute stage of hydrocephalus and in third ventricle width compared to lateral ventricle width. CSF flow as the flow-void sign could be qualitatively described. This is not very sensitive, as a flow-void sign has been seen in up to 50% of clinical failures. Cine PC MRI could be helpful even in no flow-void situation. This cine PC magnetic resonance (MR) may be helpful in determining the stoma patency and could be of value in follow-up [84]. Three-dimensional constructive interference in steady state (CISS) MR technique has been found to be sensitive to flow [85, 86]. MR ventriculography is useful in determining stoma patency after third ventriculostomy [35]. Ventriculography is helpful in providing accurate assessment of the stoma patency in the early days after surgery if EVD or Ommaya was kept during ETV. It also allows intermittent CSF drainage to relieve raised ICP.

Conclusion

The choice about the best management should be decided by many factors such as surgeon's expertise, stage and duration of disease, communicating or noncommunicating hydrocephalus, availability of resources for endoscopy, etc. Although most of the patients with hydrocephalus need surgical treatment, small-group patients in early and acute stage with mild hydrocephalus in neurologically intact and in fully conscious state can be observed with early repeat CT scans. Ventriculoperitoneal shunt is a better option in acute phase of TBM hydrocephalus in obstructive hydrocephalus, while ETV is an effective alternative in obstructed hydrocephalus in subacute or chronic phase (Fig. 30.12). Results of lumbar peritoneal shunt are better in communicating hydrocephalus.

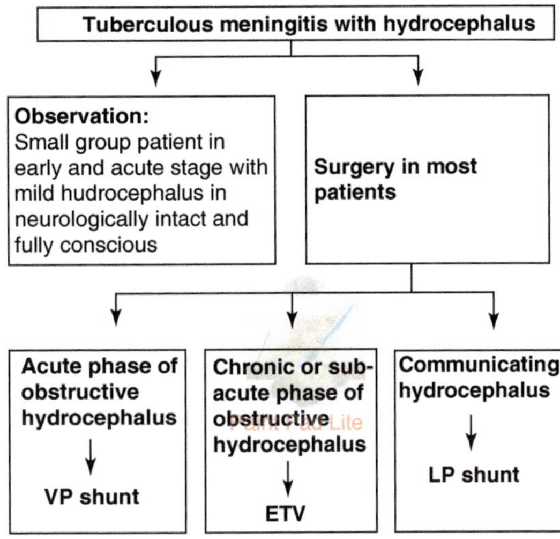

Fig. 30.12 Flowchart showing our recommendations in management of hydrocephalus in TBM

References

1. Bahr NC, Tugume L, Rajasingham R, Kiggundu R, Williams DA, Morawski B, Alland D, Meya DB, Rhein J, Boulware DR (2015) Improved diagnostic sensitivity for tuberculous meningitis with Xpert(®) MTB/RIF of centrifuged CSF. Int J Tuberc Lung Dis 19:1209–1215
2. Andronikou S, Smith B, Hatherhill M, Douis H, Wilmshurst J (2004) Definitive neuroradiological diagnostic features of tuberculous meningitis in children. Pediatr Radiol 34:876–885
3. Nagdev KJ, Bhagchandani SP, Bhullar SS, Kapgate RC, Kashyap RS, Chandak NH, Daginawala HF, Purohit HJ, Taori GM (2015) Rapid diagnosis and simultaneous identification of tuberculous and bacterial meningitis by a newly developed duplex polymerase chain reaction. Indian J Microbiol 55:213–218
4. Bhattacharyya A, Boruah DK, Handique A, Singh V, Kalita J, Misra UK, Vishnu Phadke RV (2010) Involvement of the choroid plexus in neurotuberculosis: MR findings in six cases. Neuroradiol J 23:590–595
5. Rajshekhar V (2009) Management of hydrocephalus in patients with tuberculous meningitis. Neurol India 57:368–374
6. Chan KH, Cheung RT, Fong CY, Tsang KL, Mak W, Ho SL (2003) Clinical relevance of hydrocephalus as a presenting feature of tuberculous meningitis. QJM 96:643–648
7. Raut T, Garg RK, Jain A, Verma R, Singh MK, Malhotra HS, Kohli N, Parihar A (2013) Hydrocephalus in tuberculous meningitis: incidence, its predictive factors and impact on the prognosis. J Infect 66:330–337
8. Andronikou S, Wieselthaler N, Smith B, Douis H, Fieggen AG, van Toorn R, Wilmshurst J (2005) Value

of early follow-up CT in paediatric tuberculous meningitis. Pediatr Radiol 35:1092–1099

9. Yadav YR, Mukerji G, Parihar V, Sinha M, Pandey S (2009) Complex hydrocephalus (combination of communicating and obstructive type): an important cause of failed endoscopic third ventriculostomy. BMC Res Notes 2:137
10. Yadav YR, Parihar V, Namdev H, Agarwal M, Bhatele PR (2013) Endoscopic inter laminar management of lumbar disc disease. J Neurol Surg A Cent Eur Neurosurg 74:77–81
11. Yadav YR, Parihar V, Kher Y, Bhatele PR (2016) Endoscopic inter laminar management of lumbar disease. Asian J Neurosurg 11:1–7
12. Yadav YR, Parihar V, Ratre S, Kher Y (2014) Endoscopic anterior decompression in cervical disc disease. Neurol India 62:417–422
13. Yadav YR, Parihar V, Ratre S, Kher Y, Bhatele P (2014) Endoscopic decompression of cervical spondylotic myelopathy using posterior approach. Neurol India 62:640–645
14. Yadav YR, Yadav N, Parihar V, Kher Y, Ratre S (2013) Endoscopic posterior decompression of lumbar canal stenosis. Indian J Neurosurg 2:124–130
15. Yadav YR, Parihar V, Bhatele P (2013) Endoscopic treatment of arachnoid cyst. In: Veerendra Kumar, Mukta Bhatele (eds) Lecture notes in bioengineering 2013. Proceedings of All India Seminar on Biomedical Engineering 2012 (AISOBE 2012). Springer, New Delhi, pp 29–35.
16. Yadav YR, Parihar V, Pande S, Namdev H (2014) Endoscopic management of colloid cysts. J Neurol Surg A Cent Eur Neurosurg 75:376–380
17. Yadav YR, Parihar V, Agarwal M, Sherekar S, Bhatele PR (2011) Endoscopic vascular decompression of the trigeminal nerve. Minim Invasive Neurosurg 54:110–114
18. Yadav YR, Sachdev S, Parihar V, Namdev H, Bhatele PR (2012) Endoscopic endonasal trans-sphenoid surgery of pituitary adenoma. J Neurosci Rural Pract 3:328–337
19. Yadav YR, Madhariya SN, Parihar VS, Namdev H, Bhatele PR (2013) Endoscopic transoral excision of odontoid process in irreducible atlantoaxial dislocation: our experience of 34 patients. J Neurol Surg A Cent Eur Neurosurg 74:162–167
20. Yadav YR, Parihar V, Janakiram N, Pande S, Bajaj J, Namdev H (2016) Endoscopic management of cerebrospinal fluid rhinorrhea. Asian J Neurosurg 11:183–193
21. Yadav YR, Yadav S, Sherekar S, Parihar V (2011) A new minimally invasive tubular brain retractor system for surgery of deep intracerebral hematoma. Neurol India 59:74–77
22. Yadav YR, Mukerji G, Shenoy R, Basoor A, Jain G, Nelson A (2007) Endoscopic management of hypertensive intraventricular haemorrhage with obstructive hydrocephalus. BMC Neurol 7:1
23. Yadav YR, Parihar V, Sinha M, Jain N (2010) Endoscopic treatment of supra sellar arachnoid cyst. Neurol India 58:280–282
24. Yadav YR, Basoor A, Todorov M, Parihar V (2010) Endoscopic management of large multi compartmental intraventricular arachnoid cyst extending from foramen magnum to foramen monro: case repot and review of literature. Neurol India 58:481–484
25. Yadav YR, Shenoy R, Mukerji G, Sherekar S, Parihar V (2010) Endoscopic transoral excision of odontoid process in irreducible atlanto-axial dislocation. In: Deepu Banerji, Apoorva Pauranik (ed) Progress in clinical neurosciences, vol 24. Byword Books Private Limited and Neurological society of India, New Delhi. pp 159–169
26. Gajdhar M, Yadav YR (2005) A case of thalamic abscess treated by endoscopic surgery. Neurol India 53:345–346
27. Yadav YR, Sinha M, Neha PV (2008) Endoscopic management of brain abscesses. Neurol India 56:13–16
28. Yadav YR, Yadav N, Parihar V, Khare Y, Ratre S (2015) Management of colloid cyst of third ventricle. Turk Neurosurg 25:362–371
29. Yadav YR, Nishtha Y, Vijay P, Shailendra R, Yatin K (2015) Endoscopic endonasal trans-sphenoid management of craniopharyngiomas. Asian J Neurosurg 10:10–16
30. Yadav YR, Bhagwat A, Agarwal M, Parihar V, Chandrakar S, Jain N (2011) Endoscopic treatment of neurocytoma of lateral ventricle: case report and review of literature. Chirurgia 24:173–176
31. Bhagwati S, Mehta N, Shah S (2010) Use of endoscopic third ventriculostomy in hydrocephalus of tubercular origin. Childs Nerv Syst 26:1675–1682
32. Yadav YR, Shenoy R, Mukerji G, Parihar V (2010) Water jet dissection technique for endoscopic third ventriculostomy minimizes the risk of bleeding and neurological complications in obstructive hydrocephalus with a thick and opaque third ventricle floor. Minim Invasive Neurosurg 53:155–158
33. Yadav YR, Jaiswal S, Adam N, Basoor A, Jain G (2006) Endoscopic third ventriculostomy in infants. Neurol India 54:161–163
34. Chugh A, Husain M, Gupta RK, Ojha BK, Chandra A, Rastogi M (2009) Surgical outcome of tuberculous meningitis hydrocephalus treated by endoscopic third ventriculostomy: prognostic factors and postoperative neuroimaging for functional assessment of ventriculostomy. J Neurosurg Pediatr 3:371–377
35. Singh I, Haris M, Husain M, Husain N, Rastogi M, Gupta RK (2008) Role of endoscopic third ventriculostomy in patients with communicating hydrocephalus: an evaluation by MR ventriculography. Neurosurg Rev 31:319–325
36. Singh D, Sachdev V, Singh AK, Sinha S (2005) Endoscopic third ventriculostomy in post-tubercular meningitis hydrocephalus: a preliminary report. Minim Invasive Neurosurg 48:47–52
37. Jonathan A, Rajshekhar V (2005) Endoscopic third ventriculostomy for chronic hydrocephalus after tuberculous meningitis. Surg Neurol 63:32–34

38. Figaji AA, Fieggen AG, Peter JC (2003) Endoscopic third ventriculostomy in tuberculous meningitis. Childs Nerv Syst 19:217–225
39. Yadav YR, Parihar V, Agrawal M, Bhatele PR (2011) Endoscopic third ventriculostomy in tubercular meningitis with hydrocephalus. Neurol India 59:855–860
40. Husain M, Jha DK, Rastogi M, Husain N, Gupta RK (2005) Role of neuroendoscopy in the management of patients with tuberculous meningitis hydrocephalus. Neurosurg Rev 28:278–283
41. Tandon V, Mahapatra AK (2011) Management of post-tubercular hydrocephalus. Childs Nerv Syst 27:1699–1707
42. Figaji AA, Fieggen AG (2013) Endoscopic challenges and applications in tuberculous meningitis. World Neurosurg 79(2 Suppl):S24. e9–14
43. Yadav YR, Parihar VS, Todorov M, Kher Y, Chaurasia ID, Pande S, Namdev H Role of endoscopic third ventriculostomy in tuberculous meningitis with hydrocephalus. Asian J Neurosurg. doi:10.4103/1793-5482.145100
44. Lin J, Zhang N, Sheng HS, Yin B, Wang HO, Wang MD (2011) Role of modified external ventricular drainage in the management of children with tuberculous meningitis hydrocephalus. Zhonghua Yi Xue Za Zhi 91:2488–2490
45. Lin J, Zhou H, Zhang N, Yin B, Sheng HS (2012) Effects of the implantation of Ommaya reservoir in children with tuberculous meningitis hydrocephalus: a preliminary study. Childs Nerv Syst 28:1003–1008
46. Yadav YR, Parihar V, Sinha M (2010) Lumbar peritoneal shunt. Neurol India 58:179–184
47. Yadav YR, Pande S, Raina VK, Singh M (2004) Lumboperitoneal shunts: review of 409 cases. Neurol India 52:188–190
48. Savardekar A, Chatterji D, Singhi S, Mohindra S, Gupta S, Chhabra R (2013) The role of ventriculoperitoneal shunt placement in patients of tubercular meningitis with hydrocephalus in poor neurological grade: a prospective study in the pediatric population and review of literature. Childs Nerv Syst 29:719–725
49. Peng J, Deng X, He F, Omran A, Zhang C, Yin F, Liu J (2012) Role of ventriculoperitoneal shunt surgery in grade IV tubercular meningitis with hydrocephalus. Childs Nerv Syst 28:209–215
50. Srikantha U, Morab JV, Sastry S, Abraham R, Balasubramaniam A, Somanna S, Devi I, Bangalore CA, Pandey P (2009) Outcome of ventriculoperitoneal shunt placement in Grade IV tubercular meningitis with hydrocephalus: a retrospective analysis in 95 patients. Clinical article. J Neurosurg Pediatr 4:176–183
51. Jha D, Khatri P, Choudhary A, Sethi R, Kumar S (2007) Endoscopic third ventriculostomy in prepontine-suprasellar tuberculoma with tuberculous meningitis hydrocephalus: a case report. Pediatr Neurosurg 43:42–46
52. Misra UK, Kalita J, Prabhakar S, Chakravarty A, Kochar D, Nair PP (2012) Endoscopic third ventriculostomy in tuberculous meningitis needs more evidence. Ann Indian Acad Neurol 15:233
53. Rajshekhar V (2015) Surgery for brain tuberculosis: a review. Acta Neurochir 157:1665–1678
54. Di X, Ragab M, Luciano MG (2009) Cine phase-contrast MR images failed to predict clinical outcome following ETV. Can J Neurol Sci 36:643–647
55. Figaji AA, Fieggen AG, Peter JC (2007) Endoscopy for tuberculous hydrocephalus. Childs Nerv Syst 23:79–84
56. Yadav YR, Parihar V, Pande S, Namdev H, Agarwal M (2012) Endoscopic third ventriculostomy. J Neurosci Rural Pract 3:163–173
57. Zhu XL, Gao R, Wong GK, Wong HT, Ng RY, Yu Y, Wong RK, Poon WS (2013) Single burr hole rigid endoscopic third ventriculostomy and endoscopic tumor biopsy: what is the safe displacement range for the foramen of Monro? Asian J Surg 36:74–82
58. Oertel J, Gen M, Krauss JK, Zumkeller M, Gaab MR (2006) The use of waterjet dissection in endoscopic neurosurgery. Technical note. J Neurosurg 105:928–931
59. Husain M, Singh DK, Rastogi M, Ojha BK, Chandra A, Gupta RK (2010) Intraoperative ventriculostomographic evaluation of endoscopic cerebrospinal fluid diversion and flow restoration procedures. Br J Neurosurg 24:672–678
60. Singh D, Gupta V, Goyal A, Singh H, Sinha S, Singh AK, Kumar S (2003) Endoscopic third ventriculostomy in obstructed hydrocephalus. Neurol India 51:39–42
61. Kumar A, Deopujari CE, Biyani N (2011) Utility of ventricular access in an acute deterioration after endoscopic third ventriculostomy. J Postgrad Med 57:123–125
62. Parikh D, Foroughi M, Nannapaneni R, Hatfield RH (2009) Is the routine placement of a CSF reservoir following endoscopic third ventriculostomy justified? Br J Neurosurg 23:521–523
63. Xiao B, Roth J, Udayakumaran S, Beni-Adani L, Constantini S (2011) Placement of Ommaya reservoir following endoscopic third ventriculostomy in pediatric hydrocephalic patients: a critical reappraisal. Childs Nerv Syst 27:749–755
64. Nakao N, Itakura T (2003) Endoscopic lamina terminalis fenestration for treatment of hydrocephalus due to tuberculous meningitis. Case illustration. J Neurosurg 99:187
65. Spena G, Fasel J, Nd T, Radovanovic I (2008) Subfrontal endoscopic fenestration of lamina terminalis: an anatomical study. Minim Invasive Neurosurg 51:319–323
66. ul Haq MI, Khan SA, Raja RA, Ahmed E (2012) Efficacy of endoscopic third ventriculostomy in non-communicating hydrocephalus. J Ayub Med Coll Abbottabad 24:144–146
67. Jha DK, Mishra V, Choudhary A, Khatri P, Tiwari R, Sural A, Kumar S (2007) Factors affecting the outcome of neuroendoscopy in patients with tuberculous meningitis hydrocephalus: a preliminary study. Surg Neurol 68:35–41
68. Tjemme B, Grotenhuis AJ (2002) Is the success rate of endoscopic age dependent? An analysis of the

results of endoscopic third ventriculostomy in young children. Childs Nerv Syst 18:605–608
69. Kumar A, Singh K, Sharma V (2013) Surgery in hydrocephalus of tubercular origin: challenges and management. Acta Neurochir 155:869–873
70. Cinalli G, Spennato P, Ruggiero C, Aliberti F, Zerah M, Trischitta V, Cianciulli E, Maggi G (2006) Intracranial pressure monitoring and lumbar puncture after endoscopic third ventriculostomy in children. Neurosurgery 58:126–136
71. Gu J, Xiao H, Wu F, Ge Y, Ma J, Sun W (2015) Prognostic factors of tuberculous meningitis: a single-center study. Int J Clin Exp Med 8:4487–4493
72. Güneş A, Uluca Ü, Aktar F, Konca Ç, Şen V, Ece A, Hoşoğlu S, Taş MA, Gürkan F (2015) Clinical, radiological and laboratory findings in 185 children with tuberculous meningitis at a single centre and relationship with the stage of the disease. Ital J Pediatr 41:75
73. Turgut M, Özcan OE, Özgen T, Bertan V (1993) Intradural extramedullary tuberculoma of the spinal cord -a case report. Zentralbl Neurochir 54:197–199
74. Turgut M (1997) Pott's disease. J Neurosurg 87:136–138
75. Turgut M (1997) Intradural tuberculous granuloma. Br J Neurosurg 11:264–266
76. Turgut M (2001) Spinal tuberculosis (Pott's disease): its clinical presentation, surgical management, and outcome. A survey study on 694 patients. Neurosurg Rev 24:8–13
77. Turgut M (2001) Multifocal extensive spinal tuberculosis (Pott's disease) involving cervical, thoracic and lumbar vertebrae. Br J Neurosurg 15:142–146
78. Turgut M, Özcan OE, Özgen T, Sağlam S, Bertan V, Erbengi A (1989) Tuberculomas of the craniospinal axis. Turk Neurosurg 1:34–38
79. Yadav YR, Parihar V, Kher Y (2013) Complication avoidance and its management in endoscopic neurosurgery. Neurol India 61:217–225
80. Yadav YR, Parihar V, Ratre S, Kher Y (2015) Avoiding complications in endoscopic third ventriculostomy. J Neurol Surg A Cent Eur Neurosurg 76:483–494
81. Yadav YR, Parihar V, Ratre S, Iqbal M (2016) Microneurosurgical skills training. J Neurol Surg A Cent Eur Neurosurg 77:146–154
82. Misra UK, Kalita J, Maurya PK (2011) Stroke in tuberculous meningitis. J Neurol Sci 303:22–30
83. Kalita J, Misra UK, Nair PP (2009) Predictors of stroke and its significance in the outcome of tuberculous meningitis. J Stroke Cerebrovasc Dis 18:251–258
84. Faggin R, Calderone M, Denaro L, Meneghini L, d'Avella D (2011) Long-term operative failure of endoscopic third ventriculostomy in pediatric patients: the role of cine phase-contrast MR imaging. Neurosurg Focus 30:E1
85. Doll A, Christmann D, Kehrli P, Abu Eid M, Gillis C, Bogorin A, Thiebaut A, Dietemann JL (2000) Contribution of 3D CISS MRI for pre and posttherapeutic monitoring of obstructive hydrocephalus. J Neuroradiol 27:218–225
86. Kurihara N, Takahashi S, Tamura H, Higano S, Furuta S, Jokura H, Umetsu A (2000) Investigation of hydrocephalus with three dimensional constructive interference in steady state MRI. Neuroradiology 42:634–638

Surgical Treatment of Spinal Tuberculosis Complicated with Extensive Abscess

31

Arun K. Srivastava, Jayesh Sardhara, Chaitanya Godbole, and Sanjay Behari

Contents

A.K. Srivastava, MCh • J. Sardhara, MCh
Chaitanya Godbole, MC • S. Behari (✉)
Department of Neurosurgery, Sanjay Gandhi Postgraduate Institute of Medical Sciences, Lucknow 226014, Uttar Pradesh, India
e-mail: doctorarunsrivastava@gmail.com; jayeshsardhara83@gmail.com; drchaitanyagodbole@gmail.com; sbehari27@yahoo.com

Abbreviations

AAD	Atlantoaxial dissociation
CT	Computed tomography
CVJ-TB	Craniovertebral junction tuberculosis
EMB	Ethambutol
INH	Isoniazid
MRI	Magnetic resonance imaging
PZA	Pyrazinamide
RIF	Rifampicin
TB	Tuberculosis
USG	Ultrasonography
WHO	World Health Organization

31.1 Introduction

Spinal tuberculosis (TB) accounts for about 50% of skeletal TB and 40% of all spinal infections [1, 2]. Literature suggests that one third of the world's population is infected with *Mycobacterium tuberculosis*, and each year about nine million people develop one or the other form of TB, of which a mortality of two million was reported [3]. Spinal TB has a strong correlation with the socio-economic status of the affected population. The maximum brunt is, therefore, borne by the people living in developing countries, although an increase in the incidence has been documented in developed countries in the recent era as well [4].

M. Turgut et al. (eds.), *Tuberculosis of the Central Nervous System*,
DOI 10.1007/978-3-319-50712-5_31

Besides the clinical examination, laboratory testing and radiological examination may be helpful in the diagnosis of this entity. Confirmation of the disease by identifying *M. tuberculosis* is still the gold standard for diagnosis. Anti-TB chemotherapy can yield an 80% spontaneous fusion rate; however in patients with an extensive spinal involvement, vertebral body collapse and severe deformity, the resultant neurological injury may require surgical treatment. The approach may be anterior, posterior, posterolateral or even a combination of all three. Recent data associates the best outcomes with a posterior or a combined surgical approach [1, 5]. A unique feature of spinal TB is the development of large abscesses, which in turn can have a subligamentous spread or a spread towards the spinal canal, invading the epidural space. Chemotherapy with or without surgical therapy is a safe and effective approach to treat spinal TB abscess. However, the lack of vascularity within the caseative necrotic core of the TB abscess often leads to failure of the antibiotic to penetrate this area. This may lead to a resistance to chemotherapy often mandating a surgical intervention to drain the abscess. A rapid increase in size of the abscess due to the osmotic ingression of the surrounding fluid may result in a rapid neurological deterioration. This chapter summarises the surgical management of spinal TB complicated with an extensive TB abscess and also the resultant sequel.

31.2 Pathogenesis

Pott's spine is considered as a reactivation of a haematogenous foci or a spread from the adjacent paravertebral lymph nodes. Spinal TB commonly involves ≥2 level adjacent vertebral level. The most common site of spinal TB in children is the upper thoracic spine, whereas in adults, TB commonly occurs in the lower thoracic and upper lumbar vertebrae. Disease spreads from the anterosuperior or inferior angle of the vertebral body, towards the adjacent body, and then affects the intervertebral disc. With advancing stage, it results in collapse of the vertebral bodies, often leading to kyphosis (gibbus). It may also be associated with a paravertebral 'cold' abscess. Pott's spine affecting the upper thoracic spine may track to the anterior chest wall and present as a soft tissue mass; in lower spine, it usually penetrates the inguinal ligaments or presents as a psoas abscess. Involvement of the adjacent structures in patients is frequent; the abscess can affect the perivertebral area in the thorax or abdomen, the psoas muscle or the epidural space [6]. These abscesses can become quite large before being diagnosed due to the insidious nature of this pathology [6]. Mohindra et al., have given the characteristic features of a TB abscess [7]. A TB abscess may have a history of TB affliction or there may be a low-grade indolent fever. On magnetic resonance imaging (MRI), there may be a thicker wall due to fibrosis with a low magnetisation transfer ratio due to the presence of a large number of TB bacilli in the wall, the in vivo magnetic resonance spectroscopy may reveal the presence of a lipid peak with no evidence of amino acids, the microbiological examination of the contents may yield *M. tuberculosis* and the histological examination may either yield the features of a pyogenic abscess with many acid-fast bacilli of *M. tuberculosis* (in a pure TB abscess that is often associated with immunocompromise) or the features of a tuberculoma with a central caseative necrosis with granulomas and palisading arrays of epitheloid cells, as well as Langhans and foreign body giant cells in the capsule (the latter is often associated with a good immunity) [7, 8] (Fig. 31.1).

31.3 Diagnosis

31.3.1 Ultrasonography

The abscess of the psoas region and the cervical area is well delineated with the help of an ultrasound (USG) imaging, and diagnostic/therapeutic aspiration may be carried out.

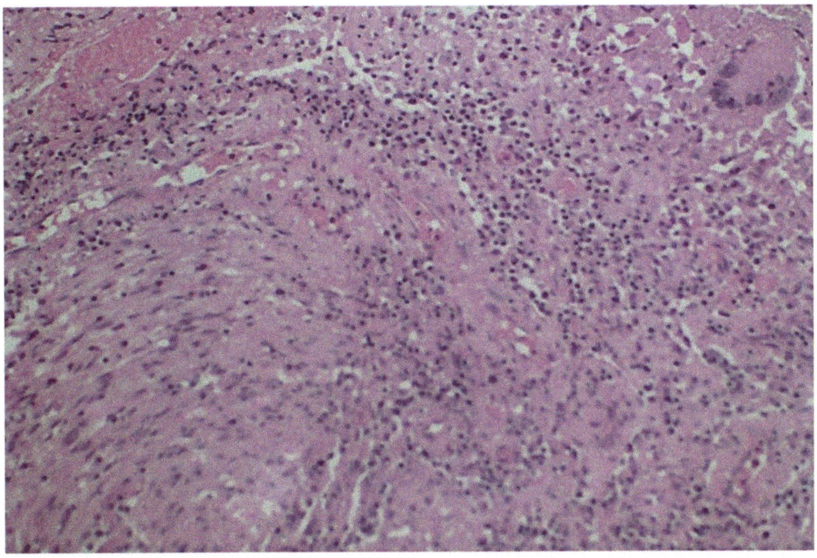

Fig. 31.1 Microphotograph showing epithelioid cell granuloma comprised of collection of epithelioid cell, lymphocytes, Langhans giant cell and necrosis (H&E ×200)

31.3.2 Plain Radiographs

These will not be of much help in the early stages of development of Pott's spine complicated with an abscess; however, in the later stages of the disease, it may reveal the bony destruction, kyphosis, scoliosis and gibbus formation in spine. An increase in the anterior prevertebral soft tissue shadow ≥7 mm at the level of the axis vertebra and ≥5 mm at the subaxial spine is an indirect evidence of the presence of granulation tissue, an abscess or soft tissue oedema in the region. This finding, therefore, often serves as a screening test that may lead to further detailed evaluation of the spine.

31.3.3 Computed Tomography

The bony delineation is clearer in comparison to an MRI and the plain radiographs. It can be used for diagnostic as well as for interventional purposes, as both the diagnostic and therapeutic computed tomography (CT)-guided aspiration of the pus and biopsy may be undertaken. Following posterior stabilisation, this helps in determining whether or not bony union has occurred by evaluating the new bone formation as well as continuation of the traversing cortical bone and bony trabeculations across the vertebral bodies and the onlay bone grafts.

31.3.4 Magnetic Resonance Imaging

MRI is the most important radiological tool; however, expertise is required to differentiate Pott's abscess from other pathologies that may reveal a similar picture, such as primary bony tumours and metastasis of the spine (that may often be associated with a necrotic core resembling a TB abscess). Caseating tuberculomas with a liquid core are often hypointense on T1-weighted images, while the central portion of the granuloma is T2 hyperintense and a peripheral hypointense ring around the central hyperintense mass is usually seen. On contrast administration, the lesion is seen as a ringlike enhancement. Adjacent perilesional oedema is seen as a hyperintense lesion on T2-weighted image. On diffusion-weighted imaging, the tuberculoma shows restriction with low intensity on apparent diffusion coefficient images [9, 10]. A high signal on T1-weighted imaging with decrease in soft tissue oedema and in the size and number of paravertebral abscesses signifies normal marrow formation within the vertebral body and the healing of vertebral body TB. The World Health Organization (WHO) recommendations for the various diagnostic procedures in the cases of Pott's spine with an abscess are summarised in Table 31.1.

Table 31.1 Recent WHO recommendations, their advantages and disadvantages for establishing the presence of tuberculous infection

Method	Use	Level of health system	Advantages	Disadvantages
Smear microscopy for acid-fast bacilli Ziehl-Neelsen's staining Fluorescent microscopy	Rapid, point-of-care test for case detection	Community	Requires moderate training, minimal infrastructure, minimal equipment	Low sensitivity
Culture On solid media In liquid media MGIT (Becton Dickinson), BacT/ALERT (BioMérieux), others	TB case detection and as a prerequisite for drug susceptibility testing	Referral laboratory	Good sensitivity	Slow time to growth in the case of solid lesions but less than 3 weeks in liquefied lesions
Chest radiograph	TB case detection	Referral	Indications and use not restricted to TB	Low specificity, low sensitivity, requires equipment, trained interpreter
Tuberculin skin test	Detection of *M. tuberculosis* infection	Community	Extensive practical and published experience	Sensitivity decreases with increasing immunocompromise, cross-reaction with BCG vaccine
Nucleic acid amplification (NAA) assay, Most recent is Xpert MTB/RIF (WHO endorsed)	TB case detection and detection of rifampicin resistance	Referral	Sensitivity between that of smear and culture, highly specific for TB	Requires moderate training and equipment; labor intensive; potential for cross-contamination among specimens
Strip-based species identification (detects TB-specific antigen in positive cultures)	Species identification (TB versus not TB) in cultures positive for mycobacterial growth	Referral laboratory (with culture)	Accurate, requires minimal training, minimal equipment, minimal consumables	
Line probe manual amplification and hybridisation –Genotype MTBDRplus (Hain Lifescience), INNO-LiPA Mycobacteria (Innogenetics)	TB case detection and drug susceptibility testing	Reference laboratory	Poor sensitivity in smear-negative specimens, relatively short time to result	Labor intensive, potential for cross-contamination, requires extensive training
Non-commercial culture and DST (drug susceptibility testing) MODS (microscopic observation drug susceptibility) NRA (nitrate reductase assay) CRI (colorimetric redox indicator assay)	TB case detection and drug susceptibility testing	Reference laboratory	Non-commercial, research	Labor intensive

Abbreviations: *TB* tuberculosis, *MGIT* mycobacteria growth indicator tube, *M. Mycobacterium*, *NAA* nucleic acid amplification, *MTB/RIF Mycobacterium*/rifampicin resistance, *WHO* World Health Organization, *MTBDR Mycobacterium tuberculosis* and drug resistance, *INNO-LiPA* line probe assay, *DST* drug sensitivity testing, *MODS* microscopic observation drug susceptibility, *NRA* nitrate reductase assay, *CRI* colorimetric redox indicator

31.4 Management

The management of an abscess associated with Pott's spine is still controversial. The debate was first started in the 1960s when Hodgson et al., [11] advocated surgical intervention and Konstam and Blesovsky [12] preferred conservative treatment. This controversial debate stimulated a series of randomised clinical trials conducted by the British Medical Research Council in the 1970s [13–16]. These trials found better results with radical decompression of the disease than with conservative management as this leads to a rapid resolution of the abscess and an early fusion [13–16]. In a multivariate analysis of spinal TB, Park et al., found better clinical scores (related to myelopathy, pain and deformity) utilising radical surgery [17].

Medical management of spinal TB includes the standard anti-TB therapy regimen, isoniazid (INH) (5 mg/kg), rifampicin (RIF) (10 mg/kg), pyrazinamide (PZA) (25 mg/kg) and ethambutol (EMB) (15 mg/kg) during the intensive phase of the disease (PZA to be continued for a duration of 3–4 months and EMB for 12 months), followed by INH and RIF during the continuation phase (the two medicines are given for a total of 18 months). Second-line treatment may be used in the cases exhibiting drug resistance to anti-TB treatment and includes ofloxacin, ciprofloxacin and cycloserine. Serial liver function tests must be done during the follow-up visits while the patient is on these medications. Interval CT and MRI scans of the spine, as well as assessment of the neurological symptomatology and signs, will determine the extent and continuation of treatment.

Surgical treatment combined with chemotherapy is a safe and effective approach to treating spinal TB and abscess. The goals of surgical intervention are to facilitate the medical management by adding radical spinal cord decompression. Prevention of further deformity with spinal stabilisation and alleviation of pain are the extra benefits obtained by surgical intervention when compared with the persistence of conservative treatment.

31.5 Craniovertebral Junction Tuberculosis

The incidence of craniovertebral junction tuberculosis (CVJ-TB) is rare (constituting 0.3–1% of patients suffering from Pott's spine). The manifestation of upper cervical myelopathy in this subset is because of atlantoaxial dissociation (AAD) and secondary basilar impression. The symptoms can rapidly progress due to the presence of associated epidural abscess or granuloma. The armamentum of the management ranges from conservative approach to radical surgery. A protocol for the management of CVJ-TB is based on the grading of severity of the disease [18]. Grade I refers to neck pain without any motor deficit; grade II refers to the presence of mild motor deficit but the patient not being dependent on others; grade III refers to a moderate motor disability with the patient being partially dependent on others for his daily needs; and grade IV refers to the persistence of severe motor deficits so that the patient is completely dependent on others for all his/her daily needs. Under the cover of anti-TB therapy, the following important factors are assessed in isolation or in combination: the above-mentioned grade, the type of AAD, instability of any other type, the presence of a large abscess causing significant cervicomedullary compression at the CVJ and the clinical and/or radiological response to anti-TB therapy at a follow-up of 3 months (Figs. 31.2 and 31.3). In the cases of minor deficits (grades I and II), the patients can be managed with conservative treatment in the form of neck stabilisation; in severe deficits (grades III and IV), however, the site of compression is usually ventral (fixed AAD and ventral paraspinal abscess) which requires ventral decompression followed by posterior fusion by various commonly practiced techniques. In patients with persistent reducible AAD, direct posterior fusion is recommended. However, significant improvement is reported even in poor-grade patients with the judicious use of the surgical options along with anti-TB therapy [19]. An important aspect of this protocol is that after the percutaneous or open drainage of a

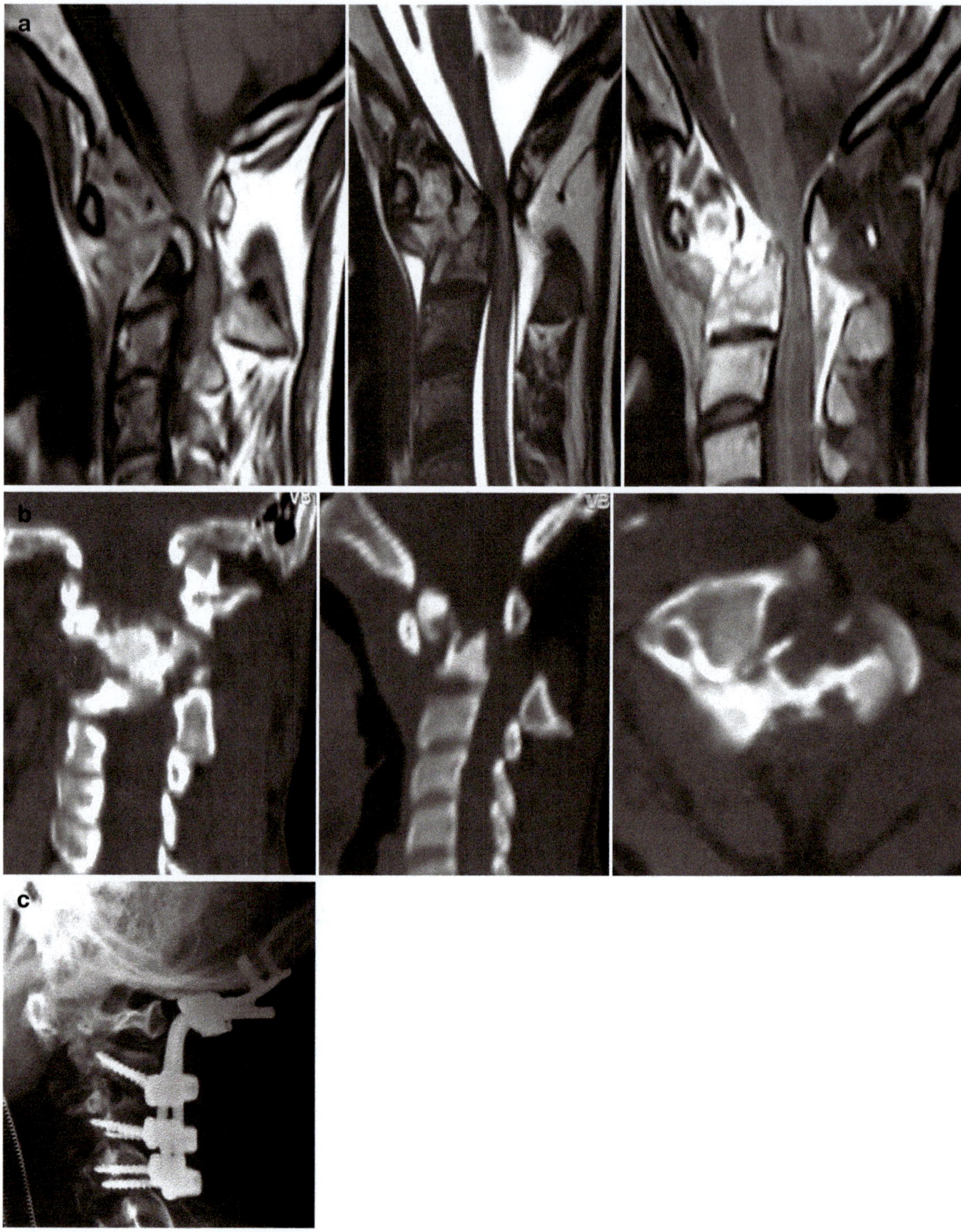

Fig. 31.2 (**a**) MRI T1, T2 and contrast images showing atlantoaxial dislocation with granulation tissue and abscess formation at the craniovertebral junction (CVJ). (**b**) Coronal, sagittal and axial CT images showing odontoid and C2 vertebral destruction and atlantoaxial dislocation due to CVJ-TB. (**c**) Postoperative lateral radiograph of the cervical spine showing posterior occipitocervical instrumentation

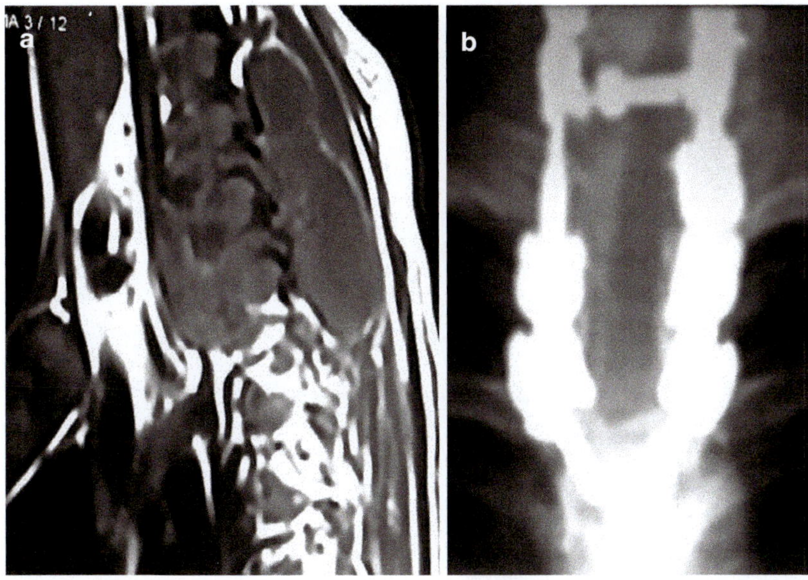

Fig. 31.3 (**a**) MRI T1 contrast showing a large TB abscess with contiguous cervical vertebral body involvement. (**b**) Anteroposterior radiograph of the same patient showing a multilevel spinal instrumentation.

CVJ-TB abscess and following continuation of anti-TB therapy, the patient should be reassessed after 3 months for persistence of reducible AAD even when the TB affliction has resolved. If there is persisting instability, then an atlantoaxial fusion is mandatory to pre-empt the appearance of delayed neurological deficits.

31.6 Cervical and Cervicodorsal Tuberculous Abscess

The cervical involvement is characterised by pain, restriction of neck movements with an extensive abscess also leading to deglutition and respiratory difficulty. The abscess formation is more severe and commoner than that seen in CVJ-TB, and its direct drainage is also easier. The drainage of an abscess may be done under USG guidance or under direct vision. Most of the surgical interventions are done from the anterior approach utilising an anterior transcervical approach (Fig. 31.4). Various studies have supported an early surgical intervention over delayed intervention in order to alleviate neuraxial compression and to prevent the development of a delayed deformity. There is not much difference in the wound healing following an early versus delayed intervention. Management options along with anti-TB therapy include a percutaneous abscess drainage or an open drainage, with or without an instrumented vertebral fusion. A cervical location that is associated with gross instability and involvement of all three vertebral columns may often require staged surgery in the form of anterior corpectomy with cage graft and second-stage posterior instrumentation and fusion [19]. The cervicodorsal region TB is also an important entity as its surgical approach differs from that utilised for a pure subaxial cervical TB. Thus, it may be accessed by a transclavicular, trans-manubrial or a posterolateral approach (Fig. 31.5).

31.7 Thoracolumbar Tuberculous Abscess

According to Osborn et al., a paravertebral abscess is present in 55–95% of the cases suffering from thoracolumbar spinal TB [20]. Gehlot et al., reported the presence of a paravertebral TB abscess in 98.5% of patients with spinal TB [21]. Mirsaedi et al., found a psoas abscess in 14.3% of these patients, and Gehlot et al., noted a psoas abscesses in 37.1% of their cases [21, 22]. Dorsolumbar spinal abscesses can be seen on plain radiographs as a paravertebral soft tissue shadow [23]. The finding of calcification within the abscess cavity is a diagnostic clue pointing towards spinal TB [24]. Plain radiographs are usually normal in the early stages of the disease.

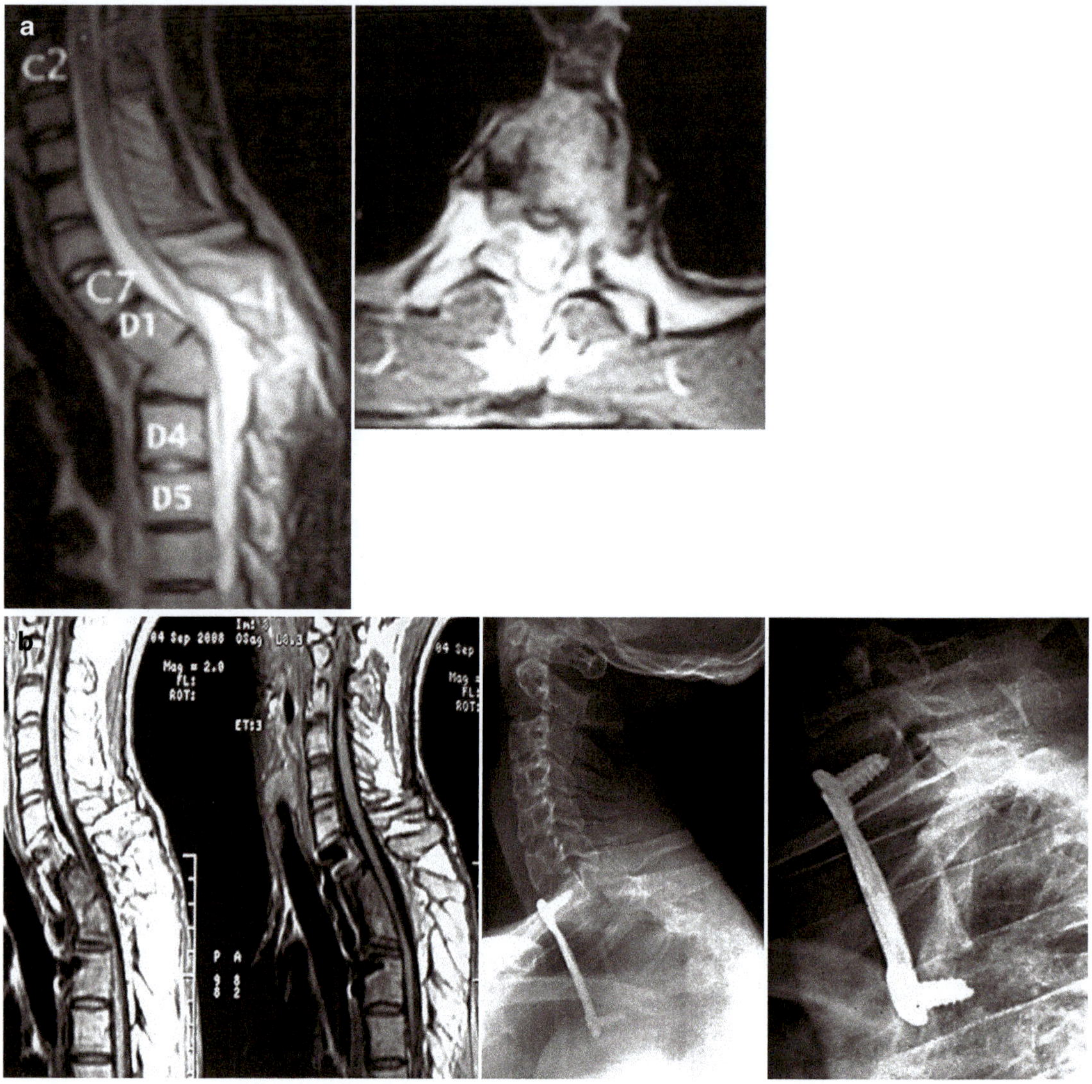

Fig. 31.4 (**a**) Sagittal and axial T2-weighted MRI of cervicothoracic junction Pott's spine with kyphosis. (**b**) Sagittal T1 MRI and plain cervicothoracic lateral view radiographs showing anterior cervical fusion with plating and a good bony alignment performed using the transclavicular approach

At this stage, a CT scan or an MRI is more sensitive in detecting early TB lesions [22].

The surgical approach for dealing with an extensive thoracolumbar paraspinal abscess can be either utilising an anterior or a posterior trajectory. The posterolateral approaches are often preferred over the ventral approaches (transthoracic or transperitoneal) as they prevent the tearing of thickened and diseased pleura, allow an easy excision of the granulation tissue and pus along the destroyed bony segments and avoid pleural and peritoneal contamination. However, for circumferential decompression and stabilisation, the anterior approach is preferable [24].

31.8 Vertebral Collapse with Spinal Instability

TB abscess formation in a single vertebral body without collapse but with cord compression and focal back pain may require only anti-TB treat-

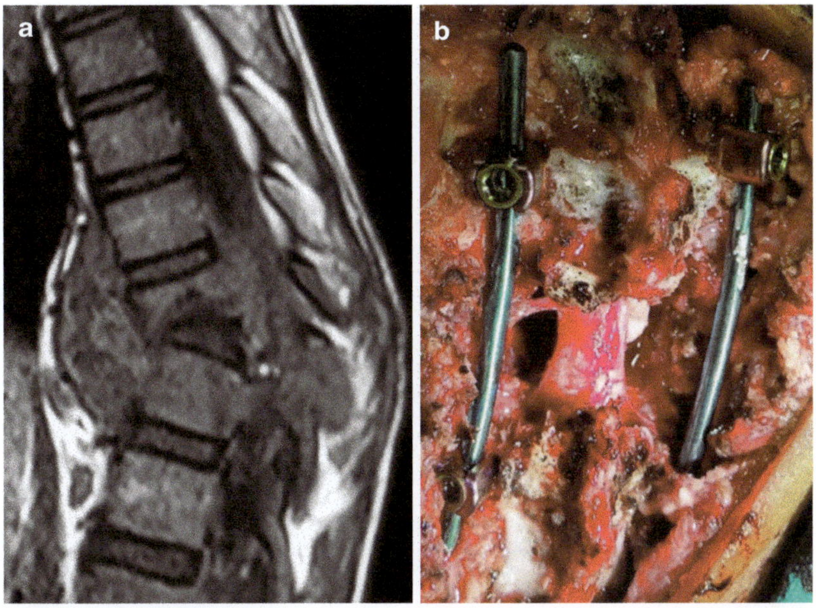

Fig. 31.5 (**a**) Thoracic Pott's spine with bony destruction and extensive anterior abscess. (**b**) Surgery utilising a lateral transpedicular-costotransversectomy extracavitary approach

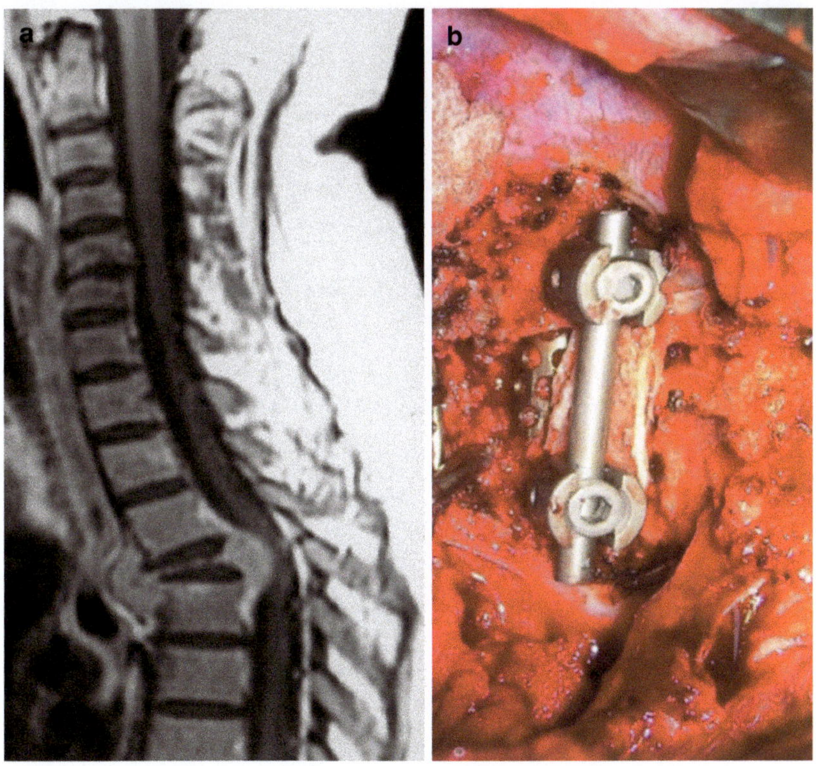

Fig. 31.6 (**a**) Thoracic Pott's spine. (**b**) Stabilisation using the transthoracic intracavitary approach

ment with follow-up evaluation utilising a detailed clinical and radiological examination (with the MRI examination being the most sensitive tool). A solitary vertebral body collapse with 50% loss of height without middle column fracture in a patient with focal pain may be treated with kyphoplasty. Patients with severe vertebral body collapse (>50%) with kyphotic deformity

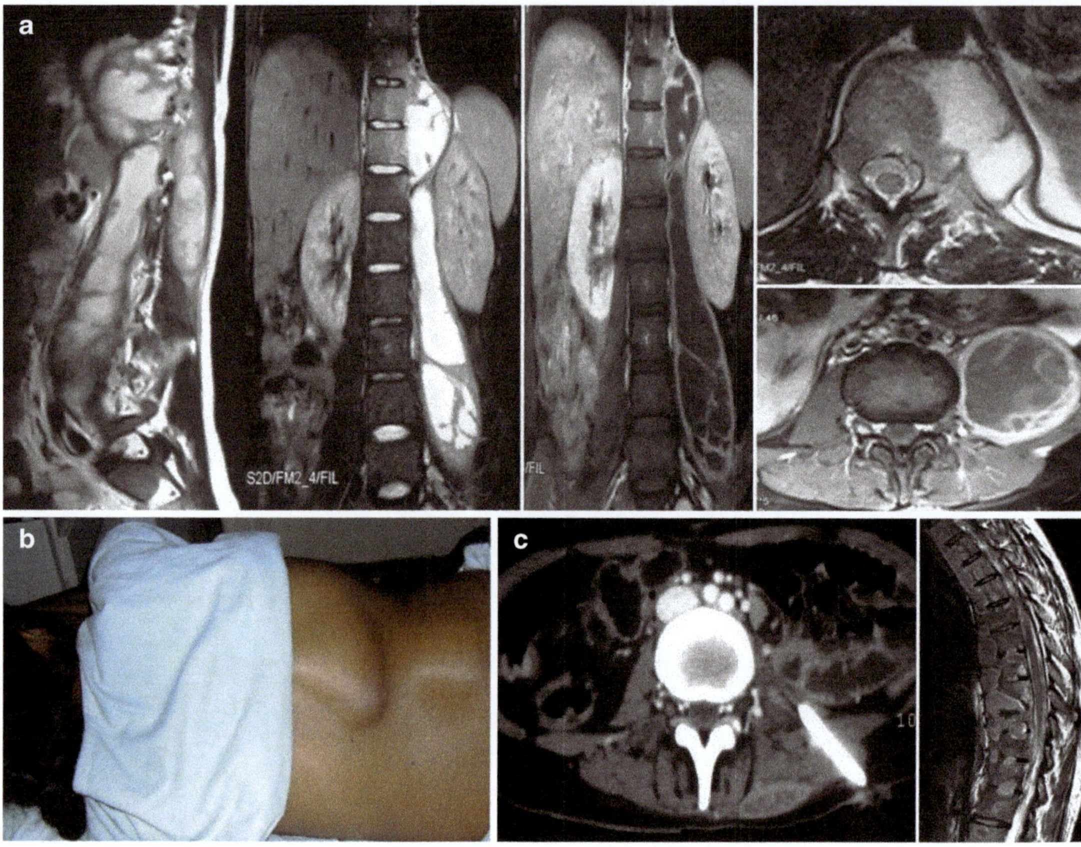

Fig. 31.7 (**a**) Parasagittal coronal and axial MRIs showing the extensive abscess complicating the thoracolumbar Pott's spine. The characteristic of the pus is in revealed in different sequences of MRI (T1/T2/T1 contrast). (**b**) The bulge due to the paravertebral abscess in the thoracolumbar region. (**c**) The CT-guided aspiration was followed by pig-tailed catheter placement. Follow-up MRI during the course of treatment after 1 year

and/or abscess formation with extension into the spinal canal and with cord compression require a corpectomy and posterior/posterolateral instrumentation and fusion (Fig. 31.6). Corpectomy with institution of an expandable cage graft may be accomplished from either a posterior transpedicular costotransversectomy route or via a transthoracic extracavitary approach (Figs. 31.6 and 31.7) depending on the location of the TB affliction and abscess within the thoracolumbar spine [19]. If the abscess formation results in a less severe deformity (Cobb's angle less than 30°) and the patient has minimal neurological disability, then a CT-guided catheter placement within the abscess cavity, avoidance of weight bearing by the spine and sustained anti-TB treatment, often helps in ameliorating the pain, instability and deformity (Fig. 31.7).

31.9 Unusual Presentations of Intraspinal Extensions of Tuberculous Abscesses

Intraspinal TB can present with or without vertebral TB. It can extend in the intraspinal space and may present with TB arachnoiditis with or without abscess formation in the loculated arachnoidal space, extradural or intradural TB granulomas, intramedullary abscess/granuloma and/or vasculitis (Fig. 31.8). It is often the cause of sudden or progressive neurological deterioration by compressive or non-compressive (ischaemic) myelopathy in patients with spinal TB. Intradural extension of TB infection is usually attributed to a haematogenous spread from outside the central nervous system. In the early stages, variable degrees of inflammatory exudates may affect the

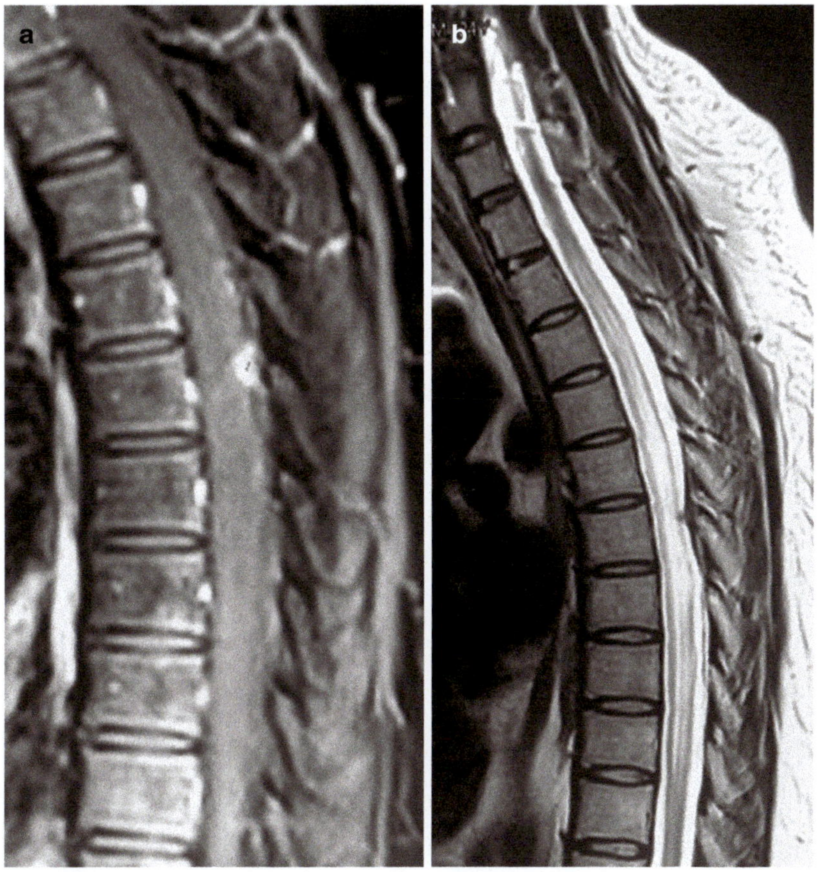

Fig. 31.8 MRI evidence of different complications of Pott's spine with extensive abscess. (**a**) Contrast MRI of same patient showing an intramedullary tuberculoma with arachnoidits. (**b**) A T2 MRI sequence showing the syrinx

meninges of the cord. The spinal cord and the nerve roots may then become oedematous and become engulfed by a gelatinous exudate [25]. Thoracic spine is the most common reported site of involvement when TB pathology is reported within the thecal sac. In occasional cases, it becomes very difficult to define whether the intradural tuberculoma is extramedullary or intramedullary [25].

Intramedullary spinal cord abscess is a very rare occurrence in the literature, since the original reported case by Hart in 1830 [26]. Abscess formation becomes manifest by the accumulation of the necrotic tissue, debris and caseous material as the disease progresses. It may then also extend to the anterior or posterior longitudinal ligament and may also spread to distant anatomical regions from the original site of the infection.

TB is the most common cause of infective arachnoiditis and resulting radiculomyelitis in almost every case. The arachnoidal membranes become thickened and cloudy with apparent adhesions [25]. Later on, owing to the abnormal cavitation within the parenchyma, syringomyelia may occur (Fig. 31.8) [27–31]. The mechanism responsible for syringomyelia is the inflammatory arachnoiditis and resulting extensive obliterative endarteritis that is usually responsible for the ischaemic necrotic cavity [27, 32]. The treatment of intramedullary abscess includes a combination of surgical and medical therapies. Surgery is indicated for the evacuation of the pus, and the use of appropriate antibiotics and corticosteroids should be considered in the treatment. Often, a thin rim of the capsule of the intramedullary TB abscess may be left in situ to avoid further damage to the spinal cord. Treatment of syringomyelia secondary to spinal TB may range from simply giving anti-TB treatment to dividing arachnoidal bands and relieving focal spinal compression. A syringo-peritoneal shunt procedure has a limited success rate due to the presence of multiple arachnoidal adhesions and lack of pressure head between the intramedullary syrinx cavity and the subarachnoid space.

Conclusion

The spine is commonly affected in the spectrum of TB disease, and most of the cases usually respond to medical treatment. Exact and early diagnosis and adequate treatment before the development of irreversible neurological deficits and spinal deformity are crucial for a satisfactory yield and good prognosis. In spite of effective and prolonged medical treatment, a TB abscess may fail to resolve. Its management demands an extensive surgical debridement and pus evacuation, not only to relieve the spinal cord compression but also to prevent further progressive spinal deformity and to alleviate the accompanying pain. Moreover, after surgery, the medical management can work more effectively in combating the disease.

References

1. Guerado E, Cerván AM (2012) Surgical treatment of spondylodiscitis. An update. Int Orthop 36:413–420
2. Joaquim Soares Do Brito MD, António Tirado MD, Pedro Fernandes MD (2014) Surgical treatment of spinal tuberculosis complicated with extensive abscess. Iowa Orthop J 34:129–136
3. McLain RF, Isada C (2004) Spinal tuberculosis deserves a place on the radar screen. Cleve Clin J Med 71:537–549
4. Luk KDK (1999) Tuberculosis of the spine in the new millenium. Eur Spine J 8:338–345
5. Ferrer MF, Torres LG, Ramirez OA, Zarzuelo MR, Gonzalez NP (2012) Tuberculosis of the spine. Asystematic review of case series. Int Orthop 36:221–231
6. Diana Afonso P, Almeida A (2011) Tuberculous spondilodiskitis: imaging features. Acta Medica Port 24:349–354
7. Mohindra S, SavardekarA GR, Tripathi M, Rane S (2016) Tuberculous brain abscesses in immunocompetent patients: a decade long experience with nine patients. Neurol India 64:66–74
8. Malik N, Behari S, Ansari MS, Jaiswal AK, Gupta P, Jain M (2011) An intramedullary tuberculous abscess of the conus in a 5-year-old child presenting with urinary dysfunction. World Neurosurg 76:592. e15–592.e18
9. Garg RK, Malhotra HS, Jain A (2016) Neuroimaging in tuberculous meningitis. Neurol India 64:219–227
10. Mohindra N, Neyaz Z (2015) Magnetic resonance sequences: practical neurological applications. Neurol India 63:241–249
11. Hodgson AR, Stock FE, Fang HS, Ong GB (1960) Anterior spinal fusion: the operative approach and pathological findings in 412 patients with Pott's disease of the spine. Br J Surg 48:172–178
12. Konstam PG, Blesovsky A (1962) The ambulant treatment of spinal tuberculosis. Br J Surg 50:26–38
13. Medical Research Council Working Party on Tuberculosis of the Spine (1973) A controlled trial of ambulant out-patient treatment and in-patient rest in bed in the management of tuberculosis of the spine in young Korean patients on standard chemotherapy a study in Masan, Korea. First report of the Medical Research Council Working Party on Tuberculosis of the Spine. J Bone Joint Surg Br 55:678–697
14. (1947) A controlled trial of anterior spinal fusion and debridement in the surgical management of tuberculosis of the spine in patients on standard chemotherapy: a study in Hong Kong. Br J Surg 61:853–866
15. (1974) A controlled trial of debridement and ambulatory treatment in the management of tuberculosis of the spine in patients on standard chemotherapy: a study in Bulawayo, Rhodesia. J Trop Med Hyg 77:72–92
16. Medical Research Council Working Party on Tuberculosis of the Spine (1976) A five-year assessment of controlled trials of inpatient and out-patient treatment and of plaster of- Paris jackets for tuberculosis of the spine in children on standard chemotherapy: studies in Masan and Pusan. Korea fifth report of the Medical Research Council Working Party on Tuberculosis of the Spine. J Bone Joint Surg Br 58:399–411
17. Park DW, Sohn JW, Kim EH, Cho DI, Lee JH, Kim KT, Ha KY, Jeon CH, Shim DM, Lee JS, Lee JB, Chun BC, Kim MJ (2007) Outcome and management of spinal tuberculosis according to the severity of disease: a retrospective study of 137 adult patients at Korean teaching hospitals. Spine 32:E130–E135
18. Behari S, Nayak SR, Bhargava V, Banerji D, Chhabra DK, Jain VK (2003) Craniocervical tuberculosis: protocol of surgical management. Neurosurgery 52:72–80
19. Kaloostian PE, Gokaslan ZL (2013) Current management of spinal tuberculosis: a multimodal approach. World Neurosurg 80:64–65
20. Osborn AG (1994) Nonneoplastic disorders of the spine and spinal cord. In: Osborn AG (ed) Diagnostic neuroradiology. Mosby, St Louis, pp 820–875
21. Gehlot PS, Chaturvedi S, Kashyap R, Singh V (2012) Pott's spine: retrospective analysis of MRI cans of 70 cases. J Clin Diagn Res 6:1534–1538
22. Mirsaeidi SM, Tabarsi P, Amiri MV, Mansoori SD, Bakhshayesh-Karam M, Masjedi MR (2003) Clinical and radiological presentation of adult tuberculous spondylitis. Tanaffos 2:59–65
23. Garg RK, Somvanshi DS (2011) Spinal tuberculosis: a review. J Spinal Cord Med 34:440–454

24. Chandra SP, Singh A, Goyal N, Laythalling RK, Singh M, Kale SS, Sharma MS, Suri A, Singh P, Garg A, Sarkar C, Tripathi M, Sharma BS, Mahapatra AK (2013) Analysis of changing paradigms of management in 179 patients with spinal tuberculosis over a 12-year period and proposal of a new management algorithm. World Neurosurg 80:190–203
25. Tanriverdi T, Kizilkiliç O, Hanci M, Kaynar MY, Unalan H, Oz B (2003) Atypical intradural spinal tuberculosis: report of three cases. Spinal Cord 41:403–409
26. Hart J (1830) A case of encysted abscess in the centre of spinal cord. Dublin Hosp Rep 5:522–524
27. Caplan LR, Norohna AB, Amico LL (1990) Syringomyelia and arachnoiditis. J Neurosurg Psychiatry 53:106–113
28. Fehling MG, Bernstein M (1992) Syringomyelia as an complication of tuberculous meningitis. Can J Neurol Sci 19:84–87
29. Kaynar MY, Kocer N, Gencosmanoglu BE, Hanci M (2000) Syringomyelia – as a late complication of tuberculous meningitis. Acta Neurochir 142:935–939
30. Savoirado M (1976) Syringomyelia associated with post-meningitic spinal arachnoiditis. Neurology 26:551–554
31. Sharif HS, Clark DC, Aabed MY, Haddad MC, al Deeb SM, Yaqub B, al Moutaery KR (1990) Granulomatous spinal infections of MR imaging. Radiology 177:101–107
32. MacDonald RL, Findlay JM, Tator CH (1988) Microcystic spinal cord degeneration causing post-traumatic myelopathy. J Neurosurg 68:446–471

Surgery for Multifocal Spinal Tuberculosis

32

Pedro Fernandes, Joaquim Soares do Brito, and Ahmet T. Turgut

Contents

P. Fernandes (✉) • J.S. do Brito
Department of Orthopedics and Trauma, Hospital de Santa Maria, Av. Professor Egas Moniz, 1649-035 Lisbon, Portugal
e-mail: pfpcm09@gmail.com; joaquimsoaresdobrito@gmail.com

A.T. Turgut
Department of Radiology, Hacettepe University School of Medicine, Ankara, Turkey
e-mail: ahmettuncayturgut@yahoo.com

Abbreviations

CT	Computed tomography
HIV	Human immunodeficiency virus
IVD	Intervertebral disk
MDR-TB	Multidrug-resistant tuberculosis
MRI	Magnetic resonance imaging
TB	Tuberculosis

32.1 Introduction

Spinal tuberculosis (TB) is one of the oldest human diseases, documented at least 5000 years ago from tombs in Africa. Spinal TB became more well known after reports by Sir Percival Pott in 1779 [1]. TB is responsible for almost 40% of all spine infections and is a frequent extrapulmonary form of the disease [1–4].

Chemotherapy was introduced to combat TB and proved successful over ensuing years. Meanwhile, human immunodeficiency virus (HIV) infections and other immunodeficiency diseases caused an increasing number of cases, especially recently [1–4]. Early diagnosis and effective treatments are essential to prevent complications associated with the disease [2, 3]. Involvement of the intervertebral disk (IVD) spaces and adjacent vertebral bodies, along with collapse of the spinal elements, vertebral instability, and progressive kyphotic deformity, is known

M. Turgut et al. (eds.), *Tuberculosis of the Central Nervous System*,
DOI 10.1007/978-3-319-50712-5_32

as Pott's disease, and the associated progressive neurological impairment with paraplegia is known as Pott's paraplegia [1]. Large abscesses can be present with or without epidural involvement [4]. Although chemotherapy is still the gold standard for treatment, the aforementioned complications can constitute possible surgical indication [1–4].

Most cases of spinal TB occur in a single vertebral body and/or two to three adjacent vertebrae [5–7]. Cases where multiple vertebral bodies at different levels of the spine are affected are known as noncontiguous spinal TB and are rare (Fig. 32.1). In general, multiple-bone noncontiguous spinal TB was believed to occur in immunocompromised patients; because of the lack of published reports, there are few guidelines for proper management [5, 8]. This chapter will address surgical treatment for multifocal spinal TB with special insight into its clinical presentation, effective management, and associated complications and outcomes.

32.2 Multifocal Spinal Tuberculosis

TB spondylitis most often involves adjacent spinal vertebrae, while noncontiguous vertebral involvement is rare [9]. Current literature reveals mostly single case reports of this rare clinical condition, with good treatment outcomes for the most part [10–14]:

- Turgut published the first case (in 2001 in the English literature) of an extensive multilevel spinal TB [13] and then highlighted the

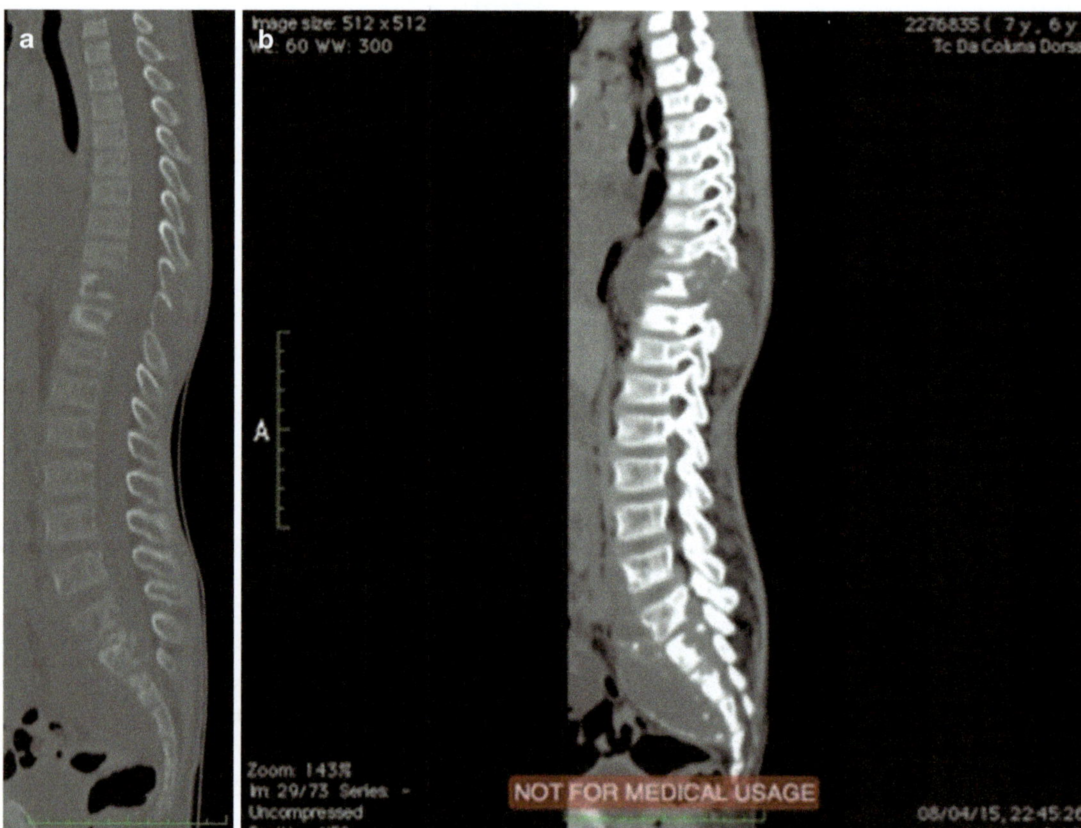

Fig. 32.1 Sagittal CT scan images (**a, b**) show noncontiguous spinal TB infection with thoracic and lumbosacral involvement in a six-year-old male patient

rarity by reporting only one case out of 694 patients [9].

- Rezai et al. reported one case of multifocal spinal TB in 20 patients; Lindahl et al. reported three patients out of 63; and in the study by Nussbaum et al., only one case out of 29 patients was reported [15–17].
- However, other authors seem to indicate that spinal TB with several foci is more frequent than reported in the literature [9]:
- Pandit et al. reported a 25% incidence of multicentricity in spinal TB. They studied bone scans from 40 spinal TB cases and reported a 25% (10 out of 40) incidence for skeletal multicentricity. Of these 40 patients, six had vertebral skip lesions, for an incidence of 15% for noncontiguous spinal TB [18].
- Polley et al. also reported a 16.3% occurrence rate for multifocal spinal TB (16 cases out of 98).

These studies have raised doubt about the actual rate of occurrence of these noncontiguous spinal TB lesions [9].

Multifocal spinal infections are by nature extensive lesions, and there is a higher incidence of neurological involvement compared to contiguous disease. This may not necessarily indicate more severe disease, but instead shows the heightened probability of complications due to the high number of levels involved [19]. Most spinal TB is of the thoracic and lumbar regions; cervical spine involvement occurs in less than 5% of all cases. TB of the cervical spine is also the most dangerous form of this disease. Mortality rates and the risk of quadriplegia are both high [20–22]. Polley et al. highlighted the higher rate of neurological impairment in cases of noncontiguous spinal TB (75%) comparing to the rest of the patients studied (58.5%) [9]. The case reported by Nussbaum et al. underwent surgery for a neurological deficit [16]. The case reported by Turgut with involvement of whole spinal segments also required surgery due to progressive quadriparesis [13]. In a newer report, Emel et al. elucidated a case of extensive noncontiguous spinal TB of the cervical, thoracic, lumbar, and sacral levels, also requiring surgery due to progressive paraparesis [10].

Multiple-bone vertebral TB is thought to occur in patients whose health is otherwise compromised due to underlying conditions such as HIV infection, steroid therapy, or other medical and/or nonmedical reasons [8]. However, some authors claim that noncontiguous multiple vertebral TB is not an overt manifestation of immunosuppression, multidrug-resistant tuberculosis (MDR-TB), or chronicity [7, 9, 19]. The real reason for an increasing rate of noncontiguous disease is not completely understood yet. This increase may be attributed to the high prevalence of TB with delayed presentation, mainly in areas where TB is endemic. Still, a likely reason may well be the increased ability to diagnose spinal TB with the use of magnetic resonance imaging (MRI) and specific protocols, which yield a full spinal study [9].

32.3 Pathophysiology

Subligamentous TB is well known to spread along the spine and into the paravertebral spaces and nearby soft tissues. TB causes osteonecrosis characterized by loss of the extracellular matrix of vertebral bone followed by collapse of the vertebrae [22]. Often, the anterior parts of two (or more) contiguous vertebrae are affected due to hematogenous spread via the bifurcation of the arteria intervertebralis, which supplies any two adjacent vertebrae [23].

To differentiate spinal TB from pyogenic osteomyelitis, look for a relative sparing of the IVDs. Mycobacteria do not have proteolytic enzymes, which are found in the bacteria, which can cause pyogenic osteomyelitis – this may spare the IVDs [24]. IVDs are avascular, which might keep them from hosting the initial site of a TB infection. Perhaps IVD involvement only begins when adjacent vertebrae are infected and the IVD loses nutritional supply [25]. Paravertebral abscesses can also distinguish Pott's disease from other infections, since the extent of these collections greatly exceeds the area of osseous involvement. These abscesses may be located anteriorly, posteriorly, laterally, or even circumferentially around the vertebrae.

The TB-abscess wall is usually thick, with irregular enhancement on both computed tomography (CT) and MRI. This radiologic finding is also diagnostic of TB spondylitis [25].

In spinal TB infections, the spinal cord may become affected via two mechanisms: the first is by direct cord compression by bone and/or the expanding abscess itself; or second, the cord may be directly affected by granulation tissue [26]. TB-caused neurological deficits in this context are generally more symmetrical and have a more gradual onset than deficits from other causes [27].

There are several proposed mechanisms to explain spinal involvement in TB infection: (1) spread through the venous system (valveless), (2) seeding via arterial pathways, (3) lymphatic spread, (4) direct infection from adjacent viscera and/or nodes, and (5) along soft tissue planes [13, 28, 29]. The venous system is probably involved in the pathological process with noncontiguous spinal TB [9]. Once a TB focus gains a foothold in the spine by arterial/venous/lymphatic means, bacilli shed into the valveless venous plexus, which allows backflow because of abdominal pressure. Thus, bacilli could travel to various levels and locations, never being filtered by the lungs or lymph system, with resulting "skip lesions," much like the mechanisms used by sarcomas in the venous sinusoids of the long bones [9]. This could explain how a patient may present with involvement of several isolated spinal levels without other overt pulmonary, visceral, or bony involvement. The less likely alternative would be multiple hematogenous arterial seedings, targeting different spinal areas preferentially [9].

32.4 Differential Diagnosis

Noncontiguous spinal TB must be distinguished from multiple metastatic spinal lesions from a systemic malignancy. Metastases will characteristically spare the IVD space, but so does spinal TB. When spinal TB involves several noncontiguous vertebrae, its appearance on imaging can be mistaken easily for metastatic disease. Two factors should distinguish spinal TB from neoplastic disease: these are the presence of paravertebral abscesses and subligamentous spread [25].

Pyogenic or, more rarely, fungal infections are other important considerations for the differential diagnosis. As mentioned, what distinguishes spinal TB from any pyogenic infection is the sparing of involvement of the IVDs [24]. Distinguishing between TB and a pyogenic spinal infection using histology and culture growth could only be done in 62.2% of cases in one study [30]. TB should be suspected, however, if the gram stain shows pus cells without pyogenic bacteria or where aerobic/anaerobic culture shows no growth of pyogenic bacteria [31].

32.5 Imaging Features

Conventional radiology still remains the cornerstone in recognition of skeletal TB, along with clinical features [24, 32]. Radiographic changes typical of Pott's disease include destruction of vertebrae and narrowing of the IVD space, both of which can be seen on plain radiographs [33].

In the adult patient with spinal TB, spinal infection begins in the vertebral somatic platform (osteomyelitis or spondylitis) and progresses to the IVD (spondylodiscitis) and then into the vertebral body above or below (Fig. 32.2). In contrast, because pediatric patients have highly vascularized IVDs, the infection may affect primarily the IVD (discitis) and secondarily the nearest vertebral bodies [34–36]. Destruction of a vertebral body inevitably leads to vertebral collapse and a secondary kyphotic spinal deformity [37–39]. Involvement of the posterior vertebral elements in spinal TB is rare but is more common with discitis from other etiologies [40]. The incidence of isolated posterior element involvement is estimated to be around 10% [41].

Spinal TB is often expressed at different vertebral levels, which can be contiguous or not [35, 37, 38]. The lumbar spine and lower thoracic spine are the most affected segments [34–37, 40, 42, 43]. Spinal TB progresses with destructive and marked osteopenia associated with lytic lesions, very little sclerosis, and poor evidence of periosteal reaction (Fig 32.3) [17]. TB infection expands into adjacent structures in 75–90% of all musculoskeletal cases. Paravertebral involvement

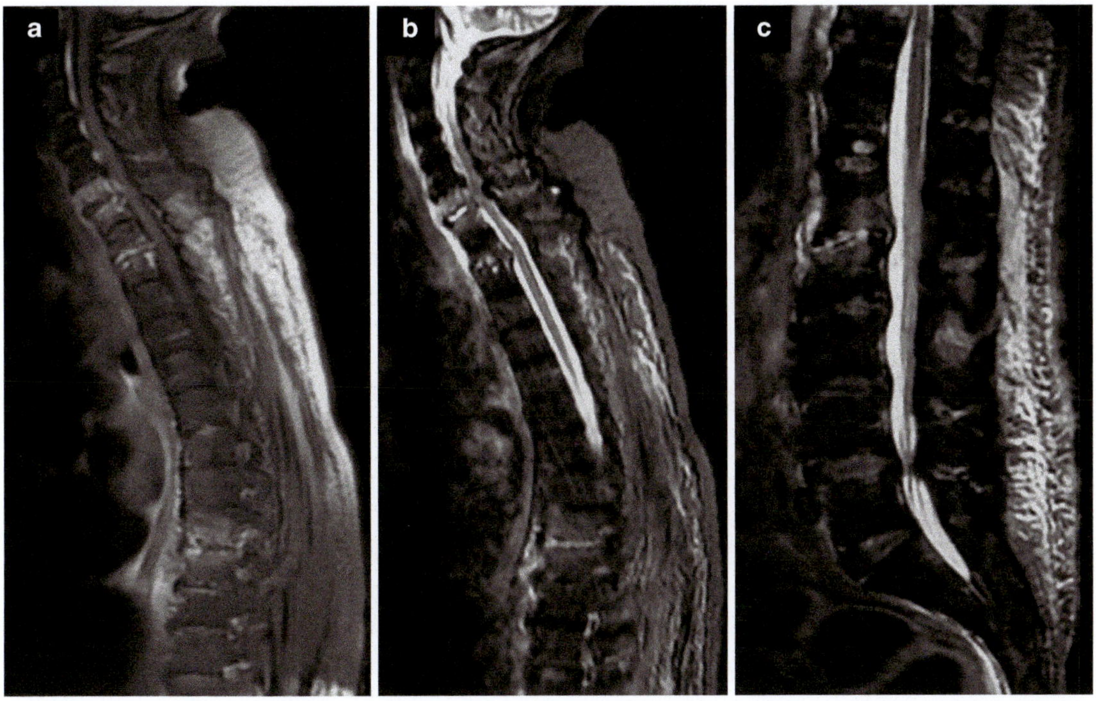

Fig. 32.2 Multiple TB spondylodiscitis at cervical, thoracic, and lumbar levels. Spinal MRI sagittal views on T1-weighted image after gadolinium injection (**a**) and on STIR sequences (**b, c**) (Courtesy of Pr. Ali Akhaddar, MD, IFAANS)

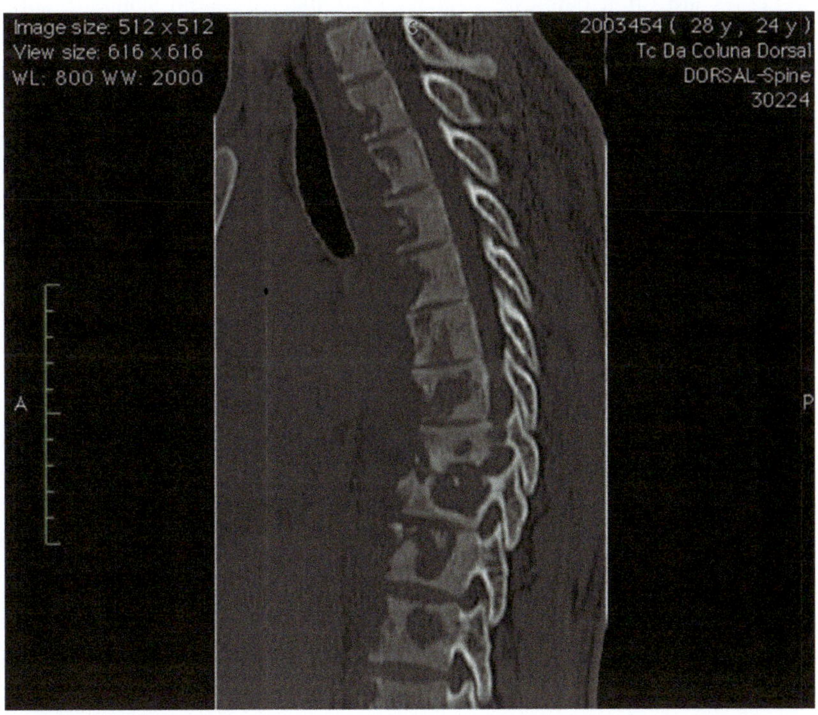

Fig. 32.3 Sagittal CT scan image showing extensive vertebral destructive lytic lesions due to contiguous TB infection. Note the lack of sclerosis and poor evidence of periosteal reaction as is characteristic in spinal TB

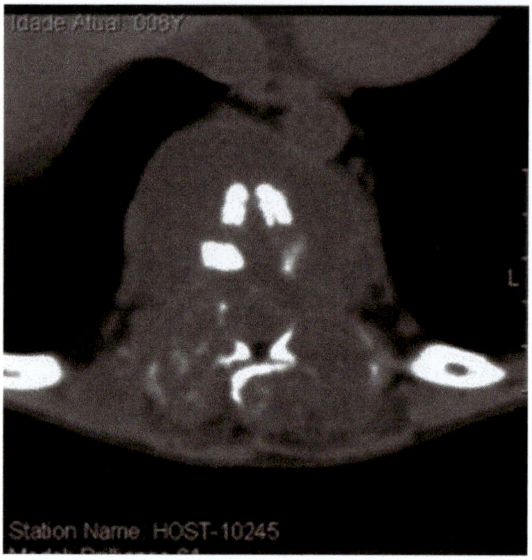

Fig. 32.4 CT scan with axial image showing paravertebral thoracic abscess as a characteristic posterior mediastinal mass, with less frequently seen extensive posterior spreading in a six-year-old child with multilevel disease

may appear in the thoracic region as posterior mediastinal masses (Fig. 32.4) and in the abdominopelvic region as iliopsoas masses [44]. These abscesses are often painless, with no systemic manifestations even in advanced stages. Calcifications may appear inside the abscess; though this is rare, it is very suggestive of TB spondylodiscitis [34, 37, 38, 45].

Paravertebral abscesses are more common in spinal TB, when compared with other etiologies. The acute nature and clinical signs/symptoms associated with pyogenic abscesses allow these to be more easily diagnosed, thereby reducing the incidence of paravertebral masses [46]. Additionally, pyogenic abscesses almost never present with calcifications [46]. Another feature, which is characteristic of spinal TB, especially with abscess formation, is anterior detachment of the lumbar segmentary vessels [34, 47]. On radiography, TB abscesses can assume a fusiform, globular, or dumbbell-shaped form, most visible in the thoracic region. When a sharp point breaks the rounded outline of an abscess shadow, lung penetration should be suspected [48].

Radiographic findings in patients with spinal TB depend on the extent and duration of infection. The first radiographs may appear entirely normal, but CT scans and MRIs are more sensitive in detecting TB lesions in their early stages [49]. An MRI can demonstrate both sparing of the IVD and any involvement of the vertebral bodies to either side of the IVD. Paravertebral/iliopsoas or epidural abscesses, nerve root compression, and/or compression of the spinal cord is also demonstrated most clearly using MRI studies (Fig. 32.5) [50].

32.6 Surgical Indications

It is well known that chemotherapy is the primary method of management of spinal TB. However, when a patient presents with kyphosis, a cold abscess, and neurological compromise (especially in an acute setting), surgical intervention can be indicated [51–53]. Unfortunately, there is no current consensus regarding standardized surgical treatment for spinal TB [51].

Although medical treatment is recognized as the gold standard, surgical procedures still hold an important place in management of spinal TB [54]. Despite this, a recent Cochrane review compared utilizing surgery and chemotherapy versus the use of chemotherapy alone and concluded that there was no significant benefit from the routine use of surgery [54]. It should be noted that patients with three or more vertebrae involved were not included in the early Medical Research Council studies. Several studies have also suggested that instability, the probability of deformity, and advancement to neurological deficit are consistent and parallel with the size of the vertebral anomalies. Complex TB lesions are also a potential indication for surgical intervention to stabilize the spine [55–57].

The accepted indications for surgical treatment have long been a need for decompression of the spinal cord despite medical treatment, posterior spinal lesions, failure of three months of nonoperative treatment, an uncertain diagnosis, or recurrence of disease [58]. In fact, according to

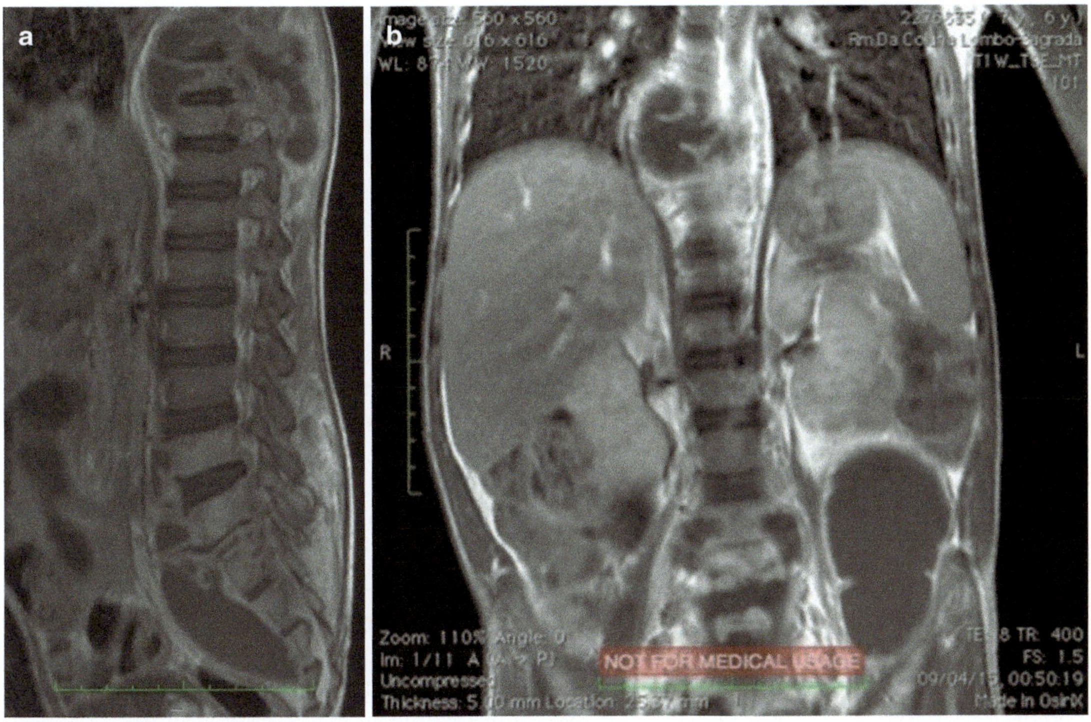

Fig. 32.5 Sagittal (**a**) and coronal; (**b**) T1-weighted MRI after gadolinium injection showing noncontiguous spinal TB with multiple thoracic left iliopsoas and pre-lumbosacral abscess with characteristic thick walls

Moon et al., surgery potentiates early healing by debriding the affected area, allowing histological assay of the disease, shortening the duration of chemotherapy, and reducing late recurrence rates [59]. Surgery also corrects or prevents spinal deformity, encourages early neurological recovery, and meets patient aesthetic demands [59].

The presence of abscesses, larger abscesses in particular, can be considered a relative indication for surgery. In 78 patients with deep-seated abscesses, as presented by Tuli, 68% of abscesses disappeared with conservative treatment, 16% regressed to a consistent size, 14% appeared calcified, and only 2% required surgical drainage because of complications [58]. In summary, lesions that present with limited destruction of the vertebrae, small abscesses, an absence of progressive spinal cord or nerve root compromise, and no MDR-TB can be treated conservatively [51]. Surgery is indicated when there is persistent pain due to instability of the spine, severe or progressing neurologic dysfunction due to spinal cord compression by paravertebral or epidural abscesses, multilevel disease involving several vertebral bodies, extensive abscess, and poor outcome following conservative treatment [47, 51].

32.7 Surgical Treatment

Treatment guidelines for noncontiguous spinal TB have been garnered from the experiences of the practitioners treating it. Surgical intervention may be indicated for patients who have severe/evolving neurological deficits despite treatment with anti-TB chemotherapy, those with persisting symptoms after adequate anti-TB therapies, and those with spinal instability and/or severe spinal deformity [60].

Surgery for multilevel, noncontiguous spinal TB most often causes more surgical trauma and a higher number of complications than surgery for single-focus TB disease. Surgical trauma inevitably resulting from the multilevel approaches must be limited by addressing the lesions with a very clear surgical plan, by using minimally invasive techniques and by utilizing partial debridement rather than more extensive surgery. Priority must be given to the most proximal lesions or the ones causing neuraxial compression, and procedures can be staged in sequence for patients with physiological deterioration [60].

There are a variety of surgical approaches for spinal TB. The approach may be anterior or posterior, or a combination of techniques, performed in several stages. Anterior radical debridement and strut graft fusion, known as the Hong Kong operation has been for a long time the standard technique. A preponderance of literature demonstrates that this approach is clinically effective though the incidence of spinal instability can be high. Complementary posterior instrumentation may be required [60].

Posterior approaches are increasingly preferred in the treatment of spinal TB. Surgeons are gaining familiarity with posterolateral thoracic approaches, pedicular subtraction osteotomies, and vertebral posterior resections. These techniques enable surgeons to perform adequate anterior debridement and provide better posterior stabilization with less morbidity [60–65].

32.8 Surgical Outcomes

There is very little published about treating noncontiguous spinal TB with surgery. In 2012, Shi et al. published a report regarding 29 cases of noncontiguous spinal TB which were treated with focal surgery [66]. A mean correction rate of 59.5% was realized with good bony fusion in the final follow-up radiographs. Zhang et al. also reported in 2012 regarding the results of posterior transforaminal thoracic debridement, limited decompression, interbody fusion, and posterior instrumentation for noncontiguous thoracic TB. Good clinical outcomes were also achieved there [61]. Huang et al. analyzed the outcomes from surgical treatment in 23 cases of noncontiguous spinal TB and concluded that both posterior and posterior-anterior surgical approaches were viable options [60]. The aforementioned techniques of posterior transforaminal debridement, interbody fusion, and posterior instrumentation as a less invasive technique are possible and efficacious for treating multilevel TB infection [60]. We have also found several case reports showing good results in noncontiguous spinal TB after surgical treatment, including cases with neurological deficits [10–14].

In patients with extensive spinal involvement, surgical treatment may cause dramatic improvement, as in the severe instances presented by Emel et al. and Turgut [10–13]. Early surgical intervention for patients with multilevel spinal TB with large abscesses (and with systemic TB) is probably recommended after ancillary support has been provided to the patient [10].

32.9 Complications

Considering that TB spinal infection is generally focused in the anterior column, an anterior approach gives direct access for debridement [67–69]. Classical anterior procedures have had problems such as higher morbidity, anesthetic complications, injuries to blood vessels, grafting failures, and inadequate fixations due to osteopenic bone [69–72]. In addition, there is evidence that a singular anterior procedure cannot appreciably correct a spinal TB deformity. Several authors have suggested that posterior instrumentation should be added in cases of multilevel spondylitis, to stop continued progression of deformation and anterior implant failure [73–75].

Alam et al. reported on a multicenter study of surgical experiences with 582 patients who had spinal TB [67]. Seven cases (1.2%) had superficial infections and four cases (0.7%) had deep infections [67]. Revision surgery was performed on six patients (1.0%), implant failure occurred in four cases (0.7%), and malpositioning of screws occurred in 12 cases (2.1%) [67]. Perioperative bleeding complications were reported in four patients (0.7%). Neurological improvement occurred in all patients except two (0.3%). There was also one patient who had a vascular injury of the thoracic aorta [67].

Although we do not have strong evidence regarding the rates of complication where there is multilevel involvement, available literature seems not to show increased rates of complication compared to single-level involvement. Problems are more dictated by the presentation of the most severe lesions, and rates can be compared with those of the contiguous presentation.

Conclusion

Multifocal spinal TB, a less frequent presentation of spinal TB, can be a diagnostic challenge and present a therapeutic dilemma. This presentation requires full spinal imaging to rule out different levels of seeding in the spine and using radiographs, CT scanning, or, more preferably, MRI. Metastatic disease or septic spondylodiscitis should be on the list of differential diagnoses, and integration of other imaging in association with blood samples can help establish a correct diagnosis.

Although multifocal spinal TB was initially considered a manifestation of an immune-compromised or debilitated host, or even a fulminant form of TB, available literature and our experiences do not support this. Most cases come from areas where TB is endemic; in fact, multifocal spinal TB may even be a rather indolent form of the disease with late presentation and concomitant significant spinal involvement.

This disease presents a therapeutic dilemma because, by itself, without the usual indications for surgical treatment, it can be treated conservatively although the threshold for cervical drainage and stabilization should be low. If one or more lesions require a surgical approach, surgery should follow a protocol for solving the neurological deficits from proximal to distal, preferably at the mechanically unstable levels first. Then less aggressive intervention can be planned with one-stage or two-stage procedures to minimize the surgical impact. It is to be expected that complications will arise when addressing more than one lesion surgically at a time, because of the risk inherent in each approach. If surgical treatment of multilevel spinal TB is successful, the outcome will be dictated by the remaining neurological deficit or any symptomatic kyphotic deformity. This is not significantly different from what is published in the literature for the treatment of contiguous spinal TB lesions.

References

1. Garg RK, Somvanshi DS (2011) Spinal tuberculosis: a review. J Spinal Cord Med 34:440–454
2. Jain AK (2010) Tuberculosis of the spine a fresh look at an old disease. J Bone Joint Surg Br 92:905–913
3. Jain AK, Dhammi IK (2007) Tuberculosis of the spine: a review. Clin Orthop Relat Res 460:39–49
4. Guerado E, Cerván AM (2012) Surgical treatment of spondylodiscitis. An update. Int Orthop 36:413–420
5. Neher A, Kopp W, Berna G, Frank J, Kohlhäufl M (2007) Advanced multifocal tuberculous spondylitis without disk involvement and with multidrug-resistant bacilli. Clin Infect Dis 45:E109–E112
6. Hong L, Wu JG, Ding JG, Wang XY, Zheng MH, Fu RQ, Sun QF (2010) Multifocal skeletal tuberculosis: experience in diagnosis and treatment. Med Mal Infect 40:6–11
7. Baba H, Tagami A, Adachi S, Hiura T, Osaki M (2013) Tuberculosis affecting multiple vertebral bodies. Asian Spine J 7:222–226
8. Zhang H, Jin D (2003) Multiple cystic tuberculous lesions in the skeleton (Jüngling Disease): a case report. Spine 28:E155–E157
9. Polley P, Dunn R (2009) Noncontiguous spinal tuberculosis: incidence and management. Eur Spine J 18:1096–1101
10. Emel E, Güzey FK, Güzey D, Bas NS, Sel B, Alatas I (2006) Non-contiguous multifocal spinal tuberculosis involving cervical, thoracic, lumbar and sacral segments: a case report. Eur Spine J 15:1019–1024
11. Hasegawa K, Murata H, Naitoh K, Nagano A (2002) Spinal tuberculosis: report of an atypical presentation. Clin Orthop Relat Res 403:100–103
12. Kim SJ, Seok JW, Kim IJ, Kim YK, Kim DS (2003) Multifocal Pott's disease (tuberculous spondylitis) incidentally detected on Tc-99 m MDP bone and Ga-67 citrate scintigraphy in a patient with diabetes. Clin Nucl Med 28:286–289
13. Turgut M (2001) Multifocal extensive spinal tuberculosis (Pott's disease) involving cervical, thoracic and lumbar vertebrae. Br J Neurosurg 15:142–146
14. Uno M, Kamijo T, Oda T, Arima K, Suzuki A, Obana M, Irimajiri S (1994) A case report of atypical tuberculous spondylitis. Kansen Shigaku Zasshi Jpn J Infect Dis 68:982–985
15. Rezai AR, Lee M, Cooper PR, Errico TJ, Koslow M (1995) Modern management of spinal tuberculosis. Neurosurgery 36:87–98

16. Nussbaum ES, Rockswold GL, Bergman TA, Erickson DL, Seljeskog EL (1995) Spinal tuberculosis: a diagnostic and management challenge. J Neurosurg 83:243–247
17. Lindahl S, Nyman RS, Brismar J, Hugosson C, Lundstedt C (1996) Imaging of tuberculosis: IV. Spinal manifestations in 63 patients. Acta Radiol 37:506–511
18. Pandit HG, Sonsale PD, Shikare SS, Bhojraj SY (1999) Bone scintigraphy in tuberculousspondylodiscitis. Eur Spine J 8:205–209
19. Kim JH, Kim SH, Choi JI, Lim DJ (2014) Atypical noncontiguous multiple spinal tuberculosis: a case report. Korean J Spine 11:77–80
20. Mousa HAL (2003) Multifocal spinal tuberculosis associated with paraplegia. Emirates Med J 21:182–185
21. Rajasekaran S, Shanmugasundaram TK, Prabhakar R, Dheenadhayalan J, Shetty AP, Shetty DK (1998) Tuberculous lesions of the lumbosacral region; a 15-year follow-up patients treated by ambulant chemotherapy. Spine 23:1163–1167
22. Meghji S, White PA, Nair SP, Reddi K, Heron K, Henderson B, Zaliani A, Fossati G, Mascagni P, Hunt JF, Roberts MM, Coates AR (1997) Mycobacterium tuberculosis chaperanin 10 stimulates bone resorption: a potential contributory factor in Pott's disease. J Exp Med 186:1241–1246
23. Bambynek C, Lemmens P, Adriaensan P (1990) Pott's tuberculous spondylitis in Belgium 1990. Acta Clin Belg 1992:277–279
24. Chapman M, Murray RO, Stoker DJ (1979) Tuberculosis of the bones and joints. In Seminars in Roentgenology, WB Saunders 14:266–282
25. Joseffer SS, Cooper PR (2005) Modern imaging of spinal tuberculosis. J Neurosurg 2:145–150
26. Turgut M (1997) Intradural tuberculous granuloma (letter). Br J Neurosurg 11:264–266
27. Hsu LCS, Leong JCY (1984) Tuberculosis of the lower cervical spine (C2 to C7). J Bone Joint Surg Br 66:1–5
28. Griffith JF, Kumta SM, Leung PC, Cheng JC, Chow LT, Metreweli C (2002) Imaging of musculoskeletal tuberculosis: a new look at an old disease. Clin Orthop Relat Res 398:32–39
29. Pande KC, Babhulkar SS (2002) Atypical spinal tuberculosis. Clin Orthop Relat Res 398:67–74
30. Buchelt M, Lack W, Kutschera HP, Katterschafka T, Kiss H, Schneider B, Kotz R (1993) Comparison of tuberculous and pyogenic spondylitis: an analysis of 122 cases. Clin Orthop Relat Res 296:192–199
31. Mousa HL (1998) Tuberculosis of bones and joints: diagnostic approaches. Int Orthop 22:245–246
32. Zahraa J, Johnson D, Lim-Dunham JE, Herold BC (1996) Unusual features of osteoarticular tuberculosis in children. J Pediatr 129:597–602
33. Bell GR, Stearns KL, Bonutti PM, Boumphrey FR (1990) MRI diagnosis of tuberculous vertebral osteomyelitis. Spine 15:462–465
34. Afonso PD, Almeida A (2011) Tuberculous spondilodiskitis: imaging features. Acta Med Port 24:349–354
35. Leonard MK, Blumberg HM (2006) Musculoskeletal tuberculosis. In: Schlossberg D (ed) Tuberculosis & nontuberculous mycobacterial infections. McGraw-Hill, New York, pp 242–264
36. Helms C, Major N, Andersson M, Kaplan P, Dussault R (2009) Spine. In: Musculoskeletal MRI. Durhan, Philadelphia, pp 293–295
37. Engin G, Acunas B, Acunas G, Tunaci M (2000) Imaging of Extrapulmonary Tuberculosis 1: (CME available in print version and on RSNA Link). Radiographics 20:471–488
38. Mukesh GH, Theresa CM, Jo-Anne OS, Jane PK, Manohar MS, Peter RM (2000) Tuberculosis from head to toe. Radiographics 20:449–470
39. Tay BK, Deckey J, Hu SS (2002) Spinal infections. J Am Acad Orthop Surg 10:188–197
40. Randy Jinkins J (2002) Magnetic resonance imaging of spinal infectious disease: pathophysiologic concepts of origin and spread. Acta Clin Croat 41:29–30
41. Vilar FC, Neves FF, Colares JKB, Fonseca BL (2006) Tuberculose vertebral (doença de Pott) associada a abscesso de psoas: relato de doiscasos e revisão da literatura. Rev Soc Bras Med Trop 30:278–282
42. Do Brito JS, Batista N, Tirado A, Fernandes P (2013) Surgical treatment of spinal tuberculosis: an orthopedic service experience. Acta Med Port 26:349–356
43. Park DW, Sohn JW, Kim EH, Cho DI, Lee JH, Kim KT, Kim MJ (2007) Outcome and management of spinal tuberculosis according to the severity of disease: a retrospective study of 137 adult patients at Korean teaching hospitals. Spine 32:E130–E135
44. Sanal HT, Kocaoglu M, Sehirlioglu A, Bulakbasi N (2006) A rare cause of flank mass: psoas abscess due to extensive primary thoracolumbar tuberculous spondylodiskitis. Am J Neuroradiol 27:1735–1737
45. Benli T, Kaya A (2005) New concepts in the treatment of Pott's disease. J Turkish Spinal Surg 16:11–34
46. Grossman RK, Yousem DM (2003) Non-degenerative diseases of the Spine. In: Neuroradiology requisites. Mosby, Philadelphia, pp 795–796
47. Do Brito JS, Tirado A, Fernandes P (2014) Surgical treatment of spinal tuberculosis complicated with extensive abscess. Iowa Orthop J 34:129–136
48. Hodgson AR, Bailey HL, Gabriel M, Shin JS (2006) The classic: tuberculosis of the spine in children. Clin Orthop Relat Res 444:16–26
49. Gehlot PS, Chaturvedi S, Kashyap R, Singh V (2012) Pott's spine: retrospective analysis of MRI scans of 70 cases. J Clin Diagn Res 6:1534–1538
50. Isada C (2004) Spinal tuberculosis deserves a place on the radar screen. Cleve Clin J Med 71:537–539
51. Yin XH, Liu SH, Li JS, Chen Y, Hu XK, Zeng KF, Zhang HQ (2015) The role of costotransverse radical debridement, fusion and postural drainage in the surgical treatment of multisegmental thoracic spinal tuberculosis: a minimum 5-year follow-up. Eur Spine J 25:1047–1055
52. Acikgoz B, Ozcan OE, Belen D, Erbengi A, Ozgen T (1991) Surgery for progressive Pott's paraplegia (tuberculous paraplegia). Paraplegia 29:537–541

53. Ferro RM, Barnaud P, Carayon A (1978) Pott's disease in African (author's transl). Medecinetropicale: revue du Corps de sante colonial 39:191–208
54. Jutte PC, Van Loenhout-Rooyackers JH (2006) Routine surgery in addition to chemotherapy for treating spinal tuberculosis. Cochrane Database Syst Rev 25:CD004532
55. Korkusuz F, Islam C, Korkusuz Z (1997) Prevention of postoperative late kyphosis in Pott's disease by anterior decompression and intervertebral grafting. World J Surg 21:524–528
56. Rajasekaran S (2002) The problem of deformity in spinal tuberculosis. Clin Orthop Relat Res 398:85–92
57. Rajasekaran S, Shanmugasundaram TK (1987) Prediction of the angle of gibbus deformity in tuberculosis of the spine. J Bone Joint Surg Am 69: 503–509
58. Tuli SM (1975) Results of treatment of spinal tuberculosis by" middle-path" regime. J Bone Joint Surg Br 57:13–23
59. Moon MS (2014) Tuberculosis of spine: current views in diagnosis and management. Asian Spine J 8:97–111
60. Huang J, Zhang H, Zeng K, Gao Q (2014) The clinical outcomes of surgical treatment of noncontiguous spinal tuberculosis: a retrospective study in 23 cases. PLoS One 9:E93648
61. Zhang HQ, Lin MZ, Shen KY, Ge L, Li JS, Tang MX, Liu JY (2012) Surgical management for multilevel noncontiguous thoracic spinal tuberculosis by single-stage posterior transforaminal thoracic debridement, limited decompression, interbody fusion, and posterior instrumentation (modified TTIF). Arch Orthop Trauma Surg 132:751–757
62. Yamasaki R, Okuda S, Maeno T, Haku T, Iwasaki M, Oda T (2013) Surgical outcomes of posterior thoracic interbody fusion for thoracic disc herniations. Eur Spine J 22:2496–2503
63. Machino M, Yukawa Y, Ito K, Nakashima H, Kato F (2010) A new thoracic reconstruction technique "transforaminal thoracic interbody fusion": a preliminary report of clinical outcomes. Spine 35:E1000–E1005
64. Zaveri GR, Mehta SS (2009) Surgical treatment of lumbar tuberculousspondylodiscitis by transforaminal lumbar interbody fusion (TLIF) and posterior instrumentation. J Spinal Disord Tech 22:257–262
65. Zhang HQ, Lin MZ, Li JS, Tang MX, Guo CF, Wu JH, Liu JY (2013) One-stage posterior debridement, transforaminal lumbar interbody fusion and instrumentation in treatment of lumbar spinal tuberculosis: a retrospective case series. Arch Orthop Trauma Surg 133:333–341
66. Shi JD, Wang ZL, Geng GQ, Niu NK (2012) Intervertebral focal surgery for the treatment of non-contiguous multifocal spinal tuberculosis. Int Orthop 36:1423–1427
67. Alam MS, Phan K, Karim R, Jonayed SA, Munir HKM, Chakraborty S, Alam T (2015) Surgery for spinal tuberculosis: a multi-center experience of 582 cases. J Spine Surg 1:65–71
68. Turgut M (2001) Spinal tuberculosis (Pott's disease): its clinical presentation, surgical management, and outcome. A survey study on 694 patients. Neurosurg Rev 24:8–13
69. Özdemir HM, Us AK, Ögün T (2003) The role of anterior spinal instrumentation and allograft fibula for the treatment of pott disease. Spine 28:474–479
70. Benli İ, Acaroğlu E, Akalin S, Kiş M, Duman E, Ün A (2003) Anterior radical debridement and anterior instrumentation in tuberculosis spondylitis. Eur Spine J 12:224–234
71. Yilmaz C, Selek HY, Gürka I, Erdemli B, Korkusuz Z (1999) Anterior instrumentation for the treatment of spinal tuberculosis. J Bone Joint Surg Am 81:1261–1267
72. Hodgson AR, Stock FE (1960) Anterior spine fusion for the treatment of tuberculosis of the spine. J Bone Joint Surg Am 42:295–310
73. Sundararaj GD, Behera S, Ravi V, Venkatesh K, Cherian VM, Lee V (2003) Role of posterior stabilisation in the management of tuberculosis of the dorsal and lumbar spine. J Bone Joint Surg Br 85:100–106
74. Talu U, Gogus A, Ozturk C, Hamzaoglu A, Domanic U (2006) The role of posterior instrumentation and fusion after anterior radical debridement and fusion in the surgical treatment of spinal tuberculosis: experience of 127 cases. J Spinal Disord Tech 19:554–559
75. Qureshi MA, Khalique AB, Afzal W, Pasha IF, Aebi M (2013) Surgical management of contiguous multilevel thoracolumbar tuberculous spondylitis. Eur Spine J 22:618–623

Concurrent Occurrence of Brain Tuberculoma Along with Spinal Cord Tuberculoma

33

Özüm Tunçyürek, Mehmet Turgut, Elif Karadeli, Yelda Özsunar, and Ahmet T. Turgut

Contents

Ö. Tunçyürek, MD (✉) • Y. Özsunar, MD
Department of Radiology, Adnan Menderes University School of Medicine, Aydın, Turkey
e-mail: ozum.tuncyurek@gmail.com; yeldaozsunar@gmail.com

M. Turgut, MD, PhD
Department of Neurosurgery, Adnan Menderes University School of Medicine, Aydın, Turkey
e-mail: drmturgut@yahoo.com

E. Karadeli, MD
Department of Radiology, Baskent University, School of Medicine, Dr. Turgut Noyan Medical and Research Center, Adana, Turkey
e-mail: elifkaradeli@gmail.com

A.T. Turgut, MD
Department of Radiology, Hacettepe University School of Medicine, Ankara, Turkey
e-mail: ahmettuncayturgut@yahoo.com

Abbreviations

ADC	Apparent diffusion coefficient
CNS	Central nervous system
CSF	Cerebrospinal fluid
CT	Computed tomography
DWI	Diffusion-weighted imaging
FLAIR	Fluid-attenuated inversion recovery
IICP	Increased intracranial pressure
MRI	Magnetic resonance imaging
RA	Rheumatoid arthritis
TB	Tuberculosis
TBM	Tuberculous meningitis

33.1 Introduction

Today tuberculosis (TB) still maintains its historical significance. It is caused by its drug-resistant forms, and the widespread occurrence of the disease within the community is closely associated with increased prevalence of diseases causing immune system deficiencies like acquired immune deficiency syndrome, known as AIDS. The increased incidence of non-pulmonary TB parallels the increase in various diseases requiring treatments which particularly suppress the immune system. Ileocecal, lymph node and central nervous system (CNS) involvement are frequent types of non-pulmonary TB.

Involvement of the CNS occurs in 1–5% of all TB patients. Every year, over one million new

M. Turgut et al. (eds.), *Tuberculosis of the Central Nervous System*,
DOI 10.1007/978-3-319-50712-5_33

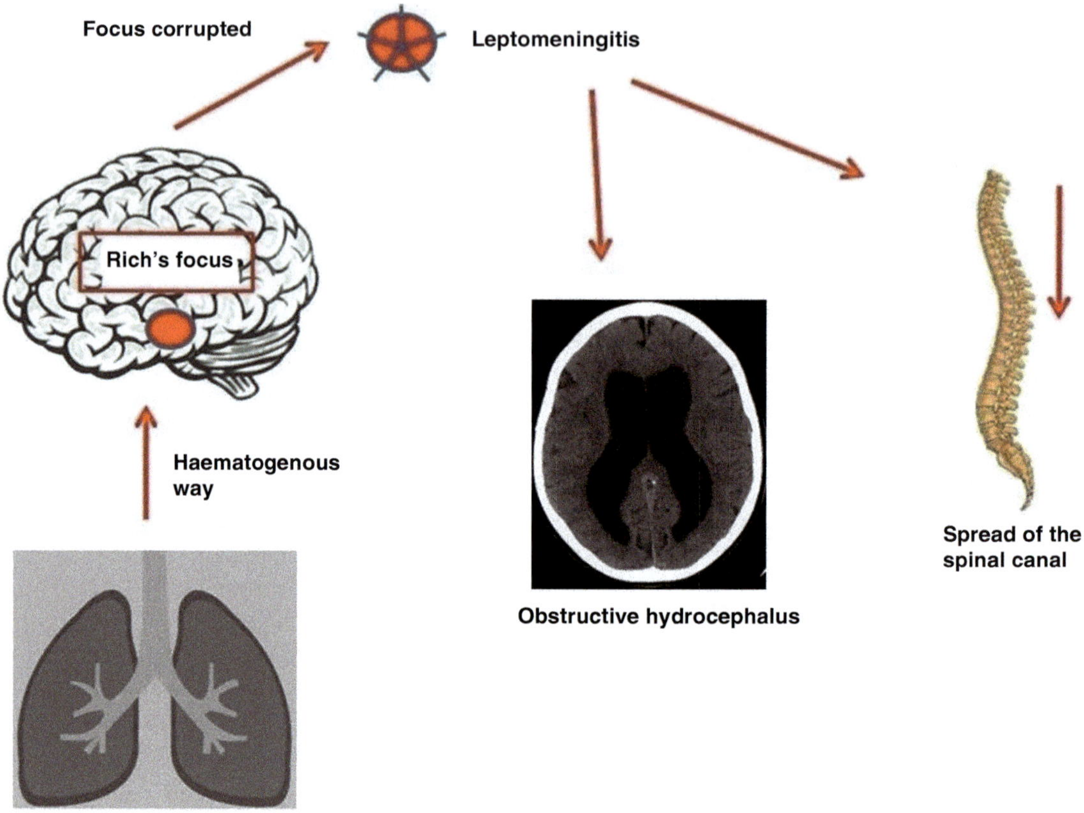

Fig. 33.1 The development of TB of the central nervous system is seen schematically

cases of TB are diagnosed. Spinal TB occurs in approximately 2% of these patients [1]. Meningitis, focal cerebritis, tuberculomas and abscesses are the most common lesions [2]. In addition, myelitis and intramedullary tuberculomas can be seen, despite being relatively rare. Fortunately, the sensitivity of magnetic resonance imaging (MRI) for depicting the lesions is high.

TB which spreads through haematogenous route results in small Rich's focus involving the subependymal portion of the brain, which is the main source of the disease. The picture of leptomeningitis occurs when the granuloma loses its integrity. This proceeds and leads to obstructive hydrocephalus (Fig. 33.1). Immune resistance is crucial, and Th1 cells play an important role in the defence mechanism against infectious process caused by intracellular TB bacteria. The developmental mechanism in immune-suppressed cases results in the formation of an abscess. Hydrocephalus, vasculitis, acute infarct and cranial nerve involvement may also be seen in these cases. Radiologically, diffusion-weighted imaging (DWI) and apparent diffusion coefficient (ADC) mapping are critical for the evaluation of acute infarct (Figs. 33.2 and 33.3). The diagnosis of concomitant brain and spinal cord tuberculoma is very important for planning of proper treatment.

33.2 Pathology

33.2.1 Tuberculous Meningitis

This condition is usually caused by the rupture of a subependymal tubercle into the subarachnoid space rather than direct haematogenous seeding.

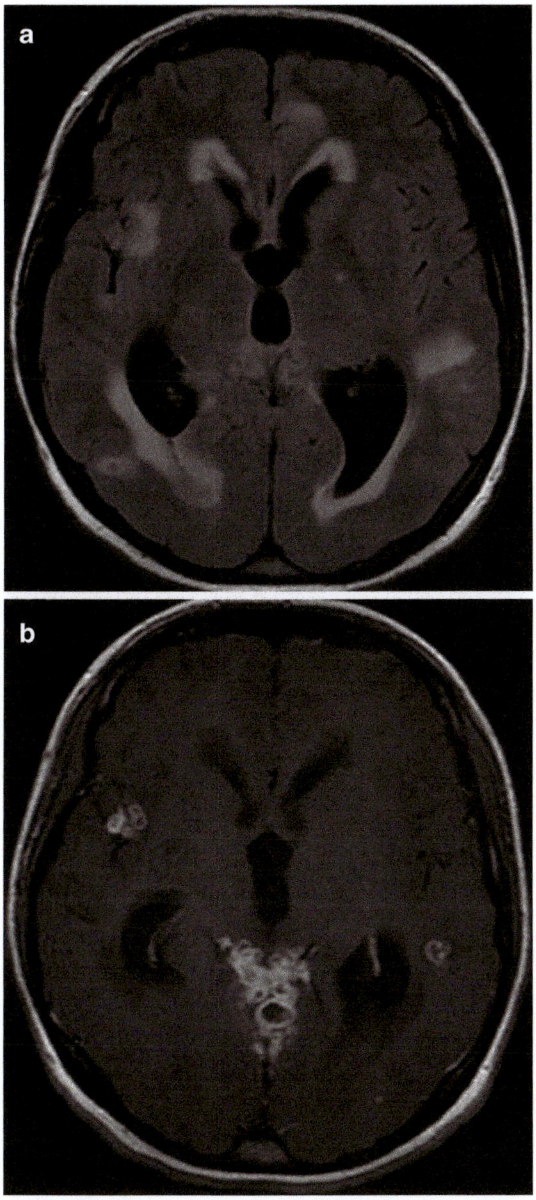

Fig. 33.2 Axial FLAIR (**a**) and contrast-enhanced T1-weighted images (**b**) show hydrocephalus and tuberculomas (Courtesy of I. Sebnem Orguc)

During childhood, meningitis is an early postprimary event, and three fourths of these individuals have a concurrently active primary complex, pleural effusion or miliary TB. Historically, Charcot ve Joffroy first defined this entity in spinal meninges [3]. Its rare cranial form is defined as TB- or syphilis-induced. On the other hand, Naffziger ve Stern [4] defined the idiopathic hypertrophic cranial pachymeningitis.

TB-induced craniospinal hypertrophic pachymeningitis was first described in 1991 by Okimura et al. [5]. In 1994, Yamashita et al. [6] reported a case with posterior fossa and high cervical spinal involvement. Clinically, symptoms of increased intracranial pressure (IICP) are seen in all these cases. In some cases, the 12th cranial nerve palsy, cerebellar ataxia and findings of myelopathy may be present. Besides TB, this entity may not only be idiopathic but also can occur in syphilis, fungal infections, sarcoidosis, Wegener's granulomatosis, rheumatoid arthritis (RA), mucopolysaccharidosis and multifocal fibrosclerosis [6]. Nevertheless, the coexistence of cranial and spinal involvement is seen in the idiopathic form and RA.

Radiologically, a hypertrophic dura mater is seen on computed tomography (CT) and MRI, where contrast enhancement is evident. Also, a T2 hyperintense rim may be seen at the periphery of the lesion that is isointense on T1- and hypointense on T2-weighted images and fluid-attenuated inversion recovery (FLAIR) images. Tuberculous meningitis (TBM) affects basal cisterns (Fig. 33.4). Importantly, the exudate in the basal cisterns can cause obstruction to CSF flow, causing hydrocephalus, and can compress certain cranial nerves.

33.2.2 Solitary Tuberculoma

The majority of solitary tuberculomas are located in the intracranial compartment. However, intradural extramedullary tuberculoma of the spinal cord is extremely rare [7]. Tuberculomas are rigid, non-vascular, caseous bulk of variable size ranging from around 1 to 4 cm. Lesions may occur on all spaces of the CNS.

Intraspinal tuberculomas are usually associated with intracranial involvement [8]. In the case series reported by Parmar et al. [9], a spinal tuberculoma and the left cerebellar tuberculoma

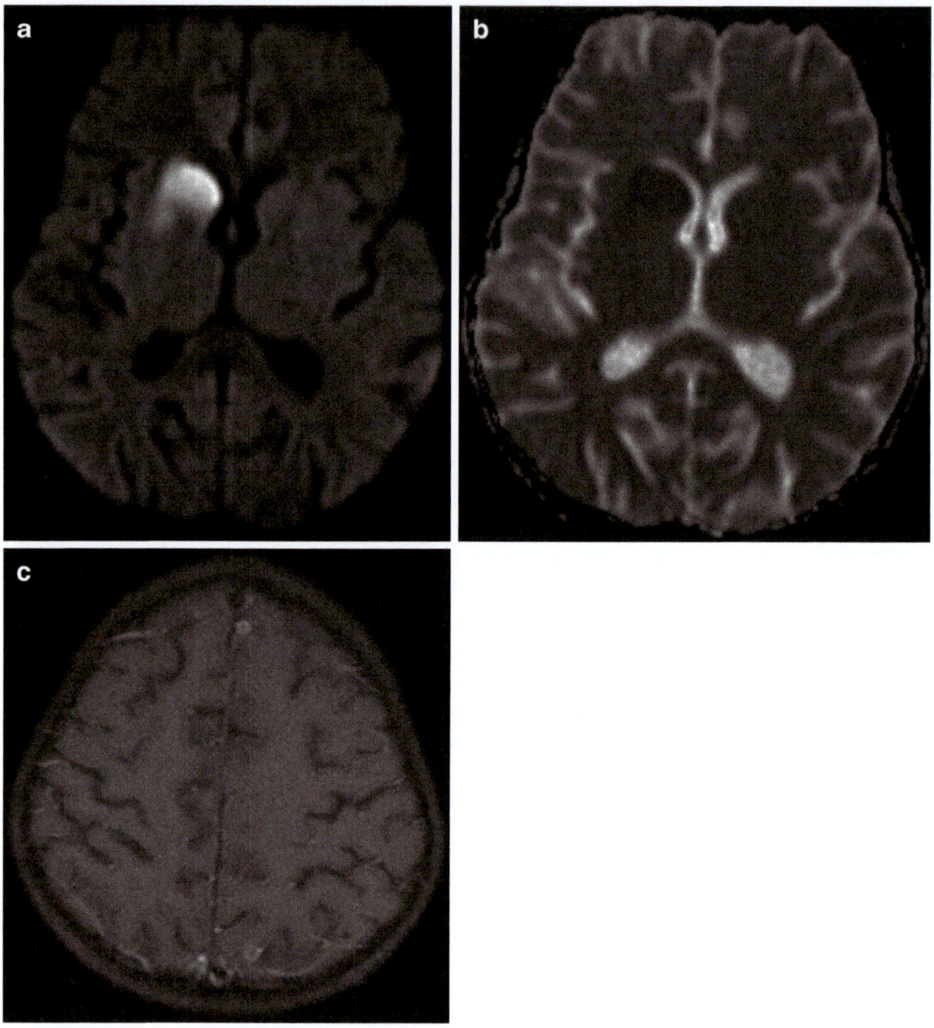

Fig. 33.3 Acute infarct in the right basal ganglia is seen hyperintense on diffusion-weighted MRI (**a**) and hypointense on ADC image (**b**). In addition, there are some tuberculomas on fat-suppressed contrast-enhanced T1-weighted image (**c**)

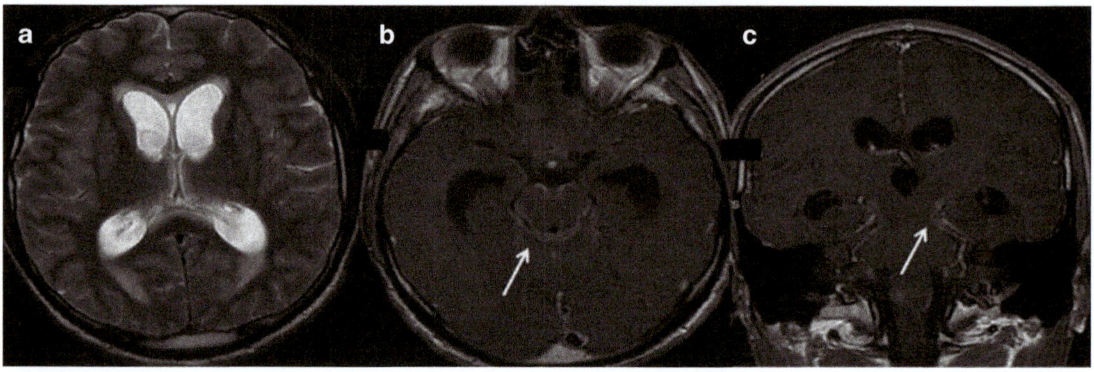

Fig. 33.4 MRI revealing TBM affecting basal cisterns (*arrow*). Hydrocephalus is seen on T2-weighted image (**a**), while pachymeningitis is seen on axial (**b**) and coronal (**c**) contrast-enhanced T1-weighted images (Courtesy of I. Sebnem Orguc)

were coexisting only in one case. In a report by Bucy and Oberhill, the lesions were also present elsewhere in the CNS in three cases out of the six cases with a spinal cord tuberculoma [10]. Multiple intracranial tuberculomas are seen at about 10–33% of the cases, whereas multiple spinal lesions are rarer [8]. Concurrent intracranial and intramedullary TBs are extremely uncommon and mostly described in immunocompromised patients [11] (Figs. 33.5 and 33.6).

In 1990, a total of three cases with concurrent intracranial and intramedullary tuberculomas were noted in a literature review by MacDonnel et al. [12]. Later, a case with both intracranial and intramedullary lesions was reported by Sharma et al. [13]. In 2007, Muthukumar et al. presented the paradoxical codevelopment of an intradural extramedullary spinal tuberculoma and multiple intracranial tuberculomas in a 21-year-old case with TBM despite the application of anti-TB therapy [14, 15]. Especially during TBM, intramedullary TB paradoxically occurs under anti-TB therapy, which is an immune response to the release of the tuberculoprotein. The destruction of bacilli increases lymphocytic proliferation, thereby enabling the inapparent tuberculomas to appear [16, 17]. Intramedullary TB develops primarily in the spinal cord or secondarily from the focus elsewhere in the body. Secondary intramedullary TBs are caused by the haematogenous inoculation of the bacilli into the cord substance or less commonly via the CSF flowing across the central canal [11]. In another report by Das et al., a patient was shown to have a cerebellar tuberculoma in addition to the cervical intramedullary lesion [11].

The imaging features of intramedullary TB lesions were shown to resemble those of intracranial lesions by Parmar et al. [9]. TB may have spinal involvement with myelitis, meningitis and arachnoiditis. In this regard, fine meningeal contrast enhancement is detected. It may involve the subarachnoid space and particularly proceed as far as the nerve roots in the lumbar region.

Although the first documented spinal TB cases date back to 5000-year-old Egyptian mummies, the first modern case of spinal TB was described in 1779 by an English surgeon Percivall Pott. Spinal TB, known as Pott's disease, accounts for half the cases of osteoarticular TB [18]. Pathophysiologically, the vertebral inoculation occurs via haematogenous route. The process then spreads to the intervertebral disc and, in some cases, to the adjacent vertebrae. Paraspinal abscesses may develop by direct spread from the vertebral lesions [18]. TB of the cervical region is the most dangerous form of the skeletal TB, and clinically the quadriplegia and death may follow. Diagnosis of Pott's disease can be missed as some cases may be asymptomatic [19].

33.3 Clinical Manifestations

The ratio of the involvement by TB of spinal cord to that of the brain is 1:42 [20]. In endemic areas, intramedullary tuberculoma is rare, and the incidence of intramedullary tuberculoma is 0.2–5% of all CNS tuberculomas [20].

In a report by Thacker et al. [21], a young girl presented with progressive paraparesis and imaging findings revealing intramedullary tuberculoma with incidentally discovered multiple intracranial tuberculoma. Besides, Tanwar et al. [22] reported a 28-year-old patient presenting with headache, vomiting, vertigo and bilateral weakness in lower extremity. In another report by Shen et al., the patients were suffering from paraplegia [23]. The most dangerous form of extrapulmonary TB is spinal TB, which can cause destruction of the vertebral body and spinal instability even paraplegia in turn [1].

33.4 Radiology

33.4.1 CT Scan

On CT, tuberculomas are irregular rounded lesions with low or high density and show ring enhancement. Also, a hypertrophic dura mater is seen in CT and contrast enhancement is evident. The radiologic differential diagnosis includes meningioma en plaque, fibroma, dural carcinomatosis, neurosarcoidosis and lymphoma [24]. Syringomyelic changes may develop at the advanced stages.

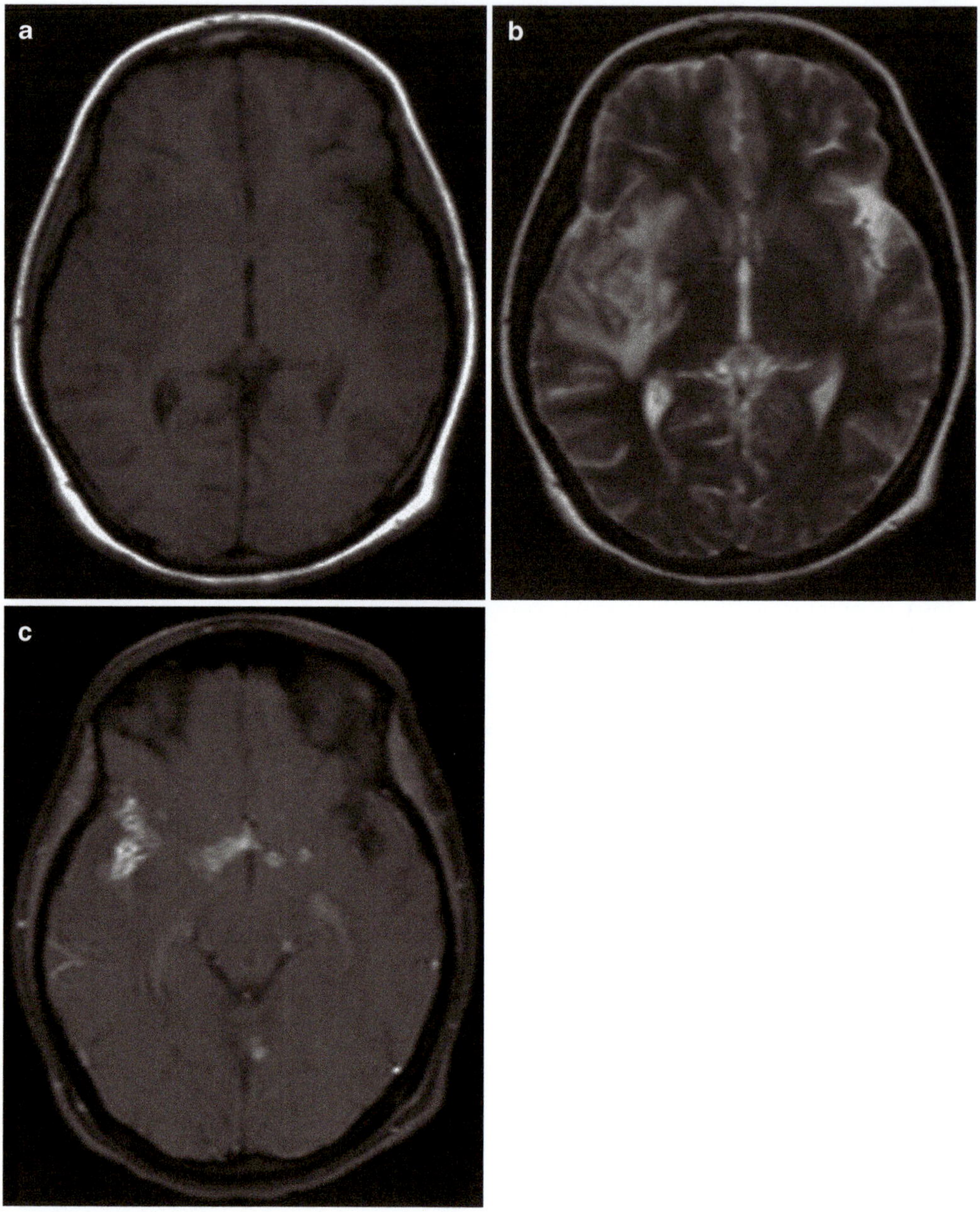

Fig. 33.5 Right temporoparietal oedema is seen as hypointense on T1-weighted image (**a**) and hyperintense on T2-weighted image (**b**). There is dense contrast enhancement due to TB in the right sylvian fissure, cistern and suprasellar cistern on fat-suppressed contrast-enhanced T1-weighted image (**c**)

33.4.2 MRI

MRI is known to be more sensitive for the detection of the disease. On MRI, a hypertrophic dura mater is seen and contrast enhancement is evident. A T2 hyperintense rim may be observed at the periphery of the lesion that is seen as isointense on T1-weighted images and

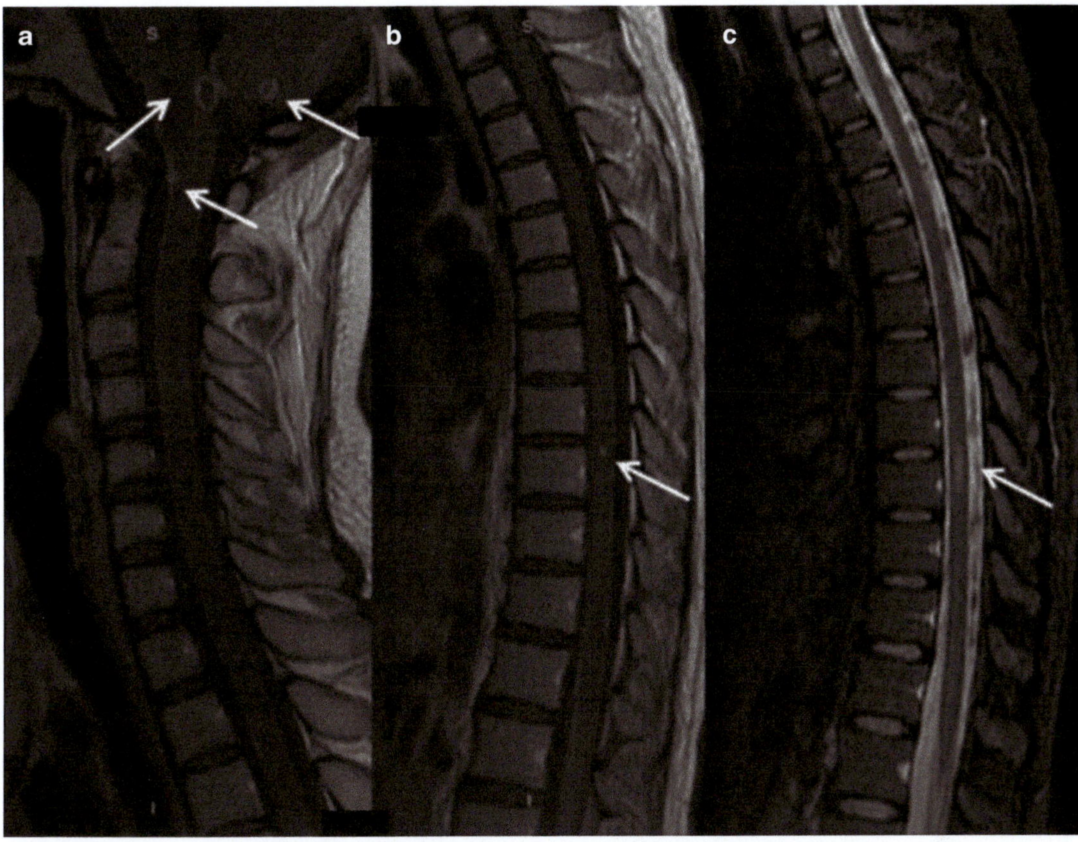

Fig. 33.6 Nodular, thick and linear intradural enhancement on sagittal contrast-enhanced T1-weighted images (**a**, **b**) and sagittal T2-weighted image (**c**), with diagnosis of cerebellar and spinal tuberculomas (*arrow*) (Courtesy of I. Sebnem Orguc)

hypointense on T2-weighted images and FLAIR images. The lesions show ring-shaped contrast enhancement. The tuberculoma depends on whether the lesion is non-caseating with a solid centre, or caseating with a liquid centre, in MRI. The non-caseating types are hypointense on T1-weighted images and/or hyperintense on T2-weighted images. Also, they show homogenous enhancement (Figs. 33.7 and 33.8). Nevertheless, the other type of tuberculoma is hypointense or isointense on both T1- and T2-weighted images and ring enhancement (Figs. 33.9 and 33.10)

In 1993, Shen et al. [23] reported a 30-year-old man with miliary TB of the lung. The patient suffered sudden paraplegia due to tuberculomas in the thoracic spinal cord, and MRI showed more tuberculomas in the cervical spinal cord, brainstem and cerebral and cerebellar hemispheres. The tuberculomas were isointense on the T1-weighted images and hyperintense on the T2-weighted images; there was marked enhancement with intravenous contrast [23]. Afterwards, Park et al. [25] and Yen et al. [26] reported 14 cases with multiple intramedullary tuberculomas. The CT or MRI of the brain was performed in four cases, where the incidence of multiple intramedullary tuberculomas concurrent with disseminated intracranial tuberculomas was 50%. Yen et al. [26] suggested that the MRI of the brain should be performed in a case of multiple intramedullary spinal tuberculomas due to the risk for the presence of early asymptomatic intracranial tuberculomas.

TB pus formation may fill the dural distance; it is seen as hyperintense on T2-weighted image and iso-hypointense on T1-weighted images. On the other hand, the dural granuloma is isointense on T2- and T1-weighted images. These granulomas have peripherally contrast enhancement [27]. In spinal cord involvement, the lesions are isointense with the spinal cord on T1-weighted images. These lesions have diffuse contrast enhancement.

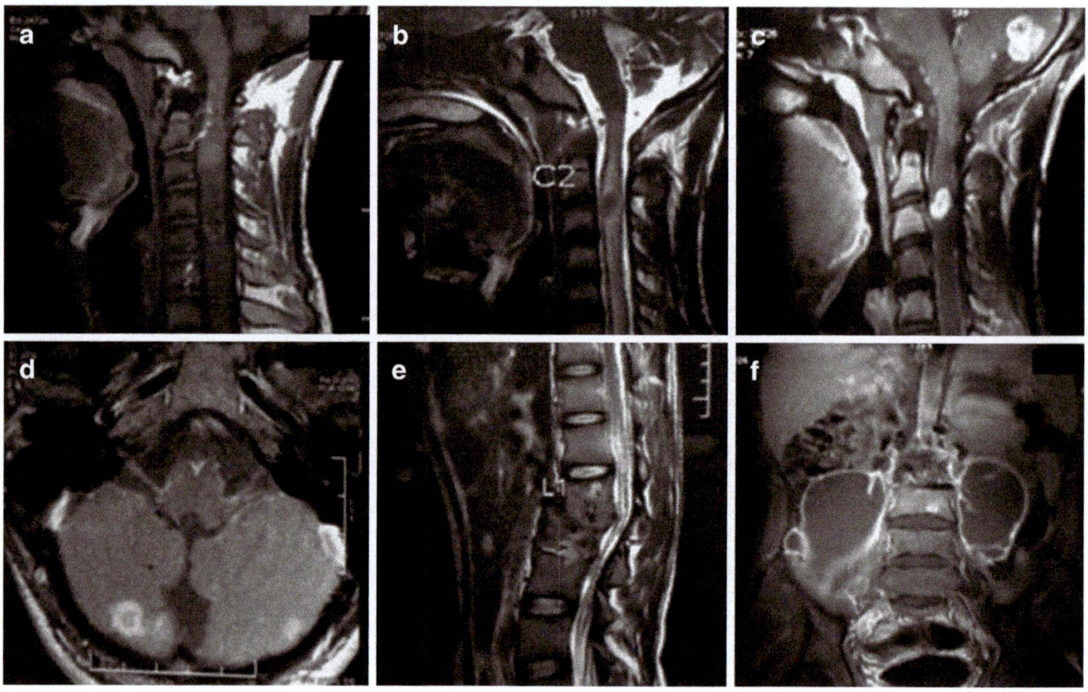

Fig. 33.7 (**a**–**f**) Well-defined and homogenous enhancement human immunodeficiency virus-positive 16-year-old male patient. Multiple tuberculomas located in the cerebellum and cervical spinal cord are seen as isointense on T1-weighted image, isointense on T2-weighted image and enhanced on contrast-enhanced T1-weighted images. In addition to these tuberculomas, there are vertebral body and disc space involvement at lumbar region and bilateral psoas abscesses. The patient presented with low back pain for 2 years and headache for 2 days, and neurological examination revealed the seventh cranial nerve involvement and paraplegia (Courtesy of YR Yadav)

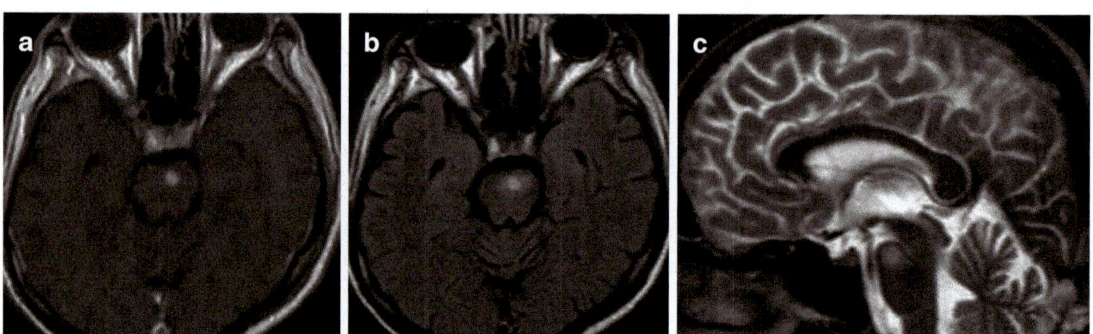

Fig. 33.8 TB granulomas are seen in the mesencephalon on axial contrast-enhanced T1-weighted (**a**), axial FLAIR (**b**) and sagittal T2-weighted (**c**) images

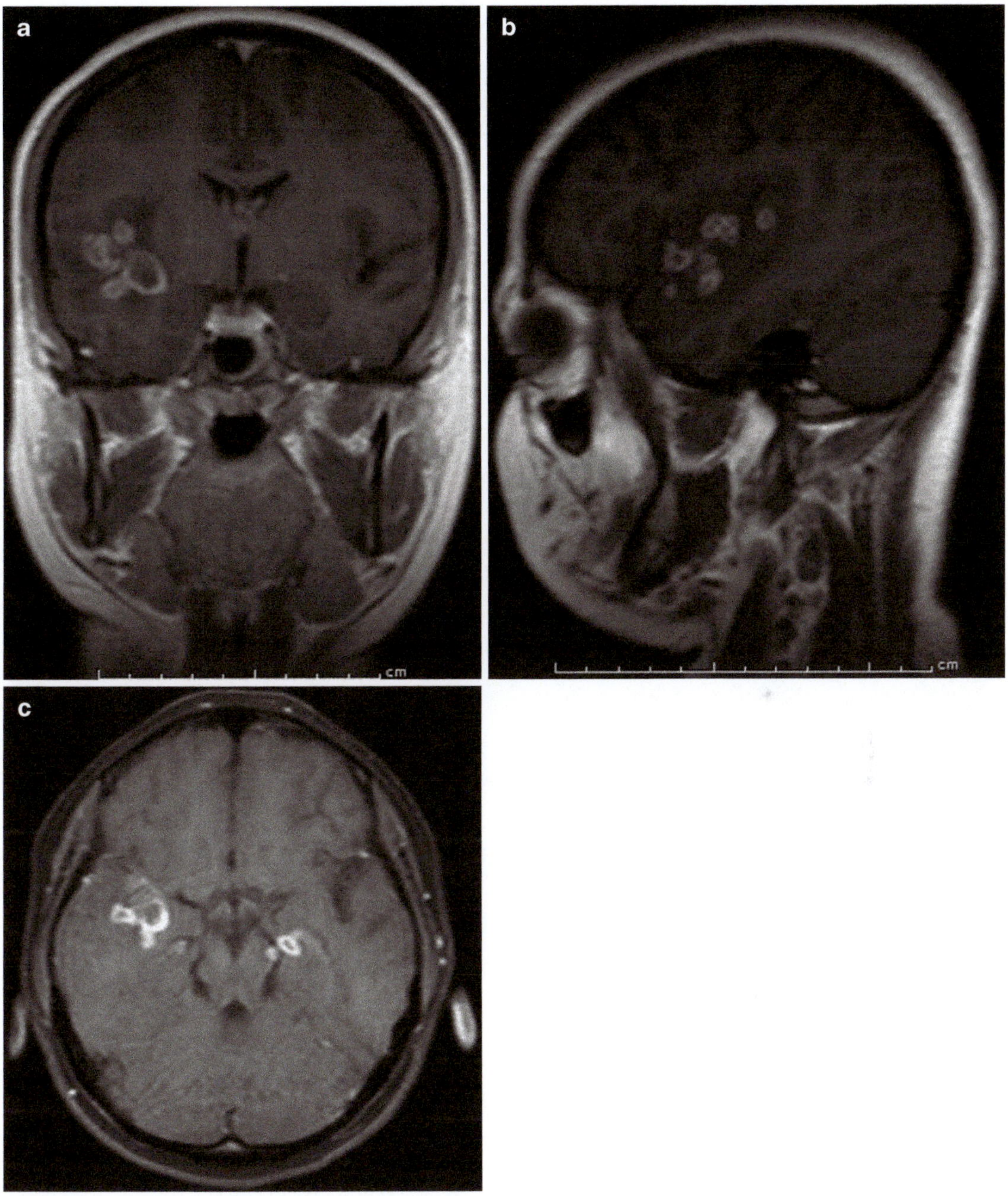

Fig. 33.9 Coronal (**a**) and sagittal (**b**) and axial (**c**) on fat-suppressed contrast-enhanced T1-weighted images show peripheral or ring enhancement multiple tuberculomas on cerebral hemispheres

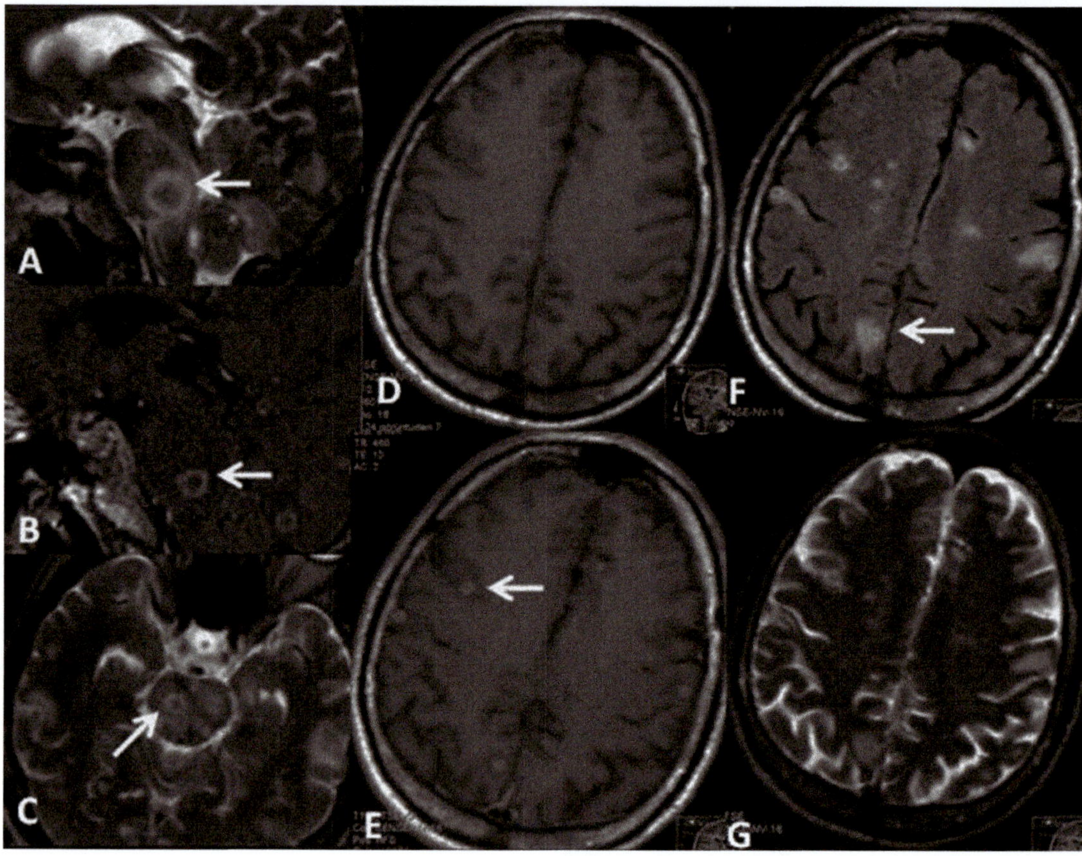

Fig. 33.10 Sagittal (**a**, **b**), axial (**c–g**), T1-weighted (**d**), contrast-enhanced T1-weighted (**b**, **e**), FLAIR (**f**) and T2-weighted (**a**, **c**, **g**) images that show ring- and *dot*-enhanced hyperintense lesions (*arrow*) were detected in a patient with headache, fever and weight loss symptoms

33.5 Differential Diagnosis

The differential diagnosis of tuberculomas (intracranial and intramedullary) includes cysticercosis, pyogenic abscess, toxoplasmosis and neoplasia (lymphoma, astrocytoma or metastatic lesion). Radiologically, the entities that should be considered in the differential diagnosis include are meningioma en plaque, leptomeningeal carcinomatosis, fibroma, dural carcinomatosis, neurosarcoidosis and lymphoma [24].

Radiologic findings of pachymeningitis are characteristic despite not being diagnostic. Chronic granulomatous infections, i.e. cryptococcus, histoplasmosis, coccidioidomycosis and syphilis, could also cause thickening of the dura. On DWI, low ADC has been found in fungal and TB abscesses similar to pyogenic abscesses. TB abscesses exhibit significantly lower magnetization transfer ratios compared with those of pyogenic abscesses. Pyogenic and TB abscesses may be differentiated by their unique metabolite pattern with recognition of amino acids in pyogenic abscesses and lipid peak in TB abscesses [28].

33.6 Medical Treatment

Medical treatment is advocated as the initial therapy for intracranial and intramedullary tuberculoma, and surgery is reserved for medical failure. In their report in 2012, Li et al. [29] discussed 23 cases that they followed between 1999 and 2008. Among these, only three cases had coexisting intracranial and spinal involvement, where the latter was noted to be at T3-4, T2-4 and C5-7 levels, respectively. Intracranial biopsy and laminectomy were performed in all cases. The Karnofsky Performance Scales of the patients during the discharge were 90, 100 and 70, respectively.

It may be important to know that in the presence of meningeal inflammation, both isoniazid and pyrazinamide reach as high concentrations as in the blood. Rifampicin penetrates the blood-brain barrier less well but still adequately.

The ethambutol level approaches 10–50% of serum levels in the patients with meningeal inflammation. Similarly, streptomycin is not detectable in normal meninges, while in patients with meningitis, CSF levels may reach up to 20% of serum concentrations [30, 31]. Most authorities recommend adjunctive corticosteroids in TBM, particularly stage 2 (objective neurologic findings) and stage 3 (stupor-coma) patients, beginning prednisone at 60–80 mg daily [32].

In the treatment of intracranial tuberculoma, corticosteroids reduce oedema and symptoms, and chemotherapy prevents the spread of the infection in cases diagnosed during the surgical intervention. Paradoxical enlargement has also been observed in isolated intracranial tuberculoma, while the patient was on anti-TB therapy. However, with continued treatment, eventual resolution of these tuberculomas occurs [33, 34].

33.7 Surgery

Concurrent occurrence of brain and spinal TB is a serious condition, where surgery should sometimes be considered for the treatment. Apparently, early diagnosis is very important. We emphasized that MRI of the cord should be performed in the case of multiple intracranial tuberculomas because of the probable presence of asymptomatic intramedullary tuberculomas. Intracranial tuberculomas that act as single space-occupying lesions with midline shifts and IICP and that fail to respond to chemotherapy should be surgically removed [35]. Hodgson achieved clinical outcomes by the 'Hong Kong operation' including debridement, excretion of the spinal cord and bone grafting, in 1964 [36]. Quian et al. [1] demonstrated the advantages of debridement: (1) debridement could promote response to chemotherapy and (2) could bring about a decompression of the spinal cord. The authors presented some disadvantages; that is, radical debridement compared to no debridement can increase the procedure time, blood loss and operative trauma.

Conclusion

Concurrent occurrence of brain and spinal TB is a serious condition. By means of the imaging features, a proper differentiation from other cases can be performed. In the most of the cases, management of cases with concurrent brain and spinal cord tuberculoma consists of anti-TB treatment and surgical removal of infection focus. Spinal involvement sometimes develops as a result of paradoxical responses of anti-TB medication. In such cases, the outcome for the treatment can be enhanced by early diagnosis.

References

1. Qian J, Rijiepu A, Zhu B, Tian D, Chen L, Jing J (2016) Outcomes of radical debridement versus no debridement for the treatment of thoracic and lumbar spinal tuberculosis. Int Orthop. doi:10.1007/s00264-016-3234-z
2. Raut AA, Naphade PS, Ramakantan R (2016) Imaging spectrum of extrathoracic tuberculosis. Radiol Clin North Am 54:475–501
3. Sylaja PN, Cherian PJ, Das CK, Radhakrishnan VV, Radhakrishnan K (2002) Idiopathic hypertrophic cranial pachymeningitis. Neurol India 50:53–59
4. Naffziger HC, Stern WE (1949) Chronic pachymeningitis; report of a case and review of the literature. Arch Neurol Psychiatry 62:383–411
5. Okimura Y, Tanno H, Karasudani H, Suda S, Ono J, Isobe K (1991) A case of hypertrophic cranial pachymeningitis (in Japan). No Shinkei Geka 19:259–262
6. Yamashita K, Suzuki Y, Yoshizumi H, Takahashi JB, Nogawa T (1994) Tuberculous hypertrophic pachymeningitis involving the posterior fossa and high cervical region – case report. Neurol Med Chir (Tokyo) 34:100–103

7. Turgut M, Ozcan OE, Ozgen T, Bertan V (1993) Intradural extramedullary tuberculoma of the spinal cord–a case report. Zentralbl Neurochir 54:197–199
8. Rhoton EL, Ballinger WE Jr, Quisling R, Sypert GW (1988) Intramedullary spinal tuberculoma. Neurosurgery 22:733–736
9. Parmar H, Shah J, Patkar D, Varma R (2000) Intramedullary tuberculomas. MR findings in seven patients. Acta Radiol 41:572–577
10. Bucy PC, Oberhill HR (1950) Intradural spinal granulomas. J Neurosurg 7:1–12
11. Das KK, Jaiswal S, Shukla M, Srivastava AK, Behari S, Kumar R (2014) Concurrent cerebellar and cervical intramedullary tuberculoma: paradoxical response on antitubercular chemotherapy and need for surgery. J Pediatr Neurosci 9:162–165
12. MacDonnell AH, Baird RW, Bronze MS (1990) Intramedullary tuberculomas of the spinal cord: case report and review. Rev Infect Dis 12:432–439
13. Sharma MC, Arora R, Deol PS, Mahapatra AK, Sinha AK, Sarkar C (2002) Intramedullary tuberculoma of the spinal cord: a series of 10 cases. Clin Neurol Neurosurg 104:279–284
14. Muthukumar N, Sureshkumar V, Ramesh VG (2007) En plaque intradural extramedullary spinal tuberculoma and concurrent intracranial tuberculomas: paradoxical response to antituberculous therapy. Case report J Neurosurg Spine 6:169–173
15. Turgut M (2007) Re: Surgery for intramedullary tuberculoma of the spinal cord: report of 2 cases (Muthukumar et al. Surg Neurol 2006;66:69–74). Surg Neurol 67:654 author reply 654-656
16. Chitre PS, Tullu MS, Sawant HV, Ghildiyal RG (2009) Co-occurrence of intracerebral tuberculoma with lumbar intramedullary tuberculoma. J Child Neurol 24: 606–609
17. Shenoy SN, Raja A (2004) Concurrent intramedullary and intracerebral tuberculomas. Neurol India 52:514–516
18. Varatharajah S, Charles YP, Buy X, Walter A, Steib JP (2014) Update on the surgical management of Pott's disease. Orthop Traumatol Surg Res 100:229–235
19. Turgut M (2001) Multifocal extensive spinal tuberculosis (Pott's disease) involving cervical, thoracic and lumbar vertebrae. Br J Neurosurg 15:142–146
20. Garcia-Monco JC (1999) Central nervous system tuberculosis. Neurol Clin 17:737–759
21. Thacker MM, Puri AI (2004) Concurrent intramedullary and intra-cranial tuberculomas. J Postgrad Med 50:107–109
22. Tanwar VS (2015) Concurrent multiple intracranial and intramedullary tuberculoma: a rare form of neurotuberculosis. J Adv Intern Med 4:25–27
23. Shen WC, Cheng TY, Lee SK, Ho YJ, Lee KR (1993) Disseminated tuberculomas in spinal cord and brain demonstrated by MRI with gadolinium-DTPA. Neuroradiology 35:213–215
24. Martin N, Masson C, Henin D, Mompoint D, Marsault C, Nahum H (1989) Hypertrophic cranial pachymeningitis: assessment with CT and MR imaging. AJNR Am J Neuroradiol 10:477–484
25. Park HS, Song YJ (2008) Multiple tuberculoma involving the brain and spinal cord in a patient with miliary pulmonary tuberculosis. J Korean Neurosurg Soc 44:36–39
26. Yen HL, Lee RJ, Lin JW, Chen HJ (2003) Multiple tuberculomas in the brain and spinal cord: a case report. Spine (Phila Pa 1976) 28:E499–E502
27. Gupta RK, Gupta S, Kumar S, Kohli A, Misra UK, Gujral RB (1994) MRI in intraspinal tuberculosis. Neuroradiology 36:39–43
28. Luthra G, Parihar A, Nath K, Jaiswal S, Prasad KN, Husain N, Husain M, Singh S, Behari S, Gupta RK (2007) Comparative evaluation of fungal, tubercular, and pyogenic brain abscesses with conventional and diffusion MR imaging and proton MR spectroscopy. AJNR Am J Neuroradiol 28:1332–1338
29. Li H, Liu W, You C (2012) Central nervous system tuberculoma. J Clin Neurosci 19:691–695
30. Donald PR, Gent WL, Seifart HI, Lamprecht JH, Parkin DP (1992) Cerebrospinal fluid isoniazid concentrations in children with tuberculous meningitis: the influence of dosage and acetylation status. Pediatrics 89:247–250
31. Ellard GA, Humphries MJ, Allen BW (1993) Cerebrospinal fluid drug concentrations and the treatment of tuberculous meningitis. Am Rev Respir Dis 148:650–655
32. Bennett JE, Dolin R, Blaser MJ (2015) Mandell, Douglas and Bennett's Principels and Practice of Infectious diseases, 8th edn. Elsevier Saunders, Canada, p 2813
33. Teoh R, Humphries MJ, O'Mahony G (1987) Symptomatic intracranial tuberculoma developing during treatment of tuberculosis: a report of 10 patients and review of the literature. Q J Med 63:449–460
34. Pauranik A, Behari M, Maheshwari MC (1987) Appearance of tuberculoma during treatment of tuberculous meningitis. Jpn J Med 26:332–334
35. Garg RK (1999) Tuberculosis of the central nervous system. Postgrad Med J 75:133–140
36. Hodgson AR, Stock FE (2006) The classic: anterior spinal fusion: a preliminary communication on the radical treatment of Pott's disease and Pott's paraplegia. 1956. Clin Orthop Relat Res 444:10–15

Paradoxical Worsening of Tuberculosis of the Nervous System During Treatment

34

Vimal Kumar Paliwal

Contents

V.K. Paliwal
Department of Neurology, Sanjay Gandhi Postgraduate Institute of Medical Sciences, Lucknow, UP 226014, India
e-mail: dr_vimalkpaliwal@rediffmail.com; drvimalkpaliwal@gmail.com

Abbreviations

CNS	Central nervous system
CSF	Cerebrospinal fluid
HART	Highly active anti-retroviral treatment
HIV	Human immunodeficiency virus
IFN	Interferon
IL	Interleukins
IRIS	Immune reconstitution inflammatory syndrome
PR	Paradoxical reaction
PR-IRIS	Paradoxical immune reconstitution inflammatory syndrome
TB	Tuberculosis
TBM	Tuberculous meningitis
TLR	Toll-like receptors
TNF	Tumor necrosis factor
TREM	Triggering receptor expressed on myeloid cells

34.1 Introduction

Paradoxical worsening or paradoxical reaction (PR), as the name suggests, is defined as the worsening of the pre-existing tuberculosis (TB) of the nervous system or appearance of newer TB lesions upon initiation of anti-TB treatment [1]. Previously thought to be rare, it is now seen in nearly half of all patients with CNS TB who

M. Turgut et al. (eds.), *Tuberculosis of the Central Nervous System*,
DOI 10.1007/978-3-319-50712-5_34

undergo treatment with anti-TB drugs [2]. The paradoxical worsening may be seen in HIV-negative as well as HIV-positive patients. However, in HIV-positive patients, paradoxical worsening of TB lesions is called immune reconstitution inflammatory syndrome (IRIS), and this paradoxical worsening is witnessed after starting highly active anti-retroviral treatment (HART) [3]. In HIV-positive patients, IRIS may be paradoxical-IRIS (PR-IRIS) or unmasking-IRIS. Paradoxical-IRIS is defined as worsening of pre-existing TB or appearance of new lesions in patients already taking anti-TB treatment after initiation of HART. Unmasking-IRIS is defined as newly appeared TB lesions in patients with HIV disease upon initiating HART in whom TB was previously not diagnosed [4]. Unfortunately, not much of research is done in HIV-negative patients with paradoxical reactions. Therefore, the case definition of paradoxical worsening of TB in HIV-negative patients is not well defined. Unlike HIV-negative patients, paradoxical-IRIS has been relatively well studied.

34.2 Paradoxical Reaction in HIV-Negative Patients

34.2.1 Case Definition

The most commonly used case definition by researchers for retrospective chart review or for prospective studies on patients with paradoxical worsening of TB includes the criteria used by Carvalho et al. [5]. The case definition for PR in immunocompetent patients is given in Table 34.1. Carvalho et al. [5] used 1 month of minimum duration of treatment with anti-TB therapy to differentiate delayed or no response to treatment from PR. However, some researchers have further classified paradoxical worsening of TB into "probable" (14–27 days after starting of anti-TB therapy) and "definite" (more than 4 weeks after initiation of anti-TB treatment) [2].

Table 34.1 Case definition of paradoxical tuberculosis in immunocompetent patients

There are four components to this case definition:
(a) The patient should have a definite or probable diagnosis of tuberculosis
(b) The clinical/radiological worsening of tuberculosis should occur at least 1 month after initiation of antitubercular treatment
(c) Prior to worsening, patient should show signs of improvement after initiation of antitubercular treatment
(d) The other causes of worsening of symptoms/signs like drug-resistant tuberculosis should be excluded

34.2.2 Epidemiology

PR can occur in pulmonary and extrapulmonary TB. Among extrapulmonary TB, PR is most frequently observed in CNS TB followed by pleural TB. The frequency of PR in CNS TB among HIV-negative patients as reported from the retrospective studies has been variable ranging from less than 1% to 32.8% [2, 5–11]. In a recently published prospective study, the frequency of PR among HIV-negative patients was found to be 56% [2]. Time to onset of PR (after initiation of anti-TB therapy) ranged from 28 days to 9 months, but majority of patients presented within 50 days. Most of the populations studied have been Asians.

34.2.3 Paradoxical Manifestations

PR may manifest as reappearance of clinical features, radiological abnormalities, or increase in cerebrospinal fluid (CSF) pleocytosis. Most common paradoxical manifestations in patients with CNS TB are reappearance of clinical features [2]. Clinical manifestations may be constitutional symptoms like fever, night sweats, new enlarged lymph nodes, or features suggestive of worsening of CNS TB like headache, vomiting, vision loss, hemiparesis, signs of meningeal irritation, or deterioration in the level of consciousness. In a prospective study of PR in CNS TB in HIV-negative patients, the clinical features that were observed in decreasing order of frequency were worsening of consciousness, seizures, hemiparesis, headache, visual impairment, third cranial nerve palsy, back pain, sixth cranial nerve palsy, and ataxic gait [2]. Rarely, PR may involve spinal cord and produce paraparesis secondary to spinal cord tuberculoma or arachnoiditis.

Neuroimaging characteristics of CNS TB-related PR in HIV-negative patients in order of decreasing frequency are deterioration of leptomeningeal enhancement, appearance of new infarcts, tuberculomas, and increase in size of persisting tuberculoma.

Leptomeningeal enhancement as a result of PR occurs at the sylvian fissures, basal regions of the brain with accumulation of thick basal exudates (Fig. 34.1). These exudates accumulate around the midbrain and pons occupying the interpeduncular cistern, cisterna ambiens, peripontine cistern, sellar area, and suprasellar cistern. These basal exudates affect the cranial nerves that traverse the base of the middle cranial fossa and produce ophthalmoplegia (third and sixth cranial nerves) [12]. Inflammation of meninges around the optic chiasma also produces vision loss and optic atrophy (Fig. 34.1) [13–15]. The basal exudate is a thick, gelatinous granulation tissue that can also produce inflammation of the major blood vessel forming the circle of Willis and may result in large artery infarcts.

The appearance of new infarcts is the second most common neuroimaging feature associated with PR in TBM. Though reported with variable

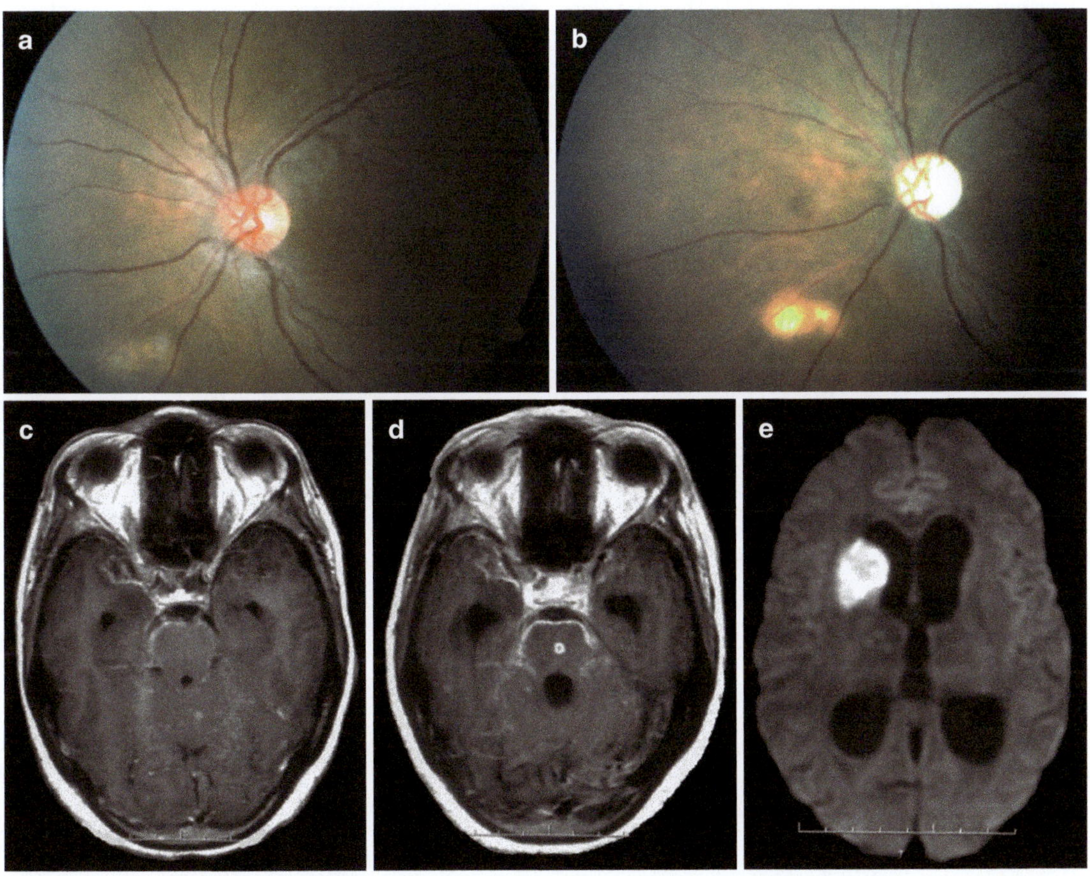

Fig. 34.1 A 25-year-old female with miliary TB shows active choroid tubercles (fluffy, raised, *light yellow*) in the inferomedial aspect of the left eye (**a**) that improved (evidenced by *glistening yellow*, sharp-circumscribed and contracted tubercles) after 3 months of anti-TB therapy (**b**). Her baseline MRI shows minimal optic chiasma and peripontine exudates (**c**). Despite improvement in fundus findings, her repeat MRI at 3 months shows extensive optic chiasmal exudates and appearance of paradoxical tuberculoma in the pons and hydrocephalus (**d**). A right paradoxical caudate infarct is also seen on diffusion-weighted image (**e**)

frequency, in a recently published study, infarcts are seen in 29% of patients at duration of 28 days to 5 months [16]. In another prospective study comprising 100 patients, only three patients developed paradoxical infarcts. On univariate analysis, stroke predictors were age greater than 25 years; involvement of cranial nerve, exudates in the sylvian fissure, posterior fossa and optic chiasma exudates; and stage III TBM [16]. Angiographic abnormalities have also been observed in few patients with TBM after starting of anti-TB therapy in the form of vasculitis or vasospasms [2, 18]. However, these findings are seen only in minority of patients. Aspirin has been shown to reduce paradoxical infarcts with a positive impact on 3-month mortality [17]. The distribution of infarcts is variable, but the periventricular area especially the basal ganglia region is most commonly involved (Fig. 34.1) [16]. However, large artery infarcts and infarcts in the posterior circulation are not uncommon.

Enlarging tuberculoma and appearance of new tuberculoma were initially thought to be the most common manifestation of PR (Figs. 34.2 and 34.3) [19]. However, in a recently reported prospective study, 20% of patients showed new tuberculoma, whereas 5% showed enlargement of pre-existing tuberculomas at duration of 28 days to 5 months and 28 days to 9 months, respectively [2]. This is in contrast to leptomeningeal enhancement that was observed in nearly one-third of all patients with PR. The increase in the size of tuberculoma is also shown to be associated with paradoxical CSF response in form of increase in polymorphonuclear cell count [20]. Clinical features associated with enlarging tuberculoma or appearance of new tuberculoma may be the worsening vision, increase in headache, new onset of seizures, and appearance of limb weakness or hemiparesis. However, the enlargement of pre-existing tuberculoma may be asymptomatic and may appear several months to more than a year after initiation of anti-TB chemotherapy (Figs. 34.2 and 34.3).

Paradoxical worsening of hydrocephalus is reported in 7–10% of patients occurring at a

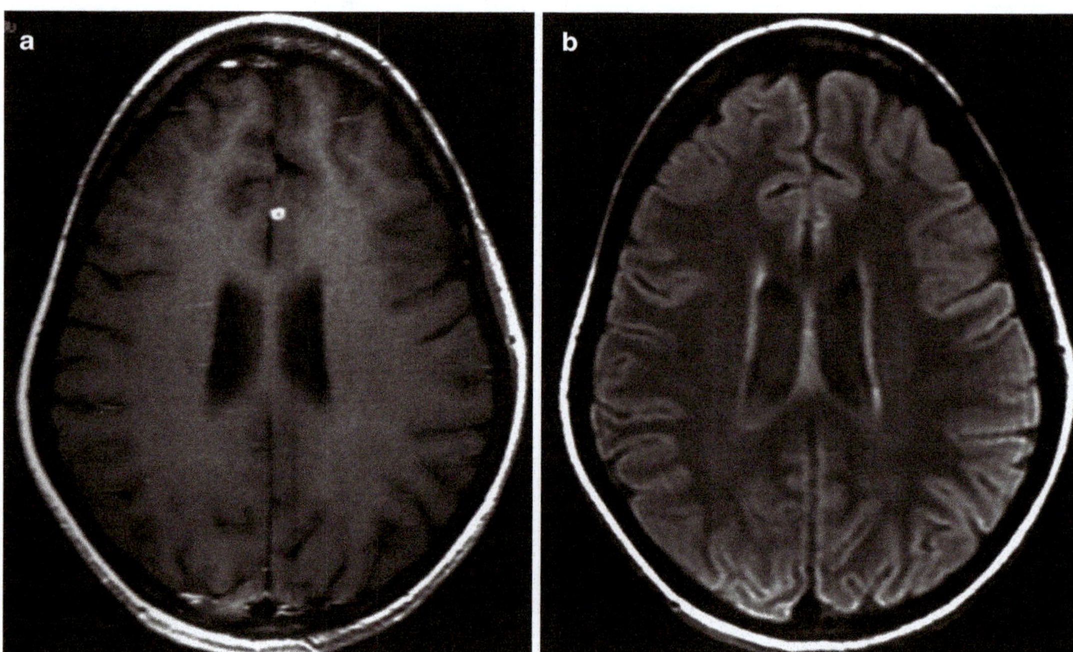

Fig. 34.2 A 30-year-old female with TBM and tuberculoma. Her baseline MRI brain shows a left paramedian frontal small tuberculoma on axial post-contrast image (**a**) with minimal perifocal edema on FLAIR image (**b**). A repeat MRI after 18 months of anti-TB therapy shows asymptomatic increase and conglomeration of left paramedian frontal tuberculoma (**c**) with increased perilesional edema (**d**)

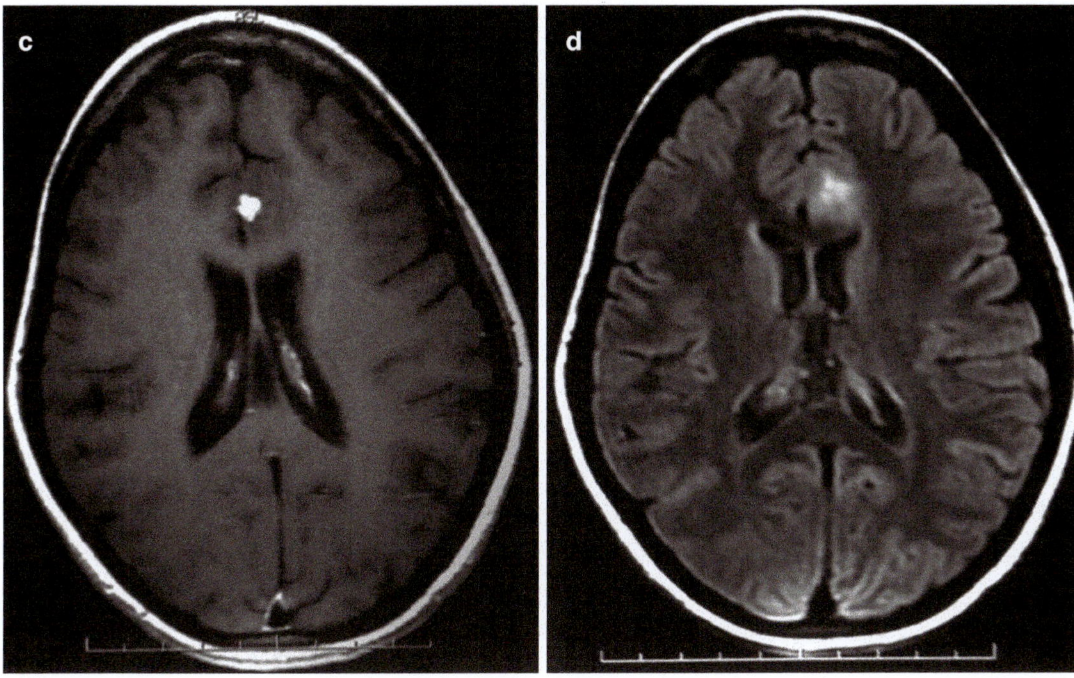

Fig. 34.2 (continued)

median duration of 28 days to 5 months after starting of anti-TB therapy [2, 21]. Paradoxical hydrocephalus is usually associated with basal exudates, tuberculoma, and infarcts and carries a poor prognosis. Usually, the hydrocephalus is communicating type but rarely it may be obstructive. Paradoxical asymmetrical dilatation of ventricles is also known which may be associated with evidence of TB ventriculitis [22]. Rarely, acute worsening of consciousness with signs of raised intracranial pressure and evidence of impending brain herniation may be seen in patients with paradoxical trapped temporal horn of lateral ventricle (Fig. 34.4). These patients may require urgent decompression of trapped ventricle by shunt surgery or urgent temporal lobectomy [22].

Paradoxical spinal cord involvement was observed in 7% of patients with TBM [2]. The observed time to paradoxical spinal cord involvement was between 28 days and 34 weeks. The involvement of the spinal cord may occur as radiculomyelopathy, myelitis, and Pott's spine. Functional abnormalities like bladder dysfunction are more common than paradoxical radiological abnormalities of the spinal cord. Paradoxical bladder dysfunction in patients with TBM was seen in 28% of patients in a prospective study that performed urodynamic study in patients with TBM [23]. Majority of these patients had lumbosacral TB arachnoiditis (Fig. 34.5) [24–26]. Other paradoxical abnormalities in the spinal cord observed in patients with TBM were spinal cord infarctions, intramedullary tuberculoma, extramedullary tuberculoma, and rarely cord myelomalacia/syringomyelia [27–32]. Many patients of TBM may also have Pott's spine which remain unnoticed due to overwhelming clinical features of TBM. Pott's spine in these patients is diagnosed only later in the course of illness when these patients become conscious or when they become mobile. These patients may be wrongly reported as paradoxical spinal cord manifestation of TBM.

Paradoxical CSF response is variably reported from 17% to 34% of patients with TBM occurring at 28 days to 7 months and 4–108 days, respectively [2, 33]. Paradoxical

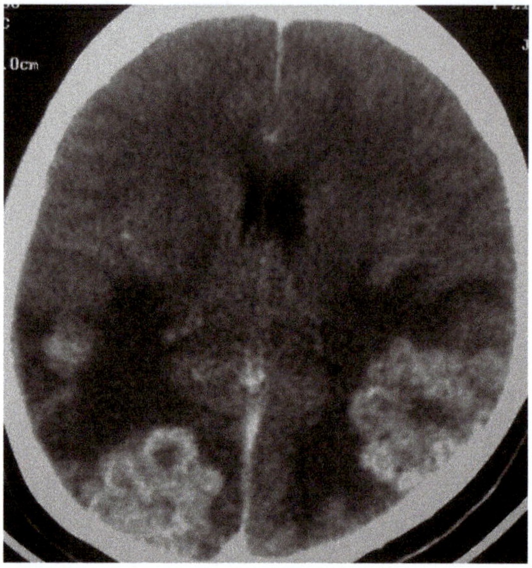

Fig. 34.3 Contrast-enhanced CT shows two large paradoxically developed tuberculomas after 3 months in a patient with TBM (Courtesy of R. K. Garg, M.D.)

manifestations of CSF may include change in cell lineage from mononuclear cells to polymorphonuclear cells, increase in cell count, and increase in CSF protein or reduction in CSF glucose [33, 34]. These CSF changes have been reported with appearance of paradoxical changes in brain tuberculoma. However, these CSF abnormalities may remain asymptomatic in majority of patients and improve over a period of time on anti-TB chemotherapy.

The recurrent PR has recently been described. Recurrent paradoxical manifestations may be seen in as high as 30% in patients with TBM [2]. The recurrent paradoxical manifestations may be in form of recurrent seizures, recurrent hemiparesis (recurrent ischemic strokes), and recurrent deterioration of consciousness. Time to recurrent paradoxical manifestations may be variable. Continued exaggerated immune response after starting of anti-TB therapy and continued antigenicity of cell wall products of *Mycobacterium tuberculosis* are hypothesized as the underlying mechanism for recurrent PR [35, 36].

34.2.4 Pathophysiology

In response to a pathogen, two types of immune responses take place in human body. One is pathogen-induced antigen-specific response that involves activation of naïve CD4 cells (Th0) which further differentiate into Th1 and Th2 cells. The Th1 cells promote inflammation by elaborating interferon gamma, activation of macrophages, and activation of other pro-inflammatory pathways. Th2 cells mainly secrete interleukin 4 and interleukin 10 and suppress inflammation and produce immunosuppression [37–39]. Regardless of specific pathogen, the immune system also has an innate immune response. The Th17 cells and regulatory T cells (Tregs) which form an important part of innate immunity have a role in pathogenesis of paradoxical responses [40]. The Th17 cells require both interleukin 6 and tumor growth factor to initiate differentiation. Once activated, they secrete interleukin 17 and interleukin 22 and thereby promote pro-inflammatory chemokines and metalloproteinases for recruitment of neutrophils for eradicating pathogens [41–43]. Tregs play a role in reducing the inflammation and preventing the resultant tissue damage [44].

Pathogenesis of PR in CNS TB in immunocompetent individuals is not clear. There are several hypothesis supported by limited evidences. It is believed that an exaggerated immune response in patients with TBM that involves both innate and acquired immunity is responsible for PR. This occurs after initiation of effective anti-TB therapy that somehow increases the CSF and peripheral lymphocytes after a time lag that co-relates with the onset of clinical/radiological manifestation of PR [45]. This presumed mechanism is similar to the one known to produce paradoxical-IRIS in HIV patients. It is also suggested that a deregulated cellular immunity results in conversion of latent TB in active TB that manifests as PR [46]. Conversion of CSF lymphocytic pleocytosis into polymorphonuclear cells has also been implicated [47]. Similarly, an elevated tumor necrosis factor (TNF-α) in the

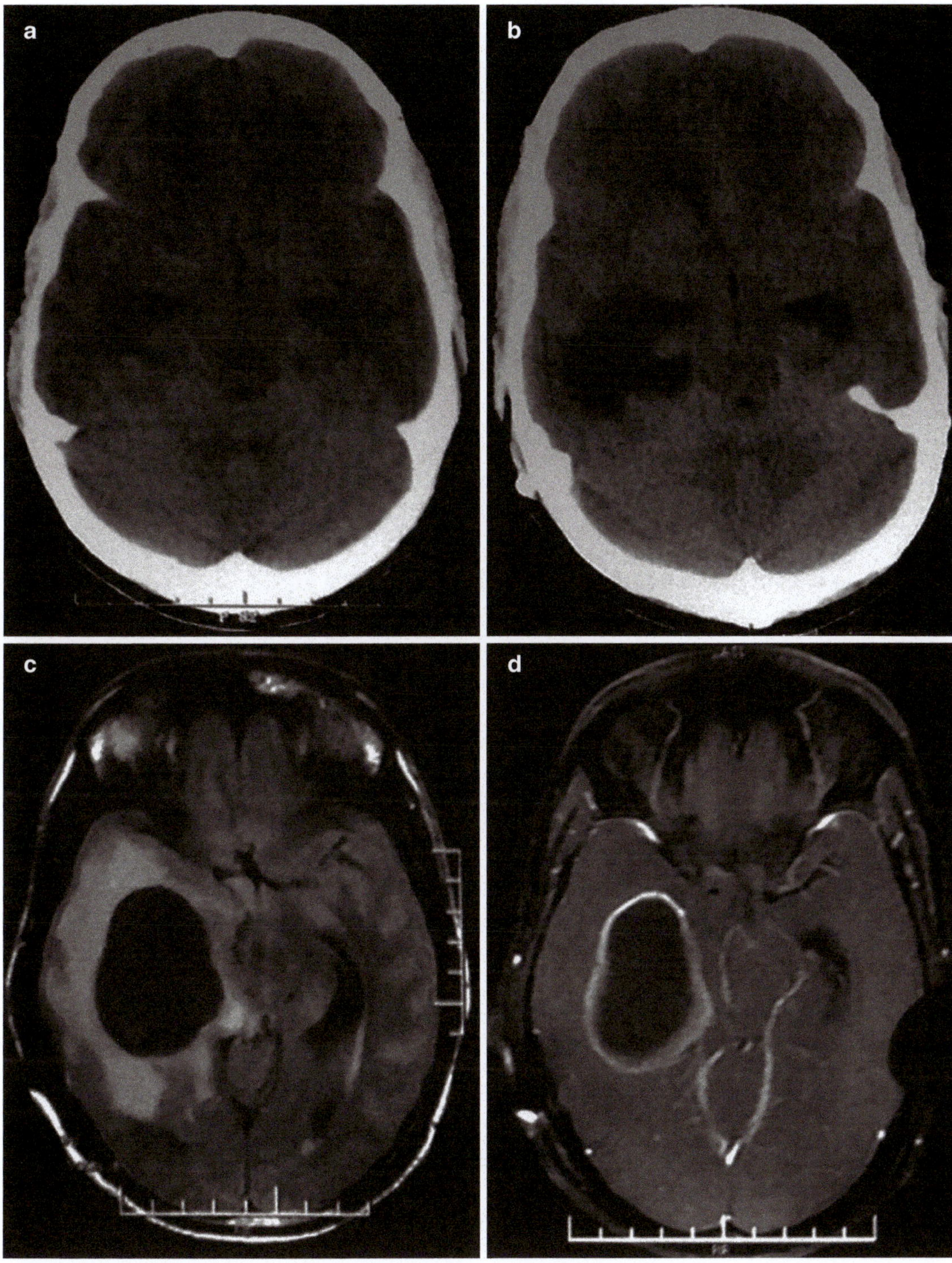

Fig. 34.4 A 18-year-old boy with TBM presented with intractable headache and papilledema and shows dilated temporal horns of lateral ventricle and small fourth ventricle suggestive of non-communicating hydrocephalus (**a**). He improved after ventriculoperitoneal shunt and anti-TB therapy along with steroids. A repeat CT head was done after 3 months due to reappearance of headache and visual obscurations. It shows paradoxical asymmetrical dilatation of right temporal horn of lateral ventricles (**b**). Two weeks later, patient presented with altered consciousness with bipyramidal signs. His cranial MRI showed trapped right temporal horn with periventricular vasogenic edema and transtentorial herniation on FLAIR images (**c**). Post-contrast T1-weighted image shows intense enhancement of ependymal lining of the right temporal horn suggestive of ventriculitis (**d**)

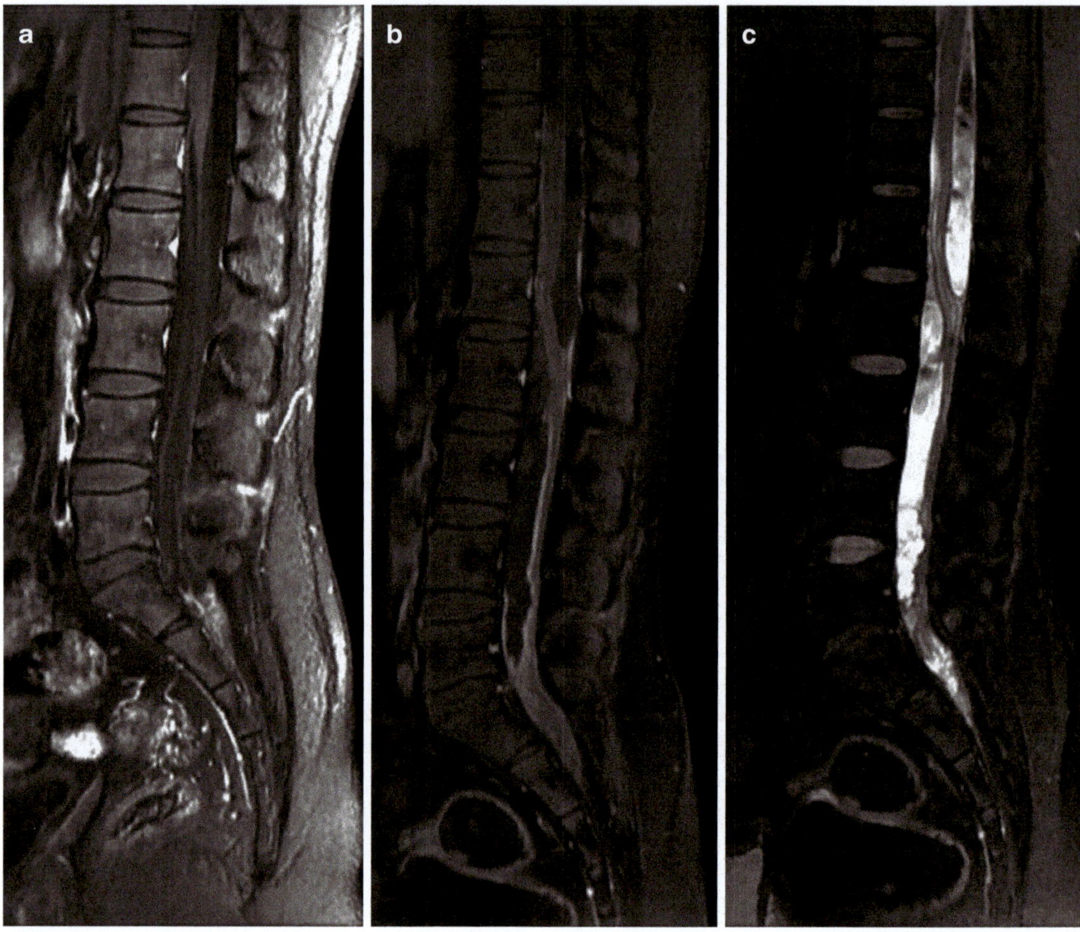

Fig. 34.5 A 36-year-old gentleman presented with TBM complicated with thick basal exudates, pontine infarct, and communicating hydrocephalus. Despite improvement of symptoms of cranial meningitis on anti-TB therapy and steroids, patient developed lower back pain with radiation to both legs and symptoms of neurogenic bladder after 4 months of initiation of anti-TB therapy. His lumbosacral MRI performed 4 months after initiation of anti-TB therapy revealed thick exudates in the epidural space opposite S1, S2 along with pachymeningeal enhancement along the cauda equina on post-contrast sagittal image. A repeat MRI of the lumbosacral spine after 18 months of anti-TB chemotherapy revealed asymptomatic paradoxical diffuse adhesive arachnoiditis with clumping and posterior displacement of cauda equina along with contrast enhancement of spinal nerve roots and increased epidural exudates opposite S1, S2 (**a**). Leptomeningeal enhancement of lumbar spinal cord is also seen (**b**). T2 fat-suppressed sagittal image shows internal septations and CSF loculations with clumped spinal nerves roots (**c**)

CSF that is responsible for initiating granulomatous inflammation is also thought to contribute to PR [48]. A role of regulatory T cells has also been hypothesized. In the early stage of infection, the frequency of regulatory T cells increases in the blood as well as at the infection site. However, these cells are discarded later in the stage of infection to prevent suppression of inflammation [48]. Despite various suggested pathways, the exact pathophysiology of PR in CNS TB in an immunocompetent host remains unclear.

34.2.5 Predictors of Paradoxical Reactions

Unlike PR-IRIS in HIV patients, the predictors of PR in immunocompetent patients are not clearly known. In a recent study, the various factors were compared between patients with definite, probable PR and no PR. These factors included age greater than 50 years, sex, stage of TBM, diabetes mellitus, use of steroids, delay in diagnosis, and disseminated TB. However, none of the factors were significantly different on univariate analysis [2]. Therefore, logistic regression methods could not be applied to determine the predictors of PR in non-HIV patients in their study.

34.2.6 Treatment

Unfortunately, there is paucity of randomized controlled trials to determine the right treatment of paradoxical manifestations in patients with CNS TB. However, the experts believe that continued treatment with anti-TB therapy and steroids generally produce recovery from PR. A study in pediatric TBM patients with adjunctive steroids showed reduced incidence of paradoxical tuberculoma [49]. However, a similar study in adults showed equal incidence of paradoxical tuberculoma in a study group who received steroids and the placebo group [20]. There are anecdotal reports of recovery of patients who developed PR despite steroids with tumor necrosis factor α inhibitors like infliximab, adalimumab, thalidomide (which is potent tumor necrosis factor α inhibitor), cyclophosphamide, and interferon-γ [50–54]. In severe life-threatening conditions, surgical treatment may have to be used. The most common surgical procedure performed is ventriculoperitoneal shunt and endoscopic third ventriculostomy as CSF divergent procedure in patients with acute hydrocephalus manifesting as PR [26]. Excision or debulking of TB abscesses or large tuberculomas and rarely temporal lobectomy are performed in patients with trapped temporal horn of lateral ventricle [26, 55]. For spinal manifestation of PR, surgical debridement of intradural extramedullary tuberculoma may be required. Excision of intramedullary tuberculoma is rarely required in medically refractory cases [56].

34.2.7 Prognosis

The outcome of patients who develop PR generally remains favorable. In a recently reported study, 61% of patients with TBM who had a definite PR and 55% with no PR improved [2]. Patients who develop infarcts, optochiasmatic arachnoiditis with associated vision loss, and optic atrophy may continue with neurological sequelae.

34.3 Paradoxical Reaction in HIV-Positive Patients

34.3.1 Case Definition

Case definitions for paradoxical-IRIS were available since 2004, initially given by French et al. [57], and later other researchers also suggested their case definitions for PR-IRIS [58, 59]. However, these case definitions were not applicable for resource-poor countries due to nonavailability of expensive laboratory methods. Therefore, a consensus-based case definition was evolved in 2008 for use in the resource-rich and resource-poor countries (Table 34.2) [4].

34.3.2 Epidemiology

Among HIV-positive patients, a meta-analysis conducted in 2010 revealed paradoxical TB-associated IRIS (that included different organ systems) in 15.7% (95% CI 9.7–24.5), and death reported were 3.2% (95% CI 0.7–9.2) among those with TB PR-IRIS [60]. In a prospective study that included patients with TBM coinfected with HIV, paradoxical TB-IRIS was seen in 47% of patients occurring at a median duration of 14 days (5–20 days) after initiation of HART [61].

34.3.3 Paradoxical Manifestations

Paradoxical manifestations of CNS TB-IRIS largely remain similar to those without HIV dis-

Table 34.2 Case definition of paradoxical tuberculosis-associated IRIS

There are three components to this case definition:
A. *Antecedent requirements*
Both requirements must be met:
Diagnosis of tuberculosis: before initiating HART, patient should fulfill WHO's diagnostic criteria for smear-positive tuberculosis, smear-negative pulmonary tuberculosis, or extrapulmonary tuberculosis
Initial response to tuberculosis treatment: the patient should have stabilized/improved on ATT before HART initiation
B. *Clinical criteria*
The onset of tuberculosis-associated paradoxical-IRIS should be within 3 months of HART initiation, reinitiation, or regimen change: one major criterion or two minor clinical criteria are required
Major criteria
New or enlarging lymph nodes, cold abscesses, or other focal tissue involvement, for example, tuberculous arthritis
New or worsening radiological features of tuberculosis (found by chest radiography, abdominal ultrasonography, CT, or MRI)
New or worsening CNS tuberculosis (meningitis or focal neurological deficit, for example, caused by tuberculoma)
New or worsening serositis (pleural effusion, ascites, or pericardial effusion)
Minor criteria
New or worsening constitutional symptoms such as fever, night sweats, or weight loss
New or worsening respiratory symptoms such as cough, dyspnea, or stridor
New or worsening abdominal pain accompanied by peritonitis, hepatomegaly, splenomegaly, or abdominal adenopathy
C. *Alternative explanations for clinical deterioration must be excluded if possible*[a]
Failure of tuberculosis treatment because of tuberculosis drug resistance
Poor adherence to tuberculosis treatment
Another opportunistic infection or neoplasm (it is particularly important to exclude an alternative diagnosis in patients with smear-negative pulmonary tuberculosis and extrapulmonary tuberculosis where the initial tuberculosis diagnosis has not been microbiologically confirmed)
Drug toxicity or reaction

Abbreviations: *ART* anti-retroviral therapy, *IRIS* immune reconstitution inflammatory syndrome

[a]It might be difficult or impossible in resource-poor settings to confirm tuberculosis drug resistance and to exclude certain other infections or neoplasia. Cases where alternative diagnoses cannot be fully excluded because of limited diagnostic capacity should be regarded as "probable paradoxical tuberculosis-associated IRIS." In these probable cases, should resolution of clinical or radiological findings of the suspected IRIS episode occur without a change in tuberculosis treatment or ART having been made, they could then be reclassified as "paradoxical tuberculosis-associated IRIS" cases

ease. However, the frequency of different manifestations may vary. The various clinical or radiological manifestations are mostly described in case reports or small case series of patients.

In a study on patients with HIV coinfected with TBM, frequency of different clinical features, radiological presentation, and CSF parameters were studied and compared with TBM patients without paradoxical-IRIS [61]. In all these patients, the HART was initiated within 2 weeks of initiation of anti-TB therapy. Forty-seven percent of patients developed paradoxical-IRIS. Clinical features in order of frequency were headache, neck stiffness, vomiting, visual disturbance, and confusion. However, the frequencies of these clinical features were not different from patients without IRIS. The mean duration of these symptoms was 19 days as compared to 9 days in patient without IRIS. They also found that the TBM-related paradoxical-IRIS patients have higher likelihood of developing extra-meningeal features and new findings on chest radiographs [61].

The radiological features of paradoxical-IRIS remain largely similar as in PR in HIV-negative patients, but the exact frequency of radiological abnormalities and the time to onset of paradoxical-IRIS after initiation of HART are not known. In a prospective study of TBM-related IRIS, 14 out of 16 patients showed cranial features of TBM, and only 2 patients had paradoxical myeloradiculitis presenting as paraparesis [47]. HIV patients with paradoxical tuberculoma enlargement have a greater perilesional edema and a higher chance of seizures and clinical deterioration secondary to mass effect.

At the time of diagnosis of paradoxical-IRIS, TBM patients may have higher neutrophil count, higher lymphocyte count as compared to baseline, lower blood/CSF glucose ratio, and higher protein levels. These are the features of recurrent CSF inflammation [47].

34.3.4 Pathophysiology

Pathogenesis of paradoxical-IRIS in HIV is mainly related to recovery of immune functions by HART. The high viral load and very low CD4 cell count are major predictors of paradoxical reactions in HIV disease. The reduced pool of CD4 cells also includes the memory T cells. After 3–6 months of initiation of HART, the CD4 T cells increase in number which means that the memory T-cell number also recovers [62]. This duration also correlates with the onset of paradoxical-IRIS. During this time, there is a greater access to interleukin 17 which further supports memory T-cell survival and expansion. Therefore, after starting HART, there is an enhanced pro-inflammatory immune environment with increase in memory T cells, expansion of interleukin 17, and high antigenic exposure due to anti-TB therapy, which together contribute to paradoxical-IRIS [63, 64]. Unlike Th17 cells, the Tregs do not recover adequately after initiation of HART [64]. Therefore, the exaggerated pro-inflammatory environment due to activation of Th17 cells is not adequately regulated, thereby resulting in greater immune-mediated injury.

Recently, Lai et al. studied differentially abundant transcripts at 0.5 week and 2 weeks after starting HART in TB co-associated HIV disease patients and prospectively followed the patients to predict the downstream activation of pro-inflammatory cytokines in those who progress to paradoxical-IRIS [65]. They found the differential transcript at 0.5 week that favored innate immune pathway in those who developed paradoxical-IRIS that was mainly represented by IL-6 cytokine pathway, upregulated type I and II IFN signaling, activation of TLR signaling, and role of macrophages. Transcriptomic signature at week 2 was also predictive of innate signaling pathways and production of pro-inflammatory cytokines (TNF-α, IL-1β, IL-6, IL-8, IL-12, IL-18, granulocyte-macrophage colony-stimulating factor, monocyte chemoattractant protein-1, and macrophage inflammatory protein-2). The signaling was carried out by TLR and IL-1/8 receptor and TREM1-induced inflammasomes and TLR. Therefore, their study also favored a major role of innate immune-mediated mechanisms responsible for paradoxical-IRIS [65].

34.3.5 Predictors of Paradoxical-IRIS in HIV Patients

A low CD4 cell count, high HIV virus load, a reduced time gap between starting of anti-TB therapy and HART, improvement in CD4 cell count and decrease in the viral load upon initiation of HART, and disseminated TB are risk factors for development of PR-IRIS in HIV patients [66]. In a prospective study, a higher baseline CSF neutrophil count, high TNF-α levels, low IFN-γ level, and positive CSF culture for *M. tuberculosis* are also found to predict the development of paradoxical-IRIS [47].

34.3.6 Treatment

A randomized placebo-controlled study of steroids in TB-IRIS patients showed significant improvement in TB-IRIS in patients who received steroids [67]. However, the study did not include patients with neurological manifestations of TB PR-IRIS. Most patients in the study were with new lung infiltrates, pleural effusion, lymphadenopathy, and cold abscess. Majority of patients with CNS manifestations of TB PR-IRIS end up receiving corticosteroids due to life-threatening nature of the illness. However, the duration of treatment remains individualized.

Timing of initiation of HART in patients with CNS TB who are receiving anti-TB therapy may be a determining factor for development of PR-IRIS. For initiating HART in patients with TB, CD4 counts may be used as a marker. The British HIV Association (BHIVA) recommends that if CD4 consistently remains >350 cells/μl, initiating HART is at physician's discretion; CD4 100–350 cells/μl, HART to be started as soon as practical but can wait until after completion of 2 months of TB treatment; CD4 < 100 cells/μl, HART to be started as soon as practical [68].

34.3.7 Prognosis

The outcome of neurological TB-related paradoxical-IRIS remains poor. In a reported series, 13% of patients died, with all-cause mortality of 25%, and 27% among survivors had severe disability. In comparison, CNS TB patients without paradoxical-IRIS had no death and 18% had severe disability.

Conclusion

Paradoxical worsening of CNS TB is more common than previously thought and may occur in nearly half of all patients upon initiation of anti-TB therapy. In HIV-positive individuals, worsening of CNS TB may occur after initiation of HART and is referred to as paradoxical-IRIS. CNS TB shows PR-IRIS more frequently than other organ systems in patients suffering from HIV. PR may present with worsening clinical features, radiological characteristics, or CSF picture. Continuation of anti-TB therapy and steroids may improve PR in majority of patients. Prognosis among paradoxical-IRIS remains poor with higher mortality and disability as compared to those patients with TBM but without paradoxical-IRIS.

References

1. Garg RK, Malhotra HS, Kumar N (2014) Paradoxical reaction in HIV negative tuberculous meningitis. J Neurol Sci 340:26–36
2. Tai ML, Nor HM, Kadir KA, Viswanathan S, Rahmat K, Zain NR, Ong KG, Rafia MH, Tan CT (2016) Paradoxical manifestation is common in HIV-negative tuberculous meningitis. Medicine (Baltimore) 95:e1997
3. Cherian A, Thomas SV (2011) Central nervous system tuberculosis. Afr Health Sci 11:116–127
4. Meintjes G, Lawn SD, Scano F, Maartens G, French MA, Worodria W, Elliott JH, Murdoch D, Wilkinson RJ, Seyler C, John L, van der Loeff MS, Reiss P, Lynen L, Janoff EN, Gilks C, Colebunders R (2008) International network for the study of HIV-associated IRIS. Tuberculosis-associated immune reconstitution inflammatory syndrome: case definitions for use in resource-limited settings. Lancet Infect Dis 8:516–523
5. Carvalho AC, De Iaco G, Saleri N, Pini A, Capone S, Manfrin M, Matteelli A (2006) Paradoxical reaction during tuberculosis treatment in HIV-seronegative patients. Clin Infect Dis 42:893–895
6. Cheng VCC, Ho PL, Lee RA, Chan KS, Chan KK, Woo PCY, Lau SKP, Yuen KY (2002) Clinical spectrum of paradoxical deterioration during anti TB therapy in non-HIV-infected patients. Eur J Clin Microbiol Infect Dis 21:803–809
7. Lorent N, Sebatunzi O, Mukeshimana G, Van den Ende J, Clerinx J (2011) Incidence and risk factors of serious adverse events during antituberculous treatment in Rwanda: a prospective cohort study. PLoS One 6:e19566
8. Cheng VC, YamWC WPC, Lau SK, Hung IF, Wong SP, Cheung WC, Yuen KY (2003) Risk factors for development of paradoxical response during antituberculosis therapy in HIV-negativepatients. Eur J Clin Microbiol Infect Dis 22:597–602
9. Geri G, Passeron A, Heym B, Arlet JB, Pouchot J, Capron L, Rangue B (2013) Paradoxical reactions during treatment of tuberculosis with extrapulmonary manifestations in HIV negative patients. Infection 41:537–543
10. Olive C, Mouchet F, Toppet V, Haelterman E, Levy J (2013) Paradoxical reaction during TB treatment in immunocompetent children: clinical spectrumand risk factors. Pediatr Infect Dis J 32:446–449
11. Sütlas PN, Unal A, Forta H, Senol S, Kirbas D (2003) Tuberculous meningitis in adults: review of 61 cases. Infection 31:387–391
12. Schoeman JF, Donald PR (2013) Tuberculous meningitis. Handb Clin Neurol 112:1135–1138

13. Anupriya A, Sunithi M, Maya T, Goel M, Alexander M, Aaron S, Mathew V (2010) Tuberculous optochiasmatic arachnoiditis. Neurol India 58:732–735
14. Sinha MK, Garg RK, Anuradha HK, Agarwal A, Parihar A, Mandhani PA (2010) Paradoxical vision loss associated with optochiasmatic tuberculoma in tuberculous meningitis: a report of 8 patients. J Infect 60:458–466
15. Sinha MK, Garg RK, Anuradha HK, Agarwal A, Singh MK, Verma R, Shukla R (2010) Vision impairment in tuberculous meningitis: predictors and prognosis. J Neurol Sci 290:27–32
16. Anuradha HK, Garg RK, Agarwal A, Sinha MK, Verma R, Singh MK, Shukla R (2010) Predictors of stroke in patients with tuberculous meningitis and its effect on the outcome. Q J Med 103:671–678
17. Misra UK, Kalita J, Nair PP (2010) Role of aspirin in tuberculous meningitis: a randomized open label placebo controlled trial. J Neurol Sci 293:12–17
18. Singh B, Garg RK, SinghMK VR, Malhotra HS, Jain A, Singh R, Kohli N, Phadke RV, Shukla R, Parihar A (2012) Computed tomography angiography in patients with tuberculous meningitis. J Infect 64:565–572
19. Anuradha HK, Garg RK, Sinha MK, Agarwal A, Verma R, SinghMK AA, Verma R, Singh MK, Shukla R (2011) Intracranial tuberculomas in patients with tuberculous meningitis: predictors and prognostic significance. Int J Tuberc Lung Dis 15:234–239
20. Thwaites GE, Macmullen-Price J, Tran TH, Pham PM, Nguyen TD, Simmons CP, White NJ, Tran TH, Summers D, Farrar JJ (2007) Serial MRI to determine the effect of dexamethasone on the cerebral pathology of tuberculous meningitis: an observational study. Lancet Neurol 6:230–236
21. Raut T, Garg RK, Jain A, Verma R, Singh MK, Malhotra HS, Kohli N, Parihar A (2013) Hydrocephalus in tuberculousmeningitis: Incidence, its predictive factors and impact on the prognosis. J Infect 66:330–337
22. Singh P, Paliwal VK, Neyaz Z, Srivastava AK, Verma R, Mohan S (2014) Clinical and magnetic resonance imaging characteristics of tubercular ventriculitis: an under-recognized complication of tubercular meningitis. J Neurol Sci 342:137–140
23. Gupta A, Garg RK, Singh MK, Verma R, Malhotra HS, Sankhwar SN, Jain A, Singh R, Parihar A (2013) Bladder dysfunction and urodynamic study in tuberculous meningitis. J Neurol Sci 327:46–54
24. Dastur D, Wadia NH (1969) Spinal meningitides with radiculo-myelopathy. 2. Pathology and pathogenesis. J Neurol Sci 8:261–297
25. Gupta RK, Gupta S, Kumar S, Kohli A, Misra UK, Gujral RB (1994) MRI in intraspinal tuberculosis. Neuroradiology 36:39–43
26. Srivastava T, Kochar DK (2003) Asymptomatic spinal arachnoiditis in patients with tuberculous meningitis. Neuroradiology 45:727–729
27. Citow JS, Ammirati M (1994) Intramedullary tuberculoma of the spinal cord: case report. Neurosurgery 35:327–330
28. Skendros P, Kamaria F, Kontopoulos V, Tsitouridis I, Sidiropoulos L (2003) Intradural, extramedullary tuberculoma of the spinal cord as a complication of tuberculous meningitis. Infection 31:115–117
29. Muthukumar N, Sureshkumar V, Ramesh VG (2007) En plaque intradural extramedullary spinal tuberculoma and concurrent intracranial tuberculomas: paradoxical response to antituberculous therapy. Case report J Neurosurg Spine 6:169–173
30. Moghtaderi A, Alavi-Naini R, Rahimi-Movaghar V (2006) Syringomyelia: an early complication of tuberculous meningitis. Trop Doct 36:254–255
31. Daif AK, al Rajeh S, Ogunniyi A, al Boukai A, al Tahan A (1997) Syringomyelia developing as an acute complication of tuberculous meningitis. Can J Neurol Sci 24:73–76
32. Pandey S, Nayak R, Mehndiratta MM (2013) Early syringomyelia in tubercular meningitis: a rare occurrence. J Neurol Res 3:46–48
33. Teoh R, O'Mahony G, Yeung VT (1986) Polymorphonuclear pleocytosis in the cerebrospinal fluid during chemotherapy for tuberculous meningitis. J Neurol 233:237–241
34. Garcia-Monco JC, Ferreira E, Gomez-Beldarrain M (2005) The therapeutic paradox in the diagnosis of tuberculous meningitis. Neurology 65:1991–1992
35. Afghani B, Lieberman JM (1994) Paradoxical enlargement or development of intracranial tuberculomas during therapy: case report and review. Clin Infect Dis 19:1092–1099
36. Kim SH, Kim YS (2009) Immunologic paradox in the diagnosis of tuberculous meningitis. Clin Vaccine Immunol 16:1847–1849
37. Mosmann TR, Coffman RL (1989) TH1 and TH2 cells: different patterns of lymphokine secretion lead to different functional properties. Annu Rev Immunol 7:145–173
38. Parkin J, Cohen B (2001) An overview of the immune system. Lancet 357:1777–1789
39. Nelms K, Keegan AD, Zamorano J, Ryan JJ, Paul WE (1999) The IL-4 receptor: signaling mechanisms and biologic functions. Annu Rev Immunol 17:701–738
40. Afzali B, Lombardi G, Lechler RI, Lord GM (2007) The role of T helper 17 (Th17) and regulatory T cells (Treg) in human organ transplantation and autoimmune disease. Clin Exp Immunol 148:32–46
41. Harrington LE, Hatton RD, Mangan PR, Turner H, Murphy TL, Murphy KM, Weaver CT (2005) Interleukin 17-producing CD41 effector T cells develop via a lineage distinct from the T helper type 1 and 2 lineages. Nat Immunol 6:1123–1132
42. Martin-Blondel G, Mars LT, Liblau RS (2012) Pathogenesis of the immune reconstitution inflammatory syndrome in HIV-infected patients. Curr Opin Infect Dis 25:312–320
43. Bettelli E, Korn T, Oukka M, Kuchroo VK (2008) Induction and effector functions of T(H)17 cells. Nature 453:1051–1057
44. Belkaid Y, Tarbell K (2009) Regulatory T cells in the control of host microorganism interactions. Annu Rev Immunol 27:551–589

45. Hawkey CR, Yap T, Pereira J, Moore DA, Davidson RN, Pasvol G, Kon OM, Wall RA, Wilkinson RJ (2005) Characterization and management of paradoxical upgrading reactions in HIV-uninfected patients with lymph node TB. Clin Infect Dis 40:1368–1371
46. Sáenz B, Hernandez-Pando R, Fragoso G, Bottasso O, Cárdenas G (2013) The dual face of central nervous system tuberculosis: a new Janus Bifrons? Tuberculosis (Edinb) 93:130–135
47. Marais S, Meintjes G, Pepper DJ, Dodd LE, Schutz C, Ismail Z, Wilkinson KA, Wilkinson RJ (2013) Frequency, severity, and prediction of tuberculous meningitis immune reconstitution inflammatory syndrome. Clin Infect Dis 56:450–460
48. Bekker LG, Maartens G, Steyn L, Kaplan G (1998) Selective increase in plasma tumor necrosis factor-alpha and concomitant clinical deterioration after initiating therapy in patients with severe tuberculosis. J Infect Dis 178:580–584
49. Schoeman JF, Van Zyl LE, Laubscher JA, Donald PR (1997) Effect of corticosteroids on intracranial pressure, computed tomographic findings, and clinical outcome in young children with tuberculous meningitis. Pediatrics 99:226–231
50. Jorge JH, Graciela C, Pablo AP, Luis SH (2012) A life-threatening central nervous system tuberculosis inflammatory reaction nonresponsive to corticosteroids and successfully controlled by infliximab in a young patient with a variant of juvenile idiopathic arthritis. J Clin Rheumatol 18:189–191
51. Lee HS, Lee Y, Lee SO, Choi SH, Kim YS, Woo JH, Kim SH (2012) Adalimumab treatment may replace or enhance the activity of steroids in steroid-refractory tuberculous meningitis. J Infect Chemother 18:555–557
52. Schoeman JF, Springer P, van Rensburg AJ, Swanevelder S, Hanekom WA, Haslett PA, Kaplan G (2004) Adjunctive thalidomide therapy for childhood tuberculous meningitis: results of a randomized study. J Child Neurol 19:250–257
53. Nandi B, Behar SM (2011) Regulation of neutrophils by interferon-γ limits lung inflammation during TB infection. J Exp Med 208:2251–2262
54. Gonzalez-Duarte A, Higuera-Calleja J, Flores F, Davila-Maldonado L, Cantú-Brito C (2012) Cyclophosphamide treatment for unrelenting CNS vasculitis secondary to tuberculous meningitis. Neurology 78:1277–1278
55. Bas NS, Güzey FK, Emel E, Alatas I, Sel B (2005) Paradoxical intracranial tuberculoma requiring surgical treatment. Pediatr Neurosurg 41:201–205
56. Shaharao VB, Pawar M, Agarwal R, Bavdekar SB (2004) Intra-medullary tuberculoma occurringduring treatment of tuberculous meningitis. Indian J Pediatr 71:107–108
57. French MA, Price P, Stone SF (2004) Immune restoration disease after antiretroviral therapy. AIDS 18:1615–1627
58. Shelburne SA, Montes M, Hamill RJ (2006) Immune reconstitution inflammatory syndrome: more answers, more questions. J Antimicrob Chemother 57:167–170
59. Colebunders R, John L, Huyst V, Kambugu A, Scano F, Lynen L (2006) Tuberculosis immune reconstitution inflammatory syndrome in countries with limited resources. Int J Tuberc Lung Dis 10:946–953
60. Müller M, Wandel S, Colebunders R, Attia S, Furrer H, Egger M, FOR iEdea Southern and Central Africa (2010) Incidence and lethality of immune reconstitution disease in HIN-infected patients starting antiretroviral therapy: systemic review and meta-analysis. Lancet Infect Dis 10:251–261
61. Pepper DJ, Marais S, Maartens G, Rebe K, Morroni C, Rangaka MX, Oni T, Wilkinson RJ, Meinties G (2009) Neurologic manifestations of paradoxical TB-associated immune reconstitution inflammatory syndrome: a case series. Clin Infect Dis 48:e96–107
62. Bucy RP, Hockett RD, Derdeyn CA, Saag MS, Squires K, Sillers M, Mitsuyasu RT, Kilby JM (1999) Initial increase in blood CD4 lymphocytes after HIVantiretroviral therapy reflects redistribution from lymphoid tissues. J Clin Invest 103:1391–1398
63. Datta S, Sarvetnick N (2009) Lymphocyte proliferation in immunemediated diseases. Trends Immunol 30:430–438
64. Schulze ZurWiesch J, Thomssen A, Hartjen P, Tóth I, Lehmann C, Meyer-Olson D, Colberg K, Frerk S, Babikir D, Schmiedel S, Degen O, Mauss S, Rockstroh J, Staszeqski S, Khayin P, Strasak A, Lohse WA, Fätkenheuer G, Hauber J, van Lunzen J (2011) Comprehensive analysis of frequency and phenotype of T regulatory cells in HIV infection: CD39 expression of FoxP31 T regulatory cells correlates with progressive disease. J Virol 85:1287–1297
65. Lai RP, Meintjes G, Wilkinson KA, Graham CM, Marais S, Van der Plas H, Deffur A, Schutz C, Bloom C, Munagala I, Anguiano E, Goliath R, Maartens G, Banchereau J, Chaussabel D, O'Garra A, Wilkinson RJ (2015) HIV-tuberculosis-associated immune reconstitution inflammatory syndrome is characterized by Toll-like receptor and inflammasome signalling. Nat Commun 6:8451
66. Mori S, Levin P (2009) A brief review of potential mechanisms of immune reconstitution inflammatory syndrome in HIV following antiretroviral therapy. Int J STD AIDS 20:447–452
67. Meintjes G, Wilkinson RJ, Morroni C, Pepper DJ, Rebe K, Rangaka MX, Oni T, Maartens G (2010) Randomized placebo-controlled trial of prednisone for paradoxical tuberculosis-associated immune reconstitution inflammatory syndrome. AIDS 24:2381–2390
68. Pozniak AL, Coyne KM, Miller RF, Lipman MCI, Freedman AR, Ormerod LP, Johnson MA, Collins S, Lucas SB, on behalf of the BHIVA guidelines subcommittee (2011) British HIV association guidelines for the treatment of TB/HIV coinfection 2011. HIV Med 12:517–524

Tuberculosis of the Nervous System in Immunocompromised Hosts

35

Mehdi Laghmari, Gedéon Thouassa, Davis Mpando, and Said Ait Benali

Contents

M. Laghmari, MD (✉)
Service de Neurochirurgie, CHU Mohammed VI, Marrakech, Morocco

Department of Neurosurgery, CHU Mohammed VI, Marrakesh, Morocco
e-mail: Me.laghmari@uca.ma

Centre Hospitalier Universitaire Mohammed VI Hopital AR-RAZI, Avenue Ibn Sina Amerchich, 2360 Marrakech, Morocco

G. Thouassa, MD • D. Mpando, MD
S.A. Benali, MD
Service de Neurochirurgie, CHU Mohammed VI, Marrakech, Morocco

Department of Neurosurgery, CHU Mohammed VI, Marrakesh, Morocco
e-mail: gedcolinthouassa@gmail.com; davismpando@gmail.com; aitbenalis@yahoo.fr

Abbreviations

AFB	Acid-fast bacilli
AIDS	Acquired immunodeficiency syndrome
ART	Antiretroviral therapy
BCG	Bacillus Calmette-Guerin
BMRC	British Medical Research Council
CNS	Central nervous system
CSF	Cerebrospinal fluid
CT	Computed tomography
DNA	Deoxyribonucleic acid
ELISPOT	Enzyme-linked immunospot assay
FRET	Fluorescence resonance energy transfer
HIV	Human immunodeficiency virus
INH	Isoniazid
IRIS	Immune reconstitution inflammatory syndrome
MRI	Magnetic resonance imaging
PCR	Polymerase chain reaction
RIF	Rifampicin
TB	Tuberculosis
TBM	Tuberculous meningitis

35.1 Introduction

Tuberculosis (TB) has become more prevalent since the emergence of the pandemic human immunodeficiency virus (HIV) infection. The complex rela-

M. Turgut et al. (eds.), *Tuberculosis of the Central Nervous System*,
DOI 10.1007/978-3-319-50712-5_35

tionship of TB in HIV described for nearly three decades is a major threat in the effort of the international community to attain the United Nations Millennium Development Goals on Health in the fight against the pandemic of HIV/acquired immunodeficiency syndrome (AIDS) [1]. In 2007 there were 2.7 million new infections and 2 million deaths from HIV infection, and at the end of 2008, an estimated 33.2 million people were reported to be infected with HIV; in the course of the same year, there were 1.37 million (15%) of TB cases associated with HIV infection, responsible for 456,000 deaths. In some African countries, the incidence of TB in patients living with HIV is around 80% [2].

In developed countries, including the United States, despite the fact that the incidence of TB has diminished significantly since 1993, the incidence of new cases of extrapulmonary locations of TB has increased exponentially [3]. The increase in these cases is correspondingly associated with those of HIV, as there is an increased sensitivity to reactivation and dissemination of TB in these patients [4].

Currently, there is a renewed interest on the extrapulmonary manifestations of TB due to their high frequency in HIV infection [5]. TB localization in the central nervous system (CNS) is quite common and is one of the expressions of severe TB. In developing countries, TB lesions represent 10–30% of intracranial expansive process [6]. CNS TB is characterized by a semiotic polymorphism, clinical, biological and morphological diagnostic criteria, which are well codified and also by the complexity and variability of its support currently the subject of great controversy [7]. In this work, we will address cases of immunodeficiency induced by HIV infection and also in patients submitted to transplants of solid organs, as these two situations increase susceptibility to the acquisition or reactivation of TB and complicate the management of the immunosuppression-induced CNS TB [8].

35.2 Central Nervous System Manifestations of TB Associated with HIV

The manifestations of CNS TB in patients infected with HIV are identical to those of uninfected patients. Tuberculous meningitis (TBM) in patients infected with HIV representing 5–15% of cases of extrapulmonary locations of TB is one of the most devastating events in terms of mortality and morbidity [9]; it occurs in people of all ages. It is more common in children, especially those under the age of 1 year [10, 11]. Forty to sixty percent of adults with extrapulmonary locations of TB have a TBM. In a study of 2025 cases, 10% of HIV-positive patients had a TBM in comparison to only 2% of patients without HIV infection [12]. The risk of TBM is greater in patients infected with HIV, with a CD4 count of lower than 100 cells/µl [13, 14]. It is the most severe presentation in terms of mortality and morbidity [15]. Mortality is often associated with a delay in diagnosis and treatment [16].

The absence of specific symptoms and signs in patients with TBM makes the early diagnosis hard. TBM is characterized by clinical polymorphism, but the most common symptoms are headache (86%), vomiting (64%) and impaired consciousness (59%) [17]. Irritation meningitis was detected in 37% of cases [17]. The involvement of basal cisterns is frequently encountered often characterized by an oculomotor palsy also by facial paralysis. This involvement of the cranial nerves is in connection with the compression of nerve trunks by thick basal exudates or intracranial hypertension, and it occurs in about 25% of cases [18]. Formidable visual complications are also described which may result in a decrease in visual acuity or even blindness but sometimes a sudden onset of ophthalmoplegia. These visual events are the consequence of the presence of exudates in the optic chiasm, but also arteritis or a compression in the visual pathways by hydrocephalus or a tuberculoma. In older people the TBM can manifest as subacute dementia syndrome with memory impairment and frontal syndrome type of behaviour [18].

TBM is sometimes manifested by an insidious onset, and a high diagnostic suspicion should be raised in children with disorders of consciousness, especially in endemic areas. The children are more probably to have nausea, vomiting and seizures; headaches are less frequent [19].

The notion of TB contagion commonly found in children (50–90%) is a critical criterion in establishing the diagnosis of paucisymptomatic form. The clinical manifestations in children are very varied; growth retardation, weight loss, irritability, lack of sleep problems, appetite, vomiting and abdominal pain are frequently seen in young children [20].

Hydrocephalus is frequently found, following cerebrospinal fluid (CSF) resorption defect due to the existence of high levels of protein. Vasospasms, thrombosis and TBM-induced haemorrhagic infarction are responsible for vasculopathies with intracranial stroke [20].

Although the clinical manifestations of the TBM is independent of HIV status of the patients, it has been reported of a frequency higher of consciousness disorders among HIV subjects as well as the existence of lymph node involvement [21, 22]. Only 15% of HIV patients are suffering from TBM triad of fever, headache and meningeal rigidity [13].

The neurological clinical picture of patients with TBM was summarized pursuant to the British Medical Research Council (BMRC) [7] which is classified into grades of the TBM as follows:

- Grade 1: patient with nonspecific symptoms and signs, without loss of consciousness or neurological deficits
- Grade 2: patient with lethargy or behavioural disorders, meningeal syndrome or minor neurological deficits such as cranial nerve palsies
- Grade 3: patient with stupor or coma, abnormal movements, convulsions or severe neurological disorders such as paresis

Specific laboratory diagnosis of TBM is established on the analysis of CSF. Biological criteria identifying CSF abnormalities induced by TBM have been well described [18].

The conventional perturbances of CSF in TBM are:

- A high-pressure CSF at lumbar puncture
- A high leukocyte count rates between 10 and 500 cells/mm^3 lymphocytic
- CSF protein of 100–500 mg/dl
- Glycorrhachia less than 40 percent of the glucose
- A positive culture of 3–6 weeks, reported in 75% of patients

However, all in all, the gold standard for laboratory diagnosis remains the identification of *Mycobacterium tuberculosis* in the CSF [11]. The best method available for the isolation of acid-fast bacilli (AFB) in CSF remains the polymerase chain reaction (PCR), although its sensitivity is controversial. The success of the microscopic study of CSF and culture of *M. tuberculosis* depends on the volume of CSF obtained during lumbar puncture. Thus, a lumbar puncture should necessarily be repeated in case of a doubt in the diagnosis. The diagnosis is confirmed after the identification of TB bacilli, and this is sometimes done after analysis of several samples; however, in 30–50% of cases, these bacilli are not found, and this is what necessitates the interest in PCR in the diagnosis, although no study has currently evaluated its effectiveness. Many authors claim to have found AFB in less than 20 cases of TBM [23]. A prospective study of the laboratory diagnosis of 107 adult patients out of 132 (81%) with clinical signs through computed tomography (CT) reported that AFB were observed in 77 cases out of 132 and grown in 94 cases out of 132 [24]. Thus, the CSF must necessarily be grown in all suspicious forms of meningitis. The value of culture is confirmed in the differential diagnosis of fungal meningitis and TBM, in which the ink and acid preparations are negative in 50% of cases, even more. However, the culture, although sensitive, is positive in about 40% of cases, and the time for the achievement of results is approximately 6 weeks [25]. The CSF of most patients with TBM contains only 100 to 102 bacilli/ml, while it takes approximately 104 bacilli/ml to obtain reliable results for the Ziehl-Neelsen and auramine; therefore in order to increase the success of the exam, the smear of CSF should have a volume of 6 ml and be analysed within 30 min of collection [24]. The nucleic acid amplification tests such as PCR assays were assessed for their efficacy in detecting the presence of bacterial DNA (deoxyribonucleic acid) in the CSF. Analysis of CSF by PCR constitutes a significant improvement in the diagnosis of TBM. CSF analyses of the PCR studies have reported a specificity of 90–100% and a sensitivity varying from 75% to 100% [26].

Several modifications of the technique PCR have been proposed to make better the sensitivity and specificity of the test. One of the more recent developments is the use of real-time PCR amplification for the detection of the product, by using fluorescence probes and the fluorescence resonance energy transfer (FRET). One of the advantages of this test is that it is the fastest and promising system; however, to date most studies have used amplification of mycobacteriophage, which detects the viable organisms in the samples. The technique is simple and does not require for expensive equipment and results are acquired within 24–48 h [27, 28]. Enzyme-linked immunospot assay (ELISPOT) is a recent test; it is for the rapid detection of specific T-cell *M. tuberculosis* [29]. The presence of AFB in smears of CSF or cultures and a positive PCR for mycobacteria or assay immunoglobulin M in the CSF were considered definitive proof of TBM. TBM "final" is defined as the isolation of one or more *M. tuberculosis* in CSF cultures and/or PCR positive.

The CT scan and magnetic resonance imaging (MRI) revolutionized the diagnosis and management of the TBM. However, these tests may be normal at the beginning of the disease. They highlight intracranial abnormalities most often associated with the complications of the TBM. Patients suffering from TBM brain complications such as hydrocephalus, focal or diffuse cerebral oedema, cerebral infarction and abscesses and intracranial tuberculoma have an indication for neurosurgery; however, complications of TBM in the brain as seen by neuroimaging, such as hydrocephalus, are significantly smaller in patients living with HIV [30].

The tuberculoma is a TB granulomatous tissue mass that has been contained and limited by the immune defences of the host. Tuberculomas of the CNS are inflammatory intracranial expansive processes, pseudotumour, usually unique but sometimes multiple and sometimes asymptomatic. The cerebral tuberculoma is a rare disease observed in 1% of all cases of TB [30] and represents 10–30% of intracranial expansive processes in TB endemic areas [31]. As for Madagascar, the central pathology service has met only two cases in 7 years [32]. The cerebral tuberculoma is a childhood of pathology. Adults 18–60 years of age are also affected, without gender predominance. Many studies point to the existence of a correlation between the appearance of a tuberculoma and HIV infection and also the presence of tuberculoma in 16–40% of patients with TBM [33].

Symptoms of tuberculoma are usually part of a very evocative context, because there is often a history of TB and clinical and radiological signs of extracerebral TB. But it is common in countries with high endemicity to observe tuberculoma as the first clinical expression of TB. Clinical expression is extremely varied and is not specific. It depends on the location of tuberculoma, its size, its mass effect relative to surrounding structures and the associated cerebral oedema. The onset is usually slow and gradual. Clinical data, although not specific, often include signs of intracranial hypertension, cerebellar syndrome, neurological signs, seizures, meningeal irritation, visual disturbances, cranial nerve involvement, consciousness disorders and rarely aphasia. Fever is observed in only 10–15% of cases [34]. However, cases of asymptomatic cerebral tuberculoma have also been reported [30].

The clinical manifestation of tuberculoma may vary in individuals infected with HIV. A small study conducted in Spain included four patients infected with HIV and having a cerebral tuberculoma, which stressed and isolated the constant presence of fever and headache, without signs of neurological focus [35].

Laboratory tests have no role in the positive diagnosis. The finding of AFB by direct examination or by removal of the tumour cultivation is positive for TBM in 30% of cases [30].

Caseating tuberculoma is the most classic form. It appears on CT scan with isodensity, discreetly hypodense compared to the brain parenchyma. After injection with a contrast, the enhancement is done either globally or in a ring, very evocative; the presence of calcification, surrounded by a hypodense central area with a peripheral ring, called "target sign" or the sign of the target, is pathognomonic of tuberculoma. The location varies, but in over half the cases, tuberculomas are located in the left cerebral hemisphere.

TB abscess is an uncommon clinical form of CNS TB, even in countries with endemic TB [36]. It represents only 4–8% of patients with CNS TB that are not affected by HIV and has been reported in only 20% of HIV patients [37]. This high frequency of TB abscess in HIV patients is probably related to the suppression of cell-mediated immunity induced by HIV, which causes the inhibition of the immune response against intracerebral TB bacilli, increasing the probability of occurrence of TB abscess, based on the granuloma [38].

The clinical presentation of TB abscess is multiple, depending on its headquarters, its volume and its mass effect in relation to nearby structures. TB abscess has a greater diameter than the tuberculomas, usually greater than 3 cm, and its clinical manifestations are usually sharper than those of tuberculoma. It generally includes, on the symptomatic level, fever, headache and focal neurological deficits. Before the AIDS era, Withener in 1978 mentioned that patients with TB abscess usually had acute clinical picture with focal neurological deficit (71%), headache (47%), fever (46%), seizures (35%) or disorders of consciousness (24%) [39].

A study in 12 patients infected with HIV with TB abscess stressed that the seizures, headache, altered consciousness and hemiparaplegia were the first symptoms most consistently frequent except in one patient who had a solitary lesion [40]. In a Mexican study in 2010, the clinical manifestations of TB abscess appeared altogether similar in immunocompetent patients and HIV patients [41].

The radiological presentation of TB abscess is the same in HIV and non-HIV patients. This is most often a uni- or multinodular lesion with a uniform capsule [42]. But it is sometimes difficult to distinguish one from another injuries especially other pyogenic abscesses. At CT, the hypodense image, circled by a fine contrast uptake, is difficult to differentiate from pyogenic abscess or some primary or metastatic tumours or a resolution lane hematoma. At the MRI, there is low signal intensity on T1 and a hyper-signal T2 in the central area with contrast enhancement in a ring as pyogenic abscesses. Parenchyma surrounding oedema usually shows less marked than in pyogenic abscess. Only spectroscopy proton MRI allows differentiating between TB abscess and pyogenic abscesses [43].

TB is a rare cause of TB radiculomyelitis or arachnoiditis. Spinal TB can be de novo or secondary to bacillary intracranial infection (TBM) or vertebral TB (Pott's disease) [44]. The extension of a TBM intracranial to the meninges of the spinal cord is the pathogenic mechanism most frequently found.

The precise incidence and prevalence of TB radiculomyelitis in most parts of the world are not well identified; however in countries with high TB endemic, these should be proportionally high.

In approximately 10% of patients suffering from extrapulmonary TB in bones, the spine is the most frequent site, representing nearly 50% of cases of bone TB. In France, in a hospital-based study, the overall incidence of vertebral osteomyelitis was estimated at 2.4/100,000 [45]. From 2002 to 2003, 1422 of 1425 patients were divided as having a definite vertebral osteomyelitis (64%), probable (24%) and feasible (12%). The *M. tuberculosis* (31%) was the main infectious agent after offending *Staphylococcus* spp. (38%) [45].

In endemic countries, spinal TB is more common in children and young adults [45]. There is no data that shows an increase in the incidence of multidrug-resistant TB in HIV patients; however, the incidence of TB radiculomyelitis would probably be proportional to the cases of HIV-associated TBM with a view that it is the primary aetiology of TB radiculomyelitis [46].

Clinical manifestations of TB radiculomyelitis have been well described since 1969 [47]. This is a clinical picture characterized by subacute onset of paraparesis, gradually settling for 1–2 months. Symptoms include neuralgia, paraesthesia, sphincter disturbances and muscle atrophy. A subsequent paralysis eventually installs, usually after a few days. It is not unusual to find lack of tendon reflexes with flaccidity of the lower limbs and the existence of plantar reflex with Babinski sign [48]. Secondary TB radiculomyelitis may occur in the acute phase of a TBM diagnosed and even treated after very variable periods. It was reported in one study, with two cases, that TB radiculomyelitis developed 7–9 years after a TBM [49]. In another study, it was mentioned that two patients had paralysis 14 and 17 years, respectively, after TBM [44]. In immunocompetent patients, the thoracic spinal cord is the most frequently involved [44, 50]. It has been shown that HIV infection does not seem to modify the clinical presentations of TB radiculomyelitis [12].

CT and MRI are important diagnostic examinations of the TB radiculomyelitis. However, MRI using sagittal and axial T1-weighted views before and after injection of the contrast agent remains by far the gold standard in the detection of patients with suspected TB radiculomyelitis, whatever the stage of the disease [46]. T2-weighted images show an inhomogeneous obliteration of the subarachnoid space and loss of the contours of the marrow in the cervical, thoracic and lumbar segments, with a tangled appearance of roots. On T1-weighted images after gadolinium injection, images appear nodular, with thickening of the meningeal space and contrast occupying the entire subarachnoid space, sheathing the roots that have an irregular contour and appear thickened and tangled. Taking spinal contrast is a strong presumption element to move towards a neuro-meningeal infection. MRI is also essential for early monitoring of treatment is worsening can be observed in rare situations, a decompression laminectomy is required. It is also essential in monitoring the evolution and in the detection of a possible syringomyelia that can remotely install.

The availability of antiretroviral therapy (ART) adds the risk of immune reconstitution inflammatory syndrome (IRIS) and TB, which complicates the diagnosis and therapeutic management of CNS TB [51]. Two forms of IRIS-related TB have been described:

- Paradoxical IRIS and TB occurs in patients diagnosed with active TB before the start of ART and have typically been responding to the TB treatment. Following initiation of ART, IRIS presents as subsequent worsening of symptoms or onset of new symptoms.
- Unmasking IRIS and TB occurs in patients who are not diagnosed with TB but have an unusual inflammatory reaction in the first 3 months after initiation of ART.

Paradoxical IRIS and TB events occur in both non-HIV-infected patients and patients infected with HIV who are not on ART [51]. The clinical expression of IRIS and TB is reflected in the appearance of a recurrent fever, exacerbation of pulmonary symptoms (worsening of pulmonary infiltrates and pleural effusions intensification), installing signs of meningeal irritation and the emergence of new tuberculoma or enlargement of those already existing.

IRIS and TB is specially severe in patients with tuberculoma, who will present new lesions or expansion of existing ones responsible for a mass effect with exacerbation of peri-lesional oedema and seizures occurring with clinical deterioration [52]. It was also observed that there is appearance of new anatomical sites of TB. In a study of 258 patients with pulmonary TB, paradoxical IRIS and TB was described in 53 (20.5%) cases just after initiation of ART and in 8 (3.1%) cases later during treatment; and 6 (10%) cases of deaths by IRIS were highlighted [52]. In the largest number of IRIS and TB affecting the CNS, the delay of onset had a median of 14 days after the start of ART [53].

The pathogenesis of IRIS and TB is variable and is attributed to a combination of factors: the release of new target antigens for destruction mycobacteria, hypersensitivity to these antigens and exaggerated immune restoration (after induced immunosuppression by TB) which occur during anti-bacillary treatment. The development of paradoxical reactions among non-HIV-infected patients is correlated with a greater increase in the number of total lymphocytes at the initiation of TB treatment. These paradoxical reactions have also been frequently highlighted in the period following the start of ART among both non-HIV-infected patients (36%) and those infected (2%) and those not under ART (7%) in a 1998 study [54].

Risk factors favouring the occurrence of paradoxical IRIS have been described [54]. These are multi-organ TB, low CD4 counts before ART and the shorter interval between initialization of TB treatment and ART. However, it is possible that other factors yet unknown may also have a share in the occurrence of IRIS and TB, such as other opportunistic infections and malignancies and the failure of TB treatment (due to non-adherence, drug resistance against TB or malabsorption of drugs against TB).

Unmasking IRIS has been less described in literature as compared to paradoxical IRIS, with few cases reported. A subset of these cases of IRIS presenting with increased intensity of clinical manifestations, particularly where there is evidence of a marked inflammatory component, in the first 3 months of the introduction of ART are designated as unmasking IRIS [54].

The diagnosis of CNS TB requires a location other than the CNS, which is easier to install.

Thus, nonspecific diagnostic investigations in the CNS, such as radiography of the chest, the tuberculin test and analysis of sputum, have a considerable interest in the diagnostic guidance of CNS TB. Studies have reported that the thorax radiography abnormalities are present in 41–60% of patients with TBM, 17–45% have a positive tuberculin test, and 50% positive sputum analysis [55]. High levels of serum interferon-gamma are highly specific for the diagnosis of TB, and its positivity is not compromised by previous BCG (bacillus Calmette-Guerin) vaccination [56]. Patients with HIV and TB having a latent phase have varying results in the test of serum interferon-gamma (Quantiferon), and a lower sensitivity is correlated with the degree of immunosuppression [57]. Culture of CSF remains the reference standard for the diagnosis of CNS TB. The advent of PCR should not be excluded in the diagnosis of CNS TB in the event of other tests' negativity. The results of studies suggest that the small test of interferon- gamma in the CSF is both highly sensitive and specific for the TBM [58]. A biological profile of CNS TB was described in a US study of 2011 [8] which includes CSF pleocytosis absent in 11–18%; there is no difference of rate between the leukocytes between patients with and without HIV, as reported by numerous studies. However, other studies describe a smaller number of leukocytes in HIV patients. In patients with CD4 counts below 50 cells/μL, pleocytosis is less common (77% versus 85.2%), and the mean number of cells present in the CSF is reduced (89 versus 246 cells/μL). No significant difference of protein or glucose levels was noted between HIV and non-HIV patients; however, some studies report lower protein levels in HIV patients. The classic triad of high protein, low glucose levels and pleocytosis was noted in 64% of cases. The colouring of the AFB had similar sensitivity for infected patients and non-HIV-infected patients, but mortality was higher among those who had a strongly smear-positive sample. The culture of AFB had not shown significant differences in sensitivity in HIV and non-HIV patients. *M. tuberculosis* was isolated in the vast majority of cases. These results are identical to the PCR.

35.3 Treatment of CNS Tuberculosis in Immunosuppression

First-line drug products for treatment recommended for all forms of TB are isoniazid (INH), rifampicin (RIF), pyrazinamide and ethambutol taken daily either individually or in combination. Since 1980, the period of 6–8 months of treatment, using a combination of four drugs in the initial phase followed by a combination of two drugs in the continuation phase, has been widely admitted. In 2004, the results of a multicentre randomized clinical trial demonstrated superior efficacy for the treatment of 6-month compared to 8-month therapy [59].

Pulmonary TB patients with associated HIV infection who are not on ART should always benefit from early initiation of ART to lower mortality, particularly in patients with CD4 cell rate of less than 50 cells/mm^3, in spite of the increased incidence of IRIS [60]. The World Health Organization advises initiation of ART after initiation of TB treatment, regardless of CD4 cell count [61]; however, the ART schedule in patients with a TBM has not been addressed in studies and may differ [7]. A study of the TBM in people infected with HIV in Vietnam compared patients who receive ART immediately on one hand and those having received 2 months later. And no major difference in mortality was stressed; however, patients who initiated ART forthwith had a higher rate of serious adverse events (grade 3 or 4). Due to the rapidity of death, the authors were incapable to determine whether these severe reactions were caused by IRIS or not [62]. Two large clinical trials of pulmonary TB in people infected with HIV and in patients with a rate less than 50 CD4 cells/mm^3 reported that initiating ART within 4 weeks after beginning TB treatment reduces mortality by 68% and 58%, respectively. In both studies, early initiation of antiretroviral therapy in people whose CD4 cell rate was below 50 cells/mm^3 was correlated with higher rates of IRIS (2.2 times and 2.5 times, respectively) [62]. In some regions of the world, individuals infected with HIV have higher rates of multidrug resistance of CNS TB, compared to HIV-negative patients, with rates ranging up to 7–12.5% [13, 63]. Patients with CNS TB and HIV have a higher mortality rate, and it is notably laborious to do the load due to the low penetration of the CNS by many second-line TB drugs [9]. For patients with multidrug resistance of TB, early initiation of ART and prolonged treatment improve the prognosis [64]. Many works have precisely suggested the participation of corticosteroids in improving morbidity and mortality among patients with IRIS [65]. In a study of 23 patients with CNS TB and IRIS, 21 (91%) received corticosteroids for an average of 58 days (range 1–49 weeks), and 16 (70%) were alive at 6 months [66]. Corticosteroids are recommended for the treatment of CNS TB, the same dosage should be used to prevent IRIS, but the long duration and slow and gradual dose reduction is recommended to avoid clinical deterioration [66].

The treatment of CNS TB in transplant patients is particularly difficult because many TB drugs interact with immunosuppressive agents. RIF, particularly, may accelerate the metabolism of cyclosporine, tacrolimus and corticosteroids and may lead to allograft rejection and higher mortality [67]. Co-administration of RIF and cyclosporine is generally avoided, although they can be used together if doses of both drugs are increased. Rifabutin can be used as an alternative to RIF, because it has less induction of cytochrome P450 and theoretically less effect on the levels of some immunosuppressive [67]. RIF and INH, optionally, can increase the catabolism of corticosteroids and therefore affect the level of immunosuppression [68]. Hepatotoxicity is an important concern in transplant patients receiving TB treatment, especially after a liver transplant. In one series, hepatotoxicity occurred in 83% of liver transplant after standard induction therapy of TB [68]. Multidrug resistance of TB is uncommon in transplant patients (reported incidence, 2%), but will likely increase as transplantation programmes develop in developing countries [69].

Conclusion

Immunosuppression increases patients' susceptibility for acquiring or reactivating TB and it complicates management. In developing world, HIV is the commonest cause of immunosuppression. It becomes very devastating when there is co-infection with TB with very high rates of morbidity and mortality worldwide. Clinical manifestations of CNS TB infection include meningitis, tuberculoma, abscess or other forms of disease. CNS TB has high morbidity and mortality and is difficult to diagnose and treat. HIV complicates the clinical presentation, diagnosis and treatment, and it is so difficult to clinically differentiate CNS TB from other potentially opportunistic infections that come with HIV. Generally HIV infection does not characteristically alter the radiographic or neurologic presentation of CNS TB; however, CSF pleocytosis is frequently absent, and patients with CD4 counts <50 cells/μL tend to have abnormal CSF findings less frequently. When a high suspicion for CNS TB is present, further CSF and ancillary testing should be performed and empirical treatment considered, especially if the patient is from an area with endemic TB or has evidence of TB outside of the CNS. ART and IRIS can affect the manifestations and outcome of CNS TB infection. Awareness of common drug interactions is of primordial importance for the successful treatment of patients with CNS TB. Patients also can benefit from the use of steroids for TBM and IRIS. With increased attention to TB diagnosis and treatment from international funding agencies, there is hope that the diagnosis and treatment of CNS TB will become easier and more effective in the near future.

References

1. Elzinga G, Raviglione MC, Maher D (2004) Scale up meeting margets in global tuberculosis control. Lancet 363:814–819
2. Granich R, Akolo C, Gunneberg C, Getahun H, Williams P, Williams B (2010) Preventing TB in people living with HIV. Clin Infect Dis 50:215–222
3. Peto HM, Pratt RH, Harrington TA, Lobue PA, Armstrong LR (2009) Epidemiology of extrapulmonary tuberculosis in the United States 1993– 2006. Clin Infect Dis 49:1350–1357
4. Rieder HL, Snider DE Jr, Cauthen GM (1990) Extrapulmonary tuberculosis in the United States. Am Rev Respir Dis 141:347–351
5. Leeds IL, Magee JM, Kurbatova EV, Rio CD, Blumberg HM, Leonard MK, Kraft CS (2012) Site of extrapulmonary tuberculosis is associated with HIV infection. Clin Infect Dis 55:75–81
6. Boukobza M, Tamer I, Guichard JP, Brunereau L, Polivka M, Leibinger F, Reizine D, Merland JJ (1999) Tuberculose du système nerveux central. Aspects IRM et évolution à propos de 12 cas. J Neuroradiol 26:172–181
7. Thwaites G, Fisher M, Hemingway C, Scott G, Solomon T, Innes J (2009) British Infection Society guidelines for the diagnosis and treatment of tuberculosis of the central nervous system in adults and children. J Infect 59:167–187
8. Nelson CA, Zunt JR (2011) Tuberculosis of the central nervous system in immunocompromised patients: HIV infection and solid organ transplant recipients. Clin Infect Dis 53:915–926
9. Daikos GL, Cleary T, Rodriguez A, Fischl MA (2003) Multidrug-resistant tuberculous meningitis in patients with AIDS. Int J Tuberc Lung Dis 7:394–398
10. Comstock GW, Livesay VT, Woolpert SF (1974) The prognosis of a positive tuberculin reaction in childhood and adolescence. Am J Epidemiol 99:131–138
11. Garg RK (2010) Tuberculous meningitis. Acta Neurol Scand 122:75–90
12. Berenguer J, Moreno S, Laguna F, Vicente T, Adrados M, Ortega A, Gonzalez-Lahoz J, Bouza E (1992) Tuberculous meningitis in patients infected with the human immunodeficiency virus. N Engl J Med 326:668–672
13. Croda MG, Vidal JE, Hernandez AV, Dal Molin T, Gualberto FA, De Oliveira AC (2010) Tuberculous meningitis in HIV-infected patients in Brazil: clinical and laboratory characteristics and factors associated with mortality. Int J Infect Dis 14:586–591
14. Dube MP, Holtom PD, Larsen RA (1992) Tuberculous meningitis in patients with and without human immunodeficiency virus infection. Am J Med 93:520–524
15. Porkert MT, Sotir M, Parrott-Moore P, Blumberg HM (1997) Tuberculous meningitis at a large inner-city medical center. Am J Med Sci 313:325–331
16. Hosoglu S, Geyik MF, Balik I, Aygen B, Erol S, Aygence TG, Mert A, Saltoglu N, Dokmetas I, Felek S, Sunbul M, Irmah H, Aydin K, Kokoglu OF, Ucmak H, Altindis M, Loeb M (2002) Predictors of outcome in patients with tuberculous meningitis. Int J Tuberc Lung Dis 6:64–70
17. Pehlivanoglu F, Yasar KK, Sengoz G (2012) Tuberculous meningitis in adults: a review of 160 cases. Scientific World Journal 169028:1–6
18. Galimi R (2011) Extrapulmonary tuberculosis: tuberculous meningitis new developments. Eur Rev Med Pharmacol Sci 15:365–386
19. Rock RB, Olin M, Baker CA, Molitor TW, Peterson PK (2008) Central nervous system tuberculosis: pathogenesis and clinical aspects. Clin Microbiol Rev 21:243–261
20. Curless RG, Mitchell CD (1991) Central nervous system tuberculosis in children. Pediatr Neurol 7:270–274
21. Thwaites GE, Duc Bang N, Huy Dung N, Thi Quy H, Tuong Oanh DT, Cam Thoa NT, Quang Hien N, Tri Thuc N, Ngoc Hai N, Ngoc Lan NT, Ngoc Lan N, Hong Duc N, Ngoc Tuan V, Huu Hiep C, Hong Chau TT, Phuong Mai P, Dung NT, Stepniewska K, Simmons CP, White NJ, Tinh Hien T, Farrar JJ (2005) The influence of HIV infection on clinical presentation, response to treatment, and outcome in adults with tuberculous meningitis. J Infect Dis 192:2134–2141
22. El Sahly HM, Teeter LD, Pan X, Musser JM, Graviss EA (2007) Mortality associated with central nervous system tuberculosis. J Infect 55:502–509
23. Garg RK (1999) Tuberculosis of the central nervous system. Postgrad Med J 75:133–140
24. Thwaites GE, Hong Chau TT, Jeremy J, Farrar JJ (2004) Improving the bacteriological diagnosis of tuberculous meningitis. J Clin Microbiol 42:378–379
25. Garcia-Mongo JC (1999) Central nervous system tuberculosis. Neurol Clin 17:737–759
26. Caws M, Wilson SM, Clough C, Drobniewski F (2000) Role of IS6110 targeted PCR, biochemical, clinical and immunological criteria for diagnosis of tuberculous meningitis. J Clin Microbiol 38:3150–3155

27. Marei AM, EL-Behedy EM, Mohtady HA, Afify RF (2003) Evaluation of a rapid bacteriophage-based method for the detection of Mycobacterium tuberculosis in clinical samples. J Med Microbiol 52:331–335
28. Albay A, Kisa O, Baylan O, Doganie L (2003) The evaluation of fast plaque TB test for the rapid diagnosis of tuberculosis. Diagn Microbiol Infect Dis 46:211–215
29. Thomas MM, Hinks TS, Raghuraman S, Ramalingam N, Ernst M, Nau R, Lange C, Kosters K, Gnanamuthu C, John GT, Marshall B, Lalvani A (2008) Rapid diagnosis of Mycobacterium tuberculosis meningitis by enumeration of cerebrospinal fluid antigen specific T cells. Int J Tuberc Lung Dis 12:651–657
30. Banzin C (1997) Tuberculose du système nerveux central. In Editions techniques Encycl Méd Chir Neurologie, Paris, p 12
31. Wasay M, Farooq S, Khowaja ZA, Bawa ZA, Ali SM, Awan S, Beg MA, Mehndiratta MM (2014) Cerebral infarction and tuberculoma in central nervous system tuberculosis: frequency and prognostic implications. J Neurol Neurosurg Psychiatry 85:1260–1264
32. Rajemiarimoelisoa CF, Randriamamonjy F, Andrianjafisamindrakotroka NS (2007) Extrapulmonary tuberculosis cases study from the surgical pathology laboratory of the university hospital center of Antananarivo Madagascar. Paper presented at the First Western Indian Ocean Pathologist Meeting, August 2007, Antananarivo, Madagascar
33. Muralidhar K, Katti MK (2004) Pathogenesis, diagnosis, treatment, and outcome aspects of cerebral tuberculosis. Med Sci Monit 10:215–229
34. Sayed EL, Adeuja AO (2006) Intracranial tuberculomas: the Hofuf, Saudi Arabia experience. Afr J Med Med Sci 35:21–27
35. Martinez-Vazquez C, Bordon J, Rodriguez-Gonzalez A, De la Fuente-Aquado J, Sopena B, Gallego-Rivera A, Martinez-Cueto P (1995) Cerebral tuberculoma: a comparative study in patients with and without HIV infection. Infection 23:149–153
36. Bottieau E, Noe A, Florence E, Colebunders R (2003) Multiple tuberculous brain abscesses in an HIV-infected patient successfully treated with HAART and antituberculous treatment. Infection 31:118–120
37. Sanchez-Portocarrero J, Perez-Cecilia E, Romero-Vivas J (1999) Infection of the central nervous system by Mycobacterium tuberculosis in patients infected with human immunodeficiency virus (the new neurotuberculosis). Infection 27:313–317
38. Farrar DJ, Flanigan TP, Gordon NM, Gold RL, Rich JD (1997) Tuberculous brain abscess in a patient with HIV infection: case report and review. Am J Med 102:297–301
39. Whitener DR (1978) Tuberculous brain abscess. Report of a case and review of the literature. Arch Neurol 35:148–155
40. Vidal JE, Penalva de Oliveira AC, Bonasser Filho F, Schiavon Nogueira R, Dauar RF, Leite AG, Lins DLM, Coeho JFGS (2005) Tuberculous brain abscess in AIDS patients: report of three cases and literature review. Int J Infect Dis 9:201–207
41. Cardenas G, Soto-Hermandez JL, Orozco RV, Silva EG, Revuelta R, Amador JL (2010) Tuberculous brain abscesses in immunocompetent patients: management and outcome. Neurosurgery 61:1081–1087
42. Kumar R, Pandey CK, Bose N, Sahay S (2002) Tuberculous brain abscess: clinical presentation, pathophysiology and treatment (in children). Childs Nerv Syst 18:118–123
43. Luthra G, Parihar A, Nath K, Jaiswal S, Prasad KN, Husain N, Husain M, Singh S, Behari S, Gupta RK (2007) Comparative evaluation of fungal, tubercular and pyogenic brain abscesses with conventional and diffusion MR imaging and proton MR spectroscopy. Am J Neuroradiol 28:1332–1338
44. Chang KH, Han MH, Choi YW, Kim IO, Han MC, Kim CW (1989) Tuberculous arachnoiditis of the spine: findings on myelography, CT, and MR imaging. Am J Neuroradiol 10:1255–1262
45. Garg RK, Somvanshi DS (2011) Spinal tuberculosis: a review. J Spinal Cord Med 34:440–454
46. Hernandez-Albujar S, Arribas JR, Royo A, Gonzalez-Garcia JJ, Pena JM, Vasquez JJ (2000) Tuberculous radiculomyelitis complicating tuberculous meningitis: case report and review. Clin Infect Dis 30:915–921
47. Wadia NH, Dastur DK (1969) Spinal meningitides with radiculo-myelopathy. 1. Clinical and radiological features. J Neurol Sci 8:239–260
48. Wadia NH (1973) Radiculomyelopathy associated with spinal meningitis (arachnoiditis) with special reference to the spinal tuberculous variety. In: Spillane JD (ed) Tropical neurology. Oxford University Press, Oxford, pp 63–69
49. Kozlowski K (1963) Late spinal blocks after tuberculous meningitis. Am J Roentgenol 90:1220–1226
50. Sharma A, Goyal M, Mishra NK, Gupta V, Gaikwad SB (1997) MR imaging of tubercular spinal arachnoiditis. Am J Roentgenol 168:807–812
51. Meintjes G, Lawn SD, Scano F, Maartens G, French MA, Worodria W, Elliott JH, Murdoch D, Wilkinson RJ, Seyler C, John L, Van Der Loeff MS, Reiss P, Lynen L, Janoff EN, Gilks C, Colebunders R (2008) Tuberculosis associated immune reconstitution inflammatory syndrome: case definitions for use in resource-limited settings. Lancet Infect Dis 8:516–523
52. Thwaites GE, Caws M, Hong Chau TT, Dung NT, Campbell JI, Phu NH, Hien TT, White NJ, Farrar JJ (2004) Comparison of conventional bacteriology with nucleic acid amplification (amplified mycobacterium direct test) for diagnosis of tuberculous meningitis before and after inception of antituberculosis chemotherapy. J Clin Microbiol 42:996–1002
53. Meintjes G, Rangaka MX, Maartens G, Rebe K, Morroni C, Pepper DJ, Wilkinson KA, Wilkinson RJ (2009) Novel relationship between tuberculosis

immune reconstitution inflammatory syndrome and antitubercular drug resistance. Clin Infect Dis 48:667–676
54. Narita M, Ashkin D, Hollender ES, Pitchenik AE (1998) Paradoxical worsening of tuberculosis following antiretroviral therapy in patients with AIDS. Am J Respir Crit Care Med 158:157–161
55. Girgis N, Sultan Y, Farid Z, Mansour MM, Erian MW, Hanna LS, Mateczun A (1998) Tuberculosis meningitis, Abbassia Fever Hospital-Naval Medical Research Unit No. 3-Cairo, Egypt, from 1976 to 1996. Am J Trop Med Hyg 58:28–34
56. Mason RJ (2010) Murray and Nadel's textbook of respiratory medicine, 5th edn. Elsevier, Philadelphia, p 754
57. Leidl L, Mayanja-Kizza H, Sotgiu G, Baseke J, Ernst M, Hirsch C, Goletti D, Toossi Z, Lange C (2010) Relationship of immunodiagnostic assays for tuberculosis and numbers of circulating CD41 T-cells in HIV infection. Eur Respir J 35:619–626
58. Juan RS, Sanchez-Suarez C, Rebollo MJ, Folgueira D, Palenque E, Ortuno B (2006) Interferon gamma quantification in cerebrospinal fluid compared with PCR for the diagnosis of tuberculous meningitis. J Neurol 253:1323–1330
59. Jindani A, Nunn AJ, Enarson DA (2004) Two 8-month regimens of chemotherapy for treatment of newly diagnosed pulmonary tuberculosis: international multicentre randomised trial. Lancet 364:1244–1251
60. Lawn SD, Torok ME, Wood R (2011) Optimum time to start antiretroviral therapy during HIV-associated opportunistic infections. Curr Opin Infect Dis 24:34–42
61. Panel on Antiretroviral Guidelines for Adults and Adolescents (2011) Guidelines for the use of antiretroviral agents in HIV-1-infected adults and adolescents. Department of Health and Human Services, Atlanta, pp 1–166
62. Torok ME, Yen NT, Chau TT, Mai NT, Phu NH, Mai PP, Dung NT, Chau NV, Bang ND, Tien NA, Minh NH, Hien NQ, Thai PV, Dong DT, Anh DT, Thoa NT, Hai NN, Lan NT, Quy HT, Dung NH, Hien TT, Chinh NT, Simmons CP, De Jong M, Wolbers M, Farrar JJ (2011) Timing of initiation of antiretroviral therapy in human immunodeficiency virus (HIV)-associated tuberculous meningitis. Clin Infect Dis 52:1374–1383
63. Patel VB, Padayatchi N, Bhigjee AI, Allen J, Bhagwan B, Moodley AA, Mthiyane T (2004) Multidrug-resistant tuberculous meningitis in KwaZulu-Natal, South Africa. Clin Infect Dis 38:851–856
64. Wells CD (2010) Global impact of multidrug-resistant pulmonary tuberculosis among HIV-infected and other immunocompromised hosts: epidemiology, diagnosis, and strategies for management. Curr Infect Dis Rep 12:192–197
65. Marais S, Scholtz P, Pepper DJ, Meintjes G, Wilkinson RJ, Candy S (2010) Neuroradiological features of the tuberculosis-associated immune reconstitution inflammatory syndrome. Int J Tuberc Lung Dis 14:188–196
66. Pepper DJ, Marais S, Maartens G, Rebe K, Morroni C, Rangala MX, Oni T, Wilkinson RJ, Meintjes G (2009) Neurologic manifestations of paradoxical tuberculosis-associated immune reconstitution inflammatory syndrome: a case series. Clin Infect Dis 48:96–107
67. Torre-Cisneros J, Doblas A, Aguado JM, San Juan R, Blanes M, Montejo M, Cervera C, Len O, Carratala J, Cisneros JM, Bou G, Munoz P, Ramos A, Gurgui M, Borrell N, Fortun J, Moreno A, Gavalda J (2009) Tuberculosis after solid organ transplant: incidence, risk factors, and clinical characteristics in the RESITRA (Spanish Network of Infection in Transplantation) cohort. Clin Infect Dis 48:1657–1665
68. Meyers BR, Papanicolaou GA, Sheiner P, Emre S, Miller C (2000) Tuberculosis in orthotopic liver transplant patients: increased toxicity of recommended agents; cure of disseminated infection with nonconventional regimens. Transplantation 69:64–69
69. Munoz P, Rodrıguez C, Bouza E (2005) Mycobacterium tuberculosis infection in recipients of solid organ transplants. Clin Infect Dis 40:581–587

Management of Multidrug-Resistant Tuberculosis Involving the Nervous System

36

Dwarakanath Srinivas and Pragyan Sarma

Contents

D. Srinivas, MS, MCh (Neurosurgery) (✉) P. Sarma, MS, MCh
Department of Neurosurgery, National Institute of Mental Health and Neurosciences (NIMHANS), Bangalore, Karnataka, India
e-mail: dwarakaneuro@yahoo.com; pragyansarma@yahoo.com

Abbreviations

ART	Antiretroviral therapy
CNS	Central nervous system
CSF	Cerebrospinal fluid
CT	Computed tomography
DST	Drug susceptibility testing
EMB	Ethambutol
INH	Isoniazid
MDR-TB	Multidrug resistant-tuberculosis
PCR	Polymerase chain reaction
PZA	Pyrazinamide
RIF	Rifampicin
TB	Tuberculosis
TBA	Tuberculous brain abscess
TBM	Tuberculous meningitis
WHO	World Health Organization
XDR-TB	Extremely drug resistant-tuberculosis

36.1 Introduction

Tuberculosis (TB) is one of the most common endemic infections encountered in developing countries and, with the advent of immunosuppression and population migration, is being increasingly reported from developed countries

M. Turgut et al. (eds.), *Tuberculosis of the Central Nervous System*,
DOI 10.1007/978-3-319-50712-5_36

[1]. Approximately 4/5 of the cases occur in areas, which are overcrowded and poverty stricken, with chronic malnutrition, while the rest is usually associated with HIV mainly in sub-Saharan Africa. Children remain at a disproportionately high risk of central nervous system (CNS) TB. In the year 2010 alone, there were a total of 8,800,000 (range, 8,500,000–9,200,000) cases and 1,100,000 (range, 900,000–1,200,000) deaths from TB. TB of CNS is one of the most devastating forms of the disease with the greatest morbidity and mortality, although only about 5% of TB infections affect the CNS [2, 3]. Hydrocephalus seen in 62–87% of patients is the most common complication of tuberculous meningitis (TBM) [4]. The tubercle bacilli are aerobic and nonmotile with a slow doubling time. It generally spreads via an airborne mechanism. For CNS-TB to occur, there is a hematogenous spread to various regions of the body including the meninges. From this "rich focus" on the meninges, the bacilli enter the subarachnoid space causing TBM. Another important feature of *Mycobacterium tuberculosis* is its ability to enter and replicate in the macrophages. Thus the microglial cells of the CNS are the main target cells. Anti-TB drugs including rifampicin (RIF) and isoniazid (INH) have been the mainstay of treatment, but in the last few years, there has been an increasing prevalence of new drug-resistant strains [multidrug resistant-tuberculosis (MDR-TB resistant to at least INH and RIF) or extremely drug resistant-tuberculosis (XDR-TB resistant to INH and RIF along with resistance to a fluoroquinolone and injectable second-line drugs)] [5]. Globally, MDR-TB accounts for 3.4% of new cases and 20% of re-treatment cases. In India, MDR-TB accounts for 2.1% of new cases and 15% of re-treatment cases [6]. XDR-TB has been reported in 69 countries worldwide and data indicates that 25,000 new cases of XDR-TB are being reported every year. This apart from increasing the mortality and morbidity of TB has also exponentially increased the cost of treatment, especially in countries that can least afford them. In this chapter we shall discuss the diagnosis and management of MDR-TB.

36.2 Clinical Features: Main Form of CNS-TB

36.2.1 Introduction

36.2.1.1 Tuberculous Meningitis

In TBM, a gelatinous thick exudate forms in the subarachnoid space with a propensity to the basal cisterns [1, 7, 8]. The grading of severity of TBM is detailed in Table 36.1: (1) hydrocephalus, due to disturbances in cerebrospinal fluid (CSF) flow; (2) infarctions, due to vasculitis of the vessels of the circle of Willis, vertebrobasilar system, middle cerebral artery, and various perforators; and (3) local inflammation and damage of adjacent brain tissue.

36.2.1.2 Tuberculoma

These arise from tubercles in the brain parenchyma and may be associated along with TBM [1, 9]. They can either be solitary or multiple. A rare manifestation is the tuberculous brain abscess (TBA), which consists of an encapsulated pus collection consisting of viable TB bacilli [9].

Table 36.1 Grading: British Medical Research Council clinical criteria for the severity of TBM

Stage/grade	Classic criterion	Contemporary criterion
I	Fully conscious and no focal deficits	Alert and oriented without focal neurological deficits
II	Conscious but with inattention, confusion, lethargy, and focal neurological signs	Glasgow Coma Scale score of 14–11 or 15 with focal neurological deficits
III	Stuporous or comatose, multiple cranial nerve palsies, or complete hemiparesis or paralysis	Glasgow Coma Scale score of ten or less, with or without focal neurological deficits

36.2.2 Clinical Features

Adult patients usually present with classical features of meningitis including fever, headache, and meningism. Other clinical features include focal neurological deficits, behavioral changes, and altered sensorium. It may be associated with a history of TB in approx. 10% of the patients. Coexistent pulmonary TB can be seen in 30–50% of the patients [10, 11]. Children usually have associated failure to thrive, weight loss irritability, decreased appetite, pain abdomen, emesis, and sleep disturbances. The progression of disease is much faster as are the chances of complications [10, 11]. On the other hand, tuberculomas and TBAs present with features such as seizures, focal deficits depending upon their location, and features suggestive of raised intracranial pressure.

36.3 Investigations and Diagnosis

36.3.1 Diagnosis

1. CSF analysis: This is the most prevalent test performed to diagnose CNS-TB. The typical CSF picture consists of lymphocytic pleocytosis (10–100 × 10^3/ml), elevated protein levels (0.5–3 g/l) along with low glucose levels (<50%) [12, 13]. Though sensitivity is high, it is nonspecific.
2. Microbiology: Identification of tubercle bacilli by microscopy and culture remains the most specific of tests to diagnose CNS-TB. However due to paucity of tubercle bacilli in CSF, its sensitivity remains quite low [13, 14]. Thwaites et al. in their study demonstrated that CSF volume (minimum 6 ml) and a longer duration of the microscopic evaluation (minimum 30 min) are independently associated with bacteriological confirmation of CNS-TB [11].
3. Molecular analysis: Since the traditional methods have significant drawback, more accurate and rapid diagnostics methods are necessary.
   (a) Antibody detection: The problem with the conventional anti-*M. tuberculosis*-specific antibody assay has been its low specificity [15–17]. This has been largely overcome through the use of measuring antibodies against a specific antigen (a 30 kDa protein) of *M. tuberculosis* (sensitivity of 92%) along with immunospot assays to detect anti-*M. bovis* BCG antibody-secreting cells (ELISPOT) [18].
   (b) Antigen detection: As antigens are released only in the presence of a host immune response, they are more sensitive. In a study, comparing dot immunobinding assay for *M. tuberculosis*-specific 14 kDa protein antigen with polymerase chain reaction (PCR) to detect IS6110, specific for *M. tuberculosis* in the CSF, the dot assay was more sensitive (75% vs. 40.5%) [19–21].
   (c) Molecular detection: While both antibody and antigen assays are cheaper and thus can be used more widely especially in low-income countries, they still not have reached a very high sensitivity and specificity levels. There are two commercially available nucleic acid amplification assays the Amplified *M. tuberculosis* Direct Test (MTD; Gene- Probe, Inc., San Diego, CA) and the Amplicor *M. tuberculosis* Test (Roche Diagnostic Systems, Inc., Indianapolis, IN). However, tests have shown that their sensitivity is only 56% and a specificity of 98% [22–24]. PCR-based assays have received a lot of attention and, in a study by Rafi et al. using IS6110 uniplex PCR assay, showed a sensitivity of 98% and specificity of 100% when compared to the culture method [25]. But in clinical TBM, the sensitivity was only 76.4% and specificity was 89.2%. However, it should be remembered that these tests are expensive and require expensive infrastructure that may not be readily available.

36.3.2 Detection of Resistance

While conventional drug susceptibility testing (DST) of cultured mycobacteria takes anywhere between 1 and 3 months, molecular tests can detect them very fast (within 2 days). They can provide a diagnosis of resistance to INH and RIF or RIF alone. The WHO in their guidelines of 2011 recommends only two molecular tests, i.e., line probe assay and Xpert *M. tuberculosis*/RIF, for diagnosis of resistance [5].

Line probe assay: Rather than relying on visualizing bacteria under a microscope, it indirectly detects the presence of *M. tuberculosis* by amplifying DNA present in the sputum by PCR [26]. It can be used both in the primary diagnosis of TB and also detecting RIF resistance. Drawbacks include it being prone to cross-contamination leading to false positives and its cost.

Xpert MTB/RIF: This can detect both *M. tuberculosis* and simultaneously RIF resistance [27]. It detects DNA sequences specific for *M. tuberculosis* and RIF resistance by PCR [28]. It identifies all the clinically relevant RIF resistance inducing mutations in the RNA polymerase beta (rpoB) gene in the *M. tuberculosis* genome in a real-time format using fluorescent probes called molecular beacons [27]. Pooled tests reveal a sensitivity of 88% and specificity of 98%. Its advantages include a high specificity and sensitivity along with the rapid results (within 2 h). However, the cost remains prohibitively expensive.

36.4 Radiology

36.4.1 Tuberculous Meningitis

About 50% of patients have chest X-rays suggestive of pulmonary TB [29]. The most common computed tomography (CT) features include hydrocephalus and enhancing basal exudates which are more common in children. Infarctions can also be seen due to vasculitis [30, 31].

36.4.2 Tuberculomas

While magnetic resonance imaging and CT have no distinguishing features to differentiate it from other ring-enhancing lesions, magnetic resonance spectroscopy has shown most promise: a large lipid CH2 peak has been used to specifically identify tuberculomas [32, 33] and also on the basis of choline/creatine ratio > 1 in tuberculoma [33, 34] (Fig. 36.1a–d).

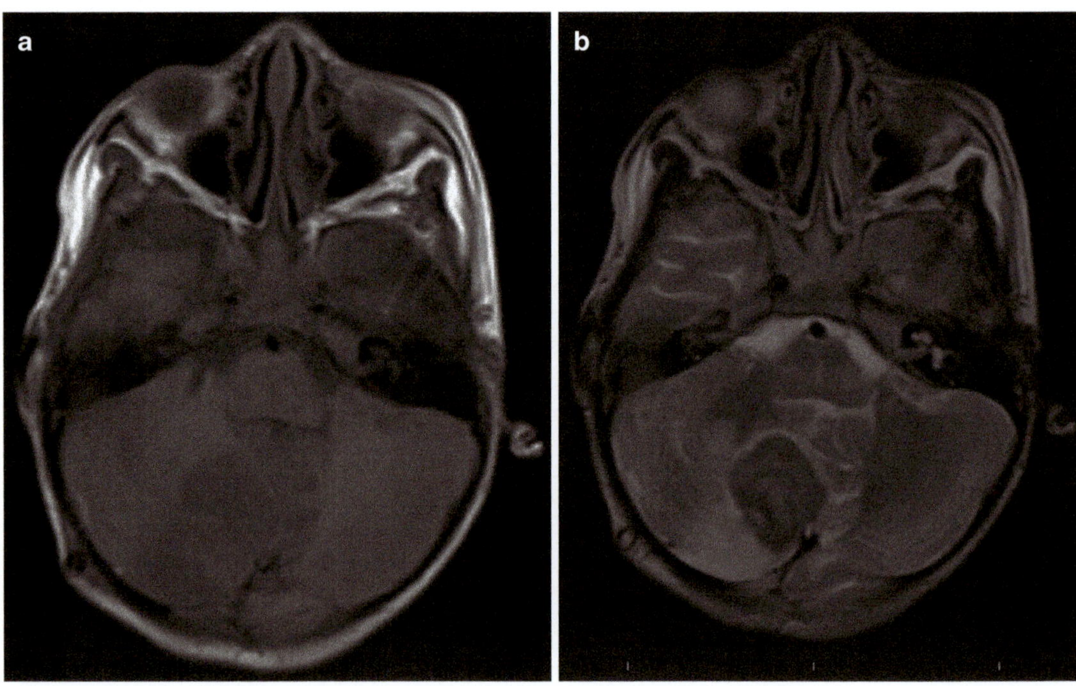

Fig. 36.1 Magnetic resonance imaging of the brain showing a lesion in the right cerebellar hemisphere. It is well marginated and hypointense in T1-weighted images (**a**), hypointense on T2-weighted images (**b**). Post-contrast images show thin peripheral rim enhancement (**c**). Magnetic resonance spectroscopy shows a large lipid-lactate peak at 1.3 ppm (**d**)

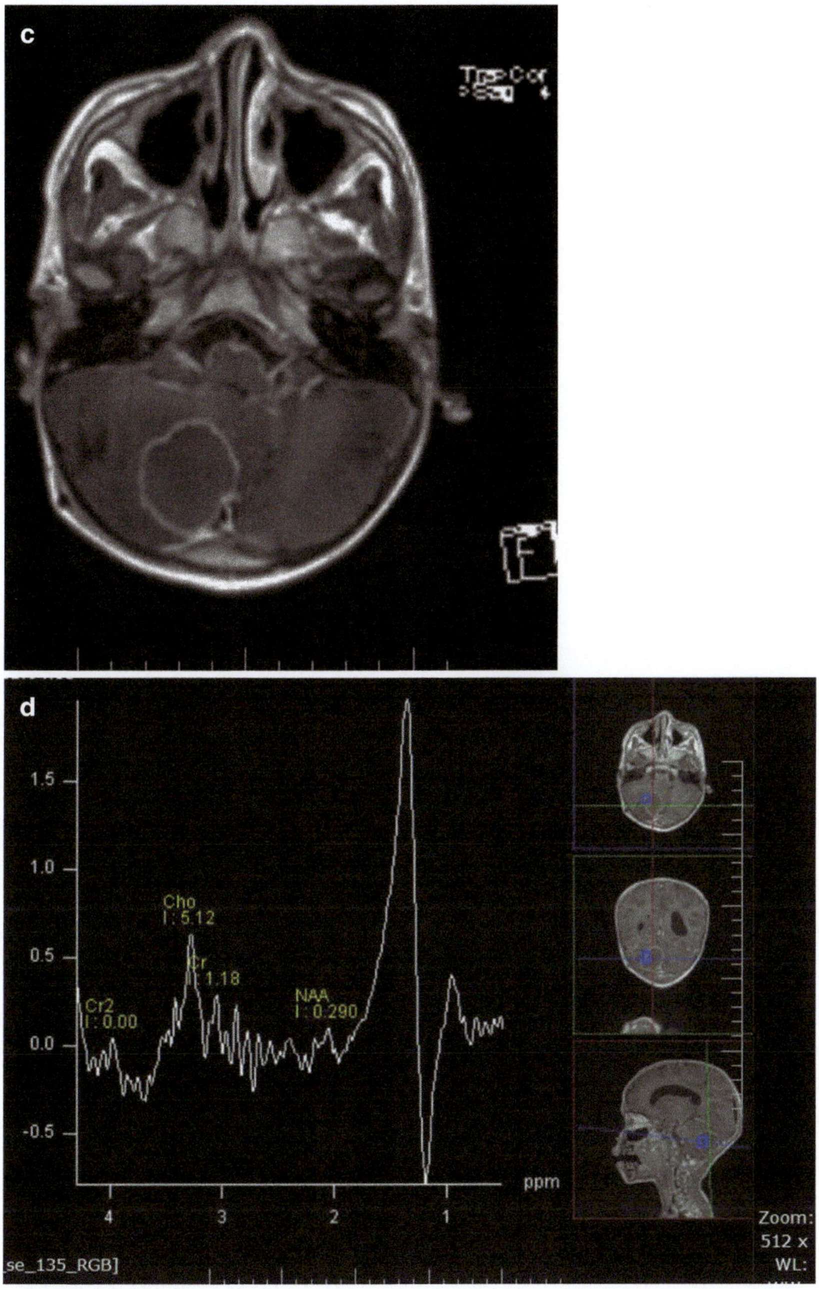

Fig. 36.1 (continued)

36.5 Management

It is important to perform sensitivity testing before starting MDR-TB as neither MDR-TB nor XDR-TB responds to first-line anti-TB chemotherapy. However, second-line anti-TB chemotherapy is both expensive and more toxic, and thus it becomes more important to perform sensitivity testing of the strain isolated. It is important to remember that most of the work has been on pulmonary TB and hardly any data exists on CNS-TB [35, 36]. However, the findings can be extrapolated from pulmonary TB. The World Health Organization (WHO) guidelines of 2011 recommend the usage of four second-line drugs along with pyrazinamide (PZA) for the regimen to be effective [5, 6]. These include a fluoroquinolone, a parenteral agent, ethionamide (or prothionamide), and cycloserine or else para-aminosalicylic acid if cycloserine cannot be used [5]. Drug susceptibility testing need not be performed for the second-line anti-TB chemotherapy, as the tests are not completely reliable [5].

36.5.1 Diagnosis of Resistance and the Routine Use of Rapid Drug Susceptibility Testing

The bane of drug susceptibility testing has been the slow culture growth of *M. tuberculosis*. Over the past few years, molecular tests have been used which are both rapid and specific. The two tests recommended by the WHO, i.e., line probe assay and Xpert MTB/RIF assay, can be used. However it is important to remember that this experience is limited to pulmonary TB and its place in CNS-TB needs analysis [28, 37].

Use of Rapid Drug Susceptibility Testing

While conventional DST of cultured mycobacteria takes anywhere between 1 and 3 months, molecular tests can detect them very fast (within 2 days). These include the line probe assay and the Xpert MTB/RIF. They provide a diagnosis of resistance to INH and RIF or RIF alone. With the emergence and increasing incidence of MDR-TB, the question arises whether rapid DST should be performed in all patients before starting anti-TB chemotherapy. The proponents of this strategy list the many benefits including early start of appropriate treatment leading to increase cure rates and decreased mortality [5]. However, there remain risks to this method that include false-positive results, increased drug toxicity to patients, and the increase in cost. The WHO guidelines have thus made the use of rapid DST conditional and recommended it be used in at least patients treated previously with anti-TB therapy and groups at higher risk of MDR-TB based on surveillance data [5].

36.5.2 Monitoring of Response

Monitoring of response is a very important part of the treatment protocol. It helps the clinicians in identifying early failures and apply corrective measures. It can also prevent spread and development of drug resistance. The WHO used data pooled from ten studies and recommended the use of sputum smear microscopy and culture rather than sputum smear microscopy alone for the monitoring of patients with MDR-TB during treatment [5]. Though the available evidence was of low quality, it is felt that adding sputum culture increases the likelihood of identifying early non-responders, though the cost remains a major factor in most countries [5, 38–40].

36.5.3 Composition of Second-Line Anti-TB Chemotherapy

A meta-analysis of three systematic reviews that included 32 studies with more than 9153 treatment episodes was performed by the Collaborative Group for Meta-Analysis of Individual Patient Data in MDR-TB [41–44]. The results of this analysis provide the best available evidence for management of MDR-TB. It is recommended that the regimen use PZA along with at least four drugs from the following subgroups (Tables 36.2 and 36.3):

Table 36.2 Classification and properties of drugs in the second anti-TB therapy regimen

Drugs	Pharmacokinetics	Pharmacodynamics	Adverse effects	Dosage
Second-line parenteral drugs				
Kanamycin Amikacin (Aminoglycosides)	*Absorption*: Highly polar cations Poorly absorbed from GIT. Absorbed rapidly from intramuscular sites Peak concentration after 30–90 min *Distribution*: Because of their polar nature, they do not penetrate into most of the cells Distribution confined to extracellular fluid *Elimination*: Mainly through the renal system. T ½ = 2–3 h	Exert mycobactericidal activity by binding to the 16S ribosomal subunit	Ototoxicity, nephrotoxicity, neuromuscular blockade, optic scotomas	15–30 mg/kg given IM or IV (maximal daily dose, 1 g), with a reduction to 10 mg/kg for patients > 60 years old. For patients with renal insufficiency, the dose and frequency should be reduced (12–15 mg/kg two or three times per week)
Capreomycin (Cyclic peptide)	*Absorption*: Given intramuscularly Peak blood levels of 20–40 mcg/mL *Distribution*: 50% of the dose excreted unaltered *Elimination*: Mainly through the glomerular filtration	Not well understood but may involve interference with the mycobacterial ribosome and inhibition of protein synthesis	Hearing loss, tinnitus, transient proteinuria, cylindruria, and nitrogen retention. Severe renal failure is rare. Eosinophilia is common. Leukocytosis, leukopenia, rashes, and fever have also been observed	15 mg/kg per day is given five to seven times per week (maximal daily dose, 1 g) The dosage may be reduced to 1 g two or three times per week 2–4 months after mycobacterial cultures become negative. For individuals >60 years of age, the dose should be reduced to 10 mg/kg per day (maximal daily dose, 750 mg). For patients with renal insufficiency, the drug should be given intermittently and at lower dosage (12–15 mg/kg two or three times per week)
Fluoroquinolones				

(continued)

Table 36.2 (continued)

Drugs	Pharmacokinetics	Pharmacodynamics	Adverse effects	Dosage
Levofloxacin	*Absorption*: Well absorbed after oral administration. Distributed widely in body tissues Peak serum levels of the drugs obtained within 1 to 3 h of an oral dose of 400 mg, with peak levels 6.4 g/ml for *levofloxacin* *Distribution* and *elimination*: The volume of distribution of quinolones is high, with concentrations of quinolones in urine; kidney, lung, and prostate tissue; stool; bile; and macrophages and neutrophils higher than serum levels. Quinolone concentrations in cerebrospinal fluid, bone, and prostatic fluid are lower than in serum	Inhibit mycobacterial DNA gyrase and topoisomerase IV, preventing cell replication and protein synthesis, and are bactericidal	Gastrointestinal (GI) side effects, nausea, and vomiting. Rare CNS side effects like mild headache and dizziness. Cardiac arrhythmias due to Qtc prolongation	500 mg daily
Gatifloxacin	Oral administration	Inhibit mycobacterial DNA gyrase and topoisomerase IV, preventing cell replication and protein synthesis, and are bactericidal	GI side effects, nausea, and vomiting Rare CNS side effects like mild headache and dizziness	400 mg/day
Ofloxacin	Oral administration	Inhibit mycobacterial DNA gyrase and topoisomerase IV, preventing cell replication and protein synthesis, and are bactericidal	GI side effects, nausea, and vomiting Rare CNS side effects like mild headache and dizziness	600–800 mg/day
Moxifloxacin	Oral administration *Elimination*: Hepatically cleared	Inhibit mycobacterial DNA gyrase and topoisomerase IV, preventing cell replication and protein synthesis, and are bactericidal	GI side effects, nausea, and vomiting Rare CNS side effects like mild headache and dizziness	400 mg daily
Oral bacteriostatic second-line drugs				

Table 36.2 (continued)

Drugs	Pharmacokinetics	Pharmacodynamics	Adverse effects	Dosage
Ethionamide/ prothionamide	The oral administration of 1 g yields peak concentrations in plasma of about 20 g/ml in 3 h, 9h is 3 g/ml T ½ = 2 hrs, drug is widely distributed	Ethionamide is also an inactive prodrug that is activated by a mycobacterial redux system. Ethionamide inhibits mycobacterial growth by inhibiting the activity of the *inhA* gene product, the enoyl-ACP reductase of fatty acid synthase II	Anorexia, nausea and vomiting, gastric irritation, severe postural hypotension, depression, drowsiness, and asthenia are common. Hepatitis is in 5%	The initial dosage for adults is 250 mg BID; it is increased by 125 mg per day every 5 days until a dose of 15 to 20 mg/kg per day is achieved. The maximal dose is 1 g daily. Children should receive 15 to 20 mg/kg per day in two divided doses, not to exceed 1 g per day
Cycloserine	Distributed throughout body fluids and tissues About 50% of a parenteral dose of cycloserine is excreted and unchanged in the urine in the first 12 h; a total of 65% is recoverable in the active form over a period of 72 h. Toxic concentrations in renal insufficiency	Cycloserine and D-alanine are structural analogs; thus, cycloserine inhibits reactions in which D-alanine is involved in bacterial cell-wall synthesis	Somnolence, headache, tremor, dysarthria, vertigo, confusion, nervousness, irritability, psychotic states with suicidal tendencies, paranoid reactions, catatonic and depressed reactions, twitching, ankle clonus, hyperreflexia, visual disturbances, paresis, and tonic-clonic or absence seizures	Adults: 250–500 mg BID
Terizidone	Oral administration, maximum concentration is achieved in 2–4 h	Terizidone and D-alanine are structural analogs; thus, inhibits reactions in which D-alanine is involved in bacterial cell-wall synthesis	Severe depression, anxiety, panic attacks, psychosis, dizziness	15–20 mg/kg daily orally
para-aminosalicylic acid	Oral administration, t 1/2 = 1 h, 80% excreted in urine	Inhibits folic acid synthesis	GI side effects, anorexia, nausea, epigastric pain, abdominal distress, and diarrhea	Adults: Daily dose of 10–12 g. Children: 150–300 mg/kg per day in 3–4 divided doses
Group 5 drugs				

(continued)

Table 36.2 (continued)

Drugs	Pharmacokinetics	Pharmacodynamics	Adverse effects	Dosage
Clofazimine	Absorption is variable through oral route; because of its lipophilic property, it gets distributed into fatty tissues	Binds to GC-rich mycobacterial DNA and also increases mycobacterial phospholipase A_2 activity and inhibits microbial K^+ transport. Weakly bactericidal	Eosinophilic enteritis Red discoloration of the skin	Daily dose is usually 100 mg
Linezolid	With oral bioavailability approaching 100%, dosing for oral and intravenous preparations is the same. Peak serum concentrations average 12–14 g/ml 1–2 h after a single 600 mg dose in adults and approximately 20 g/ml at steady state with dosing every 12 h. The half-life is approximately 4–6 h. Linezolid is 30% protein bound and distributes widely to well-perfused tissues, with a 0.6–0.7 L/kg volume of distribution	Linezolid inhibits protein synthesis by binding to the P site of the 50S ribosomal subunit and preventing formation of the larger ribosomal-fMet-tRNA complex that initiates protein synthesis	Myelosuppression, including anemia, leukopenia, pancytopenia, and thrombocytopenia	Dosage is 600 mg daily
Amoxicillin/ clavulanate	Oral administration, peak concentration after 2 h	Binds to penicillin-binding proteins and disrupts the cell wall. Penicillinase susceptible, hence mixed with clavulanate. 20% protein bound	Allergic reactions, dark urine	Daily total 4000 mg clavulanic acid- 250 mg
Thioacetazone	Orally administered	Mechanism of action – inhibits mycolic acid, cyclopropane synthase	Hypersensitivity reactions	Adults: 150 mg thioacetazone +300 mg isoniazid daily. Children: 50 mg thioacetazone +100 mg isoniazid daily
Clarithromycin	Macrolide antibiotic, clarithromycin is well absorbed orally and distributes well to tissues. It is cleared both hepatically and renally; the dosage should be reduced in renal insufficiency. Clarithromycin is a substrate for and inhibits cytochrome 3A4 and should not be administered with cisapride, pimozide, or terfenadine, as cardiac arrhythmias may occur	Inhibiting protein synthesis by binding to the 50S mycobacterial ribosomal subunit	Gastrointestinal intolerance, hepatotoxicity, headache, rash, and rare instances of hypoglycemia. Clarithromycin is contraindicated during pregnancy because of its teratogenicity in animal models	Dosage of clarithromycin is 500 mg, given morning and evening, three times a week. For the treatment of fibrocavitary or severe nodular/bronchiectatic MAC infection, a dose of 500–1000 mg is given daily. Disseminated MAC infection is treated with 1000 mg daily

Table 36.3 WHO 2011 update on regimen composition for anti-TB therapy regimen in MDR-TB

Include at least four second-line anti-TB drugs likely to be effective as well as pyrazinamide during the intensive phase of treatment
No evidence found to support the use of more than four second-line anti-TB drugs in patients with extensive disease. Increasing the number of second-line drugs in a regimen is permissible if the effectiveness of some of the drugs is uncertain
The regimen should include pyrazinamide; fluoroquinolone, a parenteral agent; ethionamide (or prothionamide); and cycloserine, or else para-aminosalicylic acid if cycloserine cannot be used
Ethambutol may be used but is not included among the drugs making up the standard regimen
Group 5 drugs may be used but are not included among the drugs making up the standard regimen

- *Second-line parenteral drug* – While all the three drugs mentioned have no significant difference between each other, kanamycin and amikacin are generally preferred due to their lower cost. Capreomycin can be used in cases resistant to kanamycin.
- *Fluoroquinolones* – These should constitute one of the main components of the second-line anti-TB therapy. Later-generation fluoroquinolones are generally preferred, while ciprofloxacin should be avoided.
- *Oral bacteriostatic drugs.*
- *Group 5 drugs.*

36.5.4 Response/Cure Rates

The cure rates in pulmonary MDR-TB vary between 60% and 70% [5]. However, in some studies, the in-hospital mortality rate in MDR-TBM was 57% and nearly 90% in human immunodeficiency virus-associated TBM [35, 36].

36.5.5 Duration of Second-Line Anti-TB Regimens

The regimens followed in various countries differ. For example, in India the Revised National Tuberculosis Control Program standardized regimen for pulmonary MRD-TB has two parts. An intensive phase lasting 6–9 months with six drugs given daily (kanamycin, ofloxacin, ethionamide, PZA, ethambutol (EMB), and cycloserine) and a continuation phase of 18 months of four drugs (viz., ofloxacin, ethionamide, EMB, and cycloserine) are used [45]. If at the end of 6 months of treatment, the culture remains positive, the intensive phase is extended for a further 3 months. The cure rates in this regimen vary from 60% to 10% in pulmonary TB [46–48]. These patients need close monitoring, as this regimen is associated with high incidence of adverse drug reactions [45].

The WHO 2011 update recommends an intensive phase of 8 months with modifications based on the response [5]. This is followed by a continuation phase lasting 12 months. The drugs to be used in the intensive phase are given in Table 36.2. In the continuation phase, the parenteral drug is omitted. In the protocol recommended, the adjusted relative risk for cure peaks at 7.1–8.5 months during the intensive phase and 18.6–21.5 months for the total treatment duration (for patients who had no previous treatment for MDR-TB [5, 39]. In patients who had previous treatment for MDR-TB, the peak was reached at 27.6–30.5 months. It is very important to keep a close surveillance as the risk of serious adverse events increases after 12 months of therapy. In XDR-TB though there are no official recommendations, some authors have recommended duration of treatment of at least 18 months for oral agents and at least 8 months after culture conversion for the injectable drug [49]. The same authors also reported that the culture conversion in XDR-TB was delayed by 1 month when compared with MDR-TB but reported an overall cure rate on 60% in pulmonary XDR-TB. They also did not find significant differences in the rate of relapse and death [49]. They also recommended respective pulmonary surgery in XDR-TB, which improved the outcome and cure rates.

36.5.6 Use of Antiretrovirals in Patients on Second-Line Antituberculosis Regimens

There has been scanty data on the utilization of antiretroviral therapy (ART) in patients with

MDR-TB. Controversies include as to whether ART should be started when there is a low CD4 count as well as the optimal time for the start of ART vis-à-vis anti-TB therapy. Based on pooled evidence from ten studies, though none of them were randomized controlled trials, the WHO recommended early commencement of ART (within 2 weeks) regardless of the CD4 status [5, 50]. This is based on the fact that several longitudinal cohort studies have shown higher cure rates and lower death rates when ART are employed early.

Conclusion

MDR-TB and XDR-TB are extremely difficult to treat. A high index of suspicion along with an early diagnosis and institution of treatment will certainly improve the outcomes in these patients. The present knowledge of management of MDR CNS-TB is mainly extrapolated from pulmonary MDR-TB. The scanty literature on MDR CNS-TB calls for more high-quality studies focusing on various aspects of composition and duration of drug regimens, management of pediatric CNS-TB, and chemoprophylaxis of contacts of MDR-TB cases.

References

1. Rock RB, Olin M, Baker CA, Molitor TW, Peterson PK (2008) Central nervous system tuberculosis: pathogenesis and clinical aspects. Clin Microbiol Rev 21:243–261
2. Ambekar S, Dwarakanath S, Pandey P, Somanna S, Chandramouli BA, Devi IB (2013) Factors influencing shunt malfunction in patients with tuberculous meningitis. Indian J Neurosurg 2:175–181
3. Kalita J, Misra UK, Ranjan P (2007) Predictors of long-term neurological sequelae of tuberculous meningitis: a multivariate analysis. Eur J Neurol 14:33–37
4. Rajshekhar V (2009) Management of hydrocephalus in patients with tuberculous meningitis. Neurol India 57:368–374
5. WHO Report (2011) Global tuberculosis control. World Health Organization, Geneva. WHO/HTM/TB/2011.16
6. Murthy J (2012) Multi-drug-resistant central nervous system tuberculosis. Neurol India 60:143–145
7. Rich AR, McCordock HA (1933) The pathogenesis of tuberculous meningitis. Bull Johns Hopkins Hosp 52:5–37
8. Donald PR, Schaaf HS, Schoeman JF (2005) Tuberculous meningitis and miliary tuberculosis: the Rich focus revisited. J Infect 50:193–195
9. Kumar R, Pandey CK, Bose N, Sahay S (2002) Tuberculous brain abscess: clinical presentation, pathophysiology and treatment (in children). Childs Nerv Syst 18:118–123
10. Sutlas PN, Unal A, Forta H, Senol S, Kirbas D (2003) Tuberculous meningitis in adults: review of 61 cases. Infection 31:387–391
11. Thwaites GE, Bang ND, Dung NH, Quy HT, Oanh DTT, Thoa NTC, Quang Hien N, Tri Thuc N, Ngoc Hai N, Thi Ngoc Lan N, Ngoc Lan N, Hong Duc N, Ngoc Tuan V, Huu Hiep C, Thi Hong Chau T, Phuong Mai P, Thi Dung N, Stepniewska K, Simmons CP, White NJ, Tinh Hien T, Farrar JJ (2005) The influence of HIV infection on clinical presentation, response to treatment, and outcome in adults with tuberculous meningitis. J Infect Dis 192:2134–2141
12. Jeren T, Beus I (1982) Characteristics of cerebrospinal fluid in tuberculous meningitis. Acta Cytol 26:678–680
13. Verdon R, Chevre S, Laissy TJP, Wolff M (1996) Tuberculous meningitis in adults: review of 48 cases. Clin Infect Dis 22:982–988
14. O'Toole RD, Thornton GF, Mukherjee MK, Nath RL (1969) Dexamethasone in tuberculous meningitis. Relationship of cerebrospinal fluid effects to therapeutic efficacy. Ann Intern Med 70:39–48
15. Behari M, Raj M, Ahuja GK, Shrinivas (1989) Soluble antigen fluorescent antibody test in the serodiagnosis of tuberculous meningitis. J Assoc Physicians India 37:499–501
16. Katti MK (2002) Assessment of antibody responses to antigens of Mycobacterium tuberculosis and Cysticercus cellulosae in cerebrospinal fluid of chronic meningitis patients for definitive diagnosis as TBM/NCC by passive hemagglutination and immunoblot assays. FEMS Immunol Med Microbiol 33:57–61
17. Katti MK, Achar MT (2001) Immunodiagnosis of tuberculous meningitis: detection of antibody reactivity to antigens of Mycobacterium tuberculosis and Cysticercus cellulosae in cerebrospinal fluid tuberculous meningitis patients by ELISA. J Immunoassay Immunochem 22:401–406
18. Quan C, Lu CZ, Qiao J, Xiao BG, Li X (2006) Comparative evaluation of early diagnosis of tuberculous meningitis by different assays. J Clin Microbiol 44:3160–3166
19. Chandramuki A, Allen PR, Keen M, Ivanyi J (1985) Detection of mycobacterial antigen and antibodies in the cerebrospinal fluid of patients with tuberculous meningitis. J Med Microbiol 20:239–247
20. Kadival GV, Samuel AM, Mazarelo TB, Chaparas SD (1987) Radioimmunoassay for detecting Mycobacterium tuberculosis antigen in cerebrospinal fluids of patients with tuberculous meningitis. J Infect Dis 155:608–611

21. Kashyap RS, Kainthla RP, Biswas SK, Agarwal N, Chandak NH, Purohit HJ, Taori GM, Daginawala HF (2003) Rapid diagnosis of tuberculous meningitis using the simple dot ELISA method. Med Sci Monit 9:MT123–MT126
22. Baker CA, Cartwright CP, Williams DN, Nelson SM, Peterson PK (2002) Early detection of central nervous system tuberculosis with the Gen-Probe nucleic acid amplification assay: utility in an inner city hospital. Clin Infect Dis 35:339–342
23. Chedore P, Jamieson FB (2002) Rapid molecular diagnosis of tuberculous meningitis using the Gen-Probe Amplified Mycobacterium tuberculosis direct test in a large Canadian public health laboratory. Int J Tuberc Lung Dis 6:913–919
24. Lang AM, Feris-Iglesias J, Pena C, Sanchez JF, Stockman L, Rys P, Roberts GD, Henry NK, Persing DH, Cockerill FR 3rd (1998) Clinical evaluation of the Gen-Probe Amplified Direct Test for detection of Mycobacterium tuberculosis complex organisms in cerebrospinal fluid. J Clin Microbiol 36:2191–2194
25. Rafi W, Venkataswamy MM, Nagarathna S, Satishchandra P, Chandramuki A (2007) Role of IS6110 uniplex PCR in the diagnosis of tuberculous meningitis: experience at a tertiary neurocentre. Int J Tuberc Lung Dis 11:209–214
26. Boehme CC, Nabeta P, Hillemann D, Nicol MP, Shenai S, Krapp F, Allen J, Tahirli R, Blakemore R, Rustomjee R, Milovic A, Jones M, O'Brien SM, Persing DH, Ruesch-Gerdes S, Gotuzzo E, Rodrigues C, Alland D, Perkins MD (2010) Rapid molecular detection of tuberculosis and rifampin resistance. N Engl J Med 363:1005–1015
27. Van Rie A, Page-Shipp L, Scott L, Sanne I, Stevens W (2010) Xpert® MTB/RIF for point-of-care diagnosis of TB in high-HIV burden, resource-limited countries: hype or hope? Expert Rev Mol Diagn 10:937–946
28. Scott LE, McCarthy K, Gous N, Nduna M, Van Rie A, Sanne I, Venter WF, Duse A, Stevens W (2011) Comparison of Xpert MTB/RIF with other nucleic acid technologies for diagnosing pulmonary tuberculosis in a high HIV prevalence setting: a prospective study. PLoS Med 8:e1001061
29. Thwaites GE, Tran TH (2005) Tuberculous meningitis: many questions, too few answers. Lancet Neurol 4:160–170
30. Yaramis A, Bukte Y, Katar S, Ozbek MN (2007) Chest computerized tomography scan findings in 74 children with tuberculous meningitis in southeastern Turkey. Turk J Pediatr 49:365–369
31. Ozates M, Kemaloglu S, Gurkan F, Ozkan U, Hosoglu S, Simsek MM (2000) CT of the brain in tuberculous meningitis. A review of 289 patients. Acta Radiol 41:13–17
32. Kent SJ, Crowe SM, Yung A, Lucas CR, Mijch AM (1993) Tuberculous meningitis: a 30-year review. Clin Infect Dis 17:987–994
33. Kingsley PB, Shah TC, Woldenberg R (2006) Identification of diffuse and focal brain lesions by clinical magnetic resonance spectroscopy. NMR Biomed 19:435–462
34. Thwaites G, Fisher M, Hemingway C, Scott G, Solomon T, Innes J, British Infection Society (2009) British Infection Society guidelines for the diagnosis and treatment of tuberculosis of the central nervous system in adults and children. J Infect 59:167–187
35. Patel VB, Padayatchi N, Bhigjee AI, Allen J, Bhagwan B, Moodley AA, Mthiyane T (2004) Multidrug-resistant tuberculous meningitis in Kwazulu-Natal, South Africa. Clin Infect Dis 38:851–856
36. Daikos GL, Cleary T, Rodriguez A, Fischl MA (2003) Multidrug-resistant tuberculous meningitis in patients with AIDS. Int J Tuberc Lung Dis 7:394–398
37. Lawn SD, Brooks SV, Kranzer K, Nicol MP, Whitelaw A, Vogt M, Bekker LG, Wood R (2011) Screening for HIV-associated tuberculosis and rifampicin resistance before antiretroviral therapy using the Xpert MTB/RIF assay: a prospective study. PLoS Med 8:e1001067
38. Migliori GB, Lange C, Centis R, Sotgiu G, Mütterlein R, Hoffmann H, Kliiman K, De Iaco G, Lauria FN, Richardson MD, Spanevello A, Cirillo DM, TBNET Study Group (2008) Resistance to second-line injectables and treatment outcomes in multidrug- resistant and extensively drug-resistant tuberculosis cases. Eur Respir J 31:1155–1559
39. Van Deun A, Maug AK, Salim MA, Das PK, Sarker MR, Daru P, Reider HL (2010) Short, highly effective, and inexpensive standardized treatment of multidrug- resistant tuberculosis. Am J Respir Crit Care Med 182:684–692
40. Suarez PG, Floyd K, Portocarrero J, Alarc6n E, Rapiti E, Ramos G, Bonilla C, Sabogal I, Aranda I, Dye C, Raviglione M, Espinal MA (2002) Feasibility and cost-effectiveness of standardised second-line drug treatment for chronic tuberculosis patients: a national cohort study in Peru. Lancet 359:1980–1989
41. Orenstein EW, Basu S, Shah NS, Andrews JR, Friedland GH, Moll AP, Gandhi NR, Galvani AP (2009) Treatment outcomes among patients with multidrug-resistant tuberculosis: systematic review and meta-analysis. Lancet Infect Dis 9:153–161
42. Johnston JC, Neal C, Shahidi NC, Sadatsafavi M, Fitzgerald JM (2009) Treatment outcomes of multidrug-resistant tuberculosis: a systematic review and meta-analysis. PLoS One 4:e6914
43. Akçakır Y (2010) Correlates of treatment outcomes of multidrug-resistant tuberculosis (MDR-TB): a systematic review and meta-analysis [MSc thesis]. McGill University Department of Epidemiology, Statistics and Occupational Health, Montreal
44. Ahuja SD, Ashkin D, Avendano M, Banerjee R, Bauer M, Bayona JN, Becerra MC, Benedetti A, Burgos M, Centis R, Chan ED, Chiang CY, Cox H, D'Ambrosio L, DeRiemer K, Dung NH, Enarson D, Falzon D, Flanagan K, Flood J, Garcia-Garcia ML, Gandhi N, Granich RM, Hollm-Delgado MG, Holtz TH, Iseman MD, Jarlsberg LG, Keshavjee S, Kim HR, Koh WJ, Lancaster J, Lange C, de Lange WC, Leimane V, Leung CC, Li J, Menzies D, Migliori GB, Mishustin SP, Mitnick CD, Narita M, O'Riordan P, Pai M, Palmero D, Park SK, Pasvol G, Peña J, Pérez-Guzmán C, Quelapio

MI, Ponce-de-Leon A, Riekstina V, Robert J, Royce S, Schaaf HS, Seung KJ, Shah L, Shim TS, Shin SS, Shiraishi Y, Sifuentes-Osornio J, Sotgiu G, Strand MJ, Tabarsi P, Tupasi TE, van Altena R, Van der Walt M, Van der Werf TS, Vargas MH, Viiklepp P, Westenhouse J, Yew WW, Yim JJ, Collaborative Group for Meta-Analysis of Individual Patient Data in MDR-TB (2012) Multidrug resistant pulmonary tuberculosis treatment regimens and patient outcomes: an Individual patient data meta-analysis of 9,153 patients. PLoS Med 9:e1001300. doi:10.1371/journal.pmed.1001300

45. Central TB Division (CTD) (2006) Directorate General of Health 2. Services, Ministry of Health and Family Welfare, Government of India. DOTS-plus guidelines. CTD, New Delhi
46. Singla R, Sarin R, Khalid UK, Mathuria K, Singla N, Jaiswal A, Puri MM, Visalakshi P, Behera D (2009) Seven-year DOTS-Plus pilot experience in India: results, constraints and issues. Int J Tuberc Lung Dis 13:976–981
47. Joseph P, Desai VB, Mohan NC, Fredrick JS, Ramachandran R, Raman B, Wares F, Ramachandran R, Thomas A (2011) Outcome of standardized treatment for patients with MDR-TB from Tamil Nadu, India. Indian J Med Res 133:529–534
48. Malla P, Kanitz EE, Akthar M, Falzon D, Feldmann K, Gunneberg C, Jha SS, Maharjan B, Prasai MK, Shrestha B, Verma SC, Zignol M (2009) Ambulatory-based standardised therapy for multi-drug resistant tuberculosis: Experience from Nepal, 2005-2006. PLoS One 23:e8313
49. Mitnick CD, Shin SS, Seung KJ, Rich ML, Atwood SS, Furin JJ, Fitzmaurice GM, Alcantara Viru FA, Appleton SC, Bayona JN, Bonilla CA, Chalco K, Choi S, Franke MF, Fraser HS, Guerra D, Hurtado RM, Jazayeri D, Joseph K, Llaro K, Mestanza L, Mukherjee JS, Muñoz M, Palacios E, Sanchez E, Sloutsky A, Becerra MC (2008) Comprehensive treatment of extensively drug-resistant tuberculosis. N Engl J Med 359:563–574
50. World Health Organization (2010 revision) Antiretroviral therapy for HIV infection in adults and adolescents: recommendations for a public health approach. Geneva, World Health Organization

Outcome of Tuberculosis of the Nervous System and Its Coverings

37

Ahmed Elsawaf

Contents

A. Elsawaf, MD, PhD
Department of Neurosurgery, Suez Canal University, Ismailia, Egypt
e-mail: ahmed_alsawaf@yahoo.com

Abbreviations

BMRC	British Medical Research Council
CNS	Central nervous system
CSF	Cerebrospinal fluid
CT	Computed tomography
EMB	Ethambutol
HIV	Human immunodeficiency virus
IICP	Increased intracranial pressure
INH	Isoniazid
LFT	Liver function test
MDR-TBM	Multidrug resistant-tuberculous meningitis
MRI	Magnetic resonance imaging
PZA	Pyrazinamide
RIF	Rifampin
RNTCP	Revised National TB Control Program
STR	Streptomycin
TB	Tuberculosis
TBA	Tuberculous brain abscess
TBM	Tuberculous meningitis
VPS	Ventriculoperitoneal shunt
WHO	World Health Organization
XDR-TBM	Extensively drug resistant tuberculous meningitis

M. Turgut et al. (eds.), *Tuberculosis of the Central Nervous System*,
DOI 10.1007/978-3-319-50712-5_37

37.1 Introduction

In spite of the decline of tuberculosis (TB) incidence within developed countries over the course of recent decades, this disease remains outstanding worldwide and is still one of the main causes of infection-related mortality across the world. According to the World Health Organization (WHO), there are about 9.2 million new TB cases and 1.7 million deaths every year [1].

TB of the central nervous system (CNS) is one of the most disastrous diseases facing neurologists or neurosurgeons. CNS-TB accounts for about 12–15% of TB cases or about 0.7% of all clinical TB [2, 3]. It usually affects young children [4–6].

The most common human immunodeficiency virus (HIV)-related infection is TB. It is also considered the most important cause of morbidity and mortality in HIV-infected individuals in the developing world [7]. Coincidence of infection with HIV and *Mycobacterium tuberculosis* was responsible for 600,000 deaths in 2004 [8]. It also increases the risk of development of reactivation TB disease from a whole life risk of 5–10% to approximately 10% per year [9–11].

37.2 Pathological Point of View

TB of the CNS can be classified as diffuse form, the common tuberculous meningitis (TBM), and localized forms, tuberculoma, and tuberculous brain abscess (TBA). Many risk factors for central nervous system TB have been identified [12]. Childhood; HIV-coinfected patients; immune-suppression conditions or the use of immunosuppressive medications; malnutrition; overcrowded populations like armies, malignancies, and alcoholism; and recent measles in children are all blamed to be risk factors for CNS-TB [13]. Studies made in developed countries have also identified that foreign-born individuals (individuals born outside of developed countries) are presented among CNS-TB cases [14, 15].

CNS-TB is caused by aerobic, acid-fast bacilli, TB bacilli. It starts by invasion of the CNS inside the macrophages and settles in the cerebral tissues or meninges as Rich nodule. Later, Rich nodule ruptures and mycobacterium bacilli release in the cerebrospinal fluid (CSF) causing cell-mediated reaction and start inflammation. Exudates can block the CSF pathway leading to hydrocephalus. Reactional vasculitis can happen and lead to luminal stenosis of the feeding cerebral arteries with serious regional ischemic infarctions.

Tuberculomas arise when Rich nodule enlarges and constitutes big inflammatory region with accompanying pressure of the adjacent cerebral tissues. It could be solitary or multiple. TB can affect any part of the CNS along the craniospinal axis with different outcomes and prognoses according to the site. Tuberculomas can appear after beginning of medical treatment for TBM [16–18]. This condition can be explained by that local tissue reactivity is dependable for a multiplicity of different paradoxical responses in intracranial tuberculomas [19]. Infected hosts develop hypersensitivity to an arrangement of mycobacterial proteins. Anti-TB drugs cause the destruction of mycobacterial structures and modify bacillar mycobacterial proteins, leading to the presence of swelling and inflammation of the focus [20, 21]; these produce a delayed hypersensitivity reaction. The intracranial microtuberculomas grow slowly and become encapsulated after a latent period resulting in paradoxical progression of existing lesions. The extension of the tuberculomas has an immunological basis [22].

TBA is an encapsulated collection of pus containing viable tuberculoma bacilli. It happens when the central necrosis part of the tuberculoma liquefies and forms pus [23]. It could be also solitary or multiple [24]. It should be differentiated from tuberculoma with central necrosis because of the difference in prognosis and therapeutic protocol [23].

37.3 Clinical Manifestations

Besides the general condition of the patient regarding chest condition (if the patient is in acute pulmonary TB), fever, night sweating, and headache, adult patients with TBM often present with the standard symptoms of meningitis such as fever, headache, and meningismus along with focal neurological deficits, behavioral changes, and alterations in consciousness [25]. There is usually a history of exposure to TB or positive tuberculin test. The presence of active pulmonary TB on chest X-ray ranges from 30 to 50% in recent series [25, 26].

Children with TBM usually present with fever, stiff neck, seizures, and abdominal symptoms such as nausea and vomiting [13, 27]. Headache is less common in children than in adults. According to the stage of presentation, neurological symptoms range from lethargy and agitation to coma. A family history of TB can be identified in approximately 50 to 60% of children, and a positive tuberculin skin test is found in approximately 30 to 50% [13, 27].

Clinical signs of patients presenting with TBM are assessed for severity based on modifications of the British Medical Research Council (BMRC) staging system [28] (Table 37.1). TBM was classified into three stages.

Clinical manifestations of tuberculoma and TBA depend on their location with focal symptoms due to pressure on adjacent eloquent centers. The patients usually present with disturbed conscious level, headache, seizures, papilledema, or other signs of increased intracranial pressure (IICP). The presentation of TBA is more acute (1 week to 3 months) than tuberculoma but slower in onset than pyogenic brain abscesses and is associated with fever, headaches, and focal neurological deficits [23].

37.4 Treatment

Medical treatment is the cornerstone of CNS-TB. Anti-TB treatment that is classified into first-line treatment includes isoniazid (INH), rifampin (RIF), rifabutin, pyrazinamide (PZA), and ethambutol (EMB). Second-line treatment includes streptomycin (STR), ciprofloxacin, kanamycin, ofloxacin, ethionamide, capreomycin, and cycloserine. According to the American Thoracic Society guidelines [29], medical protocol of management of TB includes the initial four-medicine regimen (INH, RIF, PZA, and EMB) for 3 months duration followed by two-medicine regimen (PZA and EMB) for another 9 months. Some authors recommend longer course of treatment [4, 30], while others discussed shorter treatment period of 6–9 months [31–34]. Both INH and PZA pass easily across the blood brain barrier [35–38], but INH remains the backbone of TBM treatment.

37.5 Prognostic Factors Affecting Outcome

Clinical and radiological variables affecting morbidity and mortality after CNS-TB were discussed in many articles. Many of them were found insignificant; others were found to have significant prognostic importance. Age of the patient, duration of illness, clinical stage at the time of treatment initiation (BMRC stage), vascular complication, extent of arachnoiditis, seizures, hydrocephalus, and IICP are the main factors [39].

37.5.1 Delay in Diagnosis

The duration of signs and symptoms of the disease before admission and initiation of therapy was of prognostic value in determining the outcome. The importance of early diagnosis and management is crucial as agreed by many authors that is because clinical outcome depends mainly

Table 37.1 The British Medical Research Council (BMRC) clinical criteria for assessing the severity of TBM [28]

Stage I	No definite neurological symptoms on admission or in the history before admission, with or without meningismus
Stage II	Signs of meningeal irritations with or without slight clouding of consciousness with focal neurological signs such as cranial nerve palsies or hemiparesis
Stage III	Severe clouding of consciousness or delirium, convulsions, and serious neurological signs such as hemiplegia, paraplegia, or involuntary movements

on the stage at which therapy is initiated. Some recommended that patients with the meningoencephalitis syndrome and CSF findings of low glucose levels, elevated protein levels, and pleocytosis should be treated immediately if there is evidence of TB elsewhere in the body or if rapid evaluation fails to set an alternative diagnosis [40].

In one large study evaluating TBM, the mortality rate was higher ($p < 0.001$) in patients with clinical manifestations of TBM of more than 4 weeks (80%) compared with those who had symptoms of less than 2 weeks (40%) [4]. Other studies confirmed that early anti-TB medications before the third day after hospitalization have an important protective impact on the morbidity and mortality of patients [41, 42].

37.5.2 BMRC Staging

As a role in most of neurological and neurosurgical insults, clinical condition at the initial presentation is the main predictor of outcome. The most important factor influencing the outcome of TBM is the initial clinical presentation and the neurological examination assessed by the BMRC grading system. BMRC is the standard scoring system used to assess the clinical presentation of the patients with TBM and has an important prognostic indication. The BMRC staging which was developed to establish the degree of severity of the patients with CNS-TB at the start of anti-TB treatment has been used in some studies to establish its association with the outcome [43].

Mortality is mainly influenced by presenting condition as mentioned by many authors; patients who presented conscious with only signs of meningism had a very good prognosis in comparison to comatose patients. The mortality rate was 18% for stage I TBM, 34% for stage II, and 72% for stage III according to Girgis et al. [4]. Other series mentioned 34% death of the patients who started anti-TB treatment in stage III [44, 45]. They found also that 26% at stage III and 6% of patients at stage II died before completion of therapy [31]. Stage III showed the worst prognostic outcome regarding both morbidity and mortality. In a retrospective multivariate analysis study over 108 adults with TBM over 6 years follow-up, there was no statistical difference in mortality between TBM stage I and stage II ($p = 0.915$), but patients with TBM stage III had a higher mortality rate compared with those with TBM stage I ($p = 0.014$) [46].

Table 37.2 Quito Score [44]

	Present	Absent
Impaired consciousness	2	–9
Motor deficit	4	–6
Cisternal effacement	8	–3
Cerebral infarcts	6	–2
Sum of score	20	–20

Present and absent findings can be summed up to a maximum of 20 points and a minimum of –20. This score predicts the outcome in two classes: death or serious sequelae on one side and healing or minor sequelae on the other

The weakness of BMRC is that it is a descriptive scale with overlapping features which do not include images or CSF analysis and was not built with a multivariate procedure [43, 47–51]. It is also important to consider that BMRC staging, when it was built 50 years ago, was not aimed at predicting prognosis, but to classify patients who were submitted to a new therapy (STR) in degrees of severity [43]. Another score system was developed called Quito Score. The Quito Score is easy to apply and is a good predictor of poor outcome (Table 37.2).

37.5.3 Age

Age of the patient is usually an important prognostic factor for most of CNS disorders. In TBM, age was found to correlate with poor outcomes in some studies [46, 52]. The deaths in these studies tended to be among the elderly (65.5 vs. 48.2 years, $p < 0.001$), supporting the strong relationship between age and mortality in patients with TBM. It was found that age below 40 years old was detected as an important predictor of outcome, with a significant correlation between young age and morbidity and neurological sequelae in logistic regression ($p = 0.049$) [53].

37.5.4 General Clinical Condition

General condition of the patient regarding chest condition (if the patient is in acute pulmonary TB), fever, night sweating, headache, weight loss, seizures, and meningeal signs has a prognostic indication of outcome. Cranial nerve palsy at presentation had also an important outcome prediction value regarding the development of neurological sequelae in TBM and was considered the most important by some of them [53].

37.5.5 Magnetic Resonance Imaging or Computed Tomography Scan Findings of Hydrocephalus and Leptomeningitis

Hydrocephalus is a very critical prognostic factor according to almost all studies discussing TBM. Hydrocephalus is thought to arise because of the dense inflammatory exudates in the subarachnoid space in its course from the exit site in the fourth ventricle to the absorption site in the arachnoid villi or possibly the destruction of the arachnoid villi themselves causing hydrocephalus [54]. It is a common presentation with cases of CNS-TB. Cranial computed tomography (CT) scans of the patients presenting with TBM showed hydrocephalus in 94% and basilar enhancement in 93% of patients after receiving intravenous contrast [27].

Some advise immediate CSF diversion either by ventriculoperitoneal shunt (VPS); others recommend inserting external ventricular drain for those with high protein level in CSF to be removed or changed to VP shunts after improvement of CSF parameters. In either maneuvers, the outcome is better with intervention than conservative measures in almost all cases [55, 56]. When the role of VPS has been determined to be essential for TBM-associated hydrocephalus, success rates ranged between 40 and 50%, and VPS has a complication rate of around 30% [57, 58]. Neuroendoscopy can be done with good results [59, 60].

On the other hand, some studies showed that drainage may not affect the outcome, in this study of 48 patients with TBM associated with hydrocephalus; improvement was shown after steroid therapy and medical anti-TB treatment; however, VPS, CSF drainage, and mannitol use were not associated with improved mortality [58].

37.5.6 Use of Steroids

Corticosteroids are used in the treatment of TBM as adjunctive to anti-TB medications. It works mainly as anti-inflammatory due to its effect on the immune system. It also has a role in preventing hydrocephalus and infarction. Most of the studies done assessing the role of steroids in the treatment for TBM found a significant reduction in mortality but not in morbidity in adults [46, 61]. One large placebo-controlled study on dexamethasone as adjuvant therapy of TBM identified a significant reduction in mortality but not in morbidity in adults [61]. They used an initial dose of 0.3 mg/kg/day for mild degree infection and 0.4 mg/kg/day for moderate and severe degrees, followed by a gradual taper over 6 weeks [61, 62]. Analysis on further subgroup revealed that the mortality benefit of dexamethasone occurred among all severity types of CNS-TB, but this benefit did not extend to patients coinfected with HIV [61].

Current Infectious Diseases Society of America, Centers for Disease Control and Prevention, and American Thoracic Society guidelines [29] endorse the use of steroid therapy as an adjunctive therapy joined with standard anti-TB therapy in CNS-TB. The initial dose of dexamethasone is 8 mg per day for children under 25 kg body weight and 12 mg/day for adults and children more than 25 mg kg body weight.

Regarding the effect of corticosteroids on hydrocephalus and cerebral infarction, serial magnetic resonance imaging (MRI) study was done assessing the influence of corticosteroid on hydrocephalus, cerebral infarction, and basal meningeal enhancement but found no clear effect on any of these parameters [63]. On the other hand, Schoeman et al. mentioned that steroids have no clear effect on intracranial pressure or development and extension of cerebral infarction, but still have a positive relationship to survival [64].

37.5.7 Positive CSF Ziehl-Neelsen Stain or Culture for *M. tuberculosis*

Positive CSF culture for *Mycobacterium tuberculosis* was associated with a poor prognosis, and this observation may indicate that higher concentration and burden of mycobacteria in the CSF led to an increased risk of developing consciousness disturbances, hydrocephalus, more serious TBM stages, and subsequent mortality [46, 65].

37.5.8 Cisternal Effacement

Cisternal effacement shown in CT scan on presentation is one of the indicators of high intracranial pressure in patients with TBM. It has been shown to be associated with poor prognosis in a multivariate analysis study [27].

37.5.9 Infarctions

Cerebral infarctions in patients with TBM is explained by the reactional vasculitis in the vessels of the circle of Willis, the vertebrobasilar system, and the perforating branches of the middle cerebral artery, resulting in stenosis of the vascular lumen and infarctions in the distribution of these vessels.

Cerebral infarctions are important poor outcome predictors especially those affecting basal ganglia. It was mentioned in literatures assessing cerebral infarction in childhood TBM that there is a significant association between all sites of infarction ($p = 0.0001$) other than hemispheric ($p = 0.35$) and outcome score. There was also a significant association between all types of infarction ($p = 0.0001$) other than hemispheric ($p = 0.05$) and overall poor outcome [66].

37.5.10 Presence of Tuberculoma or Tuberculous Brain Abscess

Tuberculomas TBAs may be present anywhere in the brain, but they are mostly found in the frontoparietal region and basal ganglions [67]. There was clear association between intracranial tuberculoma and hydrocephalus with about 18% incidence in TBM patients [67]. The presence of tuberculoma was detected as an independent prognostic factor on neurological sequel in the other studies ($p = 0.048$) [68].

37.6 General Outcome of CNS Tuberculosis

Nervous system TB is categorized among extrapulmonary critical illness. The Revised National TB Control Program (RNTCP) recommended 2(INH+EMB+RIF+PZA)/4(INH+RIF) regimen with extension of continuation phase for 3 months more (total 9 months). For pediatric neuro-TB, RNTCP recommends substitution of EMB with STR in the intensive phase [68].

Early recognition and treatment of CNS-TB may improve the outcome. Tuberculoma, TBA, or complications of medical anti-TB treatment itself can happen during the course of treatment. Assessment of outcome with medical treatment was tried by many authors; Smith et al. score is considered one of the most trusted for the assessment of outcome of medical treatment of TBM which recognizes five categories [69, 70] (Table 37.3).

Initial improvement of clinical symptoms usually comes gradually in most patients, and the obvious response starts sometimes after 3 to 4 weeks and may in fact briefly worsen at this initial period of management despite appropriate anti-TB therapy [25]. After starting the medication course and during the long regimen, new tuberculomas can appear or even some complications of the TBM can develop like hydrocephalus or cerebral infarcts. That is why continuous radiological follow-up should be done to follow the improvement of the condition and to check

Table 37.3 A scoring system for evaluation of the outcome of TBM by Smith et al. [70]

1	Apparently normal patients
2	Patients with slight mental abnormality or normal intelligence but with some degree of hemiparesis, minor behavioral problems, deafness, or epilepsy, with the possibility of leading relatively normal autonomous lives without assistance
3	Patients with mild sequelae that is mild mental abnormality and/or having a well-established physical impairment, being able to lead relatively normal lives with some assistance
4	Patients with severe sequelae that is severe mental abnormality and/or having a severe physical impairment being totally dependent
5	Death

the development of new tuberculomas or other complications [71]. The development of such sequelae does not necessitate the change of medical treatment or increase of the doses.

Reported mortality from TBM ranges from 22 to 27% [46, 72, 73], but reached up to 57% in some series [4]. In that large series, mortality percentage showed high dependency on the initial clinical condition: stage I showing about 18% mortality, 34% for stage II, and about 72% mortality for stage III. More than 50% of the patients who survive are left with permanent neurological sequelae [72, 73].

37.6.1 Complications of Medical Treatment

Adverse effect of anti-TB treatment can affect the compliance of the patient to medical treatment and can push the treating physician to stop the medications at least for a certain time. Of the most important complication that can lead to stoppage of medical treatment is the hepatotoxicity. It is more common in adults rather than children [74]. According to the *Guidelines for the Management of Adverse Drug Effects of Antimycobacterial Agents*, baseline liver function tests (LFTs) are obtained, and then follow-up tests should be done serially.

For asymptomatic patients with an increase in LFTs from baseline: (a) if the increase in LFTs is <3–5× normal, continue the current regimen, and monitor for symptoms of liver dysfunction [75, 76]; (b) For asymptomatic patients, if the serum transaminases increase to >3–5× normal, hold INH until levels return to baseline [75, 76].

For symptomatic patients: (a) hold all drugs, and obtain LFTs; (b) If LFTs are elevated, we have to hold drugs until symptoms resolve and the transaminases decrease to <2× normal [76, 77]. EMB and PZA should be started if drug therapy cannot be held secondary to the patient's clinical condition. STR can be used if PZA is suspected to be the cause of hepatotoxicity.

37.6.2 Multidrug Resistant-Tuberculous Meningitis (MDR-TBM)

Response to medical treatment varies significantly and depends mainly on either the patient develops resistance to medications or not. The usual delayed effect of anti-TB medications and the aggressive behavior of the disease make the identification of drug resistance late [78]. It is mentioned that one of the factors that contribute to the high mortality is the absence of standardized approach to the management of MDR-TBM and the poor CSF penetration of most MDR-TB drugs. MDR-TB is defined by resistance to both INH and RIF; it should be considered if there is a history of TB: a MDR-TB contact or a poor response to TB therapy despite adequate dosing and compliance of medications [79]. Almost 18% of the patients had MDR-TBM as mentioned in many studies [80, 81]. Risk factors for the development of MDR-TBM are inadequate initial therapy; inappropriate incomplete previous anti-TB treatment; presence of comorbid conditions like diabetes, malnutrition, and HIV; or other immunosuppressive conditions [80].

The prognosis regarding morbidity and mortality is worse in MDR-TBM cases that is why all cases suspected to be TBM should be cultured with determination of the antibiotic sensitivity pattern.

The management of MDR-TBM especially if coincident with HIV is much more complex than in the case of drug-susceptible organisms and is associated with higher treatment cost and longer treatment periods [82]. In addition, such cases show poorer patient outcome and higher mortality rates [82, 83]. Nonspecific clinical presentation especially in young children, poor diagnostics, and delays in setting up appropriate anti-TB therapy as drug susceptibility testing may require up to 10 weeks that further increase the risk of mortality or the onset of severe, irreversible neurological damage [79, 84].

37.6.3 Extensively Drug Resistant-Tuberculous Meningitis (XDR-TBM)

Of much worse prognosis is the extensively drug-resistant tuberculous meningitis (XDR-TBM) which is defined as resistance to INH, RIF, fluoroquinolones, and either capreomycin, kanamycin, or amikacin. It is not only resistant to first-line treatment but also for the second-line treatment. 5.4% of MDR-TB cases were found to have XDR-TB. Proper use of second-line drugs must be ensured to cure existing MDR-TB, to reduce its transmission and to prevent XDR-TB [80]. Seventy-three percent mortality was shown in such cases, and many of them could be discharged from the hospital because of the highly expensive long-term stay and palliative care, predisposing to spreading of such resistant organisms [85].

37.7 Outcome of Tuberculoma and Tuberculous Brain Abscess

The most common manifestation of CNS-TB is TBM [86]. Intracranial tuberculoma however is one of the usual presentations of CNS-TB that usually occurs in immune-compromised patients [86, 87]. Intracranial tuberculoma is usually presented as solitary lesion although 15–34% is multiple [17]. Tuberculomas of the craniospinal axis are the result of hematogenous spread from a primary focus elsewhere in the body, most often the lung. The incidence of associated pulmonary TB varies from 25 to 75%.

The difficulty in intracranial tuberculomas starts with diagnosis. The similarity of clinical and radiological appearance of tuberculoma to many other infectious and noninfectious cerebral disorders can delay the diagnosis and management [19, 88, 89]. In the absence of extra-neural lesions, image-guided stereotactic biopsy is preferred to open biopsy [86]. Maintaining suspicion of CNS-TB is essential to achieve an accurate diagnosis and expedite the appropriate treatment.

Tuberculomas are thought to arise from enlargement of Rich focus without rupture of this focus into the subarachnoid space, so, tuberculoma can be presented as intracranial lesion with or without TBM. It is composed of collection of inflammatory cells with central area of necrosis [23]. In a multivariate analysis study of 12 published literatures, anatomical location of tuberculoma was 58% supratentorial, 17% infratentorial, 14% thoraco-spinal, 8% cervico-spinal, and 2% lumbo-spinal [23].

Intracranial tuberculomas can appear in many patients after starting treatment of TBM, which suggest that it could be a normal pathological response to treated infection [63].

Treatment of intracranial tuberculoma is completely similar to TBM, with giving the whole regimen of anti-TB medications. The role of dexamethasone however could be more significant; beside the significant outcome regarding mortality, it has an extra-cerebral effect. It protects against severe drug-related liver toxicity and prevents life-threatening interruptions in anti-TB chemotherapy.

Surgical intervention for tuberculoma with total removal of the lesion is not much favored by many authors; it could be reserved to certain situations: for patients with life-threatening neurological involvement with intracranial hypertension and for patients with lesions that fail medical treatment and if a large lesion is not located in deep regions of the brain [90].

Arseni and Samitca reported only nine cases of intraspinal tuberculoma in a review of 219 cases of tuberculomas, of which three were intradural-extramedullary [91]. Intradural-extramedullary tuberculoma is extremely rare, with seven cases reported in literatures [91–93]. Although spinal tuberculoma shows a predilection for the thoracic region, it may occur at any level [94, 95].

CNS tuberculoma is a benign condition with a good prognosis and effective therapy options if diagnosed early. The overall outcome of management of CNS tuberculoma depends mainly on the same factors affecting the outcome. Patients presenting at an advanced disease stage had a worse outcome. For intramedullary tuberculoma, early surgical decompression is recommended and leads to complete recovery [96, 97] (Figs. 37.1 and 37.2).

This is uncommon presentation of CNS-TB. Only 57 cases of TBA were found in a review of world literature by Whitener et al. [24]. There is a high association with AIDS and development of TBA [24, 98].

TBA develops either from intracerebral TB granulomas or through the spread of TB foci from the meninges. It is characterized by an encapsulated collection of pus containing viable bacilli without evidence of the classic TB granuloma and must be distinguished from tuberculoma with central caseation and liquefaction mimicking pus [23]. TBA can arise as solitary or multiple lesions [24]. A TBA has a much thicker abscess wall than a pyogenic brain abscess [23]. Although TBA may be indistinguishable from other intracranial mass lesions, a high suspicion of TB origin can be taken if the patient has other TB extra-neural manifestations and/or lack of irregular treatment of TB, HIV case, intravenous drug abuser, immunological survey, and serology (to exclude toxoplasmosis). Single-photon emission CT and positron emission tomography scans can differentiate it from astrocytoma or lymphoma. Culture and sensitivity of the drained pus easily confirm the diagnosis [99].

The management of TBA is similar to any cerebral abscess. It starts by drainage of the abscess with confirmation of the diagnoses by culture and sensitivity of the drained pus; the complete course of anti-TB medications starts. Many trials of aspiration can be done if recollection happens.

Due to the lack of published cases on TBA, the outcome of such abscess is still not clear. In some published articles about management of few cases of TBA, the outcome with optimal management is quietly fair. Seventy-five percent had an appropriate clinical response and good outcome, and 25% patients die [99].

37.8 Outcome of Pott's Disease

Spinal TB (Pott's disease) is one of the common presentations of extrapulmonary TB. The vast majority of cases of TB vertebral osteomyelitis that involves the lower thoracic and lumbar spine reflects the consequences of thoracolumbar infection [6]. Spinal TB typically has an insidious onset and slow progression; the mean duration between onset of symptoms and clinical presentation is about 11 months in some papers (4–24 months) [100].

Pott's disease was named after Percivall Pott (1714–1788), one of the leading surgeons in London in the eighteenth century [101]. It is not considered CNS-TB; however, it is one of the important concerns of neurosurgeons. Also, spinal TB can be presented by sever myelopathic signs due to affection on the spinal cord or cranio-cervical junction which deserve urgent neurosurgical intervention in some cases. The incidence of neurological deficit in Pott's disease varies from series to series: 5–10% [102–104].

Conventional anti-TB medical treatment is the mainstay of management of Pott's disease. Indications for surgery are neurological deficit, spinal deformity with instability, severe or progressive kyphosis, retropulsed bone fragments in the canal, large abscess causing respiratory embarrassment, and no response to medical therapy.

Poor prognostic factors include neurological deficit of more than 1 year duration, myelopathic changes in the cord, poor compliance, drug resistance, and increased pretreatment kyphotic angle. Newer techniques such as sensory- and motor-evoked potentials are being studied as a prognostic marker of outcomes of Pott's paraplegia [105].

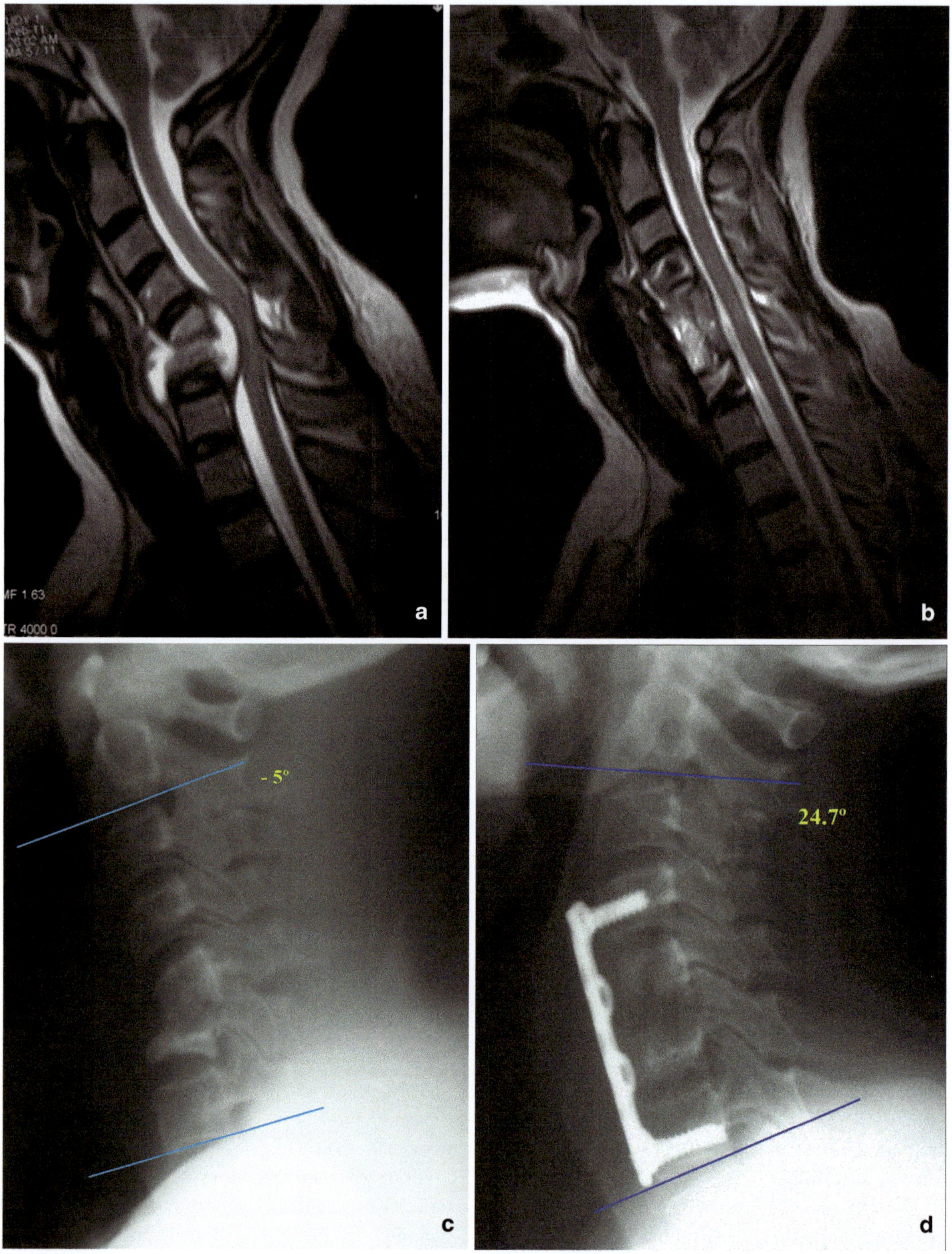

Fig. 37.1 A 30-year-old female with cervical spine tuberculosis (TB) treated by surgical decompression and fixation: (**a**) preoperative sagittal T2-WI magnetic resonance imaging (MRI) showed destruction of C5-C6 vertebral bodies with epidural collecting pus compressing the cord at that level. (**b**) Postoperative sagittal T2-WI MRI showed complete evacuation of the abscess and decompression of neural structures. (**c**) X-ray of the same patient preoperatively showing destruction of the C5-C6 vertebra with significant kyphotic angle of −5°. (**d**) Postoperative X-ray showed correction to a normal lordotic angle of 25° and good iliac crest autograft and fixation system

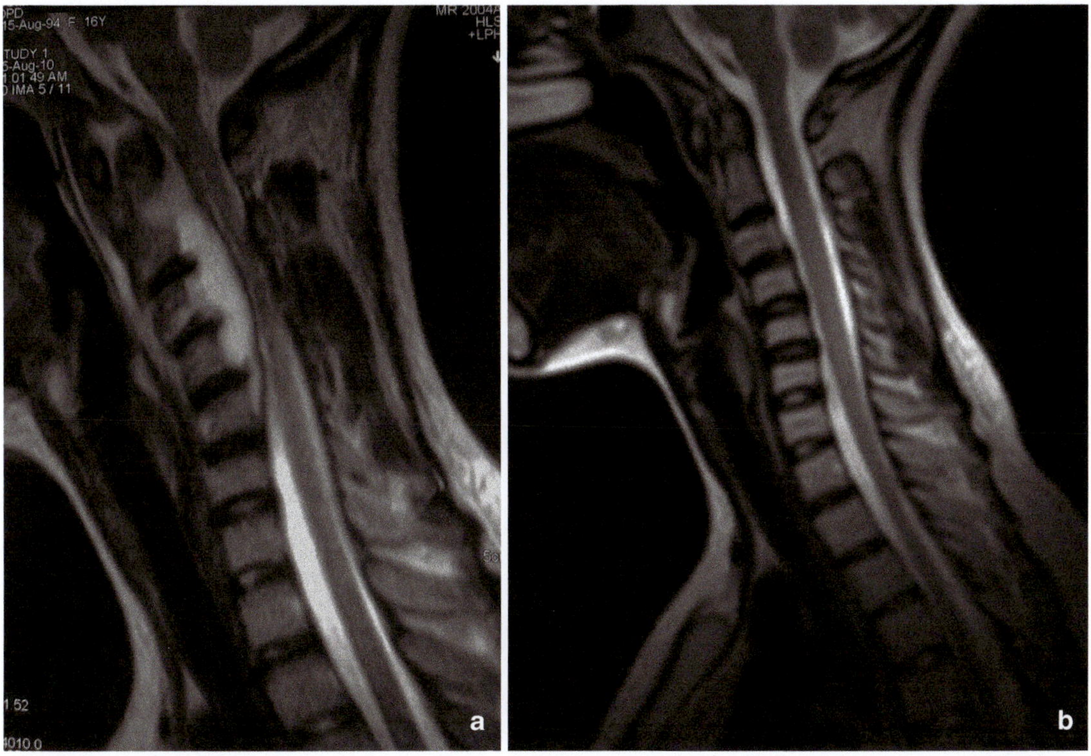

Fig. 37.2 A 16-year-old female patient treated conservatively with medical treatment only: (**a**) sagittal T2-WI MRI at first visit showing epidural abscess collection extending from C3 to C5 cervical vertebrae compressing the spinal cord at that level. (**b**) Sagittal T2-WI MRI at 1-year follow-up after medical treatment showing complete resolution of the epidural abscess with mild spastic kyphosis

Conclusion

Outcome of CNS-TB varies significantly among patients affected. Many significant factors affect the prognosis. Presenting clinical condition and response to medical treatment constitute the main influencing factors. Understanding the pathogenesis of the disease and the factors affecting it can help in the initial management and final outcome of this aggressive disorder. Many studies are still taking place to find a replacement for those patients with resistance to anti-TB treatment which significantly affects the prognosis.

References

1. WHO Report 2008 (2008) Global tuberculosis control-surveillance, planning, financing. World Health Organization, Geneva, pp 1–294
2. Prabhakar S, Thussu A (1997) CNS Tuberculosis. J Neurol India 45:132–140
3. Shanhar P, Manjunath N, Mohan KK (1991) Rapid diagnosis of tuberculous meningitis by polymerase chain reaction. Lancet i:5–7
4. Giris NI, Sultan Y, Farid Z (1998) Tuberculosis meningitis, Abbassia Fever Hospital-Naval Medical Research Unit No. 3-Cairo, Egypt, from 1976 to 1996. Am J Trop Med Hyg J 58:28–34
5. Jacobs RF, Starke JR (2003) Mycobacterium tuberculosis. In: Long SS, Pickering LK, Prober CG (eds) Principles and practice of pediatric infectious diseases. Churchill Livingstone, New York, pp 697–698
6. Rebecca W, Zafar Q, David S (1993) Cervical tuberculous vertebral osteomyelitis: case report and discussion of the literature. Clin Infect Dis 16:806–808
7. Harries A, Maher D, Graham S (2004) 2nd edn. TB/HIV 2nd edition, World Health Organization, pp 1–210
8. Kaufmann SH, McMichael AJ (2005) Annulling a dangerous liaison: vaccination strategies against AIDS and tuberculosis. Nat Med 11:33–44
9. Daley CL, Small PM, Schecter GF (1992) An outbreak of tuberculosis with accelerated progression among persons infected with the human immunodeficiency

virus. An analysis using restriction-fragment-length polymorphisms. N Engl J Med 326:231–235
10. Selwyn PA, Hartel D, Lewis VA (1989) A prospective study of the risk of tuberculosis among intravenous drug users with human immunodeficiency virus infection. N Engl J Med 320:545–550
11. Stead WW (1967) Pathogenesis of a first episode of chronic pulmonary tuberculosis in man: recrudescence of residuals of the primary infection or exogenous reinfection? Am Rev Respir Dis 95:729–745
12. Farer LS, Lowell AM, Meador MP (1979) Extrapulmonary tuberculosis in the United States. Am J Epidemiol 109:205–217
13. Yaramis AF, Gurkan M, Elevli M (1998) Central nervous system tuberculosis in children: a review of 214 cases. Pediatrics 102:E49
14. Bidstrup C, Andersen PH, Skinhoj P (2002) Tuberculous meningitis in a country with a low incidence of tuberculosis: still a serious disease and a diagnostic challenge. Scand J Infect Dis 34:811–814
15. Phypers M, Harris T, Power C (2006) CNS tuberculosis: a longitudinal analysis of epidemiological and clinical features. Int J Tuberc Lung Dis 10:99–103
16. Chambers T, Hendrickse W, Record C (1984) Paradoxical expansion of intracranial tuberculomas during chemotherapy. Lancet 2:181–183
17. Hejazi N, Hassler W (1997) Multiple intracranial tuberculomas with atypical response to tuberculostatic chemotherapy: literature review and a case report. Acta Neurochir 139:194–202
18. Yamamoto N, Kadoya S, Nakamura T (1985) A case report of intracerebral tuberculoma during anti-TB therapy (abstract). No Shinkei Geka 13:1007–1011
19. Thonell L, Pendle S, Stacks L (2000) Clinical and radiological features of South African patients with tuberculomas of the brain. Clin Infect Dis 31:619–620
20. Bas NS, Güzey K, Emel E (2005) Paradoxical intracranial tuberculoma requiring surgical treatment. Pediatr Neurosurg 41:201–205
21. Teoh R, Humphries MJ, O'Mahony G (1987) Symptomatic intracranial tuberculoma developing during treatment of tuberculosis: a report of 10 patients and review of the literature. J Med 63:449–460
22. Smith H (1987) Paradoxical responses during the chemotherapy of tuberculosis. J Infect 15:1–3
23. Kumar R, Pandey CK, Bose N (2002) Tuberculous brain abscess: clinical presentation, pathophysiology and treatment (in children). Childs Nerv Syst 18:118–123
24. Whitener DR (1978) Tuberculous brain abscess. Report of a case and review of the literature. Arch Neurol 35:148–155
25. Sutlas PN, Unal A, Forta H (2003) Tuberculous meningitis in adults: review of 61 cases. Infection 31:387–391
26. Thwaites GE, Bang ND, Dung NH (2005) The influence of HIV infection on clinical presentation, response to treatment, and outcome in adults with tuberculous meningitis. J Infect Dis 192:2134–2141
27. Farinha NJ, Razali A, Holzel H (2000) Tuberculosis of the central nervous system in children: a 20-year survey. J Infect 41:61–68
28. Medical Research Council, Streptomycin in Tuberculosis Trials Committee (1948) Streptomycin treatment of tuberculous meningitis. Lancet 1948:582–596
29. American Thoracic Society, Center for Disease Control and Prevention, and Infectious Diseases Society of America (2003) Treatment of tuberculosis. MMWR Recom Rep 52:1–77
30. Goel A, Pandya SK, Satoskar AR (1990) Whither short-course chemotherapy for tuberculous meningitis? Neurosurgery 27:418–421
31. Donald PR, Schoeman JF, Van Zyl LE (1998) Intensive short course chemotherapy in the management of tuberculous meningitis. Int J Tuberc Lung Dis 2:704–711
32. Jacobs RF, Sunakorn P, Chotpitayasunonah T (1992) Intensive short course chemotherapy for tuberculous meningitis. Pediatr Infect Dis J 11:194–198
33. Phuapradit P, Vejjajiva A (1987) Treatment of tuberculous meningitis: role of short-course chemotherapy. Q J Med 62:249–258
34. VanLoenhout-Rooyackers JH, Keyser A, Laheij RJ (2001) Tuberculous meningitis: is a 6-month treatment regimen sufficient? Int J Tuberc Lung Dis 5:1028–1035
35. Ellard GA, Humphries MJ, Allen BW (1993) Cerebrospinal fluid drug concentrations and the treatment of tuberculous meningitis. Am Rev Respir Dis 148:650–655
36. Ellard G, Humphries M, Gabriel M (1987) Penetration of pyrazinamide into the cerebrospinal fluid in tuberculous meningitis. Br Med J Clin Res Ed 294:284–285
37. Kaojarern S, Supmonchai K, Phuapradit P (1991) Effect of steroids on cerebrospinal fluid penetration of anti-tuberculous drugs in tuberculous meningitis. Clin Pharmacol Ther 49:6–12
38. Phuapradit P, Supmonchai K, Kaojarern S (1990) The blood/cerebrospinal fluid partitioning of pyrazinamide: a study during the course of treatment of tuberculous meningitis. J Neurol Neurosurg Psychiatry 53:81–82
39. Balasubramanian R, Ramachandran R (2000) Management of non-pulmonary forms of tuberculosis: review of TRC studies over two decades. Indian J Pediatr 67:S34–S40
40. Leonard J, Des Prez R (1990) Tuberculous meningitis. Infect Dis Clin North Am 4:769–787
41. Bernaerts A, Vanhoenacker FM, Parizel PM (2003) Tuberculosis of the central nervous system: overview of neuroradiological findings. Eur Radiol 13:1876–1890
42. Brooks J, Daneshvar M, Haberberger R (1990) Rapid diagnosis of tuberculous meningitis by

frequency-pulsed electron-capture gas-liquid chromatography detection of carboxylic acids in cerebrospinal fluid. J Clin Microbiol 28:989–997
43. Marshall G, Blacklock JS, Cameron C (1948) Streptomycin treatment of tuberculous meningitis. Lancet 17:582–596
44. Fernando A, Moreira J, Rivera J (2012) Tuberculous meningitis: do modern diagnostic tools offer better prognosis prediction? Indian J Tuberc 60:5–14
45. Lu CH, Chang WN, Chang HW (2001) The prognostic factors of adult tuberculous meningitis. Infection 29:299–304
46. Hsu P-C, Yang C-C, Ye J-J (2010) Prognostic factors of tuberculous meningitis in adults: a 6-year retrospective study at a tertiary hospital in Northern Taiwan. J Microbiol Immunol Infect 43:111–118
47. Alarcon F, Escalante L, Perez Y (1990) Tuberculous meningitis. Short course of chemotherapy. Arch Neurol 47:1313–1317
48. Karstaedt AS, Valtchanova S, Barriere R (1998) Tuberculous meningitis in South African urban adults. QJM 91:743–747
49. Misra U, Kalita J, Srivastava M, Mandal S (1996) Prognosis of tuberculous meningitis: a multivariate analysis. J Neurol Sci 137:57–61
50. Porkert MT, Sotir M, Parrott-Moore P (1997) Tuberculous meningitis at a large inner-city medical center. Am J Med Sci 313:325–331
51. Verdon R, Chevret S, Laissy JP (1996) Tuberculous meningitis in adults: review of 48 cases. Clin Infect Dis 22:982–988
52. Hosoglu S, Ayaz C, Geyik MF (1998) Tuberculous meningitis in adults: an eleven-year review. Int J Tuberc Lung Dis 2:553–557
53. Pehlivanoglu F, Yasar KK (2010) Prognostic factors of neurological sequel in adult patients with tuberculous meningitis. Neurosciences 15:262–267
54. Goel A (2004) Tuberculous meningitis and hydrocephalus. Neurol India 52:155
55. Sil K, Chatterjee S (2008) Shunting in tuberculous meningitis: a neurosurgeon's nightmare. Childs Nerv Syst 24:1029–1032
56. Palur R, Rajshekhar V, Chandy MJ (1991) Shunt surgery for hydrocephalus–9.in tuberculous meningitis: a long-term follow-up study. J Neurosurg 74:64
57. Agrawal D, Gupta A, Mehta V (2005) Role of shunt surgery in pediatric tubercular meningitis with hydrocephalus. Indian Pediatr 42:245–250
58. Lamprecht D, Schoeman J, Donald P (2001) Ventriculo-peritoneal shunting in childhood tuberculous meningitis. Br J Neurosurg 15:119–125
59. Husain M, Jha DK, Rastogi M (2005) Role of neuroendoscopy in the management of patients with tuberculous meningitis hydrocephalus. Neurosurg Rev 28:278–283
60. Yadav YR, Jaiswal S, Adam N, Basoo A (2006) Endoscopic third ventriculostomy in infants. Neurol India 54:161–163
61. Thwaites GE, Nguyen DB, Nguyen HD (2004) Dexamethasone for the treatment of tuberculous meningitis in adolescents and adults. N Engl J Med 351:1741–1751
62. Thwaites GE, Tran TH (2005) Tuberculous meningitis: many questions, too few answers. Lancet Neurol 4:160–170
63. Thwaites GE, Macmullen-Price J, Tran TH (2007) Serial MRI to determine the effect of dexamethasone on the cerebral pathology of tuberculous meningitis: an observational study. Lancet Neurol 6:230–236
64. Schoeman JF, Van Zyl LE, Laubscher JA (1997) Effect of corticosteroids on intracranial pressure, computed tomographic findings, and clinical outcome in young children with tuberculous meningitis. Pediatrics 99:226–231
65. Wang JT, Hung CC, Sheng WH (2002) Prognosis of tuberculous meningitis in adults in the era of modern antituberculous chemotherapy. J Microbiol Immunol Infect 35:215–222
66. Andronikou S, Wilmshurst J, Hatherill M (2006) Distribution of brain infarction in children with tuberculous meningitis and correlation with outcome score at 6 months. Pediatr Radiol 36:1289–1294
67. Sonmez G, Ozturk E, Sildiroglu H (2008) MRI findings of intracranial tuberculomas. Clin Imaging 32:88–92
68. Central TB Division, DGHS, Ministry of Health & Family Welfare, Govt. of India (1997). RNTCP technical guidelines for tuberculosis control. Revised National Tuberculosis Control Programme 2:14–22
69. Freiman I, Geefhuysen J (1970) Evaluation of intrathecal therapy with streptomycin and hydrocortisone in tuberculous meningitis. J Pediatr 76:895–901
70. Smith AL (1975) Tuberculous meningitis in childhood. Med J Aust 1:57–60
71. Andronikou S, Wieselthaler N, Smith B (2005) Value of early follow-up CT in pediatric tuberculous meningitis. Pediatr Radiol 35:1092–1099
72. Karande S, Gupta V, Kulkarni M (2005) Prognostic clinical variables in childhood tuberculous meningitis: an experience from Mumbai, India. Neurol India 53:191–196
73. Thilothammal N, Krishnamurthy PV, Banu K (1995) Tuberculous meningitis in children – clinical profile, mortality and morbidity of bacteriologically confirmed cases. Indian Pediatr 32:641–647
74. Starke JR (1992) Current chemotherapy for tuberculosis in children. Infect Dis Clin North Am 6:215–238
75. American Thoracic Society (1994) Treatment of tuberculosis and tuberculosis infection in adults and children. Am J Respir Crit Care Med 149: 1359–1374
76. Patel AN, McKeon J (1995) Avoidance and management of adverse reactions to anti-tuberculosis drugs. Drug Saf 12:1–25

77. Obrien RJ (1991) Hepatoxic reaction to antituberculous drugs: adjustments to therapeutic regimen. JAMA 265:3323
78. Patel V, Padayatchi A, Bhigjee J (2004) Multidrug-resistant tuberculous meningitis in KwaZulu-Natal, South Africa. Clin Infect Dis 38:851–856
79. Padayatchi N, Bamber S, Dawood H (2006) Multidrug-resistant tuberculous meningitis in children in Durban, South Africa. Pediatr Infect Dis J 25:147–150
80. Chander B, Vidyanidhi G, Manisha J (2008) Multi drug resistant tuberculous meningitis in pediatric age group. Iran J Pediatr 18:309–314
81. Venkataswamy MM, Rafi W, Nagarathna S (2007) Comparative evaluation of Bactec 460tb system and Lowenstein-Jensen medium for the isolation of M. tuberculosis from cerebrospinal fluid samples of Tuberculous meningitis patients. Indian J Med Microbiol 25:236–240
82. Wells CD, Cegielski JP, Nelson LJ (2007) HIV infection and multi-drug resistant tuberculosis; the perfect storm. J Infect Dis 196:86–107
83. Gandhi NR, Moll A, Sturm AW (2006) Extensively drug-resistant tuberculosis as a cause of death in patients co-infected with tuberculosis and HIV in a rural area of south Africa. Lancet 368:1575–1580
84. Sofia M, Maniscalco M, Honore N (2001) Familial outbreak of disseminated multidrug resistant tuberculosis and meningitis. Int J Tuberc Lung Dis 5:551–558
85. Pietersen E, Ignatius E, Streicher EM (2014) Long-term outcomes of patients with extensively drug-resistant tuberculosis in South Africa: a cohort study. Lancet 5:1230–1239
86. Dubé P, Holtom D, Larsen A (1992) Tuberculous meningitis in patients with and without human immunodeficiency virus Infection. Am J Med 93:520–524
87. Mutasem A, Bo X, Yan C (2008) Central nervous system tuberculomas: a review article. Am J Infect Dis 4:168–173
88. Martinez-Vazquez C, Bordon J, Rodriguez-Gonzalez A (1995) Cerebral tuberculoma: a comparative study in patients with and without HIV infection. Infection 23:149–153
89. Zavascki AP, Dias AE, Cruz RP (2006) Intracranial tuberculomas in an immunocompetent patient mimicking brain metastasis of unknown origin. Infection 34:181–182
90. Rajsekhar V, Chandy M (1993) CT-guided stereotactic surgery in the management of intracranial tuberculomas. Br J Neurosurg 7:665–671
91. Arseni C, Samitca DC (1960) Intraspinal tuberculous granuloma. Brain 83:285–292
92. Ohaegbulam SC (1977) spinal extras osseous extradural tuberculoma. Tubercle 58:97–99
93. Slade HW, Glazer N (1955) Extramedullary spinal tuberculoma, report a case with unusual clinical and laboratory findings. J Pediatri 46:288
94. Compron JS, Dorsch NWC (1984) Intradural-extramedullary tuberculoma of the cervical spine. Case report. J Neurosurg 60:200–203
95. Dastur HM, Shah MD (1968) Intramedullary tuberculoma of the spinal cord. Indian Pediatr 5:468–471
96. Li H, Liu W, You C (2012) Central nervous system tuberculoma. J Clin Neurosci 19:691–695
97. Turgut M, Ozcan OE, Ozgen T (1993) Intradural extramedullary tuberculoma of the spinal cord – a case report. Zentralbl Neurochir 54:197–199
98. Dechamenoit G, Boni NG, Santini JJ (1993) Tuberculous abscess of the cerebellum. Neurochirurgia 39:326–329
99. Vidal JE, de Penalva o AC, Bonasser F (2005) Tuberculous brain abscess in AIDS patients: report of three cases and literature review. Int J Infect Dis 9:201–207
100. Ramani PS, Sharma A, Jituri S (2005) Anterior instrumentation for cervical spine tuberculosis: an analysis of surgical experience with 61 cases. Neurol India 53:83–89
101. Flamm ES (1992) Percivall Pott: an 18th century neurosurgeon. J Neurosurg 76:319–326
102. Omari B, Robertsopn JM, Nelson RJ (1989) Pott's disease, a resurgent challenge to the thoracic surgeon. Chest 95:145–150
103. Ozbarlas S, Gulsen H, Erdem M (2014) Surgical treatment of Pott's disease. Turk J Bone Joint A Surg 1:35–38
104. Rezai AR, Lee M, Cooper MR (1995) Modern management of spinal tuberculosis. Neurosurgery 36:87–97
105. Misra UK, Kalita J (2004) The role of sensory and motor evoked potentials in the prognosis of Pott's paraplegia. Clin Neurophysiol 115:2267–2273

Part VII

Tuberculosis in Humans

An Overview of Tuberculosis: What You Need to Know

38

Kristina Galic

Contents

K. Galic, MD
Department of Lung Diseases, University Clinical Hospital Mostar, School of Medicine,
University of Mostar, Bijeli Brijeg bb, 88000 Mostar, Bosnia and Herzegovina
e-mail: kgkristinagalic@gmail.com

Abbreviations

AIDS	Acquired immunodeficiency syndrome
BAL	Bronchoalveolar lavage
CNS	Central nervous system
CXR	Chest X-ray
DOTS	Directly observed therapy short course
DST	Drug susceptibility testing
EMB	Ethambutol
FDC	Fixed drug combination
HIV	Human immunodeficiency virus
ICD	International Classification of Diseases
IFN-γ	Interferon gamma
INH	Isoniazid
LJ	Löwenstein Jensen
MDG	Millenium Development Goals
MDR-TB	Multidrug resistant-tuberculosis
MGIT	Mycobacterial growth inhibitor tubes
PCR	Polymerase chain reaction
RIF	Rifampicin
RR-TB	Rifampicin resistant-tuberculosis
STAG-TB	The Strategy Technical Advisory Group Tuberculosis
STR	Streptomycin
TB	Tuberculosis
TBB	Transbronchial biopsy
TDR-TB	Total drug resistant-tuberculosis

M. Turgut et al. (eds.), *Tuberculosis of the Central Nervous System*,
DOI 10.1007/978-3-319-50712-5_38

TNF	Tumor necrosis factor
VR	Vital registration
WHA	World Health Assembly
WHO	World Health Organization
XDR-TB	Extensively drug resistant-tuberculosis
ZN	Ziehl-Neelsen

38.1 Introduction

Tuberculosis (TB) is an infectious disease caused by *Mycobacterium tuberculosis*. It can affect any organs, usually the lungs. Other strains of *Mycobacterium*, such as *M. bovis* and *M. africanum*, are exceptionally appearing as pathogens in Europe.

TB is transmitted among people through the air. The source of infection is human, from persons who have pulmonary TB or TB of the larynx. Other clinical forms of TB are not contagious. Patients with pulmonary TB are contagious if, when they cough, there are up to 10,000 bacilli in 1 ml of sputum. When patients with pulmonary TB cough, sneeze or spit, they expel germs into the air. For infection to occur, only a few of these germs need to be inhaled.

The risk of infection in a person living in close contact with a diseased person is 30%. Health care professionals who work with patients with TB and employees of microbiological laboratories that diagnose TB are at greater risk. The incubation period lasts 4–12 weeks, from infection to the presence of radiopaque lesions on the lung. Infection usually remains latent and can persist for a lifetime. Only about 3% of infected people develop the disease within 3 years. Progression of infection to the disease is significantly higher in immunocompromised patients, such as those with acquired immunodeficiency syndrome (AIDS), cancers and diabetes mellitus. One-third of the world's population has latent TB; that is, people who have been infected by *M. tuberculosis* but do not yet have the disease and cannot transmit it.

In active TB disease, the symptoms (e.g., fever, night sweats, cough, weight loss) may be mild for a long time. This can lead to failure in seeking care and results in further transmission of *M. tuberculosis*. Without adequate therapy, more than two-thirds of people with TB disease will die.

38.2 Epidemiology

TB was mentioned thousands of years ago as the most common infective disease. Hippocrates called TB "phthisis" and concluded that it is was the most widespread fatal disease of his time [1]. The period of greatest TB infection was in the nineteenth century, when it took the largest number of lives, often young.

Robert Koch, in 1882, discovered the cause of TB, a rod-shaped bacterium, *M. tuberculosis*. The major step in the fight against TB in the modern age was his lecture on Friday, March 24, 1882, in Berlin, where he described *M. tuberculosis*. His work was published on April 10, 1882, in the journal *Berliner Klinische Wochenschrift* and was translated into many world languages [2]. From that time, he began research on drugs to combat the disease. In the second half of the twentieth century TB treatment became successful, with several drugs used in combination, the control of patients' treatment, and long enough therapy. However, since the last two decades of the twentieth century, the incidence of TB cases has been growing again, and the disease has now returned, associated with the new disease, AIDS.

The big problem in TB treatment is a new form of the disease, multidrug resistant-tuberculosis (MDR-TB). TB is also more commonly associated with diseases such as diabetes, malignant disease, renal disease and congenital and acquired immunodeficiencies. The highest rates of TB are in Africa, Southeast Asia, and parts of South America. Developing countries, in contrast to industrialized countries, have a higher rate of the disease. Rising numbers of MDR-TB represent a major threat that is going out of control. Despite the measures taken by the World Health Organization (WHO), the infection is spreading rapidly. In 1993, the WHO declared TB a global emergency, concerned because of the extent of

TB as a problem in most developing countries [3, 4]. In the last two decades of the twentieth century, global strategies for TB control have been recommended for acceptance and adaptation in all countries. The phenomenon of MDR-TB forms of the disease led to the introduction of new measures in the therapy of TB; namely the directly observed therapy short course (DOTS) strategy [5].

38.2.1 Risk Factors for Developing Diseases

TB is a disease related to poverty, and this could explain its appearance in different population groups. Risk factors such as poverty, lack of food, financial problems, and difficult psychosocial circumstances are the major determinants of TB [6, 7]. Also, there are vulnerable groups, which include those with human immunodeficiency virus (HIV) infection, homeless people, migrants and refugees, alcohol abusers, and prisoners. Because of their increased risk these groups are more likely to develop active disease. In these patients TB may not be diagnosed, representing a danger for spreading infection in the community [8]. A common aggravating factor is the fear of stigmatization, which is an important reason for poor compliance with treatment. The most sensitive groups have to be identified in every region so that intervention aimed at the needs of difficult to reach groups can be implemented [9]. HIV/AIDS-positive patients have an extremely high risk of contracting TB. So, the HIV status of every newly diagnosed TB patient has to be checked, according to current recommendations. The percentage of TB patients who know their HIV status has increased in the past 10 years, reaching a peak of 46% in 2012 [10].

The world prison population is currently about 8–10 million people. The median incidence rate ratio for TB in inmates versus the general population was reported to be 23. Treatment that was not sufficiently long, and interrupted treatment, significantly increased the development and spread of MDR-TB, thus creating TB reservoirs, a factor that threatens the whole community, through prison officials, visitors, and former prisoners [11–13].

38.3 Directly Observed Therapy Short Course

Directly observed therapy short course (DOTS) was launched in 1994–1995. It was based on five crucial components: (1) political commitment with increased and continual financing, (2) case detection among people presenting with symptoms in clinics through quality-assured bacteriology, (3) standardized and supervised treatment along with patient support, (4) an effective drug supply and management system, and (5) a standard monitoring and evaluation system ("Framework-WHO, 1994, IUATLD, 1996") [14, 15].

To accelerate efforts and reach the international targets set in the context of the Millenium Development Goals (MDG), in 2006 the WHO launched an enhanced global strategy named the Stop TB Strategy. This new strategy aimed to ensure universal access to high-quality health services and patient-centered care for all individuals with TB, through additional efforts addressing the challenges emerging in the new century [16, 17].

The principles of DOTS were incorporated as the first component of the 2006 Stop TB Strategy, together with five additional components: (1) address TB/HIV, MDR-TB, and the needs of vulnerable populations, (2) contribute to health system strengthening based on primary health care, (3) engage all care providers, (4) empower TB patients and encourage community engagement and (5) enable and promote research [16].

The WHO extended the DOTS program in 1998 to include the treatment of MDR-TB (called "DOTS-Plus"). The scope of this plan was to address the MDG challenge and pursue the other international targets in order to halve the 1990 TB prevalence and mortality rate by 2015 and eliminate TB as a public health problem by 2050 (<1 case per 1 million population) [18]. Despite all these efforts and the resulting achievements described above, including the reaching of the TB-relevant target in the MDG, global control is progressing slowly, with a decline in incidence of 2% per year on average.

The new post-2015 Global TB Strategy approved by the 67th World Health Assembly in May 2014, aims at "ending the global TB epidemic" by 2035 This implies a reduction of mortality for 95% by decreasing incidence for 90% (<10 TB cases/100,000 population) to 2035 in comparison with 2015, and the suppression of any "catastrophic cost" for TB-affected families [19].

The most important aspect of treatment was the introduction and the routine use of new technologies for the quick detection of resistant strains and the development of special diagnostic algorithms, which were particularly useful for high-risk patients. Despite the implementation of these all measures, TB is still one of the world's biggest health problems.

38.4 TB Mortality

TB mortality among HIV-negative patients can be directly measured by using data from national Vital registration (VR) systems. VR systems have high coverage, and causes of death are accurately coded according to the newest revision of the International Classification of Diseases (ICD-10). For estimating TB deaths, mortality surveys can be used. Most countries with a high incidence of TB lacked national or sample VR systems in 2014, and few mortality surveys were done. In the absence of VR systems or mortality surveys, TB mortality can be estimated as a product of TB incidence and the case fatality rate, or it can be based on mortality data from countries with VR systems. TB deaths in HIV-positive people are difficult to estimate even when VR systems exist, because deaths among HIV-positive people are coded as HIV deaths, and contributory causes (such as TB) are mostly not recorded. Africa is the part of the world, where is the greatest need to introduce or implement VR systems where causes of death are classified according to the ICD system.

The fight against TB has resulted in a yearly death rate in 2013 of approximately half that in comparison with the rate in 1990. In 2014 1,510,000 people were killed by TB (1.1 million HIV-negative and 0.4 million HIV-positive), among them 890,000 men, 480,000 women, and 140,000 children [19]. Worldwide, TB ranks alongside HIV as a one of the leading causes of death. In 2014 there were 1.2 million deaths from HIV, including 0.4 million TB deaths among HIV-positive people.

38.5 Immunopathogenesis of TB Disease

The development of an infection by *M. tuberculosis* depends on the initial relationship between the pathogen and the host cell, most often the macrophage. The surface characteristics of both entities will strongly affect the outcome. Mycobacteria are gram-positive, but their wax-rich cell walls confer on them unique features. Because of this, they are classified as acid-fast bacilli. *M. tuberculosis* is capable of binding to a variety of host cell receptors, including Fc receptors and complement receptors (both with or without prior opsonization), the macrophage mannose receptor, surfactant protein receptors, and CD14. Having gained entry into the macrophage with its variety of its surface molecules, *M. tuberculosis* faces the problem of establishing residence inside a primary host effector cell. The manipulation of the nutritional requirements of *M. tuberculosis*, coupled with the immune status of the host, dramatically alters the course of infection and could open up potential avenues for therapeutic intervention [20].

Although interferon-gamma (IFN-γ) is a major cytokine involved in the control of *M. tuberculosis* infection, many others cytokines, such as interleukin 12 (IL-12) and tumor necrosis factor (TNF), participate in the activation of the immunological system. TNF can synergize with IFN-γ to activate macrophages. TNF is also the cytokine most responsible for organizing granulomas. However, as with many infections, the synthesis of TNF must be precise, as too much synthesis leads to increased cellular accumulation, and to compromised lung function and damaged tissue.

CD4+ T cells are important in the host defence. The importance of this T-cell subset in controlling acute mycobacterial infections has long been proposed. Despite the intraphagosomal location of mycobacteria, it is known that CD8+ T cells have an important role in the successful immune response to the organism. A better understanding of the relationship between *M. tuberculosis* and its host will ensure very important new guidelines for the fight against this disease, which is still of major importance [21].

38.6 Clinical Course

Clinically, TB has a wide range of symptoms. The disease can affect any organ system; however, it usually affects the lungs (60–80%). Extrapulmonary TB is present in 20% of cases, of which 13% are specific pleuritis and 1–4% specific lymphadenitis, while sporadic central nervous system (CNS), genitourinary, osteoarticular, and intestinal TB are also observed. In HIV-positive patients the clinical presentation is atypical and extrapulmonary TB is present in up to two-thirds of patients.

According to sputum positivity, localization of the disease, drug resistance, and recurrence or relapse of the disease, the WHO recommended the following definitions of TB cases [22] (for use since March 2013):

Bacteriologically confirmed case of TB: "*A patient from whom a biological specimen is positive by smear microscopy, culture or WHO-approved rapid diagnostic test (such as Xpert Mycobacterium tuberculosis/RIF). All such cases should be notified, regardless of whether TB treatment is started.*"

Clinically diagnosed case of TB: "*A patient who does not fulfil the criteria for bacteriologically confirmed TB but has been diagnosed with active TB by a clinician or other medical practitioner who has decided to give the patient a full course of TB treatment.*"

Case of pulmonary TB: "*Any bacteriologically confirmed or clinically diagnosed case of TB involving the lung parenchyma or the tracheobronchial tree. Miliary TB is classified as pulmonary TB because there are lesions in the lungs. TB intra-thoracic lymphadenopathy (mediastinal and/or hilar) or TB pleural effusion, without radiographic abnormalities in the lungs, constitutes a case of extrapulmonary TB. A patient with both pulmonary and extrapulmonary TB should be classified as a case of pulmonary TB.*"

Case of extrapulmonary TB: "*Any bacteriologically confirmed or clinically diagnosed case of TB involving organs other than the lungs, e.g. abdomen, genitourinary tract, joints and bones, lymph nodes, meninges, pleura, skin.*"

New case of TB: "*A patient who has never been treated for TB or has taken anti-TB drugs for less than one month.*"

Retreatment cases of TB: "*A patient who has been treated for 1 month or more with anti-TB drugs in the past. Retreatment cases are further classified by the outcome of their most recent course of treatment into four categories. Relapse patients have previously been treated for TB, were declared cured or treatment completed at the end of their most recent course of treatment, and are now diagnosed with a recurrent episode of TB (either treatment).*"

Treatment after loss to follow-up patients: "*They have previously been treated for TB and were declared 'lost to follow-up' at the end of their most recent course of treatment.* "

Case of multidrug resistant-tuberculosis (MDR-TB): "*TB that is resistant to two first-line drugs: isoniazid (INH) and rifampicin (RIF).*"

Case of RIF resistant-tuberculosis (RR-TB): "*A patient with TB that is resistant to RIF detected using phenotypic or genotypic methods, with or without resistance to other anti-TB drugs.*"

Treatment after failure: "*The patients have previously been treated for TB and their most recent course of treatment failed i.e. they had a positive sputum smear or culture result at month 5 or later during treatment.*"

38.7 Diagnostic Tests in Tuberculosis

38.7.1 Screening Test

The WHO has developed guidelines on TB screening, according to The Strategic and Technical Advisory Group TB (STAG-TB) [23]. Screening is defined as: "*the presumptive identification of unrecognized disease or defect by the application of tests, examinations, or other procedures which can be applied rapidly.*" Screening tests distinguish well persons who probably have a disease from persons who have not. Screening tests are not diagnostic. Persons with a positive or suspected positive result must visit their doctors for diagnosis and, eventually, therapy [24].

There are two key goals of systematic screening for active disease: (1) thorough early detection and therapy achieve a better outcome for patients suffering from TB and (2) by shortening the duration of TB infectiousness, the incidence and transmission of TB is significantly decreased [25].

Persons whose are positive at screening should be subjected to confirmatory testing to establish a TB diagnosis, with any reference tests or new tests that are available. Persons whose are negative at screening would not be tested with any confirmatory tests.

38.7.2 Index Tests

Chest X-ray (CXR) as a screening test means one posterior-anterior CXR recording. There are three different types of recording: conventional CXR (producing a 36 × 43 cm film), digital, and mass miniature radiography [26]. CXR classification systems can distinguish any abnormality versus a normal recording. Among abnormal CXRs only abnormalities suspicious of TB would qualify as a positive screening result [27]. Sequential (or serial) screening has two steps. In the first step persons are screened for symptoms, and CXR screening, as a second step, is performed only for symptom positive persons. Parallel screening means both screening steps are available, and persons having symptoms and/or abnormalities on chest X-ray have conditions that suggest a further diagnostic test. For example, this is practiced in TB prevalence studies, in order to ensure that the sensitivity is as high as possible. Parallel screening also avoids the need for laboratory diagnostics to be performed in all respondents [28].

38.7.3 Reference Tests

Tests with high specificity, considering mycobacterial culture and mycobacterium speciation, are the reference tests for bacteriologically confirmed TB. Cultures on liquid medium are the most sensitive. Before the automated reading of mycobacterial growth inhibitor tubes (MGIT) culture was available, culture on solid medium Löwenstein Jensen (LJ) was the basis of culture tests, and can still be the only available test in settings with limited resources. MGIT culture increases the recovery of mycobacteria by 11–18% compared with LJ culture, but MGIT culture can have lower specificity because of higher contamination rates [29, 30]. The Ziehl-Neelsen (ZN) method shows a wide variation of sensitivity, between 50% and 70% in most studies [31]. Direct ZN microscopy has a specificity of 98%. In comparison with culture, the sensitivity of the nucleic acid amplification test Xpert MTB/RIF test is 92%, and specificity is 99% in smear-positive and smear-negative patients [32]. Serological tests are not recommended as diagnostic tests in TB [33]. Before choosing the best diagnostic algorithm, the TB prevalence, test availability, and logistic conditions should be considered (e.g., X-ray or Xpert *Mycobacterium tuberculosis*/RIF availability). A systematic review to determine screening tests in HIV-infected persons has been published recently. Due to the increase in the prevalence of TB and its close association with

AIDS, there has been research into new methods for quickly discovering TB in clinical samples, new systems for culture and sensitivity testing TB, and amplification methods, polymerase chain reaction (PCR). Rapid tests such as PCR confirmed the diagnosis of TB in 1–2 days, while current substrates AST-streptomycin (STR), INH, RIF, etambutol (EMB) (SIRE) confirmed the diagnosis in 7–10 days [34].

38.8 Radiological Diagnosis of TB

Given the most common sites of pulmonary TB, X-ray and computed tomography of the heart and lungs is a basic diagnostic method for the detection of pulmonary TB. The primary infection shows infiltrative lesions in the parenchyma of the middle and lower lung fields, with regional lymphadenitis (which occurs most commonly 3 months after infection) and calcified-primary complex or Ghon's complex.

38.8.1 Postprimary Infection

There are three basic radiological signs of postprimary pulmonary TB: ulcers, caverns, and fibrosis. Radiologically, these signs manifest as multiple infiltrates with areas of destruction in the typical radiological images of caverns (Fig. 38.1).

Hematogenous dispersion of TB leads to radiological signs of miliary TB and hematogenous dissemination to other organ systems (e.g., CNS, bones and kidneys) (Fig. 38.2).

Radiologically visible pleural effusion, with or without signs of destruction of lung parenchyma, is the second most common radiological sign of TB. A special entity is tuberculoma a solitary peripheral nodule that is usually peripherally linked to a pleura.

Late radiological manifestations of TB in the lung generally represent its complications, and they include aspergilloma, arterial pseudoaneurysms, bronchiectasis, bronchial artery pseudoaneurysm, bronchopleural fistula, pulmonary artery pseudoaneurysm/Rasmussen aneurysm, empyema and fibrothorax.

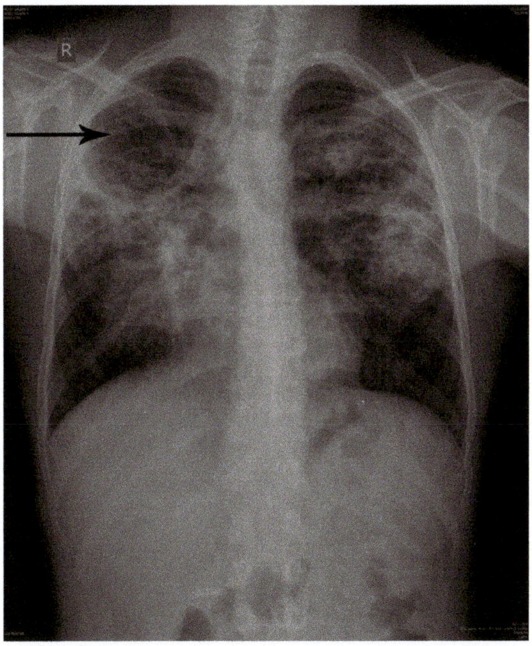

Fig. 38.1 Massive pulmonary tuberculosis (TB) with bronchogenic dissemination shows multiple infiltrates with areas of destruction in the typical radiological images of caverns on both sides of the lung

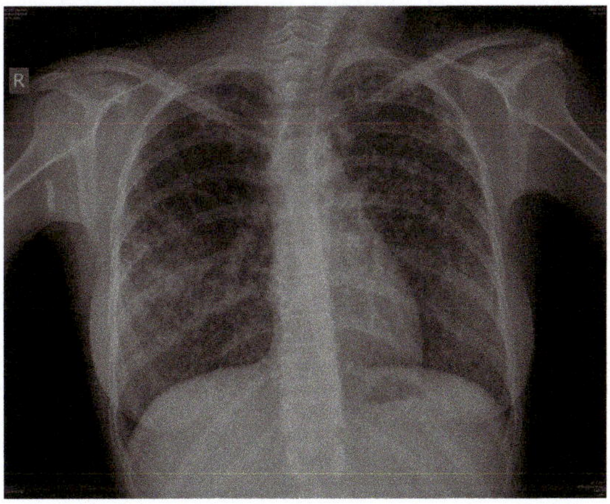

Fig. 38.2 Miliary pulmonary TB shows diffuse micronodular lesions (like grains of millet in the lung parenchyma)

38.8.2 Bronchoscopy as a Diagnostic Test for Tuberculosis

Bronchosopy is a very important diagnostic method in patients with clinical or radiological suspicion of TB who are not able to produce sputum, or those patients with negative sputum smear microscopy results. In some studies, bronchoalveolar lavage (BAL) showed a sensitivity of 60% and a specificity of 100%. Bronchoscopy is a credible method for the diagnosis of pulmonary TB, with a low incidence of complications. The combination of transbronchial biopsy (TBB) and BAL increases the sensitivity of this method and clarifies the differential diagnosis with other diseases [35].

38.9 Anti-Tuberculosis Drugs

Global TB control has achieved the greatest success with the implementation of the DOTS strategy worldwide. The essential first-line anti-TB drugs include INH, RIF, EMB, pyrazinamide and STR. Second-line anti-TB drugs include aminoglycosides (kanamycin, amikacin), quinolones (ciprofloxacin, ofloxacin, levofloxacin), ethionamide or prothionamide, cycloserine, para-aminosalicylic acid and a polypeptide (capreomycin).

The WHO recommends the use of a fixed dose combination of anti-TB drugs, although these combinations have not been systematically evaluated [35]. The doses of the first and second-line anti-TB drugs are presented in Tables 38.1a and 38.1b.

The second-line anti-TB drugs are useful for treating disease that is resistant to first-line treatment (i.e., MDR–TB).

An initial phase treatment with a combination of several first-line anti-TB drugs serves to take care of the drug-resistant organisms and to provide "a quick kill" to decrease the bacillary load. As the final, that results in decreased the number of "persisters" in the focus.

For those TB patients with known positive HIV status and for all TB patients living in HIV prevalent settings, daily TB treatment, at least during the intensive phase and also during the continuation phase, is recommended.

While standard anti-TB therapy needs to be used for all new TB cases, when retreatment is required for relapse, starting with first-line therapy and drug susceptibility testing (DST) is recommended. If DST is not applicable and the patient has had a good clinical and radiological response for 2–3 months of therapy, or if DST confirms that there is no resistant disease, first-line therapy could be continued and given for 7 months [36]. When fully supervised first-line therapy fails, or if DST shows that a patient has MDR-TB, then second-line drugs have to be included for this patient. If patients do not respond on MDR treatment or they show extensively drug resistant tuberculosis (XDR-TB) on DST, they need to be treated with salvage regimens.

Third-line drugs may be useful, but they have doubtful or non-proven efficacy. The third line anti-TB drugs are rifabutin, macrolides, linezolid, thioacetazone, thioridazine, arginine, vitamin D and bedaquiline. These drugs, apart from

Table 38.1a Anti-TB drugs (first line) and their recommended doses for adults

	Recommended dose			
	Daily		3 times per week	
Drug	Dose and drug (mg/kg body weight)	Maximum (mg)	Dose and drug (mg/kg body weight)	Daily maximum (mg)
Isoniazid	5 (4–6)	300	10 (8–12)	900
Rifampicin	10 (8–12)	600	10 (8–12)	600
Pyrazinamide	25 (20–30)	–	35 (30–40)	–
Ethambutol	15 (15–20)	–	30 (25–35)	–
Streptomycin	15 (12–18)		15 (12–18)	1000

Notes: (1) Patients over 60 years old may not be able to tolerate more than 500–750 mg daily, so some guidelines recommend reduction of the dose to 10 mg/kg per day in these patients. (2) Patients weighing less than 50 kg may not tolerate doses above 500–750 mg daily (*WHO Model Formulary 2008*, www.who.int/selection_medicines/list/en/)

Table 38.1b Second-line anti-TB drugs and their recommended doses for adults

Drugs	Daily dose (mg/kg)	Route	Maximum daily dose
Kanamycin	15	IM	Up to 1 g
Amikacin	15	IM	Up to 1 g
Ethionamide	10–15	Oral	Up to 1 g
Cycloserine	10	Oral	Up to 1 g
Para-aminosalicylic acid	250	Oral	Up to 1 g
Ofloxacin	15–20	Oral	800–10,000 mg
Levofloxacin	7.5–10	Oral	750–1000 mg
Moxifloxacin	7.5–10	Oral	400 mg

IM intramuscular

rifabutin, are not very effective. Rifabutin is effective, but because of its high price, it is not on the WHO list for most developing regions.

38.10 Challenges in the Prevention and Treatment of Tuberculosis Today

Patients with MDR-TB are often unsuccessfully treated, with approximately 50% of MDR-TB patients worldwide being treated successfully. In 2015 the treatment success target of ≥75% with MDR-TB patients was achieved by 43 of the 127 countries and regions that investigated outcomes for the 2012 cohort, including three high-MDR-TB-burden countries (Estonia, Ethiopia, and Myanmar). Extensively drug resistant-tuberculosis (XDR-TB) was reported by 105 countries in 2015, representing about 9.7% of all reported TB cases in those countries [37].

After the development of RIF in the 1960s, no new anti-TB drugs were registered until 2012 and 2013. A new drug, bedaquiline, which was approved by the US Food and Drug Administration in 2012, is recommended by the WHO for the therapy of selected MDR-TB cases [37]. The European Medicines Agency approved bedaquiline in 2013 and this drug is now available for use in MDR-TB therapy in Europe [38]. Early diagnosis, motivation of patients to comply with treatment, and the implementation of the DOTS strategy are crucial for preserving the efficacy of anti-TB therapy and disease control.

Conclusion

TB has, for centuries, represented a major health problem. Since 1882, when Robert Koch discovered *M. tuberculosis*, there has been research on drugs for TB. During the 20th century the WHO implemented a number of guidelines for preventive measures and for the therapy of this disease, including the DOTS strategy, which led to a fall in the incidence of TB. However, in the last two decades of the 20th century, the number of TB cases again grew, associated with the new disease, AIDS. In some parts of the world, such as Africa, TB associated with AIDS is one of the leading causes of death. Also, a new form of the disease, MDR-TB, has become a big problem. Additional measures by the WHO, implemented in the health care systems of the relevant countries, as well as research on new drugs, will be necessary, in the future, for better control of the disease.

References

1. Grle SP (2004) Tuberculosis rechallenge to medicine at the beginning of the third millennium. University Hospital for Lung Diseases Jordanovac, Ministry of Health Republic of Croatia
2. Santic Z, Galic K (2013) Epidemiology of tuberculosis during the period 1703-2011: honoring the World Tuberculosis Day. Mater Soc 25:291–294
3. Zumla A, Mwaba P, Huggett J, Kapata N, Chanda D, Grange J (2009) Reflections on the white plague. Lancet Infect Dis 9:197–202
4. World Health Organization (WHO) (1994) TB: a global emergency, WHO report on the TB epidemic. WHO/TB/94.177
5. Global tuberculosis report 2015 (2015) World Health Organization
6. Nadjane Batista Lacerda S, Cristina de Abreu Temoteo R, Maria Ribeiro Monteirode Figueiredo T, Darliane Tavares de Luna F, Alves Nunes de Sousa M, Carlos de Abreu L, Luiz Affonso Fonseca F (2014) Individual and social vulnerabilities upon acquiring tuberculosis: a systematic literature review. Int Arch Med 7:35
7. Lönnroth K, Castro KG, Chakaya JM, Chauhan LS, Floyd K, Glaziou P, Raviglione MC (2010) Tuberculosis control and elimination 2010–50: cure, care, and social development. Lancet 375:1814–1829

8. Hwang LY, Grimes CZ, Beasley RP, Graviss EA (2009) Latent tuberculosis infections in hard-to-reach drug using population detection, prevention and control. Tuberculosis 89:S41–S45
9. Sulis G, Roggi A, Matteelli A, Raviglione MC (2014) Tuberculosis: epidemiology and control. Mediterr J Hematol Infect Dis 6(e):20140
10. World Health Organization (2012) WHO policy on TB/HIV collaborative activities:guidelines for national programmes and other stakeholders
11. World Health Organization (2013) Tuberculosis in prisons: a major health problem: in Global Tuberculosis Report 2013. WHO/HTM/TB/2013.11
12. Baussano I, Williams BG, Nunn P, Beggiato M, Fedeli U, Scano F (2010) Tuberculosis incidence in prisons: a systematic review. PLoS Med 7(e):1000381
13. Dara M, Chadha SS, Vinkeles Melchers NV, van den Hombergh J, Gurbanova E, Al-Darraji H, van der Meer JB (2013) International Union against tuberculosis and lung disease. Time to act to prevent and control tuberculosis among inmates. Int J Tuberc Lung Dis 17:4–5
14. International Union against Tuberculosis and Lung Disease (IUATLD) (1996) Tuberculosis guide for low income countries, 4th edn. IUATLD, Paris
15. World Health Organization (1994) WHO tuberculosis programme: framework for effective tuberculosis control. WHO/TB/94.179
16. World Health Organization (2006) The stop TB strategy. WHO/HTM/TB/2006.368
17. Onozaki I, Raviglione MC (2010) Stopping tuberculosis in the 21st century: goals and strategies. Respirology 15:32–43
18. World Health Organization (2006) Stop-TB Partnership. The global plan to stop TB 2006–2015: actions for life towards a world free of tuberculosis. Int J Tuberc Lung Dis 10:240–241. WHO/HTM/STB/2006.35
19. World Health Organization (2013) Global strategy and targets for tuberculosis prevention, care and control beyond 2015. WHO/HTM/TB/2013.2
20. Collins HL, Kaufman SH (2001) The many faces of host responses to tuberculosis. Immunology 103:1–9
21. Kaufmann SHE (2000) Is the development of a new tuberculosis vaccine possible? Nat Med 6:955–960
22. World Health Organization (2013) Definitions and reporting framework for tuberculosis – 2013 revision. WHO/ HTM/TB/2013. 2
23. Stop TB Department World Health Organization (2011) Draft meeting report of the Scoping meeting for the development of guidelines on screening for active TB. WHO
24. Wilson J, Jungner G (1968) Principles and practice of screening for disease. In: Originally appearing in: commission on chronic illness (1957) Chronic illness in the United States, volume I. Prevention of chronic illness. Harvard University Press, Cambridge, p 45
25. Lonnroth K (2012) DRAFT: systematic screening for active tuberculosis. Proposed principles and recommendations. Proposed outline and draft principles and recommendations for discussion in the technical consultation to review evidence on screening for active TB, May 2012
26. Kerley P, Major T (2014) Technique in mass miniature radiography. Br J Radiol 15:346–347
27. Den Boon S, White NW, van Lill SW, Borgdorff MW, Verver S, Lombard CJ, Bateman ED, Irusen E, Enarson DA, Beyers N (2006) An evaluation of symptom and chest radiographic screening in tuberculosis prevalence surveys. IntJTuberc Lung Dis 10:876–882
28. World Health Organization (2010) Tuberculosis prevalence surveys: a handbook, 2nd edn. World Health Organization, Geneva
29. Whitelaw A, Sturm WA (2009) Microbiological testing for Mycobacterium tuberculosis. In: Schaaf HS, Zumla AI (eds) Tuberculosis. A comprehensive clinical reference. Saunders, Philadelphia, pp 164–168
30. Somoskovi A, Kodmon C, Lantos A, Bartfai Z, Tamasi L, Fuzy J, Magyar P (2000) Comparison of recoveries of Mycobacterium tuberculosis using the automated BACTEC MGIT 960 system, the BACTEC 460 TB system, and Lowenstein-Jensen medium. J Clin Microbiol 38:2395–2397
31. Steingart KR, Henry M, Ng V, Hopewell PC, Hopewell PC, Ramsay A, Cunningham J, Urbanczik R, Perkins M, Aziz MA, Pai M (2006) Fluorescence versus conventional sputum smear microscopy for tuberculosis: a systematic review. Lancet Infect Dis 6:570–581
32. Boehme CC, Nicol MP, Nabeta P, Michael JS, Gotuzzo E, Tahirli R, Gler MT, Blakemore R, Worodria W, Gray C, Huang L, Caceres T, Mehdiyev R, Raymond L, Whitelaw A, Sagadevan K, Alexander H, Albert H, Cobelens F, Cox H, Alland D, Perkins MD (2011) Feasibility, diagnostic accuracy, and effectiveness of decentralised use of the Xpert MTB/RIF test for diagnosis of tuberculosis and multidrug resistance:a multicentre implementation study. Lancet 377:1495–1505
33. Getahun H, Kittikraisak W, Heilig CM, Corbett EL, Ayles H, Cain KP, Grant AD, Churchyard GJ, Kimerling M, Shah S, Lawn SD, Wood R, Maartens G, Granich R, Date AA, Varma JK (2011) Development of a standardized screening rule for tuberculosis in people living with HIV in resource-constrained settings: individual participant data. Meta-analysis of observational studies. PLoS Med 8:e1000391
34. Ruch-Gerdes S, Domehl C, Nardi G, Gismondo MR, Hans-Martin W, and Pfyffer GE (1999) Multicenter evaluation of the mycobatera growth indicator tube for testing susceptibility of Mycobacterium tuberculosis. J Clin Microbiol 37:45–48
35. Jacomelli M, Silva PR, Rodrigues AJ, Demarzo SE, Seicento M, Figueiredo VR (2012) Bronchoscopy for the diagnosis of pulmonary tuberculosis in patientswith negative sputum smear microscopy results. J Bras Pneumol 38:167–167
36. International Standards for Tuberculosis Care (ISTC) (2009) 2nd ed The Hague, Tuberculosis coalition for technical assistance
37. World Health Organization (2013) The use of bedaquiline in the treatment of multidrug resistant tuberculosis: Interim PolicyGuidance. WHO/HTM/TB/2013.6
38. Ryan NJ, Lo JH (2014) Delamanid: first global approval. Drugs 74:1041–1045

Part VIII

Further Insights into Tuberculosis

In Vitro and Animal Models of Tuberculosis of the Nervous System

39

Onur Yazici, Ahmet T. Turgut, and Mehmet Turgut

Contents

O. Yazici
Department of Chest Diseases, Adnan Menderes University School of Medicine, Aydin, Turkey
e-mail: dronur_yazici@hotmail.com

A.T. Turgut, MD
Department of Radiology, Hacettepe University School of Medicine, Ankara, Turkey
e-mail: ahmettuncayturgut@yahoo.com

M. Turgut, MD, PhD (✉)
Department of Neurosurgery, Adnan Menderes University School of Medicine, Aydın, Turkey
e-mail: drmturgut@yahoo.com

Abbreviations

BBB	Blood-brain barrier
CNS	Central nervous system
CoMTb	Conditioned medium from *M. tuberculosis*-infected human monocytes
CSF	Cerebrospinal fluid
HBHA	Heparin-binding hemagglutinin adhesin
HIV	Human immunodeficiency virus
iNOS	Inducible nitric oxide synthetase
MAPK	Mitogen-activated protein kinase
MMP	Matrix metalloproteinase
TB	Tuberculosis
TBM	Tuberculous meningitis
TIMP	Tissue inhibitor of metalloproteinase

39.1 Introduction

Tuberculosis (TB) of central nervous system (CNS) is a grave and deadly disease, constituting approximately 1% of all TB cases. In this disorder with high mortality and morbidity, children and human immunodeficiency virus (HIV)-infected individuals are more affected. The rarity of the disease together with the variability of the symptoms leads to difficulties in making the diagnosis. Although various suggestions have been reported related to the occurrence mechanism of the disease, the mechanism is not entirely understood yet [1]. It is considered that *Mycobacterium tuberculosis* should pass through

M. Turgut et al. (eds.), *Tuberculosis of the Central Nervous System*,
DOI 10.1007/978-3-319-50712-5_39

the blood-brain barrier (BBB) and create the parenchymal and meningeal tuberculoma, and then these tuberculomas should rupture and bacilli should pass to the subarachnoidal space for the occurrence of TB of CNS [2–5]. In vitro and animal models have been used from the past to present in various studies for understanding the pathogenesis of TB of CNS.

39.2 In Vitro Models

The in vitro models are relatively cost free and easy to use models, but they have various limitations. The reason for this is that the in vitro systems use one or more cell lines grown in one or more compartments and, thus, their inability to simulate the complex interactions among various cell types and additionally not resembling a living in vivo system. Nevertheless, these models can be very helpful for understanding how various microorganisms interact with the organism.

In previous studies, *M. tuberculosis* was shown to invade endothelial cells in various in vitro studies [6, 7]. Afterward, the studies in human autopsies have supported this finding [8]. Bermudez et al. [6] showed that *M. tuberculosis* invaded A549 pulmonary epithelial cells with an efficiency of 2–3% of the initial inoculum, despite its insufficiency in the invasion of endothelial cells in the bilayer alveolar wall model, consisting of epithelial and endothelial cells. However, they also showed that the bacteria invading the A549 epithelial cells were taken in by the endothelial cells with an efficiency of 5–6% of the initial inoculums [6]. Moreover, they showed that both free and intracellular (inside the infected monocytes) *M. tuberculosis* bacilli were able to pass across the bicellular, monolayer – epithelial and endothelial cells – formations [6].

Recently, Menozzi et al. [9] showed that 28-kDa heparin-binding hemagglutinin adhesin (HBHA), which is required for dissemination of the bacilli out of the lungs, induced the reorganization of the active filament network in adjacent endothelial cells, but did not affect the tight junctions. When HBHA is combined with the colloidal gold particles, it acts as the mediator for these particles to be attached to the membranes of the Hep-2 and A549 epithelial cells. Once attached, the particles are taken inside within the membrane-bound vacuoles and migrate inside the A549 cells toward the basal side. These observations clearly suggest that *M. tuberculosis* induces the receptor-mediated endocytosis and the epithelial transcytosis of HBHA. This can represent the mechanism for dissemination of *M. tuberculosis* independent of macrophages, leading to systemic infection.

In normal physiological circumstances, the CNS is separated from the systemic circulation by the BBB [10]. Typically, this barrier consists of specialized and tightly apposed human brain microvascular endothelial cells [10]. The basal sides of these endothelial cells are supported by astrocytes [10]. The transcellular movement from the BBB is limited due to the small number of endocytic vesicles and the absence of endothelial fenestration. The paracellular transport is also limited due to the presence of tight junctions in endothelial cells. These properties make the BBB impermeable to large molecules, hydrophilic molecules, and circulatory pathogens.

The exact entry mechanism of *M. tuberculosis* to the CNS by passing through the BBB has not been fully elucidated to date. While some authors have suggested that free bacilli directly pass through the endothelial barrier, others have considered that bacilli enter via the macrophages [6, 9, 11]. Various in vitro studies have shown that free *M. tuberculosis* invades the endothelial cells [3, 4].

Using an in vitro model, Jain et al. [11] constituted for investigating the meningitis-forming bacteria, created a monolayer human brain microvascular endothelial cell line, and infected these cells with various mycobacterium strains. They showed that *M. tuberculosis* H37Rv and CDC1551 strains invaded and breached this layer consisting of endothelial cells much more efficiently when compared to *M. smegmatis* [11]. This result supported the suggestion that free mycobacteria can pass through the specialized endothelial cells. Nevertheless, while brain microvascular endothelial cells were used in the model that they created, the cells forming the brain side of the BBB – primarily astrocytes – were not included in this model. Therefore, what kind of resistance these cells create during the transport of the mycobacterium to the brain parenchyma is not clear. Together with the experiments using microarray profiling and selected *M. tuberculosis* transposon mutants, the results of this study suggested that specific *M. tuberculosis* genes might be required for invasion and breaching [11]. The model created by Jain et al. is a significant study for understanding the interactions of mycobacteria with endothelial cells [11].

TB of CNS is a disease characterized by extensive tissue inflammation. This inflammation is driven by the molecules known as matrix metalloproteinase (MMP). MMPs are the enzymes that degrade the extracellular matrix. Information about the regulation of these enzymes in CNS is limited. Green et al. [12, 13] demonstrated that microglia secreted MMPs in high concentrations in a simplified CNS cell model of TB. They determined elevated levels of MMP-1, MMP-3, MMP-8, and MMP-9 in cerebrospinal fluid (CSF) of patients with TB disease [12, 13]. They also showed the presence of MMP-1, MMP-3, and MMP-9 in tuberculoma of the CNS, but the specific tissue inhibitor of metalloproteinase-1 was not present in this tubercle [12, 13]. In this study, analysis of all of the MMPs demonstrated that conditioned medium from *M. tuberculosis*-infected human monocytes (CoMTb) stimulated greater MMP-1, MMP-3, and MMP-9 gene expression in human microglial cells than direct infection [12, 13].

Moreover, Green et al. [14] stimulated the human microglial cell line by using the CoMTb in a cellular model of TB of CNS. CoMTb upregulated the microglial secretion of MMP-1 and MMP-3 in a dose- and time-dependent manner. By phospho-array profiling, it was shown that the highest increase in kinase activity was in p38 mitogen-activated protein kinase (MAPK) [14]. They concluded that the monocyte-microglial network-dependent MMP-1 and MMP-3 gene expression and secretion were p38 MAPK-dependent in TB [14]. Therefore, they suggested that p38 was a potential target for the treatment of TB of CNS [14].

39.3 Animal Models

39.3.1 History and First Studies

The first information related to the pathogenesis of tuberculous meningitis (TBM) was obtained as the result of the studies performed by Rich and McCordock [5, 15] (Table 39.1). In their study using guinea pigs and rabbits, they concluded that the meninges did not get infected by the hematogenous spread of the TB bacilli, and for formation of TBM, the bacilli should be inoculated to the CNS directly [5].

Table 39.1 Summary of different experimental models described in the literature for pathogenesis of TBM and TB granuloma to date

Researcher	Year	Experimental Model	Main Topic of Study
Rich and McCordock [5]	1930	Guinea pig Rabbit	Pathogenesis of TBM
Tsenova et al. [16]	1977	Rabbit	A drug study for TBM
Mazzolla et al. [17]	2002	Mice	Different immune response in TBM between two types of mice
van Well et al. [18]	2007	Mice	Pathogenesis of TBM
Olin et al. [19]	2008	Mice	The role of inducible nitric oxide synthase in clinic of TBM
Rock et al. [20]	2008	Mice	Pathogenesis of TBM
Be et al. [2]	2008	Mice	Invasion and survival of *M. tuberculosis* in the CNS
van Leeuwen et al. [21]	2014	Zebrafish	Early pathogenesis of TBM and granulomas

Abbreviations: *CNS* central nervous system; *TBM* tuberculous meningitis

Rich and McCordock [5] challenged the sensitized and nonsensitized guinea pigs and rabbits by giving them *M. tuberculosis* and *M. bovis* intravenously, respectively. Although acute exudative meningitis did not develop in any animal, several or diffuse granulomatous lesions formed in the brain parenchyma or meninges of all animals. Thus, they suggested that these foci had developed throughout the initial bacteremic phase around the deposited bacteria in the brain parenchyma and meninges [5].

By performing a series of postmortem investigations, Rich and McCordock [5] reported that a meningeal focus was present at the site that the bacilli had entered the subarachnoidal space and had formed TBM in almost all cases. Depending on these seminal observations and subsequent studies to a great extent, it has generally been considered that a caseating vascular focus known as "Rich focus" is present in the cerebral cortex and the meninges, and this focus is the key pathway for the TB bacilli to pass to the subarachnoidal space [22–25].

Nevertheless, the information that Rich and McCordock had reported as the result of their studies was not able to explain the relationship of miliary TB with TBM [5]. Donald et al. [23] analyzed the original reports together with the subsequent essays. Depending on the increasing probability of development of "Rich focus" in disseminated TB, and since the likelihood of unexpected rupture of this focus that causes TBM clinically increases, they concluded that disseminated TB plays a significant role in development of TBM in children. The mechanism of initial invasion of this barrier by the bacilli while the meninges and the brain parenchyma are being protected from the systemic circulation anatomically and physiologically has not been fully understood.

39.3.2 Studies with Intracranial Injections

In addition to the animal models which had emerged with the experiments of Rich and McCordock related to the TB of CNS in guinea pigs and rabbits, new animal models were developed by conducting studies for investigation of the neuropathogenesis of *M. tuberculosis* [5]. Tsenova et al. [16] described a rabbit model in which they made intracranial injections of *M. bovis* Ravenel, which is virulent in rabbits, for creating acute mycobacterial meningitis (Table 39.1). In this rabbit model, they were able to produce an acute inflammatory response in CSF and to grow live bacteria within CSF [16]. In this model, they were also able to show the clinical features of TBM in rabbits, to identify granulomatous meningitis by histopathological examination, and to display the live mycobacteria in the other organs [16]. In that study, the mortality was observed after a follow-up period of 8 days [16]. Although this model mimicked many clinical and pathological features of TBM in humans, the progression of the disease was much faster when compared to the human TBM. Related to this rapid course in this model in which acute meningitis had developed, Tsenova et al. [16] reduced the concentration of intracranially injected *M. bovis* Ravenel and created a subacute TBM model. In this modified model, the clinical features were manifested at the third week following inoculation, and on the 28th day, mortality or neurological disability occurred in almost all rabbits [16]. This model showed similarities to the acute model concerning the subjects of producing an inflammatory response and growing live bacilli in other organs [16]. Then, the investigators used the same model for assessment of the efficacy of a recombinant polypeptide vaccine, for showing the significance of TNF alpha in the progression of TBM, and for evaluation of potential roles of thalidomide and its analogues in the course of TBM [16].

By inoculating *M. bovis* Bacillus-Calmette Guerin Montreal via intracerebral injections in BALB/c and DBA/2 mice, Mazzolla et al. [17] demonstrated that mononuclear cellular infiltration and microglial activation developed, mycobacteria grew, and the number of mycobacteria increased throughout 21 days following infection, in 2002 (Table 39.1). Nevertheless, they did not discuss the clinical signs of the disease and the mortality rates in their report [17]. More recently, van Well et al. [18] developed a murine model for studying TBM

(Table 39.1). The virulent *M. tuberculosis* laboratory strain H37Rv was inoculated intracranially to the C57BL/6 mice. In this model, they showed that a neuroinflammatory response leading to lymphocytic infiltration around meninges and in perivascular areas was formed [18]. Besides, they were able to acquire the bacilli from the mouse brain homogenates, but not from the CSF [18]. They did not report any neurological sign of meningitis in their study and did not record any mortality within the 24-week study period [18].

Olin et al. [19] inoculated intracerebrally the FVBN mice with the *M. tuberculosis* H37RV strain. Although an inflammatory infiltration was determined histopathologically, no mouse displayed the clinical features of the disease and none developed mortality [20]. Depending on the previously performed studies, Olin et al. [19] considered that the murine model of TBM did not reflect the seriousness of the disease in humans and that inducible nitric oxide synthetase (iNOS), expressed by the active microglial cells, was its cause. Thus, they created a model by infecting the iNOS−/−mice by *M. tuberculosis* [19] (Table 39.1). They demonstrated that severe clinical findings developed and granulomatous lesions containing TB bacilli were formed around the meninges in iNOS −/− mice in this model [19]. In healthy mice, however, these results were not present [19].

Since the immune system of pigs was very similar to that of humans, Rock et al. [20] developed a model of human TB in pigs, and they observed the development of TBM in some animals (Table 39.1). Nevertheless, this model was replaced by the murine model due to various implementation difficulties encountered while working with infected pigs. They were able to show significant lymphocytic infiltration around meninges and perivascular infiltration of the parenchyma following intracranial inoculation of *M. tuberculosis* H37Rv in FVB/N mice [20]. Also, they were able to determine the formation of granuloma inside the parenchyma and the presence of the bacilli inside the granuloma [20]. Nevertheless, they also did not observe any mortality within the 3 months of the study [20], as did in the study of Well et al. [18].

Van Leeuwen et al. [21] developed zebrafish model of *M. marinum* infection both to get more information about the role for early pathogenesis of Rich focus which is a characteristic feature in TBM and to get detailed information about early pathogenesis of TBM (Table 39.1). In this study, they regulated to define optimal inoculation ways (intraperitoneally, intravenously, and direct CNS injection) that caused to TBM at different maturation phases of zebrafish [21] (Table 39.1). Firstly, in this model, it is analyzed if TBM grew in mature zebrafish or not [21]. The adult zebrafishes that have the BBB and fully developed immune system were successfully infected to *M. marinum* that is a close relative of *M. tuberculosis*. After 8 weeks' time that a year-old zebrafishes are infected with *M. marinum*, granuloma formation has been shown in abdominal organs of all fishes [21]. Granuloma formation in the brain and meninges which are closely related to each other has been determined for 5 in 26 fishes (approximately 20%) [21]. It has been seen that granulomas in the area, which affected the meninges and submeningeal space, are multifocal, variable sized (50–300 cm in diameter), and quite limited [21]. Although minimal lymphocytic inflammation and gliosis have been seen on brain tissue under meningeal granulomas, any clear infection has been observed on parenchyma [21]. There were uniform population of foamy macrophages and epithelioid on these granulomas and rarely accompanied by lymphocytes [21]. Congestion of brain parenchymal blood vessel and meninges has been seen around these granulomas [21]. Briefly, granulomas formed on meninges and brain that are related to each other after intraperitoneal infection on adult zebrafishes which have a full immune system. So, it is demonstrated as a natural and representative model of zebrafish–*M. marinum* infection for TBM pathogenesis study [21]. Afterward, they characterized the initial phases of zebrafish infection by using different routes of bacteria inoculation. After infection, on three different inoculation routes on zebrafish embryos, it has been seen bacterial infiltration and clustering of infected phagocyte (parenchyma, hindbrain ventricle, caudal vein) [21]. After local and systemic infection with the formation of bacterial clusters, there has been a brain infection on most of zebrafish embryos which have an innate immunity [21]. All clusters were including a population that consisted of foamy macrophage and both mycobacterium and epithelioid [21]. These clusters weren't affected because of the BBB. In an interesting way, no differences were observed when embryos were infected before or after early formation of the BBB, and this indicated that bacteria can comparatively cross this barrier with high efficiency [21]. In 70% of the cases that are formed by infection via the bloodstream resulted in the formation of early granulomas in brain tissue [21]. Infiltrates were placed in the proximity of blood vessels in these zebrafish embryos [21].

One of the important virulence factors of both *M. marinum* and *M. tuberculosis* is ESX-1 locus. As a result of infection of embryos with an *M. marinum* ESX-1 mutant, small clusters and scattered isolated phagocytes with high bacterial loads occurred on brain tissue [21]. This was also shown on former studies [26]. Nevertheless, on this study, it is indicated that bacterial migration wasn't effected from bloodstream to brain parenchymal. In this study, it is indicated that zebrafish model is accessible and reproducible both to analyze early CNS granuloma formation pathogenesis and to describe the factors in this process. In addition, it is indicated that the formation of BBB didn't have an effect on the early granuloma formation [21].

Its small size, the ease of breeding and genetic manipulation and the big similarities with the human immune system and BBB are the great advantages of zebrafishes. When combined with fluorescent tools, the transparency of the zebrafish embryos could allow real-time imaging of host-pathogen interactions in infectious diseases, including TBM.

39.3.3 Study with Related Genes

Other investigators have described murine and animal models of TBM developing after administration of *M. tuberculosis* into the CSF by direct intracisternal inoculation [16, 17, 19, 20]. However, TB of CNS in humans is the consequence of the passage of *M. tuberculosis* from blood to the CNS. Therefore, Be et al. [2] created IV challenge hematogenous spreading *M. tuberculosis* infection in Balb c mice to develop a murine model for investigating the invasion of CNS by *M. tuberculosis* and the genes which have roles in the pathogenesis of TB of CNS. They described the mycobacterial genes that were present in the pathogenesis of TB of CNS and absent in the lungs in this model, which was developed for investigating the CNS invasion [2]. *M. tuberculosis* genes Rv0311, Rv0805, Rv0931c, Rv0986, and MT3280 were identified as genes having specific roles in CNS invasion and for surviving there [2].

Conclusion

In sum, the rabbit model has been the model that mimics the human disease most, if we look at the animal models developed for TBM until now. Although this model demonstrates the clinical and histological findings of the disease precisely, the lack of availability of some immunological tools in rabbit studies makes the ongoing trials for creating a murine model for TB of CNS worthwhile. Zebrafish model is especially suitable for characterization of the early steps in the formation of brain granulomas, their immunological composition, and the effect of bacterial virulence factors in the context of TBM. So far the pathogenesis of TB of CNS has not been fully understood yet, in spite of all conducted studies with in vitro and animal models. New studies with in vitro and animal models are required concerning development, clinical course, prognosis, and therapeutic response of the disease.

References

1. Armand-DeLille PF (1903) Role des poisons du bacille de Koch dans la meningite tuberculeuse et la tuberculose des centres nerveux: etude experimentale et anatomo-pathologique. Universite de Paris, Paris
2. Be NA, Lamichhane G, Grosset J, Tyagi S, Cheng QJ, Kim KS, Bishai WR, Jain SK (2008) Murine model to

study the invasion and survival of Mycobacterium tuberculosis in the central nervous system. J Infect Dis 198:1520–1528
3. Drevets DA, Leenen PJ, Greenfield RA (2004) Invasion of the central nervous system by intracellular bacteria. Clin Microbiol Rev 17:323–347
4. Lemierre A, Ameuille P (1938) Granulieconse'cutive al'injectionintraveineuse volonteire d'une e'mulsion de bacilles de Koch. Bull Mem Soc Med Hop Paris 54:286–295
5. Rich AR, McCordock HA (1933) The pathogenesis of tuberculous meningitis. Bull Johns Hopkins Hosp 52:5–37
6. Bermudez LE, Sangari FJ, Kolonoski P, Petrofsky M, Goodman J (2002) The efficiency of the translocation of Mycobacterium tuberculosis across a bilayer of epithelial and endothelial cells as a model of the alveolar wall is a consequence of transport within mononuclear phagocytes and invasion of alveolar epithelial cells. Infect Immun 70:140–146
7. Birkness KA, Deslauriers M, Bartlett JH, White EH, King CH, Quinn FD (1999) An in vitro tissue culture bilayer model to examine early events in Mycobacterium tuberculosis infection. Infect Immun 67:653–658
8. Hernández-Pando R, Jeyanathan M, Mengistu G, Aguilar D, Orozco H, Harboe M, Rook GA, Bjune G (2000) Persistence of DNA from Mycobacterium tuberculosis in superficially normal lung tissue during latent infection. Lancet 356:2133–2138
9. Menozzi FD, Reddy VM, Cayet D, Raze D, Debrie AS, Dehouck MP, Cecchelli R, Locht C (2006) Mycobacterium tuberculosis heparin-binding haemagglutinin adhesin (HBHA) triggers receptor-mediated transcytosis without altering the integrity of tight junctions. Microbes Infect 8:1–9
10. Rubin LL, Staddon JM (1999) The cell biology of the blood-brain barrier. Annu Rev Neurosci 22:11–28
11. Jain SK, Paul-Satyaseela M, Lamichhane G, Kim KS, Bishai WR (2006) Mycobacterium tuberculosis invasion and traversal across an in vitro human blood-brain barrier as a pathogenic mechanism for central nervous system tuberculosis. J Infect Dis 193:1287–1295
12. Green JA, Dholakia S, Janczar K, Ong CW, Moores R, Fry J, Elkington PT, Roncaroli F, Friedland JS (2011) Mycobacterium tuberculosis-infected human monocytes down-regulate microglial MMP-2 secretion in CNS tuberculosis via TNFalpha, NFkappaB, p38 and caspase 8 dependent pathways. J Neuroinflammation 8:46
13. Green JA, Elkington PT, Pennington CJ, Roncaroli F, Dholakia S, Moores RC, Bullen A, Porter JC, Agranoff D, Edwards DR, Friedland JS (2010) Mycobacterium tuberculosis upregulates microglial matrix metalloproteinase-1 and -3 expression and secretion via NF-kappaB- and Activator Protein-1-dependent monocyte networks. J Immunol 184:6492–6503
14. Green JA, Rand L, Moores R, Dholakia S, Pezas T, Elkington PT, Friedland JS (2013) In an in vitro model of human tuberculosis, monocyte-microglial networks regulate matrix metalloproteinase-1 and -3 gene expression and secretion via a p38 mitogen activated protein kinase-dependent pathway. J Neuroinflammation 10:107
15. Rich AR, McCordock HA (1929) An enquiry concerning the role of allergy, immunity and other factors of importance in the pathogenesis of human tuberculosis. Bull Johns Hopkins Hosp 44:273–382
16. Tsenova L, Sokol K, Freedman VH, Kaplan G (1998) A combination of thalidomide plus antibiotics protects rabbits from mycobacterial meningitis-associated death. J Infect Dis 177:1563–1572
17. Mazzolla R, Puliti M, Barluzzi R, Neglia R, Bistoni F, Barbolini G, Blasi E (2002) Differential microbial clearance and immunoresponse of Balb/c (Nramp1 susceptible) and DBA2 (Nramp1 resistant) mice intracerebrally infected with Mycobacterium bovis BCG (BCG) FEMS. Immunol Med Microbiol 32:149–158
18. van Well GT, Wieland CW, Florquin S, Roord JJ, van der Poll T, van Furth AM (2007) A new murine model to study the pathogenesis of tuberculous meningitis. J Infect Dis 195:694–697
19. Olin MR, Armien AG, Cheeran MC, Rock RB, Molitor TW, Peterson PK (2008) Role of nitric oxide in defense of the central nervous system against Mycobacterium tuberculosis. J Infect Dis 198:886–889
20. Rock RB, Olin M, Baker CA, Molitor TW, Peterson PK (2008) Central nervous system tuberculosis: pathogenesis and clinical aspects. Clin Microbiol Rev 21:243–261
21. van Leeuwen LM, van der Kuip M, Youssef SA, de Bruin A, Bitter W, van Furth AM, van der Sar AM (2014) Modeling tuberculous meningitis in zebrafish using *Mycobacterium marinum*. Dis Model Mech 7:1111–1122
22. Blacklock JWS, Griffin MA (1935) Tuberculosis meningitis: problems in pathogenesis and treatment. J Pathol Bacteriol 40:489–502
23. Donald PR, Schaaf HS, Schoeman JF (2005) Tuberculous meningitis and miliary tuberculosis: the Rich focus revisited. J Infect 50:193–195
24. Horne NW (1951) Tuberculous meningitis: problems in pathogenesis and treatment. Edinburgh Med J 58:413–429
25. MacGregor AR, Green CA (1937) Tuberculosis of the central nervous system, with special reference to tuberculous meningitis. J Pathol Bacteriol 45:613–645
26. Volkman HE, Clay H, Beery D, Chang JCW, Sherman DR, Ramakrishnan L (2004) Tuberculous granuloma formation is enhanced by a mycobacterium virulence determinant. PLoS Biol 2:e367

Conclusion

Tuberculosis is one of the few infectious diseases that have resisted eradication despite the development of many modern biologic and imaging diagnostic tools in addition to effective antituberculous drugs. Still widely spread around the world, neurotuberculosis is a complex and potentially devastating disease especially in patients with neurological disabilities and in those diagnosed and treated tardily.

With these in mind, the aim of this richly illustrated book is to provide the reader with a frame of symptoms and signs of this particular infectious disease in an effort to suspect and confirm the diagnosis of neurotuberculosis at the earliest stage and therefore prevent late effects on different divisions of the central nervous system and its coverings.

Antituberculous therapy is the cornerstone of appropriate treatment for central nervous system tuberculosis. However, in many patients diagnosis remains under question, or medical regimens are not effective, and serious complications needing surgical intervention may occur. Finally, close coordination of care between neurosurgeons, neurologists, biologists, radiologists, and infectious diseases consultants is increasingly important in the management of many patients harboring this complicated multifaceted problem.

M. Turgut et al. (eds.), *Tuberculosis of the Central Nervous System*,
DOI 10.1007/978-3-319-50712-5

Author Index

M. Turgut et al. (eds.), *Tuberculosis of the Central Nervous System*,
DOI 10.1007/978-3-319-50712-5

D

G

K

L

M

O

P

U

V

X

Subject Index

M. Turgut et al. (eds.), *Tuberculosis of the Central Nervous System*,
DOI 10.1007/978-3-319-50712-5

N

Q

R

S

U

V

CPI Antony Rowe
Chippenham, UK
2017-09-04 22:13